Focused Issues in Family Therapy

Series Editor

D. Russell Crane, Brigham Young University, Provo, UT, USA

More information about this series at http://www.springer.com/series/13372

Tai Mendenhall · Angela Lamson
Jennifer Hodgson · Macaran Baird
Editors

Clinical Methods
in Medical Family Therapy

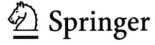

Editors
Tai Mendenhall
Department of Family Social Science
University of Minnesota
Saint Paul, MN, USA

Jennifer Hodgson
Department of Human Development
and Family Science
East Carolina University
Greenville, NC, USA

Angela Lamson
Department of Human Development
and Family Science
East Carolina University
Greenville, NC, USA

Macaran Baird
Family Medicine and Community Health
University of Minnesota Medical School
Minneapolis, MN, USA

ISSN 2520-1190   ISSN 2520-1204   (electronic)
Focused Issues in Family Therapy
ISBN 978-3-030-09853-7   ISBN 978-3-319-68834-3   (eBook)
https://doi.org/10.1007/978-3-319-68834-3

© Springer International Publishing AG, part of Springer Nature 2018
Softcover re-print of the Hardcover 1st edition 2018
This work is subject to copyright. All rights are reserved by the Publisher, whether the whole or part of the material is concerned, specifically the rights of translation, reprinting, reuse of illustrations, recitation, broadcasting, reproduction on microfilms or in any other physical way, and transmission or information storage and retrieval, electronic adaptation, computer software, or by similar or dissimilar methodology now known or hereafter developed.
The use of general descriptive names, registered names, trademarks, service marks, etc. in this publication does not imply, even in the absence of a specific statement, that such names are exempt from the relevant protective laws and regulations and therefore free for general use.
The publisher, the authors and the editors are safe to assume that the advice and information in this book are believed to be true and accurate at the date of publication. Neither the publisher nor the authors or the editors give a warranty, express or implied, with respect to the material contained herein or for any errors or omissions that may have been made. The publisher remains neutral with regard to jurisdictional claims in published maps and institutional affiliations.

Printed on acid-free paper

This Springer imprint is published by the registered company Springer International Publishing AG part of Springer Nature.
The registered company address is: Gewerbestrasse 11, 6330 Cham, Switzerland

Tai Mendenhall
I dedicate this book to my incredible wife, Ling. Thank you for loving me for who I am, and for supporting me in all of the ways that you do along this always-exciting, sometimes-exhausting, never-boring, and forever-evolving career path. You inspire me every day, and I love you with all of my heart. I also want to thank my family—my parents (Vince and Diann, Tom and Suzette), sisters and brothers-in-law (Tiffany and Jeff, Carrie and Patrick), niece (Jessa), and nephew (Kadin)—for cheering me on. Thank you to my mentors—Drs. Bill Doherty, Pauline Boss, Wayne Caron, Wayne Denton, Pete Harper, Paul Rosenblatt, Hal Grotevant, and others—for believing in me over the years, even (especially!) during times when I was not so sure. And to my students, my patients, and their families: I thank you for keeping me humble, and for teaching me more than I have ever taught you.

Angela Lamson
To the love of my life, Brad Lamson, thank you for supporting me through the many nights and weekends away from you and Carter in order to get this book to completion. I am so grateful that

you helped me to carve out an hour each day to walk with you and talk about our day, visions for our future, and the joys of raising a teenager. God could not have created a better husband for me or a better father for our son. Carter Lamson, thank you for your hugs of reassurance throughout my writing of this book. My favorite conversation with you was the day that we discussed how you were my best biopsychosocial-spiritual innovation, and you are. I love you, son! I want to thank my coeditors—Tai, Jennifer, and Mac—for your passion for this field and for your late night messages when I needed them most. Thank you to my parents, mother-in-law, siblings, dearest friends, extended family, and godchildren, who kept wondering what topic I was writing about next and for giving me virtual hugs to charge forward. Mom, Dad, Marty, and Patty—a special thank you to you for believing in me and instilling in me your love and a work ethic to want more for this world. A very big thank you to the ECU administrators (especially Chancellor Steve Ballard, Dr. Paul Gemperline, and Dr. Cynthia Johnson) and our wonderful MFT/MedFT faculty (Drs. Brimhall, Didericksen, Dosser, Hill, Hodgson, Jensen, Krepps, Markowski, Rappleyea, Roberts, Tyndall, and White) over the years who had the forward thinking to allow us to create such an incredible PhD program. I also must extend deep gratitude to my numerous personal and professional mentors, to the students who have grown this field beyond my imagination, and to the patients and families who have welcomed me into their lives and reminded me that the human soul can endure incredible pain and still find space for hope and resilience.

Jennifer Hodgson
I dedicate this book to my amazing husband, Steve, who is 100% in my corner as a working mom. I also dedicate it to my three children,

Lauren, Ava Lynn, and Brennon. They are the reason behind how hard I work. My goal is to leave behind a better healthcare system for them. I also want to send a special thank you out to my family, colleagues, and students. My family inspires my work ethic. I am grateful for their love and support. I could also not forget my mentors and colleagues who have made it possible for me to focus on my scholarship and who have added depth and breadth to the advancement of medical family therapy as a field. Lastly, to my students and patients, you show me new ways to think about health and wellness. You demonstrate what courage and commitment are in the work that you do. It is such a privilege to be in your company and revel in your wisdom and grit.

Macaran Baird
While indebted to numerous mentors and professional colleagues, I dedicate this book to my wife, Kris. You have literally and metaphorically traveled with me during my professional and personal journey for over 48 years. And to my children: Macavan; his wife, Shannon Lundeen; and their two sons, Paxton and Harlan, and to Trina-Marie Baird and her husband, Todd Guttman, as well as his extended family. All of you have shared generously your love, trust, and commitment to me while also improving the lives of others. I could not have contributed to this book without you. In particular, I dedicate the legacy of this book to Macavan, whose courage, gentle intelligence, and love is a legacy in itself.

Tai Mendenhall, Angela Lamson, Jennifer Hodgson, & Macaran Baird
We dedicate this book to all of the families and loved-ones for whom we hope our collective efforts will benefit.

Foreword

This is at least the third generation of books defining and shaping the field of medical family therapy (MedFT). The pioneering text, *Medical Family Therapy: A Biopsychosocial Approach to Families with Health Problems*, by Susan McDaniel, Jeri Hepworth, and William Doherty in 1992 reviewed the developmental history, medical interface, and clinical scope and context of a newly named field. Its foreword by Donald Block, MD, forecast that the field would survive, adapt, and expand even as he recognized inherent flaws in the U.S. healthcare system. A notable second text, *Medical Family Therapy: Advanced Applications*, by Jennifer Hodgson, Angela Lamson, Tai Mendenhall, and D. Russell Crane in 2014 offered a more detailed view of this expanding field. Its separate sections on training, research, policy, and finance revealed a maturing of MedFT with distinct practical demonstrations of doctoral training programs, research in existing integrated settings, policy options that support this type of integrated care, and insights into sustainable financial models that recognize MedFT's economic value.

In just a few years, this field has grown in both breadth and depth. It is no longer a rare experience to see a MedFT provider in action or to be identified with this formal title on staffing lists at a hospital or clinic. Trainees can choose from several PhD programs specifically tailored to MedFT. In short, the field is now an established part of our medical infrastructure. This new text, *Clinical Methods in Medical Family Therapy*, joins others in clarifying practice strategies in MedFT that improve the lives and experiences of patients and families who face serious, chronic, and/or debilitating illnesses and injuries.

My own connection to MedFT is both professional and personal. As a family physician who was trained in family therapy as a resident, I grew up professionally by striving to integrate family therapy into family medicine, into any kind of primary care and, eventually, into larger care systems before we had a concise name for this field. We just did our best with like-minded colleagues to create teams that integrated systems thinking, family therapists, physicians, and clinicians of all types. We looked for research opportunities and tested our ideas across many care contexts with little financial or administrative support. Over time, more sophisticated clinicians linked with fully trained research professionals to create increasingly credible scholarship. Policies and payment models evolved that created opportunities to move beyond fee-for-service reimbursement for clinical care, which opened doors to broader teams in both primary care and specialty services. Currently, there may be more medical family therapists in specialty services with bundled payment such as oncology and cardiology than in primary care practices. As an early participant, I marvel at how we have collectively grown in the academic and applied clinical field of MedFT.

Over the past decade, my personal connection as a patient with intermittently life-threatening illnesses has given me insight into how the impact of serious illness can land powerfully on family members just as much as it might for an individual patient with a medically defined disease. I have survived several cardiac events, cardiac surgery, and—finally—acute leukemia. I acquired a new awareness that my journey as a patient was more direct as I had my own medical procedures and interventions, medication side effects, chest pain, etc. Perhaps these experiences were more dramatic and, thus far, survivable—but they left a relatively small post-illness legacy of loss and sadness for me as a patient. During my own illnesses, it was clear to me that my wife and two children suffered more emotionally with feelings of powerlessness in the face of said illnesses and my need for intense expert care. Had I succumbed, they would have been left with the aftermath—not me. They provided me tremendous emotional and physical support, but I had the good fortune of being directly involved in my own survival by being a fully engaged patient. They could listen, support, worry, lie awake at night, and help in innumerable ways, but they could not directly affect my disordered body and organ systems. I was less exhausted in the journey than they were. Family education, therapeutic discussions not yet labeled as medical family therapy, and friends helped them recover as I healed. Fortunately, we have all recovered emotionally from those experiences during an era prior to the wider availability of MedFT.

Just as we are finishing this text, I have been alerted again to the need for and benefit of formally trained, fully established care teams that include MedFTs. Our son, a nonsmoker at age 41, was recently diagnosed with stage IV adenocarcinoma of the lung with metastases. He is under the expert care of a noted oncology center and is receiving state-of-the-art medical care that we hope will prolong his life. His wife and two young children were quickly introduced to the expanded oncology team, including a medical family therapist and an experienced family-life educator. At the care visit, this team helped my son's family and all of us grapple with this sudden awful illness with a greater sense of empowerment and stability than would have been possible a decade earlier. We have already discussed hope, mortality, how to maintain a purposeful daily life, and how we can help each other the most. As we manage our shock and grief, we already know that we will all have help in this journey. Now, I more fully comprehend that sense of helplessness and deep sadness sitting within us while we family members strive to maintain hope and gratefulness for each day that we have together. The therapist and team helped us to engage these thoughts and feelings rather than hide from them. With this help, I know that we and, especially, our grandchildren will understand the journey, survive it, and move ahead someday with greater capacities to cope with tragedies that life brings our way unexpectedly from time to time.

I am grateful that our family is facing this challenge during a time when MedFT is a routine part of care in a place where the other components of excellent treatment are already established. This gratitude is welcomed by us, as it will be for other families in the future. It is about time that healthcare is delivered at the family (versus exclusively at the individual) level. Patients return from our offices to their homes, communities, and support systems. That is where change happens, and that is where we need to focus our interventions, research, and care. MedFTs are doing groundbreaking work in these areas across clinical, training, research, and policy levels.

This text describes clinical methods useful in a variety of settings and medical specialties (spanning across primary, secondary, tertiary, and other unique care environments and clinical populations) that can be used by current and future generations of MedFTs and others assisting families who are facing medical challenges. Its grounding in research-informed applications, clear illustrations of diverse treatment teams, engaging examples and discussions regarding common care challenges, and articulate illustrations of MedFT clinical, teaching, supervisory, research, and policy efforts across a continuum of scope and sophistication serve to confirm how far this field has come. And as healthcare practice(s) continues to grow and evolve, it is my hope that healthcare providers—therapists, medical providers, and other professionals—will continue to advance MedFT into the uncharted territories that lie before us.

Macaran Baird
Department of Family Medicine and Community Health
University of Minnesota Medical School
Minneapolis, MN, USA

References

Hodgson, J., Lamson, A., Mendenhall, T., & Crane, D. (Eds.). (2014). *Medical family therapy: Advanced applications*. New York, NY: Springer.

McDaniel, S., Hepworth, J., & Doherty, W. (1992). *Medical family therapy: A biopsyhosocial approach to families with health problems*. New York, NY: Basic Books.

Preface

Introduction to Clinical Methods in Medical Family Therapy

Medical family therapy (MedFT) represents a rapidly growing field in health care that purposefully interweaves patients and their families' physical, psychological, social, and spiritual worlds. It does this with both scientific rigor and systemic training at its foundation. Originally coined in the 1990s, MedFT challenged outdated orthodoxies like mind-versus-body and nature-versus-nurture (McDaniel, Hepworth, & Doherty, 1992). The field has since served to bridge multiple facets of the healthcare system together, including collaborative and integrated behavioral healthcare (IBHC) research, training, policy, and practice (McDaniel, Doherty, & Hepworth, 2014; Hodgson, Lamson, Mendenhall, & Crane, 2014). Since these early beginnings, MedFT has grown in its visibility, scope, and influence across training programs, healthcare contexts, research, and policy discussions around the world. MedFTs are now serving as leaders in educational, research, policy, and clinical service settings wherever it is taught, studied, advocated, and provided. Its empirically rooted definition—aligning with efforts by Tyndall, Hodgson, Lamson, White, and Knight (2010)—is a field that is grounded in

> a BPSS [biopsychosocial-spiritual] perspective and marriage and family therapy, but also informed by systems theory. The practice of MedFT spans a variety of clinical settings with a strong focus on the relationships of the patient and the collaboration between and among the healthcare providers and the patient. MedFTs are endorsers of patient and family agency and facilitators of healthy workplace dynamics. (pp. 68–69)

Guided by our passion to grow the field, we engaged the editor of *Contemporary Family Therapy* (Dr. Russell Crane) in 2010 to co-construct a special issue on MedFT. This then led to an exciting collaboration in 2014 to assemble an edited text through Springer called *Medical Family Therapy: Advanced Applications*. This landmark volume synthesized contemporary advancements in MedFT training, research, policy, and financial models (Hodgson, Lamson, Mendenhall, & Crane,

2014). It has been well-received by colleagues in practice, research, policy think tanks, and teaching/training sites—and serves as a go-to reference for practitioners, administrators, scholars, supervisors, and students/trainees alike.

This new text, *Clinical Methods in Medical Family Therapy*, serves to highlight MedFTs in action across a variety of specialized healthcare settings. Alongside our own shared and respective areas of expertise, we have recruited and engaged skilled and innovative colleagues (including practitioners, theorists, supervisors, leaders, administrators, researchers, policy makers, and up-and-coming professionals)—most of whom identify as family therapists and/or medical family therapists—to describe the applications of MedFT within and across a myriad of care contexts and foci.

Layout of the Text

This edited book begins (Chapter 1) by providing a brief history and description of MedFT's evolution, as well as the interweaving of our own relationships with one another and with our worlds as MedFTs. In this chapter, we introduce Hodgson, Lamson, Mendenhall, and Tyndall's (2014) five-level *MedFT Healthcare Continuum* and then use the continuum as a guiding framework for each of the remaining chapters. This continuum serves to assist MedFTs in understanding the scope (breadth), sophistication (depth), and application of specific knowledge and skill sets at different levels. Respective levels do not represent sequential or chronological steps en route to an ultimate goal (i.e., *Level 5*); instead, they serve as anchors onto which you, as our readers, can position and conceptualize the MedFT work that best fits your aims.

We then divide the book into four distinct sections, wherein authors introduce research-informed practice and applications of MedFT across (a) primary care, (b) secondary care, (c) tertiary care, and (d) unique care environments and clinical populations. Contexts described in primary care include MedFT in *Family Medicine* (Chapter 2), MedFT in *Pediatrics* (Chapter 3), and MedFT in *Internal Medicine* (Chapter 4). Contexts described in secondary care include MedFT in *Intensive Care* (Chapter 5), MedFT in *Obstetrics and Gynecology* (Chapter 6), MedFT in *Emergency Medicine* (Chapter 7), MedFT in *Oncology* (Chapter 8), and MedFT in *Psychiatry* (Chapter 9). Contexts described in tertiary care include MedFT in *Hospice and Palliative Care* (Chapter 10), MedFT in *Endocrinology* (Chapter 11), and MedFT in *Alcohol and Drug Treatment* (Chapter 12). Contexts representing unique care environments and clinical populations include MedFT in *Community Health Centers* (Chapter 13), MedFT in *Community Engagement* (Chapter 14), MedFT in *Disaster Preparedness and Trauma Response Teams* (Chapter 15), MedFT in *Spiritual Care* (Chapter 16), MedFT in *Employee Assistance Programs* (Chapter 17), and MedFT in *Military and Veteran Health Systems* (Chapter 18).

Each chapter begins with a description of the unique context that it is oriented to (e.g., health foci targeted and treated, conditions under which care is provided). The authors provide a case example (vignette) to illustrate commonplace challenges that MedFTs see and engage with as part of their work with patients, families, and colleagues. They describe the makeup of care teams tailored for the chapter's focused environment (e.g., members trained in a unique discipline or specialty) and highlight fundamental knowledge and practical skill sets that are essential for MedFTs positioned therein. The *MedFT Healthcare Continuum* (Hodgson et al., 2014) and research-informed practices are used to depict diverse ways in which MedFTs can function in each care context. To further assist you in applying the content of each chapter, the authors offer reflection questions that encourage personal deliberations, collective (small-group) discussion, and/or further exploration regarding specialized content and practical applications. The authors also present resources that are specific to chapter foci (e.g., literature, websites, organizations, measures/instruments), and asterisked readings in their reference lists to denote significant publications worthy of review.

In our conclusion (Chapter 19), we describe new and emerging directions in MedFT and IBHC. We offer descriptions of field leaders' efforts as they—to use Mac Baird's often-cited adage (Baird, 1995)—build ships as they sail them. Their accounts frame MedFT as a field still very much evolving, charging forward into and across new and uncharted treatment sites and contexts. We are frequently asked what types of job opportunities exist for MedFTs. Therefore, the premise behind this chapter is to feature those who are successfully leading careers in MedFT in the following areas: (a) interdisciplinary research; (b) training innovations and health specializations; (c) faculty appointments in primary, secondary, and tertiary care departments; and (d) policy and leadership.

This edited text represents a timely undertaking. MedFT is becoming a mainstream and widely recognized field, as evidenced by (a) the advent and growth of new MedFT training programs; (b) increasing numbers of couple/marriage and family therapy (C/MFT) students aligning their studies and clinical placements to medical/healthcare settings; and (c) increasing numbers of behavioral health workforce members across a myriad of disciplines (e.g., C/MFT, psychology, social work, counseling) entering medical schools and other healthcare facilities. Our intent with this book is to recognize and advance the work of MedFT's leaders while at the same time inspire new professionals and students who are preparing to engage in and further advance this work across a diverse range of care contexts, populations, and job markets.

Tai Mendenhall
Angela Lamson
Jennifer Hodgson
Macaran Baird

References

Baird, M. (1995). Building the ship as we sail it. *Family Systems Medicine, 13*, 269–273. https://doi.org/10.1037/h0089066.

Hodgson, J., Lamson, A., Mendenhall, T., & Crane, D. (Eds.). (2014). *Medical family therapy: Advanced applications*. New York, NY: Springer.

Hodgson, J., Lamson, A., Mendenhall, T. & Tyndall, L. (2014). Introduction to Medical family therapy: Advanced applications. In J. Hodgson, A. Lamson, T. Mendenhall, and D. Crane (Eds.), *Medical family therapy: Advanced applications* (pp. 1–9). New York, NY: Springer.

McDaniel, S., Doherty, W., & Hepworth, J. (2014). *Medical family therapy and integrated care* (2nd ed.). Washington, DC: American Psychological Association.

McDaniel, S., Hepworth, J., & Doherty, W. (1992). *Medical family therapy: A biopsyhosocial approach to families with health problems*. New York, NY: Basic Books.

Tyndall, L., Hodgson, J., White, M., Lamson, A., & Knight, S. (2010). *Medical family therapy: Conceptual clarification and consensus for an emerging profession* (Unpublished doctoral dissertation). East Carolina University, Greenville, NC.

Acknowledgments

The editors would like to send a special thank you to the following individuals for their time and boundless energy in serving as junior editors for this text:

Catherine Futoransky (University of Minnesota)
Jessica Goodman (East Carolina University)
Therese Nichols (University of Minnesota)
Olivia Riser (East Carolina University)
Erin Sesemann (East Carolina University)
Julie Smith (East Carolina University)

And to the following colleagues for their valuable consultations, recommendations, and guidance:

Caanan Crane, PhD, LMFT (Oklahoma Baptist University)
CAPT Brenda Gearhart, LCSW-C, BCD
Chad Lamson, MBA, RN (AxoGen, Inc.)
Tiffany M. Martin, MS, PA-C (Forsyth Medical Center, NC)
Bret Roark, PhD (Oklahoma Baptist University)
Doug Smith, CEO (Greene County Health Care, Inc.)

Contents

1 **The Beginning of Us: A Conversation Among Friends About Our MedFT Family**................................ 1
Angela Lamson, Jennifer Hodgson, and Tai Mendenhall

Part I Medical Family Therapy in Primary Care

2 **Medical Family Therapy in Family Medicine** 17
Jennifer Hodgson, Lisa Trump, Grace Wilson, and Diego Garcia-Huidobro

3 **Medical Family Therapy in Pediatrics** 61
Keeley Pratt, Catherine Van Fossen, Katharine Didericksen, Rola Aamar, and Jerica Berge

4 **Medical Family Therapy in Internal Medicine** 87
Jennifer Harsh and Rachel Bonnema

Part II Medical Family Therapy in Secondary Care

5 **Medical Family Therapy in Intensive Care** 113
Angela Lamson and Jessica Goodman

6 **Medical Family Therapy in Obstetrics and Gynecology** 147
Angela Lamson, Kenneth Phelps, Ashley Jones, and Rebecca Bagley

7 **Medical Family Therapy in Emergency Medicine** 181
Rosanne Kassekert and Tai Mendenhall

8 **Medical Family Therapy in Oncology** 207
Talia Zaider and Peter Steinglass

9 **Medical Family Therapy in Psychiatry** 231
Kenneth Phelps, Jennifer Hodgson, Alison Heru, and Jakob Jensen

Part III Medical Family Therapy in Tertiary Care

10 Medical Family Therapy in Palliative and Hospice Care 263
Jackie Williams-Reade and Stephanie Trudeau

11 Medical Family Therapy in Endocrinology 293
Max Zubatsky and Tai Mendenhall

12 Medical Family Therapy in Alcohol and Drug Treatment 321
Kristy Soloski and Jaclyn Cravens Pickens

Part IV Medical Family Therapy in Unique Care Contexts and Populations

13 Medical Family Therapy in Community Health Centers 357
Jennifer Hodgson, Angela Lamson, Rola Aamar, and Francisco Limon

14 Medical Family Therapy in Community Engagement 401
Tai Mendenhall, William Doherty, Elizabeth "Nan" LittleWalker, and Jerica Berge

15 Medical Family Therapy in Disaster Preparedness and Trauma-Response Teams 431
Tai Mendenhall, Jonathan Bundt, and Cigdem Yumbul

16 Medical Family Therapy in Spiritual Care 463
Jonathan Wilson, Jennifer Hodgson, Eunicia Jones, and Grace Wilson

17 Medical Family Therapy in Employee Assistance Programs 497
Calvin Paries, Angela Lamson, Jennifer Hodgson, Amelia Muse, and Glenda Mutinda

18 Medical Family Therapy in Military and Veteran Health Systems 537
Angela Lamson, Meghan Lacks, Erin Cobb, and Grace Seamon

19 Innovations in MedFT: Pioneering New Frontiers! 583
Jennifer Hodgson, Tai Mendenhall, Angela Lamson, Macaran Baird, and Jackie Williams-Reade

Index 603

About the Authors

Rola Aamar is a postdoctoral scholar in the medical family therapy program at East Carolina University (ECU). Her clinical interests include medical and behavioral mental health disparities among underserved and minority populations and patient-centered treatment of comorbid medical and mental health conditions. Her research agenda is focused on factors associated with obesity in children and families, as well as the relationship between treatment alliance and treatment for childhood obesity and adult chronic illnesses. As a postdoctoral scholar, Dr. Aamar helped establish clinical practice protocols that increase patients' knowledge about health behaviors to promote better outcomes for both mental health and medical diagnoses.

Rebecca Bagley is a clinical associate professor at East Carolina University's (ECU) College of Nursing. She currently serves as the nurse-midwifery program director while continuing a faculty practice in labor and delivery and at ECU Women's Medical Clinic. She has experience in full scope midwifery, including women's health throughout the lifespan, in private practice, in public health, and in the academic setting. She serves on the board of the Association of Professors of Gynecology and Obstetrics (APGO) and is a site visitor for the Accreditation Commission for Midwifery Education (ACME).

Macaran Baird is professor and head of the University of Minnesota Medical School's Department of Family Medicine and Community Health. He began his medical career in 1978 as a rural physician and family therapist. He and Dr. Bill Doherty coauthored *Family Therapy and Family Medicine* in 1983, which launched his academic and leadership career. Dr. Baird has since held positions in Oklahoma, New York, and Rochester, MN. His leadership involvement has also included service on the Robert Wood Johnson Foundation's (RWJF) Depression in Primary Care National Advisory Council and as cochair of the Institute of Medicine's (IOM) *Report on Health and Behavior*. He is a past president of the Society of Teachers of Family Medicine (STFM) and was a recipient of the American Academy of Family Physician's (AAFP) Thomas Johnson Award for career contributions in family medicine education. Dr. Baird's principal research and clinical foci center on the integration of behavioral health and primary care and in identifying social and care system factors that inhibit and/or contribute to positive outcomes for patients and families.

Jerica Berge is an associate professor, researcher, and behavioral medicine provider in the Department of Family Medicine and Community Health at the University of Minnesota (UMN) Medical School. She is a clinical member of the American Association for Marriage and Family Therapy (AAMFT) and an AAMFT-approved supervisor. Dr. Berge's research expertise is in measuring and analyzing risk and protective factors for childhood and adolescent obesity. She conducts epidemiological research, mixed-methods studies, and randomized controlled trials to reduce childhood obesity disparities. Dr. Berge is the codirector of the Healthy Eating and Activity Across the Lifespan (HEAL) Center, which facilitates integration across research, clinical practice, policy, and community to promote a culture of health.

Rachel Bonnema is an associate professor in the Department of Internal Medicine at the University of Nebraska Medical Center (UNMC). She is an associate program director for the internal medicine residency at UNMC and directs the women's health elective for fourth year medical students, internal medicine residents, and obstetrics/gynecology residents. Her clinical area of interest is women's health, and her academic focus remains in medical education—particularly in women's health, professional development, and communication skills.

Jonathan Bundt is a board-certified expert in crisis response and traumatic stress. He has worked in the behavioral science and mental health fields for over 30 years, specializing in disaster and crisis, preparedness, response, and recovery. Jonathan operates his own consulting company, called Masa Consulting, which specializes in the integration of behavioral science into risk and threat mitigation of workplace violence. In his early career, he rose to the rank of chief inspector in the National Israeli Police Force, wherein he worked in the field of anti- and counter-terrorism training and response. Jonathan's work in the United States began in 1995 as a mental health professional for the Hennepin County Sheriff's Office, Minneapolis Police Department (SWAT), as a trainer and on-scene support advisor where he specialized in training crisis/hostage negotiators and critical incident response. He has been involved in responding to over 3000 local, regional, and national incidents of crisis, violence, and risk mitigation. He regularly provides consultation and training services to the private sector, hospitals, EMS, police and fire departments, and the MN State Departments of Corrections, Public Health, Human Services, Public Safety, and Emergency Management.

Erin Cobb is a doctoral candidate in the medical family therapy program at East Carolina University. She is currently completing an internship in behavioral medicine at Dartmouth Family Medicine Residency/Concord Family Health Center. Her dissertation explores disordered eating among veterans and military service members. She has served as a MedFT researcher and clinician in a variety of contexts, ranging from eating disorder treatment in pediatric primary care to mobile mental health services for homeless veterans.

Katharine Didericksen is an assistant professor of human development and family science in East Carolina University's (ECU) medical family therapy and marriage and family therapy programs. She is an American Association for Marriage and Family Therapy (AAMFT) clinical fellow and approved supervisor. Dr. Wickel Didericksen's primary research interests focus on pediatric obesity within family contexts, the relationship(s) between poverty and health, and community-engaged research.

William Doherty is a medical family therapist and professor in the Department of Family Social Science at the University of Minnesota (UMN). He is also the director of the UMN's Citizen Professional Center. Along with Susan McDaniel and Jeri Hepworth, Dr. Doherty pioneered the conceptual and clinical development of the field of MedFT. He works actively on citizen professional projects to bring democratic engagement to health care.

Catherine Van Fossen is a doctoral student in the human development and family science program and couple and family therapy specialization in the Department of Human Sciences at The Ohio State University. Her primary interests include how integrated care models meet the needs of minority and underserved populations and assessing family functioning in pediatric primary care to determine MedFT need and involvement.

Diego Garcia-Huidobro is an assistant professor at Pontificia Universidad Católica de Chile Department of Family Medicine and adjunct faculty at the University of Minnesota (UMN) Medical School's Department of Family Medicine and Community Health. He completed medical school and residency training at Pontificia Universidad Católica de Chile and then a PhD in family social science and postdoctoral training from the UMN. Dr. García-Huidobro conducts transdisciplinary community-based participatory translational research focused on how family and other psychosocial factors influence health outcomes and on how family interventions can promote healthier behaviors to prevent chronic illnesses.

Jessica Goodman is a doctoral student in medical family therapy at East Carolina University (ECU). She is a preclinical fellow with the American Association for Marriage and Family Therapy (AAMFT) and has worked as a MedFT across dental, emergency department, employee assistance, inpatient, primary care, and traditional care settings. Jessica's current research focuses on frequent utilization of the emergency department, alongside policy and advocacy efforts in family therapy.

Jennifer Harsh is an assistant professor in the Department of Internal Medicine at the University of Nebraska Medical Center (UNMC), wherein she directs the behavioral medicine and resident wellness programs in the Division of General Internal Medicine. She is actively involved in providing patient and family care across both outpatient and inpatient internal medicine settings, supervising MedFT interns, teaching behavioral health providers and internal medicine residents, and conducting research. Her investigative interests currently include the use of novel approaches to assess medical providers' well-being and integrating MedFT into general hospital settings.

Alison Heru is an interim chair and professor of psychiatry at the University of Colorado Denver, wherein she established and directs the psychosomatic medicine psychiatry fellowship. Dr. Heru is the treasurer of the Association of Family Psychiatrists. She has presented and published on multiple topics, including family therapy, culture and family, and medical student mistreatment. She has authored four books about families, most recently *Working with Families in Medical Settings*. Dr. Heru publishes a monthly column in *Clinical Psychiatry News* called "Families in Psychiatry." She is a member of the Group for the Advancement of Psychiatry (GAP) and chair of GAP's Family Committee.

Jennifer Hodgson is a professor at East Carolina University (ECU) in the Department of Human Development and Family Science. She is the director for the doctoral program in medical family therapy and coeditor of the 2014 text *Medical Family Therapy: Advanced Applications* with Angela Lamson, Tai Mendenhall, and D. Russell Crane. Dr. Hodgson is a clinical member of the American Association for Marriage and Family Therapy (AAMFT) and an AAMFT-approved supervisor. She has numerous presentations, publications, and funded grants in the areas of MedFT and integrated behavioral healthcare. Dr. Hodgson has held national leadership positions for her profession and in the Collaborative Family Healthcare Association (CFHA).

Jakob Jensen is an assistant professor at East Carolina University (ECU) in the Department of Human Development and Family Science. He is also an affiliated member of ECU's Center for Applied Psychophysiology. Dr. Jensen has several national and international publications and presentations about romantic/social relationships, issues in aging, and psychophysiological stress. He currently provides supervision to doctoral-level MedFT students at a psychiatric inpatient hospital facility.

Ashley Jones is an assistant professor of clinical neuropsychiatry and adjunct assistant professor of clinical obstetrics and gynecology at the University of South Carolina (USC) School of Medicine. She is a board-certified psychiatrist with special interests in reproductive psychiatry. She serves as the associate program director for USC's general psychiatry residency and director of Adult Resident Outpatient Clinics within the Outpatient Psychiatry Clinic. Additionally, Dr. Jones supervises residents practicing in an integrated psychiatry-ob-gyn clinic, wherein comprehensive treatment is delivered to prenatal and postpartum women and their families.

Eunicia Jones is a doctoral student in the medical family therapy program at East Carolina University (ECU). Niecie has worked in several clinical, research, and teaching settings focused on identity and development. She has worked primarily with teens and adults on issues such as trauma, grief, and life transitions and uses methods that focus on spirituality and narrative construction. Niecie is a past fellow of the American Association for Marriage and Family Therapy's (AAMFT) Minority Fellowship Program, which has helped to further her research with racial and ethnic minorities. She plans to continue doing clinical and academic work using spirituality as a tool for change and growth.

Rosanne Kassekert (recently retired) served as the director of the behavioral science education program at Health Partners Institute of Education's family medicine residency at Regions Hospital in Saint Paul, MN. She worked actively in the conduct of critical care and residency education for 27 years. She was an active member of the Society for Teachers of Family Medicine (STFM) and, along with supervising resident physicians, mentored graduate students in both social work and MedFT. Rosanne also worked at Regions Hospital's Emergency Medicine Department crisis intervention program for 14 years, wherein she evaluated and triaged patients experiencing mental health trauma and other illnesses.

Meghan Lacks is the director of integrated care at a federally qualified health center (FQHC) in North Carolina. Dr. Lacks is responsible for the implementation of integrated care in over 30 primary care clinics, and she provides support, training, and supervision to clinicians working as behavioral health consultants in these clinics. She earned both her master's degree in marriage and family therapy and Ph.D. in medical family therapy from East Carolina University. She completed a predoctoral internship with the Association for Marriage and Family Therapy (AAMFT) serving as a research and policy analyst for military initiatives. Dr. Lacks completed her doctoral dissertation on the biopsychosocial-spiritual (BPSS) health of active duty women. She also conducted research on integrated care with military couples.

Angela Lamson is a professor at East Carolina University (ECU) in the Department of Human Development and Family Science. She is also the associate dean for research in the College of Health and Human Performance and coeditor of the 2014 text *Medical Family Therapy: Advanced Applications* with Jennifer Hodgson, Tai Mendenhall, and D. Russell Crane. Dr. Lamson is a clinical member of the American Association for Marriage and Family Therapy (AAMFT) and an AAMFT-approved supervisor. Dr. Lamson has served as the program director for the medical family therapy doctoral program and marriage and family therapy master's program at ECU, as division president for the North Carolina Association for Marriage and Family Therapy, and as member of the Elections Council for AAMFT. In addition, she is on the Executive Committee for the Alliance of Military and Veteran Family Behavioral Health Providers at the national level. Dr. Lamson's teaching, funding, and publications have been devoted to MedFT and integrated care, particularly in the areas of trauma, chronic illness, loss, and compassion fatigue in the lives of individuals, couples, families, and providers. Her training and research initiatives have been housed in community health, primary care, specialty care, and military bases.

Francisco Limon is the behavioral health director at Greene County Health Care (GCHC) in the state of North Carolina. Dr. Limon is a clinical fellow of the American Association of Marriage and Family Therapy (AAMFT) and a member of the Collaborative Family Healthcare Association (CFHA). His research interests include health disparities in the areas of depression and diabetes in underserved populations, acculturation stress, and program development and evaluation.

Elizabeth "Nan" LittleWalker is a Native American member of the Ho-Chunk Nation; she has lived and served in the Twin Cities of St. Paul and Minneapolis for more than 30 years. As a dedicated stakeholder and leader in the community, Nan has worked as an educator, volunteer, American Indian advisor and liaison, outreach worker, and advocate for programs and initiatives oriented to the advancement of Native people. She is one of the founding members of the Interfaith Action of Greater Saint Paul/Department of Indian Work's Family Education Diabetes Series (FEDS), which was developed through community-based participatory research (CBPR) methods in partnership with biomedical and behavioral health providers at the University of Minnesota (UMN). Through these and related efforts, Nan is very knowledgeable regarding Minnesota's American Indian community and its respective tribes, their religious and spiritual belief systems, family and clan organizations, and service organizations and providers.

Tai Mendenhall is an associate professor and medical family therapist in the couple and family therapy program at the University of Minnesota (UMN) in the Department of Family Social Science. He is also an adjunct professor and clinician in the UMN Medical School's Department of Family Medicine and Community Health, an associate director of the UMN's Citizen Professional Center, and the director of the UMN's Medical Reserve Corps' Mental Health Disaster-Response Teams. Dr. Mendenhall is a coeditor of the 2014 text *Medical Family Therapy: Advanced Applications* with Drs. Jennifer Hodgson, Angela Lamson, and D. Russell Crane. He is a clinical member of the American Association for Marriage and Family Therapy (AAMFT) and an AAMFT-approved supervisor. He works actively in the conduct of integrated health care and community-based participatory research (CBPR) focused on a variety of public health issues.

Amelia Muse is the director of operations at the Center of Excellence for Integrated Care, a program of the Foundation for Health Leadership and Innovation in North Carolina. She graduated from East Carolina University (ECU) with a PhD in medical family therapy and a certificate in quantitative methods for social and behavioral sciences. In her role at the Center of Excellence for Integrated Care, Dr. Muse assists health systems in integrating physical and behavioral healthcare services.

She has clinical experience in community mental health, rural primary care, and occupational health.

Glenda Mutinda is a medical family therapy doctoral student at East Carolina University (ECU). She is currently completing her research, clinical, and teaching fellowship at St. Mary's Family Medicine Department in Grand Junction, Colorado.

Calvin Paries is the director of the employee assistance/health and wellness program for Centura Health, a large health system in Colorado and Western Kansas. He earned his doctorate in occupational health/EAP and is a certified employee assistance professional (CEAP). Dr. Paries has worked in the EAP field for over 25 years, serving in senior management positions in both regional and large national EAP and wellness companies. He has worked as a consultant for several large organizations and has run numerous internal hospital-based employee assistance programs focusing on integrated care and outcome-based counseling.

Kenneth Phelps is an associate professor of clinical neuropsychiatry and adjunct associate professor of clinical pediatrics at the University of South Carolina (USC) School of Medicine. With a doctorate in medical family therapy, he also serves as the director for the Palmetto Health, University of South Carolina Outpatient Psychiatry Clinic. Dr. Phelps has prior clinical experience in labor and delivery, neonatal intensive care units, pediatric intensive care units, and other pediatric settings.

Jaclyn Cravens Pickens is an assistant professor and director of the addictive disorders and recovery studies (ADRS) program at Texas Tech University (TTU). Her administrative role at TTU has included the development of an online/distance education offering of the undergraduate minor in ADRS, which provides the educational requirements for the licensed chemical dependency counselor (LCDC) designation in Texas. She teaches both undergraduate- and graduate-level courses in addiction recovery. Dr. Cravens Pickens' area of research focuses on the impact of technology and the Internet on couples and families, including process addictions related to technology use.

Keeley Pratt is an assistant professor in the human development and family science program, couple and family therapy specialization, in the Department of Human Sciences at The Ohio State University. She also is an assistant professor at The Ohio State University's Wexner Medical Center in the Department of Surgery, wherein she oversees the behavioral health and family therapy programming for adult weight management and bariatric surgery patients. Dr. Pratt is an American Association for Marriage and Family Therapy (AAMFT) clinical fellow and approved supervisor. Her research interests include the assessment of family factors to predict successful outcomes in child and adult weight management programs, designing family-based weight management interventions for children in pediatric obesity treatment, and couples interventions in adult weight management and bariatric surgery programs.

Grace Seamon is a graduate of the East Carolina University's marriage and family therapy program. She works as a clinical specialist on two military installations.

Kristy Soloski is an assistant professor in the marriage and family therapy program at Texas Tech University (TTU). She is an associate licensed marriage and family therapist and a licensed chemical dependency counselor in the state of Texas. Dr. Soloski was a fellow of the American Association for Marriage and Family Therapy (AAMFT) Minority Fellowship Program for 3 years, where she received specialized training in the delivery of culturally competent mental health and substance abuse services to underserved populations. She has designed and taught coursework on adolescent substance use. Dr. Soloski's area of research examines factors related to the trajectory of binge drinking from adolescence onward, including the gene-environment interaction. She is also presently examining how a biological versus environmental narrative on addiction impacts people's perceptions of and attitudes toward substance users.

Peter Steinglass is president emeritus of the Ackerman Institute for the Family, director of the Ackerman Institute for the Family's Center for Substance Use and the Family, and clinical professor of psychiatry at Weill Cornell Medical College. He is a board-certified psychiatrist whose multi-decade research career has focused on family factors influencing the onset and clinical course(s) of substance use disorders and chronic medical illnesses. These efforts included a series of studies with colleagues at the Memorial Sloan-Kettering Cancer Center, a part of which has been Dr. Steinglass's pioneering work in the use of multifamily discussion groups for families dealing with major medical illnesses.

Stephanie Trudeau is a doctoral candidate at the University of Minnesota (UMN) in the Department of Family Social Science's couple and family therapy program. Her clinical and research interests include family medicine, family coping with chronic illness and end of life, provider well-being, and integrated behavioral healthcare model design, development, and evaluation.

Lisa Trump is a marriage and family therapist at Stone Arch Psychology and Health Services in Minneapolis, MN. She completed her doctoral education at the University of Minnesota (UMN) in the Department of Family Social Science, specializing in couple and family therapy and medical family therapy. Dr. Trump's clinical work and research focuses on the biopsychosocial-spiritual (BPSS) health of military couples, patients' and families' coping with—and management of—chronic illnesses, and integrated behavioral healthcare. She has published in our field's top journals and has presented her work across both local and national forums and conferences.

About the Authors

Jackie Williams-Reade is an associate professor at Loma Linda University in the marriage and family therapy (MFT) doctoral program. She is a clinical fellow and approved supervisor with American Association for Marriage and Family Therapy (AAMFT). Dr. Williams-Reade received her MedFT training through her MS at Seattle Pacific University and her PhD from East Carolina University. She completed her internship and postdoc at Johns Hopkins University where she conducted NIH-supported research on the application of pediatric palliative care to adolescents with complex conditions. She is interested in the application and advancement of MedFT in pediatric specialty care settings and utilizing qualitative research to privilege patient and family voices in healthcare.

Grace Wilson is a behavioral science faculty member at the Great Plains family medicine residency program. She is a former fellow in the Society of Teachers of Family Medicine's (STFM) behavioral science/family systems educator fellowship. In her role as a behaviorist, Dr. Wilson facilitates interdisciplinary cross-training of family medicine residents alongside MedFT interns and supervises the delivery of integrated behavioral health services in a community-based primary care clinic. Her clinical and research interests center on infertility, pregnancy, trauma, and couple relationship.

Jonathan Wilson is an assistant professor at Oklahoma Baptist University in the Department of Behavioral and Social Sciences. He cofounded Oklahoma's first advanced clinical training certificate in medical family therapy and has various publications and presentations in MedFT and integrated behavioral healthcare. He has also held leadership positions for the Oklahoma's Association for Marriage and Family Therapy.

Cigdem Yumbul is a doctoral student in the couple and family therapy program at the University of Minnesota (UMN), Twin Cities. She is currently completing an autoethnographic dissertation regarding behavioral health relief efforts provided to affected communities following the 2014 Soma Mining Massacre in Turkey. As a psychotherapist, Cigdem works with individuals, couples, and families—primarily targeting issues related to trauma, loss, and grief—at the Bude Psychotherapy Center in Istanbul, Turkey. She is a member of the Turkish Psychological Association and continues to actively participate in psychosocial support efforts delivered to individuals and communities impacted by mass trauma.

Talia Zaider is assistant attending psychologist and director of the Family Therapy Clinic at Memorial Sloan Kettering Cancer Center (MSKCC) in New York, NY. Her research has focused on identifying and addressing the support needs of couples and families in the context of cancer care. She leads an interdisciplinary outpatient clinic that serves couples and families under care at MSKCC, and is leading an effort to advance the roles of inpatient oncology nurses to deliver family-centered supportive care in acute care settings. She has served as a coinvestigator on randomized controlled trials testing psychosocial support interventions for couples and families coping across early- and advanced-stage disease.

Max Zubatsky is an assistant professor in the medical family therapy program at Saint Louis University. He is an American Association for Marriage and Family Therapy (AAMFT) clinical fellow and approved supervisor. Dr. Zubatsky is a coinvestigator on two Health Resources and Service Administration (HRSA)-funded grants for behavioral health workforce training of MedFTs and primary care training and enhancement for family medicine residents. In addition, he directs the Memory Clinic, which is a comprehensive geriatrics clinic at Saint Louis University's Center for Counseling and Family Therapy.

Chapter 1
The Beginning of Us: A Conversation Among Friends About Our MedFT Family

Angela Lamson, Jennifer Hodgson, and Tai Mendenhall

From the very beginning of our (Tai, Angela, Jennifer) efforts in planning this book, we identified ideas that we wanted to convey through *Chapter 1*. Sometimes even the best laid plans lead to unanticipated routes, and sometimes those routes bring even better—more purposeful—results. This chapter, while formulated first, was the last to be written. In the name of transparency, we started our contributions to this book by writing our respective—other—chapters. As we were rounding into the halfway mark, and while at the same time experiencing several influential changes in our lives, a clearer vision for this chapter came to us. We recognized that many of you, as our readers, might be new to medical family therapy (MedFT) and would thereby need some perspective about our field's history. While we wanted you to be informed about this history, we also wanted to offer something beyond just a history lesson—especially since the foundation of MedFT had already been described through other books and manuscripts (e.g., Doherty, McDaniel, & Hepworth, 1994; Hodgson, Lamson, Mendenhall, & Crane, 2014; McDaniel, Doherty, & Hepworth, 2014; McDaniel, Hepworth, & Doherty, 1992; Tyndall, Hodgson, Lamson, White, & Knight, 2012, 2014). In one of our many conference calls, we decided to construct an academic snapshot of MedFT (i.e., a cliff notes version) and then follow that content up with an opportunity for you to learn more about our own personal journeys that lead us to the field. Our hope is that these stories invite you into our love for MedFT and inspire you to build upon this field's impressive history over the days and years to come.

A. Lamson (✉) · J. Hodgson
Department of Human Development and Family Science, East Carolina University, Greenville, NC, USA
e-mail: lamsona@ecu.edu

T. Mendenhall
Department of Family Social Science, University of Minnesota, Saint Paul, MN, USA

An Academic Snapshot

The most current definition of MedFT that we align with was constructed in 2010 through a modified Delphi study that included contributions from many of the field's leading experts (Tyndall, Hodgson, Lamson, White, & Knight, 2010). From that effort, MedFT was defined as a field grounded in a

> BPSS [biopsychosocial-spiritual] perspective and marriage and family therapy, but also informed by systems theory. The practice of MedFT spans a variety of clinical settings with a strong focus on the relationships of the patient and the collaboration between and among the health-care providers and the patient. MedFTs are endorsers of patient and family agency, and facilitators of healthy workplace dynamics. (p. 68–69)

As first introduced in our text's *Preface*, we adopted this definition because it is research informed and was developed through the input of many diverse voices, rather than constructed from our own biases regarding what MedFT represents or reflects. We anticipate that this definition will change over time to keep up with the dynamic nature of MedFT that now exists across research, training, supervision, leadership, administration, and policy—all of which are contexts that extend beyond those aligned with the clinical settings as cited in this definition.

While researchers within and outside of the field may have their own version(s) of what MedFT is or should be, its foundation is unquestioned: MedFT stemmed from many of the founders of family therapy, spanning a wide variety of disciplines. Brilliant minds from nearly seven decades ago were integrating their training in biology with family therapy (e.g., Gregory Bateson, Murray Bowen, Ludwig von Bertalanffy), and while nearly two decades would pass until more recognition was given to the ways in which physical health influences psychosocial well-being (e.g., Edgar Auerswald, Salvador Minuchin, Lyman Wynne), the systemic lens of family therapy never wavered. One of the most powerful voices that MedFTs align with is that of George Engel (1977, 1980), a visionary who took a bold risk to describe the importance of stepping out of the medical model and into a biopsychosocial (BPS) model that was grounded in systems theory. This innovative vision gave way to new energy all over the United States (and beyond), whereby MedFTs began collaborating in health-care contexts, and medical providers began to recognize the value of family therapy when integrated into the medical system (Bloch, 1984; Doherty & Baird, 1983; Hepworth & Jackson, 1985; McDaniel & Campbell, 1986; Rolland, 1984).

In 1992, McDaniel, Hepworth, and Doherty wrote the field's primer text, *Medical Family Therapy: A Biopsychosocial Approach to Families with Health Problems*. This book called attention to the need for a family-centered behavioral health model of care and opened the gates for a new field. At about that same time, a group of family nurses (Bell, Wright, & Watson, 1992) wrote a pointed article concerning the title of MedFT, particularly addressing a lack of recognition for nurses when the name was narrowed to "medical" family therapy. While the term remained, researchers have worked hard to honor nurses' contributions to the success of MedFT—both directly and indirectly (e.g., Anderson, Huff & Hodgson, 2008; Marlowe & Hodgson, 2014; Martin, White, Hodgson, Lamson, & Irons, 2014). Informed by the invaluable contribution by Wright, Watson, and Bell (1996) called *Beliefs: The Heart of Healing in Families and Illness*, we (Angela, Jennifer, and Tai) work to train MedFTs to assess for spiritual domains of health and incorporate these into treatment plans when appropriate (Hodgson, Lamson, & Reese, 2007). Acknowledgments regarding the importance of using a biopsychosocial-spiritual (BPSS) framework in the practice of MedFT—as advanced through the pioneering work of Engel (1977, 1980) and Wright et al. (1996)—are illustrated in every chapter of this text.

A new generation of MedFTs emerged with the new millennia, as did recognition for the ways in which a growing number of medical diagnoses influence relational health—biologically, psychologically, socially, and spiritually. To cite all of the work in MedFT since 2000 would not be possible, but many of these publications are referenced in the remaining chapters of this text. Some of the pivotal markers indicating a critical need for MedFT in health care include the burgeoning of accredited training programs and internship sites in MedFT (highlighted in Chapter 19), the development of MedFT core competencies (Tyndall, Hodgson, Lamson, White, & Knight, 2014), and more recently the creation of the MedFT Healthcare Continuum (Hodgson, Lamson, Mendenhall, & Tyndall, 2014). This continuum places MedFT skills and knowledge across five levels of application that range in both proficiency and intensity. It suits any context that promotes relational and BPSS health and offers a range of skills appropriate for a wide variety of health-care professionals who are invested in family-centered care and integrated behavioral health-care models.

The value of the MedFT Healthcare Continuum (Hodgson et al., 2014) is strengthened when considered in context of other historical works in our field, such as the five levels of primary care/behavioral health collaboration advanced by Doherty, McDaniel, and Baird (1996). Together, MedFTs are able to map a level of collaboration (suitable to their context, needs of patients/families, and/or unique relationships with each provider) in tandem with their MedFT knowledge and skill sets to build a successful and sustainable model of care (see Lamson, Pratt, Hodgson, & Koehler, 2014, for a detailed explanation of how Doherty et al.'s (1996) levels interface with Hodgson et al.'s (2014) continuum). Workplace opportunities for which MedFT skills and knowledge are embedded are now far reaching; these include primary, secondary, and tertiary health-care contexts, as well as a variety of others that stretch beyond the bricks and mortar of traditional health-care environments. Further, the roles and corresponding skills of MedFTs in health-care settings continue to evolve, offering greater opportunities for MedFT in research, teaching, supervision, leadership, administration, and policy. The exponential growth of MedFTs in the workforce over the past decade is a sign that this field will only continue to grow. Throughout the remaining chapters in this text, attention is given to the roles and contexts that have emerged over the past two decades (especially) and the research, knowledge, and fundamental skills needed for MedFTs situated in each unique setting/population.

As authors and editors, we take great pride in the remaining chapters of this text, as first-, second-, and third-generation MedFTs have come together to honor the past, present, and future of this incredible field. Each of us found this field through our own serendipitous routes—whether it was through a passion to be involved in health care, via personal experiences, or both. In constructing this chapter, we wanted to share with you how we found MedFT and how it became our chosen career. Our stories represent a homage to our mentors, filled with gratitude for colleagues and students, and an invitation for professionals to join us in this amazing field.

Our Family Photo

By Angela Lamson

My story began well before I ever identified as a MedFT. There were two pivotal narratives that had a presence in my childhood, but their influence did not really hold their value until I began my life in academia. One significant narrative relates to a legacy of strong women in my family and, not coincidentally, in my professional life. My grandmother was born with significant abnormalities in both of her hips, so much so that her pediatrician had confidence that she would not live a long life and would most certainly never bear children. This remarkable woman recently died at the age of 90 and had given birth to eight children. One of these children is my mother, another very strong woman. Through the legacy of these two women, a message was engraved onto my heart that I, too, would become a woman who exceeded in what others might not expect of me. I was the first person on both sides of my family to receive an education from a university—earning a bachelor's, master's, and Ph.D. degree.

A second narrative was passed onto me from my father, a man of many talents in home and commercial building. He took me and my siblings to job sites when we were children, and I remember how he once shared the incredible importance of the foundation for any home or building. He felt strongly that a structure was not sound if the foundation was not first attended to. While I may not have given much thought to my dad's lesson as a child, his words have had a powerful narrative for me as a professional, a wife, and a mother. I have translated his words over time and began to see their connection to my self-of-therapist. I soon realized that if my own foundation (beliefs, values, biases) was not well attended to, the structure of what I do (in any role) was not likely to be sound. I felt so connected to this lesson from my father that I co-wrote a pedagogical chapter about how MedFTs are able to evaluate the role of their own foundation (also considering the ways in which BPSS factors influence our outlook on life and relationships) in relation to the development of their theory of change. This work is called the *Building Your Home Project* (Lamson & Meadors, 2007) and is shared annually with my marriage and family therapy (MFT) and MedFT students.

These two narratives set my purpose into motion, heavily influencing my career (in which I advocate for marginalized groups, champion health care, train students for a better health-care workforce, and lead investigations on research and grants for underserved populations). To describe my steps toward MedFT, I should share two key experiences that occurred during my master's program. If either of these two had not occurred, I am fairly certain that my present-day career would be much different. First, in the early fall of my first year as a Human Development and Family Studies master's student, I met Jennifer Bernasek (now Jennifer Hodgson). We met while working as waitresses at a restaurant near the campus. Later that year, we had offices near one another and found ourselves talking about the family therapy program. It is interesting how some things never change (my office is now two doors down from Jennifer, and we still talk daily about our ongoing research, grants, training programs, and policy-oriented initiatives).

My other pivotal experience during this time was having the opportunity to help care for a centenarian. She was in great health but longed for a friend to read to and talk with her. While visiting this young woman, I was asked to help feed dinner to her 70+ year-old son-in-law who had been an esteemed physician earlier in his career. He had diagnosed himself with Alzheimer's disease, and his BPSS struggle was evident. I went on to conduct my dissertation research on the role(s) of Alzheimer's disease in the life of caregivers under the mentorship of Dr. Harvey Joanning. The people I have described were placed in my life so purposefully—all of whom have shaped who I have become as a MedFT trainer, researcher, supervisor, clinician, and advocate.

In 1998, during my last year of my Ph.D. program, I was at an American Association for Marriage and Family Therapy (AAMFT) annual conference in Dallas, TX, and had decided to go to the showcase for accredited programs to learn about potential job opportunities. I remembered standing in front of a display for a program that was well-known to do some MedFT training when I felt a hand on my elbow. That hand belonged to Dr. Mel Markowski, who gently guided me over to the East Carolina University (ECU) display. He then shared his vision with me for a future MedFT doctoral program at ECU. He says that he remembers me literally jumping up and down with excitement. While I do not remember the jumping, I do recall my heart skipping a few beats. I was 25 years old at the time and somehow in a discussion about creating a Ph.D. program at a university that had only a dozen or so doctoral programs on campus. Another subtle issue was that it would be the first of its kind in the nation. Drs. Mel Markowski and David Dosser were brave enough to hire me for the job, whereupon it became my duty to find another courageous soul to come on board to create this program. Mel and I began a large recruitment campaign—but serendipity took over when Jennifer Hodgson reentered my life.

From 2000 to 2003, Jennifer and I worked tirelessly along with many other colleagues and administrators to create the Ph.D. program, all the while working toward tenure. We received permission to start the program 4 months after I became a mother. We took in our first doctoral students in the fall of 2005 and graduated our first cohort in 2008. Due to a series of unfortunate events, our first Ph.D. program director had to step down from his role, which meant another big change in my life.

I simultaneously became the program director for our master's program, program director for our doctoral program, and clinic director of our ECU Family Therapy Clinic—while still maintaining a teaching and research workload. With the incredible support and investment from Jennifer and our MFT team, we went on to earn accreditation with the Commission on Accreditation for Marriage and Family Therapy Education (COAMFTE) for the doctoral program (as the first medical family therapy Ph.D. program).

Thinking back on my life with Jennifer (at ECU) over the past 17 years is similar to what life is like when growing up with a sibling. Our children have literally grown up together, and she and I have collaborated on so many projects that people sometimes call us by one another's name (that happened early on in our careers, and we have actually received mail with "Angela Hodgson" and "Jennifer Lamson" on the envelopes). From the start, Jennifer and I worked hard to introduce one another to people that we knew had a heart for BPSS and relational health. We sought out a community that would afford us a sense of belonging—something that she and I call "matched energy."

At my first Collaborative Family Healthcare Association (CFHA; then the Collaborative Family Healthcare Coalition) conference, Jennifer introduced me to her mentor, Dr. Susan McDaniel, who then introduced me to her colleagues Drs. William (Bill) Doherty, Mac Baird, Don Bloch, Bill Gunn, Jeri Hepworth, John Rolland, and Dave Seaburn. They then introduced me to their colleagues, all of whom have been essential mentors to me over the years. I have learned more from my conversations with these champions than I can ever describe, but I must particularly punctuate my gratitude to Bill Doherty. He has given his time to me so selflessly, and the life lessons and lessons as a professional that he has passed onto me are priceless. His legacy is one of a kind.

Part of meeting incredible mentors, like Bill, is meeting their amazing mentees. While attending a conference in North Carolina in 2002, I had the chance to meet a doc intern who was at Wake Forest University School of Medicine. This intern had so much energy for MedFT that any attendee at that conference had no choice but to want to be on the MedFT innovation train with him. Tai Mendenhall was the name of that intern. He quickly became part of my professional family; another sibling was in the mix. Jennifer, Tai, and I went on to present at many conferences with one another for years, but had not really published together until more recently. When we decided to make a commitment to do this, we decided to "go big or go home." We worked on a special issue of medical family therapy in the journal of *Contemporary Family Therapy* and are now finishing our second book together. We see ourselves as a generation of MedFTs who are grateful to all of the founding fathers and mothers who were influential in developing MedFT and have made it our vision to grow the potential opportunities for the next generation. While MedFT began as a subdiscipline often most closely aligned to family therapy, it is now recognized as a field that has made its mark in training, research, practice, supervision, and policy initiatives.

When I think about why I chose MedFT to begin with, it was because I believed that health, illness, loss, and trauma occur in the context of families. No matter if it was my work with children and their families who experienced Hurricane Floyd; couples who had experienced a miscarriage or stillbirth; providers struggling with compassion fatigue who worked in pediatrics, the NICU or PICU; families facing a chronic illness; or the couples receiving integrated behavioral health care in a family medicine clinic on a military base, I recognized that biological, psychological, social, and spiritual health are interwoven and have the capacity to change the trajectory of a life and, thus, a system. I have learned a lot of lessons throughout the past two decades, especially—such as my belief that everyone seeks a sense of belonging (so find a community that strengthens you!). Equally important is that if you are in a position to be a champion or an ambassador, then fulfill that role to the best of your ability.

Our charge as MedFTs is not an easy one. We have a country and world that faces incredible health disparities and treatments that come with an extraordinary expense to their families and communities. MedFTs are relational health experts and, as such, must push to tear down silos across health care. We must provide best practices for families, conduct ethical and responsible research that makes an impact on the lives of families and health care, offer training that is current and relevant to the domestic and global health-care needs of patients and populations, and construct policy briefs that make a real difference in the delivery of health care. My hope is that this book triggers for each reader the possibility of growing the future of MedFT.

By Jennifer Hodgson

Like Angela, I too was a first-generation college student. The first in my family to achieve my bachelor's to doctoral degrees. I was the only person on both sides to have a master's and doctoral degree until a maternal cousin achieved her doctorate in veterinary medicine a decade later. I felt tremendous pressure to complete college, but the kind of pressure that excited me to keep going. Secretly, I wanted to be a physician. I liked the idea of helping people to feel better and live healthier lives. However, I did not have a role model for a career in health care, so it seemed out of reach. I was a natural musician and loved computers, so I thought one of those career paths would be my lane. However, my heart always found its way back to helping people and being around others during their times of greatest struggle. It would be the marriage of my admiration for health care and compassion for people in need that would lead me to medical family therapy. However, it would take several life events to help to carve that pathway.

It was a graduate student who was teaching my "Introduction to Psychology" course at the University of Akron who inspired me to be an academician. She looked like she was having so much fun teaching that I wanted to do that as well. From that day, forward, I could not get enough of what the field of psychology had to offer. Everything was new to me, and everything was a missing puzzle piece. I loved research, statistics, writing, presenting, and learning from the faculty who I cherish today (Richard Haude, Charlie Waehler, and Linda Subich). They took a chance on me. And while they were grooming me for a career in psychology, they could tell I saw things a bit differently. Dr. Subich shared in a quiet moment how there was a field called marriage and family therapy (MFT) that she thought would fit my philosophy of health a bit better. I met with the program director for the MFT program later that week and, within 10 minutes, knew I had found my professional home. My grounding in psychology was critical to my success, and I am forever grateful for that beginning.

During my master's program, the faculty member who recruited me into the program, Anthony Health, left his position to join a family medicine residency program as their director of behavioral medicine. I was curious about his new job and why he would leave family therapy to pursue it. He offered me the opportunity to shadow him one day in his new role, and I was smitten. It was like someone had turned the light on; I could see how all the parts of my academic past fit together neatly. I had already known I wanted a Ph.D., so that I could teach in a university setting, but now I knew what I wanted to focus on. However, it was not until I was applying to doctoral programs that I learned about Bill Doherty and his research in MedFT at the University of Minnesota. While life events directed me to Iowa State University for my doctoral studies, I was determined to find a way to get training in MedFT.

As a doctoral student, I was encouraged by my faculty to follow my passion. Chuck Cole, Linda Enders, and Harvey Joanning encouraged me to identify ways to get MedFT training even though it was not available at Iowa State University. So, I shadowed a behavioral medicine provider in a family medicine residency program in Des Moines, IA. It was there I received opportunities to guest lecture the residents and affirm my interests. I learned that if I wanted to be a MedFT, then I would need to get intensive training. I learned of a summer institute at the University of Rochester run by Susan McDaniel, Dave Seaburn, Pieter Leroux, and Tom Campbell (to name a few). I contacted Dave to see if they offered scholarships, and he said sadly they did not. So instead, I saved my graduate assistantship pennies and bought a ticket the following summer. It was transformative, and I knew that I would return there for more training. Later that year, I applied for their doctoral internship in MedFT and trained under Barbara Gawinski, Dave Seaburn, Susan McDaniel, Nancy Ruddy, Cleve Shields, and countless others. After I completed by internship, I applied for their newly established postdoctoral fellowship in MedFT and worked under Susan McDaniel's supervision. I will forever be grateful to her and to the whole Rochester team.

My first academic job after completing my postdoctoral fellowship was at Nova Southeastern University (NSU). There, I helped teach courses toward a certificate in families, systems, and health to their master's and doctoral family therapy students. During that time, I coedited the CFHA newsletter with Don Block. Don was a family psychiatrist and major innovator in the field of family therapy. He was a founding member of CFHA. He took me under his wing and taught me so much about the organization and the numerous opportunities that would lie ahead for MedFTs. Many of my former students at NSU are now major players in MedFT. I loved my experience at NSU and all my colleagues there. However, the next step in my career path would take everything I had learned thus far and apply it in full force.

One day out of the blue, Angela Lamson called me and shared with me how Dr. Mel Markowski, a professor at East Carolina University, had a vision to start the first doctoral program in MedFT. (Please read, above, how we met in Angela's section. I love that story.) She asked me to apply for their open position because she wanted someone to help her with this task. However, being a loyalist, I told Angela I could not leave NSU as I had only been there a year and a half. A month later, Mel Markowski called himself and asked me again to consider applying. He further described his vision for the doctoral program, and I realized that it was the opportunity I needed professionally. Shortly after arriving in August of 2000, Angela and I started writing the doctoral program proposal. By 2005 we were taking in our first cohort of doctoral students. The administration at ECU took a chance on two junior faculty, and it has paid off with a nationally awarded and well-established accredited program with 24 graduates to date!

During my time at ECU, I had the privilege of retaining relationships with many of my mentors. I became more involved in the Collaborative Family Healthcare Association (CFHA) where I have met so many pivotal innovators in integrated behavioral health care, too many to name here. One year after having my third baby, I received a call from Frank deGruy, stating that they wanted to nominate me to serve as president of CFHA. This was such a tremendous honor. However, I only agreed to do it because Randall Reitz was the executive director at the time, and I knew we would be a great team (and we were). Many of my most cherished relationships have formed through my work with CFHA and at the American Association for Marriage and Family Therapy (AAMFT) conferences. These communities have afforded me the opportunities to collaborate with Tai Mendenhall and Angela Lamson along a professional journey together to advance our shared passion for MedFT.

In my career thus far, I have been able to thrive as a researcher, educator, administrator, supervisor, and clinician. I have held major officer positions at the state and national levels and have become passionate about policy reform to help advance parity among the mental health professions and health professions. I am particularly interested in policies that advance integrated behavioral health care and family-centered models of care. My research and funding portfolio is rich with studies and grants showing my interest in advancing the biopsychosocial and spiritual health of individuals, couples, families, and communities. In some ways, I feel like I am just getting started despite having achieved full professor in 2012 and accomplishing many of my professional goals. I think it is because I love what I do and who I work with (Mel Markowski [retired], David Dosser [retired], Angela Lamson, Damon Rappleyea, Andy Brimhall, Kit Didericksen, Jake Jensen, Erin Roberts, and countless other colleagues, administrators, and students all across the ECU campus). ECU gives me the support I need as a woman, mother, academician, and innovator. While I never know where life will take me next, I am forever grateful to all those who have taught me so much about following your passion and living your dream.

By Tai Mendenhall

People often ask me why I chose medical family therapy (MedFT) as my career path. Sometimes they pose these queries in ways that are straightforwardly "academic." They are sensitive to larger trends about how behavioral health care—broadly defined—is becoming more visible and integrated into U.S. health systems and are interested in what drew me in. Other times people ask me about MedFT with what sounds like an almost aghast curiosity: "Why do you want to work in a hospital?", "Don't you see horrible things there?", and "Aren't the hours really bad?"

Accordingly, my answers are sometimes straightforward and professional (e.g., I highlight the merits of integrated care and how research supports it as an effective way to treat this, that, or the other thing). Other times my answers are more personal. I talk about my "calling" to work in a medical environment and about wanting to contribute to a larger mosaic of healing and care within teams of interdisciplinary colleagues working with and alongside patients and families. I talk about growing up watching my father—a research surgeon—perform operations at any hour of the day or night, and discussing in graphic detail a myriad of things over dinner that others might consider unpleasant. I maintain that working long hours is natural for me because I watched all of my parents and grandparents do it. I joke about how my doctoral internship in a psychiatry residency aligned well with my innate tendencies to be a workaholic, or reflect about how health care is so welcoming to those who get bored with routines or a 40-hour week. But in truth, it was for all of these reasons—and many others—that I chose MedFT. Or maybe it chose me.

I began my master's degree in marriage and family therapy (MFT) with an indefatigable want to connect the dots between my clients' (we call them "patients" in medical environments) and their families' lives. Having learned all about systems thinking during my undergraduate days, I saw family therapy's inclination to advance treatment in ways that embrace this complexity as a natural next step. When I first began to see patients and families in clinical work, I was drawn most to the especially difficult cases (other students and colleagues called them the "tough families," the "heart-sink" patients, etc.). Being—as I have always been—an adrenaline junky (e.g., motorcycles, bridge jumping), many said students and colleagues did not find this surprising. But the draw was not something grounded in any kind of personal excitement or voyeuristic appeal; it was a natural extension of the very systems thinking that drew me to MFT in the first place.

"Difficult" cases are, by their nature, systemically complex. I thereby found, early on, where the limits and boundaries of my baseline MFT training were. Collaborating with social workers, probation officers, school teachers, addictions counselors, physicians (of all stripes), psychiatrists, psychologists, and others directly involved in the lives of my patients and their families served to humble my heretofore espoused notions that MFT was the "best" way to care for people. I came to understand, instead, how MFT fits into a complex constellation of many other fields that are also very good at what they do. And, more importantly, I came to value—cherish, even—the work that we can do together.

With these understandings, though, grew a frustration with the limited scope of my training at the time. I wanted to learn more about "medicine" in a broad sense and about how to purposefully integrate and collaborate within and across interdisciplinary teams. I thereby knew that my doctoral training could not simply be more-of-the-same in MFT—but at the time, I did not know how it could be anything else. And just as I was beginning to change course so that I could pursue medical school (with the intent, afterward, to connect MFT with biomedical care), I learned about a burgeoning idea—a "subspecialty" at the time—called medical family therapy.

I chose my Ph.D. program so that I could work with Dr. William (Bill) Doherty in Minnesota. He, along with colleagues Drs. Susan McDaniel and Jeri Hepworth, was pioneering MedFT as a way to engage families struggling with health problems. They were bridging disciplines that had heretofore not talked to each other very much. I could not have possibly been at a better place at a better time.

Alongside his mentorship, Bill got me into a family medicine residency housed within Regions Hospital and Ramsey Family Physicians Clinic in Saint Paul, MN. It was through this work that I met—and had the privilege to train with—local leaders in integrated health care. Rosanne Kassekert, LICSW, Milt Cornwall, MD, and Pete Harper, MD, pushed me so far out of my comfort zone that I often did not know where I was—but, at the same, I knew that this was exactly where I needed to be. Through the Collaborative Family Healthcare Association (CFHA), Bill introduced me to Drs. Susan McDaniel and Jeri Hepworth. He also introduced me to Drs. Mac Baird, C.J. Peek, Sandy Blount, Rusty Kallenberg, Frank deGruy, and others—all who were working together to promote efforts in the respective fields they represent (e.g., family medicine, family therapy, psychology) to do the same. I was excited, inspired, and honored to join their cause.

As a new and, honestly, hyper-engaged member of CFHA, I soon—and finally—met Drs. Jennifer Hodgson and Angela Lamson. They were a couple of years ahead of me in terms of their doctoral training and early career steps, but I nevertheless felt close to them as like-minded colleagues who were (are) advancing MedFT as the next generation of scholars, clinicians, and supervisors trained by some of MedFT's most influential founders. By the time I completed the internship requirements of my doctoral program at Wake Forest University's School of Medicine (with Dr. Wayne Denton), our collegiality had evolved into close friendships.

Over the next several years, Angela, Jennifer, and I worked hard together in advancing MedFT's visibility and scope. We (I, as a new faculty member at the University of Minnesota's Medical School, and they, as pioneers of East Carolina University's first-ever doctoral program in MedFT) presented together at almost every annual conference for CFHA, the American Association for Marriage and Family Therapy (AAMFT), and other local and national forums. We trained students and colleagues about ways to effectively prepare for MedFT through didactic content (e.g., clinical methods/strategies, psychopharmacology, health-care administration, payment policies, health maintenance organizations, medical terminology). We shared wisdom—often learned the hard way—about how to enter medical contexts as a behavioral health provider without being a bull-in-a-china-shop about it. We began describing MedFT's applications in and beyond the arenas of family medicine (i.e., as its most established "home"). All of this then led to our leading a special issue for the journal *Contemporary Family Therapy*. This effort enabled us to connect formally with colleagues all over the country to bring MedFT to light across contemporary training, research, policy, and financial foci. In 2014 we—with colleague Dr. Russell Crane—extended this effort with a textbook entitled *Medical Family Therapy: Advanced Applications*.

Now—with one of CFHA's most visible and beloved physician leaders and MedFT advocates, Dr. Mac Baird—we have constructed *Clinical Methods in Medical Family Therapy*. This new text highlights MedFT's ever-growing presence, reach, and contributions across a myriad of primary, secondary, tertiary, and other care settings. We see it as a landmark confirmation of how the work we are doing in integrated behavioral health care is helping to ease suffering, advance agency, enhance communion, and empower patients and families in our care.

Closing Thoughts

By reading about our journeys into MedFT, we hope it is clear that our stories are still far from over. We (Angela, Jennifer, and Tai) see ourselves as continuing to advance what our mentors first put into motion. These professional paths are ones that have been less traveled. It has taken inner passion, grit, and resilience to stay on a course that continues to tear down the silos between biological, psychological, social, and spiritual health and health care. Our paths were made possible through a community of mentors willing to serve as both champions for the next generation of learners and ambassadors for their own patients who received relational and BPSS health care.

It is up to us to continue this legacy. As such, we offer through this book a series of chapters that describe ways that MedFT functions across primary, secondary, tertiary, and other care contexts. Our authors first introduce the uniqueness of each setting and present a clinical vignette that represents the unique population(s) they serve. They then describe treatment teams and possible collaborators, fundamental knowledge and skills, and research-informed practices associated with that context. They present the MedFT Healthcare Continuum to depict ways in which MedFTs can function across a range of foci (breadth) and sophistication (depth). At the conclusion of each chapter, our authors offer pointed reflection questions and specific clinical measures/instruments, resources, and organizational links to further prepare MedFTs for their upcoming work and contributions.

Finally, it is important to note that many of the contributing authors in this book were (or are) our own students. As MedFT's newest generation, they are charging into uncharted territories in health care that are defined by ever-changing political and organizational uncertainties. We are confident that they will continue to grow and innovate in this work long after we are gone. This, to be sure, is one of the most rewarding things about what we are doing. All of us believe in MedFT's vision, and we are contributing to it in ways that are collectively greater than what any one of us—or any single generation of us—could. It is an honor and a privilege to be a part of this movement.

References

Anderson, R. J., Huff, N. L., & Hodgson, J. L. (2008). Medical family therapy in an inpatient psychiatric setting: A qualitative study. *Families, Systems, & Health, 26*, 164–180. https://doi.org/10.1037/1091-7527.26.2.164

Bell, J. M., Wright, L. M., & Watson, W. L. (1992). The medical map is not the territory; or, "medical family therapy"-watch your language. *Family Systems Medicine, 10*, 35–39. https://doi.org/10.1037/h0089250

Bloch, D. (1984). The family therapist as health care consultant. *Family Systems Medicine, 2*, 161–169. https://doi.org/10.1037/h0091652

Doherty, W. J., & Baird, M. A. (1983). *Family therapy and family medicine: Towards the primary care of families*. New York, NY: Guilford.

Doherty, W. J., McDaniel, S. H., & Baird, M. A. (1996). Five levels of primary care/behavioral healthcare collaboration. *Behavioral Healthcare Tomorrow*, October 1996. Also appears as Doherty (1995), The why's and levels of collaborative family healthcare. *Family Systems Medicine, 13*, 275–281. https://doi.org/10.1037/h0089174

Doherty, W. J., McDaniel, S. H., & Hepworth, J. (1994). Medical family therapy: An emerging arena for family therapy. *Journal of Family Therapy, 16*, 31–46. https://doi.org/10.1111/j.1467-6427.1994.00775.x

Engel, G. L. (1977). The need for a new medical model: A challenge for biomedicine. *Science, 196*, 129–136. https://doi.org/10.1126/science.847460

Engel, G. L. (1980). The clinical application of the biopsychosocial model. *American Journal of Psychiatry, 137*, 535–544. http://ajp.psychiatryonline.org/

Hepworth, J., & Jackson, M. (1985). Health care for families, models of collaboration between family therapists and family physicians. *Family Relations, 34*, 123–127. https://doi.org/10.2307/583765

Hodgson, J., Lamson, A., Mendenhall, T., & Crane, D. (Eds.). (2014). *Medical family therapy: Advanced applications*. New York, NY: Springer.

Hodgson, J., Lamson, A., & Reese, L. (2007). The biopsychosocial-spiritual interview method. In D. Linville, K. Hertlein, and Associates (Eds.), *Therapist's notebook for family healthcare* (pp. 3–12). New York, NY: Hayworth Press.

Lamson, A. L., & Meadors, P. (2007). Building your home project. In D. Linville, K. Hertlein, and Associates (Eds.), *Therapist's notebook for family healthcare* (pp. 225–232). New York, NY: Haworth Press.

Lamson, A. L., Pratt, K., Hodgson, J., & Koehler, A. (2014). MedFT supervision in context. In J. Hodgson, A. Lamson, T. Mendenhall, and D. Crane (Eds.), *Medical family therapy: Advanced applications* (pp. 125–146). New York, NY: Springer.

Marlowe, D., & Hodgson, J. (2014). Competencies of process: Toward a relational framework for integrated care. *Contemporary Family Therapy, 36*, 162–171. https://doi.org/10.1007/s10591-013-9283-1

Martin, M. P., White, M. B., Hodgson, J. L., Lamson, A. L., & Irons, T. G. (2014). Integrated primary care: A systematic review of program characteristics. *Families, Systems & Health, 32*, 101–115. https://doi.org/10.1037/fsh0000017

McDaniel, S. H., & Campbell, T. L. (1986). Physicians and family therapists: The risks of collaboration. *Family Systems Medicine, 4*, 4–8. https://doi.org/10.1037/h0090176

McDaniel, S. H., Doherty, W. J., & Hepworth, J. (2014). *Medical family therapy and integrated care*. Washington DC: American Psychological Association.

McDaniel, S. H., Hepworth, J., & Doherty, W. J. (1992). *Medical family therapy: A biopsychosocial approach to families with health problems*. New York, NY: Basic Books.

Rolland, J. (1984). Toward a psychosocial typology of chronic and life-threatening illness. *Family Systems Medicine, 2*, 245–262. https://doi.org/10.1037/h0091663

Tyndall, L., Hodgson, J., Lamson, A., White, M., & Knight, S. (2010). *Medical family therapy: Conceptual clarification and consensus for an emerging profession (unpublished doctoral dissertation)*. Greenville, NC: East Carolina University.

Tyndall, L., Hodgson, J., Lamson, A., White, M., & Knight, S. (2012). Medical family therapy: A theoretical and empirical review. *Contemporary Family Therapy, 34*, 156–170. https://doi.org/10.1007/s10591012-9183-9

Tyndall, L., Hodgson, J., Lamson, A., White, M., & Knight, S. (2014). Charting a course in competencies. In J. Hodgson, A. Lamson, T. Mendenhall, and D. Crane (Eds.), *Medical family therapy: Advanced applications* (pp. 33–53). New York, NY: Springer.

Wright, L. M., Watson, W. L., & Bell, J. M. (1996). *Beliefs: The heart of healing in families and illness*. New York, NY: Basic Books.

Part I
Medical Family Therapy in Primary Care

Chapter 2
Medical Family Therapy in Family Medicine

Jennifer Hodgson, Lisa Trump, Grace Wilson, and Diego Garcia-Huidobro

The practice of family medicine is dedicated to using innovative approaches to provide holistic care for patients of all ages, addressing all organ systems and diseases (Hudon et al., 2012). In fact, primary care has become the gateway to behavioral health, expanding medical care to also include screening for and treating behavioral healthcare needs (Substance Abuse and Mental Health Services Administration [SAMHSA], 2016). The task of sorting through and differentiating between biological, psychological, social, and spiritual problems can be messy and challenging, however, because they all relate to the onset and trajectory of the illness (Hodgson, Lamson, Mendenhall, & Tyndall, 2014). Addressing one area of health (e.g., physical health) without recognition or acknowledgement of other interacting forces (e.g., mental health, spirituality) will likely result in failed interventions and frustrated patients and providers (Hatala, 2012). The great need for family medicine providers who will coordinate continued care in a comprehensive manner (i.e., with interdisciplinary teams addressing different aspects of one's health) is becoming increasingly evident (Phillips et al., 2014).

Like most medical specialties, there are opportunities in family medicine to not only collaborate with providers in independent practice settings, but also during

---

J. Hodgson (✉)
Department of Human Development and Family Science, East Carolina University, Greenville, NC, USA
e-mail: hodgsonj@ecu.edu

L. Trump
Stone Arch Psychology and Health Services, Minneapolis, MN, USA

G. Wilson
Great Plains Family Medicine Residency Program, Oklahoma City, OK, USA

D. Garcia-Huidobro
Department of Family Medicine and Community Health, University of Minnesota Medical School, Minneapolis, MN, USA

their residency training years. Residency settings provide collaborators, patients, and families with unique strengths and challenges that inspire important models of integrated behavioral healthcare (IBHC) to emerge. Residents have the opportunity to practice while learning innovative and empirically supported treatments and models. However, with the benefits come the challenges as patients and collaborators struggle with continuity of care concerns related to scheduling issues (e.g., residents off-site or in the hospital for rotations) and turnovers of resident physicians every 3 years. The following case vignette provides one example of someone with MedFT knowledge and skills and illustrates how they integrated into a family medicine residency clinic. It involves a family medicine resident in her final year of training, Dr. Cheryl Robbins, and a behavioral health provider trained in MedFT, Martha Lewis, working together to support a patient and family through challenges related to Alzheimer's disease.

Clinical Vignette
[Note: This vignette is a compilation of cases that represent treatment in family medicine. All patients' names and/or identifying information have been changed to maintain confidentiality.]

Mary is a 72-year-old widowed African American mother of two who is accompanied to her appointment by her oldest daughter, Tisha (age 46), and grandson, Ronnie (age 20). Her husband died 20 years ago of lung cancer, and she has been living independently ever since. Two years ago, her grandson moved in with her to help with some minor caregiver duties and household tasks. Once living with her, he noticed that on occasion, she would display signs of memory impairment such as forgetting calendar events, conversations with family members, names of people she has met multiple times, left her car running in the driveway with the door open, and even most recently left food cooking on the stove until it set-off the smoke detector. Thankfully, Ronnie was home each time and could contain these situations safely. However, he is increasingly worried about leaving Mary alone to the point of transferring colleges so he could obtain his degree online. He never complained about caring for his grandmother but recently has shared with his family that he is starting to get irritable and resentful about his quality of life.

Mary is a patient at a family medicine clinic close to her home; she has received care from several different residents over the years. She was diagnosed with mild cognitive impairment 5 years ago but refused to come see anyone after her "favorite" doctor had graduated. Her grandson believed that this was an excuse because Mary knew her memory is getting worse and did not want anyone to diagnose her with Alzheimer's disease. One event that finally alerted Ronnie's mother to the severity of the situation was when Mary looked at one daughter and insisted she was the other. She got angry when they tried to correct her and would not go to church with the one she thought was not supposed to take her. It scared her family and they scheduled a visit with Dr. Cheryl Robbins, a third-year family medicine resident. Dr. Robbins read Mary's chart ahead of the scheduled visit. There was a phone call message from the patient's daughter indicating the family was concerned about memory loss issues and that the patient would probably not bring it up on her own. Dr. Robbins immediately sent and internal email to Martha Lewis, one of the behavioral health providers (BHP), and requested that she attend all or some of the visit to help assess for a possible cognitive impairment and family members' concerns.

Upon entering the exam room, the family was anxiously awaiting the visit. Mary was smiling and sitting on the exam table, however, quite relaxed. She agreed to all requests by Dr. Robbins and Martha, and even agreed to have a cognitive functioning screener administered, which showed that she was in the severe cognitive impairment range. The family asked Dr. Robbins outside the exam room how they will know if Mary needs a higher level of care. They felt tremendous guilt as they promised her they would care for her in her own home until her death. However, the level of caregiving she was beginning to need was exceeding Ronnie's ability and the daughters both had full-time jobs that they could not afford to quit.

Dr. Robbins and Martha scheduled a family meeting to discuss the options with Mary and her family. They held several family meetings to develop a care plan that everyone could get behind, including signs and symptoms that would tell everyone when it was time for Mary to receive more services and where. Everything was written down for Mary so when she became confused, she could read it to understand why certain safety precautions were being taken. Dr. Robbins and Martha also met with Mary and members of her family separately to help ensure that Mary's biological, social, psychological, and spiritual needs were addressed, as well as those of the involved family members as some were also managing their own health issues (e.g., depression, irritable bowel syndrome, multiple sclerosis). Dr. Robbins and Martha communicated through the electronic health record (EHR) email system where they were able to bring one another up to date on any developments. When the time came to recommend that a care facility would be more beneficial to Mary's quality of life, Mary and her family were prepared. Thankfully, even though Dr. Robbins graduated at the end of the year and Mary transitioned to another resident, Martha stayed on her team. This was comforting to Mary and helped provide good continuity of care.

What Is Family Medicine?

The initiation of family medicine as a medical specialty shares much in common with the establishment of IBHC as a service and the development of medical family therapy (MedFT) as a field. All were designed in response to a fragmented healthcare system. Their intent was to redesign a healthcare system that at the time was responding only to the rapid advancements in science about *parts* of the person versus understanding the *whole*. In the 1960s, researchers were getting increasingly good at honing in on specific parts of the mind and body, but the translation of this research into practice left the connections between them ignored. Subsequently, reimbursement policies were developed that lacked sensitivity to how the practice of healthcare (mind and body) would impact the patient's whole health, family, community, etc. According to Taylor (2006), "The initial promise of Family Medicine was that we would rescue a fragmented health care system, put it together again, and return it to the people" (p. 184).

It has been documented that American adults prefer to access the primary care system as an entry point for addressing their mental health needs (Kessler & Stafford, 2008; Reiss-Brennan et al., 2016; Strosahl, 1994). Since the 1970s, this desire has made primary care the nation's de facto mental healthcare system (deGruy, 1996; Regier, Goldberg, & Taube, 1978; Regier et al., 1993; Strosahl, 2005). Interestingly, researchers found that up to 70% of primary care visits have a psychosocial component (Fries et al., 1993; Gatchel & Oordt, 2003), but unfortunately many mental health disorders go undiagnosed and/or untreated (Bitar, Springer, Gee, Graff, & Schydlower, 2009; Kessler, Chiu, Demler, & Walters, 2005; Kessler & Stafford, 2008; McCann & le Roux, 2006; Reiss-Brennan et al., 2016). Mental health impairments have been shown to impact one's overall functioning (especially at home and in social relationships), and even more so than common physical disorders (Druss et al., 2009). Another population in need of behavioral healthcare are patients who seek care for medical symptoms of which up to 84% have no organic cause and typically include expensive and sometimes unnecessary testing (Kroenke & Mangelsdorff, 1989). Primary care providers are recognizing these concerns; in a 2011 national survey, 63% of urban and suburban and 71% of rural physicians working in primary care claimed that inadequate access to mental health services, and patients' inability to have the cost covered, affects their patients' health negatively (Goldstein & Holmes, 2011). Due to cost, days missed from work, and/or stigma (among other factors), patients are often forced to choose one or the other service (i.e., medical or mental health), but not both. What physicians and physician extenders have available and easily accessible are their prescription pads; not all have as extensive training in mental health issues. Many also do not have behavioral health providers on-site to provide colocated or integrated behavioral healthcare. While not all mental health disorders or patients with behavioral health issues require psychotropic intervention (Kessler et al., 2005), all patients have people outside of their healthcare team who influence their healthcare decisions in positive and/or challenging ways. Therefore, it seems logical that primary care providers need behavioral health providers, like MedFTs, who are trained to focus on relational and systemic issues, deliver research-informed interventions collaboratively, and understand the medical complexities of their patients, leading to positive biopsychosocial-spiritual (BPSS) outcomes (Engel, 1977, 1980; Wright, Watson, & Bell, 1996).

McDaniel, Doherty, and Baird are pioneers in the field of integrated healthcare. All three held jobs in family medicine at the time that they wrote about their vision for a new field: medical family therapy. They wrote numerous peer-reviewed publications and well-known textbooks explaining how to apply MedFT skills in family medicine and other primary care settings, alongside common medical concerns that MedFTs would encounter (e.g., Doherty & Baird, 1983, 1987; McDaniel, Campbell, Hepworth, & Lorenz, 2005; McDaniel, Hepworth, & Doherty, 1992; McDaniel, Doherty, & Hepworth, 2014). Others would follow and continue to write about opportunities for MedFTs in family medicine (e.g., Hodgson, Fox, & Lamson, 2014; Marlowe, Hodgson, Lamson, White, & Irons, 2012; Reitz & Sudano, 2014; Tyndall, Hodgson, Lamson, White, & Knight, 2014), and in fact, family medicine is the more commonly published collaborative partnership field with the MedFT field to date.

Treatment Teams in Family Medicine

As presented in the clinical vignette, either in outpatient or inpatient family medicine settings, teamwork is the rule rather than the exception. As family medicine providers work in ambulatory and hospitalized settings, this creates great opportunities for integrated care between primary, secondary, and tertiary care. Although beneficial for patients, this is also complex. Services to be coordinated might be dispersed, collaboration across settings of care frequently require a high amount of time and personal effort, and not all providers value or understand a need for collaboration (nor know how to delegate and work as a team). To effectively do this, MedFTs require the ability to navigate multiple styles of caring for patients as well as the willingness to take an additional step to ensure patient safety and well-being. MedFTs must also balance this task with efforts to take care of themselves.

Because family medicine is a medical specialty with a broad spectrum of care, MedFTs need to be versatile in helping patients and family members that are going through a wide variety of medical conditions. In this section, we highlight key contributors to the treatment team, in addition to behavioral health providers such as MedFTs, who are relevant in family medicine.

Family medicine providers. Although family doctors are not the only medical specialists working in primary care, these physicians are commonly found in primary care clinics. Family doctors are either medical doctors (MDs) or doctors in osteopathic medicine (DOs). During their 3-year training, family medicine *interns* and *residents* have inpatient and outpatient rotations (supervised by *preceptors*), including adult and pediatric medicine and obstetrics and gynecology, making them capable to provide care for a wide range of patients. Family medicine providers could also have *fellowship training*, which includes additional years of clinical experience focused on a specific area of interest (e.g., adolescent medicine, emergency medicine, palliative care, sports medicine, geriatrics). During residency, family doctors oftentimes receive training in family systems, so they are more likely to have a family orientation in the care that they provide. They frequently serve as the primary care provider (PCP) for patients. PCPs are the clinicians that provide preventive and medical care for patients over time. In addition, they interact with other specialists, such as behavioral health providers, gastroenterologists, and surgeons as needed. Regardless of the setting where family medicine providers work, they collaborate with a wide range of medical providers. Other primary care medical specialists are pediatricians, who serve children and adolescents, internal medicine physicians focusing in adults and elders, obstetrics and gynecology doctors who take care of high-risk pregnancies and women's health, and psychiatrics who provide care for people with behavioral health conditions.

Nurses, physician assistants, and medical assistants. These providers are close allies of family medicine providers. They are focused in helping patients and families obtain, maintain, and recover their health. Nurses have a wide range of skills and specialties foci, such as neonatal, pediatrics, adult/gerontology, women's health, psychiatry/mental health, and community/public health. According to their training and licensing, they could be registered nurses (RNs) or nurse practitioners (NPs). RNs are nurses who have graduated from a nursing program and have met the licensing requirements of the state. Their scope of practice varies according to the local legislation but usually is centered in supporting and educating patients achieving their clinical goals. NPs have completed additional training and are capable of diagnosing and treating multiple acute and medical illnesses.

Physician assistants (PAs) are licensed healthcare professionals who practice medicine independently or, most commonly, under the collaboration and supervision of physicians. Their training is shorter compared to physicians (usually 2 or 3 years of graduate education without residency or fellowship training). PAs have a wide scope of practice, which is regulated by each state, but frequently include preventive care, diagnosing and treating common health problems, interpreting laboratory exams, prescribing medications when needed, and assisting physicians during surgery. Because of their ability to provide continuity of care, nurses and PAs frequently serve as patients' PCPs.

Medical assistants (MAs) support the work of other healthcare providers. After completing their 2-year training, MAs are responsible for taking vital signs, administering immunizations, taking X-rays, and other routine clinical and administrative duties (e.g., scheduling appointments, filling medical records, etc.), under the direct supervision of other health providers.

Behavioral health providers. Behavioral health providers in primary care may include MedFTs, "traditional" family therapists, social workers, psychologists, counselors, and psychiatric nurses. All provide mental health services and collaborate with PCPs and other clinical providers to provide comprehensive and integrated patient care. MedFTs are the ideal behavioral health providers to work in family medicine settings, as they bring unique skills to the different settings of family medicine. As shown in the vignette, MedFTs have a deep understanding of the medical conditions that patients and their families are dealing with. They know about medications' effects (including side effects) and are trained to cross disciplinary boundaries to activate and support patients, their family members, and the healthcare team to work together to improve health and well-being.

Dieticians. Registered dieticians help patients in their dietary and nutritional care. They assess nutritional requirements and eating lifestyle and help patients in setting and achieving weight and nutritional goals. Most of the time, they guide and support patients dealing with overweight/obesity and other medical conditions that require changes in a patient's diet (e.g., diabetes, malnutrition).

Pharmacists. In primary care, registered pharmacists educate patients in how to use medications, alongside what side effects and interactions with other prescriptions the said medications may have with what a patient is taking. Pharmacists also help patients to mitigate and/or cope with side effects or drug interactions (e.g., adjusting timing of dosages). In deciding which medications to prescribe, on-site pharmacists often collaborate with prescribers, particularly in complex cases. Depending in their training and scope of practice, pharmacists can also support administering immunizations and certain prescriptions.

Physical therapists. These providers help patients to improve their physical condition, such as reducing pain, and to restore and/or improve mobility and functionality. Physical therapists have different specialty areas, such as cardiovascular, pediatric, geriatric, neurological, and sports physiotherapy.

Fundamentals of Care in Family Medicine

MedFTs working in family medicine must be familiar with a myriad of content, including common problems presented within this care context, populations generally seen, and tests and procedures frequently advanced. They must also attend activity to issues of patient/family diversity and health disparities.

Common Problems Addressed in Family Medicine

The Centers for Medicaid and Medicare Service (CMS, 2013) reported that the ten most common diagnostic codes in family medicine include abdominal pain, acute respiratory infections, back and neck pain, chest pain, diabetes mellitus without complications (type 2), general medical examination, headache, hypertension, pain in the joint, pain in the limb, other forms of heart disease, and urinary tract infection/cystitis. Because family medicine physicians see patients across the lifespan with a wide variety of medical conditions, a MedFT working in this setting should be aware of basic medical diagnoses, tests, and procedures to best collaborate with providers and communicate with patients. For this chapter, we will focus on the most common problems of diabetes mellitus, hypertension, chronic pain, and preventive care.

Diabetes mellitus. Diabetes is an endocrine chronic condition that affects the body's ability to process insulin. It is one of the most common diagnoses made by family medicine providers, affecting approximately 22 million Americans (Pippitt, Li, & Gurgle, 2016). Type 1 diabetes is an autoimmune disease that usually presents during childhood, while type 2 diabetes is caused by insulin resistance and is most common in obese patients. Uncontrolled diabetes can have a number of serious complications, including blindness, kidney failure, limb amputation, and vascular and heart disease (Pippitt et al., 2016). According to Siu (2015), family medicine providers usually follow the United States Preventive Services Task Force (USPSTF) recommendation to screen all adults age 40–70 years who are overweight or obese. They also screen other patients who have risk factors such as a close relative with type 2 diabetes, women who have had gestational diabetes, or patients from a high-risk ethnicity (American Diabetes Association [ADA], 2015). Screening is done through a finger-stick hemoglobin A1C blood test; the results of this test indicate the patient's approximate blood glucose levels over the last 3 months (Pippitt et al., 2016). The typical goal of diabetes treatment is to achieve an A1C <7.0%, while a less stringent goal of <8.0% may be appropriate for individuals if achieved without adverse events (ADA, 2016).

For patients with diabetes, experts recommend a comprehensive, collaborative approach to treatment (George, Bruijn, Will, & Howard-Thompson, 2015). Pharmacological treatment of diabetes may involve oral medications to control blood sugar, such as metformin or insulin management (George et al., 2015; Petznick, 2011). These medications sometimes have poor adherence from patients. Metformin, a frequently used oral agent for treatment of diabetes, can have uncomfortable gastrointestinal side effects for patients, and insulin frequently requires complicated dosing instructions and frequent self-monitoring of blood sugar. MedFTs can be helpful utilizing a motivational interviewing approach to improve patient adherence (Rollnick, Miller, & Butler, 2008) and helping with patient education about their medications. There are also significant lifestyle changes recommended for diabetes patients, including changes to diet, exercise, and weight management (George et al., 2015), and patients with diabetes are at a higher risk for depression (Nouwen et al., 2010). A MedFT can assist patients in their recommended lifestyle dietary changes and provide screening and brief intervention for depression as necessary.

Hypertension. Hypertension, or blood pressure greater than 140/90 mmHg, is another common chronic diagnosis in primary care. It is a major preventable contributor to diseases and death in the United States (Oza & Garcellano, 2015). About 33% of adults in the United States have hypertension. According to Piper, Evans, Burda, et al. (2014), the USPSTF recommends screening for high blood pressure in all adults ages 18 years and over, even if they have no known history of hypertension. Patients with this condition are at higher risk for myocardial infarction (heart attack), renal failure, and death (Oza & Garcellano, 2015).

Patients identified as having high blood pressure benefit from both pharmacological treatment and lifestyle changes. The goal of treatment is to achieve a blood pressure less than 150/90 mmHg in adults over age 60, and 140/90 mmHg in patients 30 to 59 years of age (Langan & Jones, 2015). One major dietary recommendation for patients with hypertension is to reduce sodium (salt) and to follow the Dietary Approaches to Stop Hypertension (DASH) diet, which gives specific recommendations for daily nutrient intake, including 27% of calories from fat, 18% of calories from protein, 30 g of fiber, and 1500 mg of sodium (Sacks et al., 2001). Other key lifestyle recommendations include moderate to vigorous activity for 40 minutes, three times per week, and tobacco cessation (Oza & Garcellano, 2015). There is some mixed evidence indicating that relaxation techniques can be successful for lowering blood pressure; transcendental meditation and biofeedback techniques may modestly lower blood pressure (Brook et al., 2013). MedFTs should familiarize themselves with relaxation and mindfulness techniques to teach patients in this population and to help them adhere with the dietary, physical activity, and pharmacological treatments.

Chronic pain. There are more than 50 million Americans who experience chronic pain (Jackman, Purvis, & Mallett, 2008). Chronic pain may include pain due to osteoarthritis, strained muscles or bulging or ruptured disks in the lower back region, digestive conditions like irritable bowel syndrome, or other known or unknown causes. Although pain can be an important indicator of acute injury, chronic pain is burdensome and difficult to manage. One major problem in treating chronic pain lies with opioid pharmacological agents; they are sometimes abused or diverted and have a high risk of overdose. According to Dowell, Haegerich, and Chou (2016), the Centers for Disease Control and Prevention (CDC) recently released new recommendations for prescription of opioid medications in the treatment of chronic pain, focusing on mitigating their risks with a patient-centered approach to care. The CDC recommends use of short-acting medications, frequent follow-ups, and use of compliance measures such as pill counts, urine drug screening, and checking state registries for patients' histories of refilling controlled medications (Dowell et al., 2016).

Experts of treating chronic pain in primary care recommend that patients should be assisted in setting realistic goals for functioning. The primary goal for treatment should not be complete resolution of the patient's pain; it should instead be improved quality of life while decreasing pain (Jackman et al., 2008). There are many nonpharmacological treatments for chronic pain that can be used in addition to (or instead of) opioids. Lifestyle changes, including tobacco cessation and weight loss, are recommended (Hayes, Naylor, & Egger, 2012). There are also benefits from exercise, physical therapy, biofeedback, cognitive behavioral therapy, and relaxation. Complementary and alternative medicine approaches such as acupuncture, massage, and mindful mediation may benefit patients as well (Jackman et al., 2008). MedFTs can be instrumental in engaging patients in self-management goals, establishing realistic expectations, and working with patients and family members on living a fulfilling life alongside their pain.

Preventive care. One major goal of primary care is to provide patients with ongoing preventive care. Family medicine providers follow the recommendations of the USPSTF, which provides guidelines for preventive medicine. Guidelines are based on age and gender, and they are targeted at improving the overall population health and preventing serious diseases and complications (USPSTF, 2016). In children, preventive care typically includes periodic well-child visits and administration of immunizations. In adults, preventive care recommendation include a variety of tests, from less invasive, such as blood pressure testing, to much more involved, such as colonoscopies, pap smears, and mammograms.

MedFTs working in primary care can help to expand this definition of preventive care to go beyond physical health, taking a more biopsychosocial-spiritual view instead. There are many behavioral health concerns that they can provide screening for, including depression, anxiety, ADHD, and others. They can also engage patients in their healthcare decision making by using techniques such as motivational interviewing to assess patient health goals and monitor progress in those areas.

Depression and anxiety. Two of the most prevalent mental health diagnoses are major depressive disorder and anxiety (which includes generalized anxiety disorder, social anxiety disorder, specific phobias, and others). Many patients experiencing symptoms of depression and anxiety will present to their physician first, rather than through the traditional mental health system (Petterson, Miller, Payne-Murphy, & Phillips, 2014). Although recommendation from the USPSTF is to screen adult patients for depression, they add the caveat that physicians should not be screening all patients unless they have a system for follow-up in place (Siu, 2016). Many physicians feel uncomfortable addressing psychopathology in patients due to lack of knowledge about community resources and increasing time pressures. MedFTs working in primary care are instrumental in the screening and treatment of depression. For patients who screen positive, the MedFT can either provide follow-up care for patients or refer them to community health resources. Although there is not an analogous screening recommendation for anxiety disorders, generalized anxiety disorder is a prevalent concern among patients that can have implications for exacerbations of health problems such as insomnia and hypertension. MedFTs can provide screening, brief intervention, and referrals to treatment as appropriate.

Populations Served in Family Medicine

Patients served in family medicine include all ages across the lifespan, from infants to the elderly.

Children. About 70% of family medicine providers provide care for children in their practices; overall, family medicine providers spend about 10% of their time caring for children, and they are responsible for about 16–21% of all child healthcare visits (Makaroff et al., 2014). MedFTs can be helpful both for well-child visits and for childhood chronic illnesses, such as asthma, ADHD, and obesity. For well-child visits, MedFTs may use a behavioral health screening tool such as the Pediatric Symptom Checklist (PSC), which assesses for internalizing symptoms such as depression and anxiety, attention difficulties, and externalizing symptoms such as anger outbursts and behavioral difficulties (Gardner et al., 1999). MedFTs can also help monitor child development and attainment of milestones and screen for developmental difficulties, learning disorders, or autism spectrum disorders. Finally, MedFTs can also provide parenting guidance.

For children with chronic health conditions, MedFTs can be an important part of the treatment team's intervention. The National Health Interview Survey found that 6.8% of children in the United States have asthma (CDC, 2016). Evidence has shown that behavioral intervention for asthma can be beneficial, including self-management training, such as through the development of an asthma action plan, breathing training, and exercise or physical activation programs. Systemic factors, such as parental smoking, can also be modified; if the MedFT is able to work with the patient's parents to quit smoking, there may be a beneficial effect on the child's health and symptoms. ADHD is also a common childhood illness, affecting about 11% of American children (Visser et al., 2014). The symptoms of ADHD first appear between ages 3 and 6 years old, and the average age at first diagnosis is 7 years. In addition to helping with screening and early identification of symptoms, MedFTs can provide behavioral intervention to children and their families who are facing ADHD. Pharmacological treatment of ADHD, typically stimulant medication, has a number of side effects, including poor appetite, irritability, anxiousness, and sleep problems (Felt, Biermann, Christner, Kochhar, & Van Harrison, 2014). Effective behavioral treatments include parent training, classroom management, and peer interventions.

Finally, another example of a problem increasing in the pediatric population is obesity. Growing numbers of children are presenting to their primary care doctor with weight difficulties; 12.1% children 2–5 years of age, 18.0% of children 6–11 years of age, and 18.4% of adolescents 12–19 years of age meet the diagnostic criteria for obesity (National Institute of Diabetes and Digestive and Kidney Diseases, 2012). The American Medical Association expert recommendations suggest that family medicine providers should address diet and exercise habits with families at least once a year (Rao, 2008). Further, they urge that families need to make changes together to improve children's health. MedFTs, with their solid foundation in systems theory and family therapy, as well as their experience and awareness of behavioral intervention, are particularly suited to aid physicians in these recommendations. Further, they may be able to help establish collaboration with a nutritionist, coordinating care and communication between members of the treatment team.

Adults. Family medicine providers care for adults across a wide range of health conditions, as well as services particular to women's health (which includes gynecological care and maternal/fertility treatment services). When adults are needing more specialty care (e.g., gastroenterology, endocrinology, dermatology, cardiology, specialty mental healthcare), family medicine providers refer to indicated professionals and expand the team accordingly. Residents pursuing their family medicine specialization are trained to deliver babies, but not all may offer this service as a part of their practice. Overall, primary care systems, such as family medicine, are typically the first point of contact for adults. However, patients' type of insurance and coverage may limit their access to certain primary care systems or providers. Some insurers will permit patients to seek specialty care without a referral from their primary care provider.

Elderly. At the other end of the spectrum, family medicine providers also treat patients who are at the end of their lifespan. In addition to helping geriatric patients who have the conditions previously described, there are other considerations that may be beneficial to this population. Physicians and MedFTs can partner with geriatric patients and their families to assess their goals for maintaining functional abilities and aging in place and can connect them with community resources or assistive technology that may assist them in reaching these goals. Further, MedFTs can help family medicine providers as they aid their patients in end-of-life planning, completion of advanced directives, and entry into hospice. They also can aid in screening for cognitive decline, such as by administering the Mini-Mental Status Exam or a similar test of cognitive functioning. Although depression is common in older adults, there is often a stigma associated with therapy that is a significant barrier to traditional treatment of depression in this generation (Conner et al., 2010). For these patients, an integrated behavioral healthcare format may help them overcome stigma and be more willing to receive help for their condition.

Common Tests and Procedures in Family Medicine

Tests and procedures often advanced in family medicine vary considerably; those most common are described below.

Tests. Family medicine providers utilize many common tests (see Table 2.1) in the diagnosis and management of illnesses and diseases in their patients. The presented lab tests and interpretations are intended to be evaluated by primary care providers or other professional types with training in this area. The American Academy of Family Physicians (AAFP) recommends education in urinalysis, vaginal smears, stool microscopy, skin scraping microscopy, post-vasectomy semen analysis, blood draws for labs sent to outside laboratories, finger-stick glucose, finger-stick A1c, urine pregnancy test, rapid strep antigen, rapid influenza test, and occult blood testing of stool or emesis. Some family medicine practices have labs available in the clinic so that patients can have their needs met all in one place, whereas others have to refer patients to outside laboratories for testing. It is important that MedFTs know and understand some of the more common labs run in a primary care setting as some indicate that a patient's health is improving or deteriorating. For example, if a patient's blood pressure is higher than normal (140/90 mmHg), it is an opportunity to stop and try to identify potential causes of

Table 2.1 Common Tests and Procedures in Family Medicine

Test	Normal Limits	Purpose/Description of Test	Basic Interpretation of Abnormal Findings
Vitamins			
B12	200–900 pg/mL	B12 is a vitamin used in the metabolism of every cell in the body; it is particularly important in the production of red blood cells.	Deficiency may result in anemia but also could explain altered mental status and be confused with dementia.
Vitamin D	30–80 ng/mL	Vitamin D is essential for calcium absorption and bone formation.	Low levels may cause bone softening leading to fractures and increased mortality; in addition, low levels could explain depression-like symptoms.
Endocrine function			
TSH (thyroid-stimulating hormone), T_3 (triiodothyronine), T_4 (thyroxine)	TSH: 0.4 to 4.0 mIU/L T3: 100–200 ng/dL T4: 4.5–12 ug/dL	TSH is a hormone produced by the pituitary gland that stimulates the production of thyroid hormones (T_3 and T_4); these labs are used to measure the functioning of the thyroid gland.	High levels of TSH and low levels of T4 and T3 can explain symptoms attributed to hypothyroidism, such as fatigue, weight gain, reduced sexual drive, and difficulty with concentration and memory that could be easily attributed to depression. On the contrary, low levels of TSH and high levels of T4 and T3 can explain anxiety, mood swings, mania or hypomania, impaired concentration, irritability, and insomnia, due to hyperthyroidism and not a primarily mental health problem.
Glucose	70–100 mg/dL	Measures circulating glucose.	Low levels of blood glucose could provoke nausea, dizziness, altered vision, and disturbed mental status; if a patient is experiencing hypoglycemia, this requires urgent medical care. On the contrary, high levels of blood glucose indicate the body's incapacity to manage healthy glucose levels; high levels indicate diabetes or other metabolic problems (e.g., glucose intolerance); extremely high levels (greater than 500 mg/dL) require urgent medical care.

(continued)

Table 2.1 (continued)

Test	Normal Limits	Purpose/Description of Test	Basic Interpretation of Abnormal Findings
Hemoglobin A1c (A1c)	<5.7%	Evaluates how much hemoglobin (molecule in the red blood cells) has been glycosylated ("covered with sugar"); it is a measure of average blood glucose in the last 3 months.	Chronic hyperglycemia is related to stroke, coronary artery disease, neuropathy, renal failure, and increased mortality; for patients with diabetes, treatment goals could be having A1cs under 6.5 or 7%, depending on the patient; higher levels require treatment adjustment to improve diabetes control.
Liver function			
Albumin	3.4–5.4 g/dL	In general, this panel of lab tests measure how the liver and their associated organs (e.g., gallbladder, bile ducts) are working.	In asymptomatic patients, high levels of these tests could reflect damage to the liver or its associated organs.
ALP (alkaline phosphatase)	44–147 IU/L		
ALT (alanine aminotransferase)	10–40 IU/L		
AST (aspartate aminotransferase)	10–34 IU/L		
Total bilirubin	0.3–1.9 mg/dL		
Kidney function			
BUN (blood urea nitrogen)	6–20 mg/dL	These lab tests evaluate how well the kidney is eliminating these molecules.	High levels of creatinine might explain acute or chronic kidney failure but also high intensity exercise or other medical conditions; high BUN levels result in mental status changes including disorientation and confusion that require acute medical care.
Creatinine	0.6–1.3 mg/dL		
CBC (complete blood count)			
RBC (red blood cell) count	Male: 4.7–6.1 million cells/mcL Female: 4.2–5.4 million cells/mcL	RBCs carry oxygen to the body organs; these tests evaluate the counts of red blood cells (RBC), the % of red blood cells in the blood sample (hematocrit), and the amount of hemoglobin (molecule inside the RBC that carries the oxygen).	Low levels of these exams could be related to anemia (which has many causes); symptoms of this condition include profound fatigue, loss of mental acuity, and reduced ability to perform simple tasks like reading; high levels are rare and could be explained by dehydration, living at a high-altitude location, or bone marrow diseases.
Hematocrit	Male: 40.7–50.3% Female: 36.1–44.3%		
Hemoglobin	Male: 13.8–17.2 gm/dL Female: 12.1–15.1 gm/dL		

(continued)

Table 2.1 (continued)

Test	Normal Limits	Purpose/Description of Test	Basic Interpretation of Abnormal Findings
WBC (white blood cell) count	4500–10,000 cells/mcL	WBC are the body's defense against infection(s); common types of WBCs are leukocytes and lymphocytes.	Low levels (leukopenia or lymphopenia) could be explained by viral and other infections (including HIV), bone marrow diseases, cancer, autoimmune disorders, or as medication side effects; high levels of WBC (leukocytosis or lymphocytosis) can be explained by an active infection, drug reactions, bone marrow diseases (e.g., leukemia), and other immune disorders; as a CBC is ordered by a provider, MedFTs could encourage patients to follow-up with their PCP.
Platelet count	150,000–450,000/dL	Platelets play an important role in the blood clot formation.	Extremely low platelet levels (thrombocytopenia) produce excessive bleeding (internal and external) and could be explained by multiple reasons that require an evaluation by the provider who ordered the test; high levels are very uncommon.

this dysregulation (e.g., being in a hurry, having smoked a cigarette, having drunk coffee). If blood pressure remains high in several opportunities, the client could have hypertension and should be referred to his/her PCP for a diagnosis. If the client has been diagnosed with hypertension, this could be an opportunity to address stress management, lifestyle changes, and medication adherence and/or hold a family conference to expand support.

Procedures. Most family medicine providers perform at least some outpatient procedures in their offices. In the AAFP's 2015 Member Census, family medicine providers most commonly reported performing skin procedures such as biopsies (74.7%), musculoskeletal injections (68.4%), spirometry (35.7%), endometrial sampling (31.1%), X-ray (26.1%), and colposcopy (16.5%). Although MedFTs do not participate in the performance of these procedures, they can play an important role with patient care in this area. Informed consent for treatment requires patients' understanding of a procedure, alongside its anticipated benefits and potential risks. The MedFT can assist doctors in ensuring that patients have an understanding of their procedure in a way that matches the patient's level of health literacy. MedFTs can also help patients who are anxious about treatments and procedures by assisting them in relaxation and mindfulness exercises as they are waiting for their procedure to be performed.

Sensitivity to Diversity and Health Disparities

Primary care is designed to meet the needs of all populations, including those who are underserved, by providing them with a medical home where they can have many of their needs met in one location. According to the 2015 AAFP Member Census, 59% of family physicians accept Medicaid (AAFP Member Census, 2015). At a national level, the Family Medicine for America's Health Project is a collaborative effort of multiple organizations, including the AAFP and the Society for Teachers of Family Medicine (STFM), designed to improve practice models and payment so that more patients can have their healthcare needs met through primary care (Kozakowski et al., 2016).

Despite these efforts, significant health disparities still exist. Members of marginalized groups including ethnic minorities, lesbian, gay, bisexual, transgender, and queer (LGBTQ) populations, migrant and seasonal farm workers, and low socioeconomic status patients frequently experience poorer health outcomes and numerous barriers to care compared to more privileged populations (Purnell et al., 2016). Access to mental healthcare is even more fragmented (Cook et al., 2014). Despite changes in education standards, biases still exist among healthcare providers that exacerbate these problems (Blair et al., 2013; Chapman, Kaatz, & Carnes, 2013). Experts have recommended various solutions for these problems, including programs that impact social determinants of health (Thornton et al., 2016) and integrated care (Sanchez, Ybarra, Chapa, & Martinez, 2016; Vander Wielen et al., 2015). Emerging evidence suggests that integrated healthcare helps reduce healthcare disparities for Latinos (Bridges et al., 2014), people with severe mental illnesses (Kelly, Davis, & Brekke, 2015), underserved urban (Wrenn, Kasiah, & Syed, 2015), and rural populations (Ranson, Terry, Glenister, Adam, & Wright, 2016).

MedFTs can help family medicine physicians in their efforts to address problems with diversity and health disparities. In a general way, integrated care reduces the stigma of behavioral healthcare and increases access by providing services in the primary care office (Sanchez et al., 2016; Vander Wielen et al., 2015). MedFTs can also assist providers in delivering culturally appropriate care. One way to do this is through Galanti's (2014) four Cs—that is, inquiring about what the patient calls their illness, what are their concerns about it, what do they believe caused it, and what do they believe will cure it. Conversations like these can help providers understand patients' culturally bound health beliefs. They can also reveal areas of poor health literacy. Although healthcare providers often fail to recognize poor health literacy, it is a serious problem with implications for patient morbidity (Caplan, Wolfe, Michaud, Quinzanos, & Hirsh, 2014) and mortality (Bostock & Steptoe, 2012). MedFTs working in integrated behavioral healthcare are the perfect people to help bridge gaps in health literacy, because they have both the experience of working in a healthcare setting as well as the lack of a medical degree; they are adept at helping translate medical jargon into terms a layperson can easily understand.

2 Medical Family Therapy in Family Medicine

Table 2.2 MedFTs in Family Medicine: Basic Knowledge and Skills

MedFT Healthcare Continuum Level	Level 1	Level 2	Level 3
Knowledge	Somewhat familiar with family medicine as a medical specialty and its background and collaboration with MedFTs, as well as unique and overlapping skills/roles, and the team's overall structure. Limited knowledge about BPSS impacts of a few common population health conditions seen at family medicine clinics. Rarely engages professional members, patients, and support system members collaboratively. Basic understanding regarding strategies for a healthy lifestyle when living with someone with a health condition. If conducting research and/or policy/advocacy work, on rare occasions will collaborate with other disciplines related to family medicine and consider relational and/or BPSS aspects of health and well-being.	Can recognize the disease processes and differentiate between some of the more common ones and other comorbid BPSS health conditions and impacts. Familiar with benefits of couple and family engagement in health-related adjustments and/or lifestyle maintenance but tends to refer more than provide this service. Knowledgeable about how to use the electronic health record system or other forms of secured communication to collaborate with various team members. Is an occasional contributor to discussions about research design and policy/advocacy work that include relational and/or BPSS aspects of health and well-being.	Working knowledge of specific team members (e.g., allopathic and osteopathic physicians, nurse practitioners, physicians assistants, nurses, medical office assistants, phlebotomists, pharmacists, nutritionists, physical therapists, other behavioral health disciplines, etc.) and medical terminology with regard to medications and EHR charting (e.g., prn, qd, BGL, TSH), as well as common comorbid conditions to family medicine illnesses (e.g., hypertension, hyperlipidemia, diabetes mellitus, cardiopulmonary obstructive pulmonary disease). Broad range of knowledge about research-informed family therapy and BPSS interventions; able to and usually will conduct couple and family therapy and incorporate BPSS health factors into treatment with minimal need to refer out due to limited expertise. When work permits, is knowledgeable and consistency committed to conducting research and constructing policy/advocacy work that identifies and intervenes on behalf of individuals, couples, families, and healthcare teams toward the advancement of BPSS health and well-being.

(continued)

Table 2.2 (continued)

MedFT Healthcare Continuum Level	Level 1	Level 2	Level 3
Skills	Able to recognize at a basic level the BPSS dimensions of health and apply a BPSS lens to practice, research, and/or policy/advocacy work. Can discuss (and psycho-educate) basic relationships between biological processes, personal well-being, and interpersonal functioning. Demonstrates minimal collaborative skills with family medicine and other related healthcare providers; prefers to work independently, but, when care is complex enough, will contact /refer to other providers about additional services.	Knowledgeable about how to apply systemic interventions in practice and does it occasionally; capable of assessing patients and support system members present for background health issues such as family history and risk-related factors. Demonstrates adequate and occasional collaborative skills through (a) written and verbal communication mediums that are understandable to all team members and (b) coordination of referrals to specialty behavioral health providers and communication with the patient's primary care provider. Conducts separate treatment plan from other providers involved in the patient's care; goals and interventions can overlap with—or be informed by—a family medicine team, but BPSS goals and collaboration with the team is not consistently done.	Able to and usually will integrate respective team members' expertise and counsel into treatment planning. When done can successfully conduct a systemic assessment of a patient and family with competencies in assessing for BPSS aspects of family medicine illnesses and/or comorbid diseases and resources within the family. Usually engages other professionals within and outside of the practice who are actively involved in the patient's care. Skilled with standardized measures to track patients' individual and relational strengths and challenges (e.g., PHQ9, GAD7, Relationship Dynamics Scale). Attends and contributes to team meetings to help shape BPSS treatment plans for patients.

Family Medicine Across the MedFT Healthcare Continuum

The family medicine setting lends itself well to all applications of MedFT across the healthcare continuum (see Tables 2.2 and 2.3; Hodgson et al., 2014). If fact, many of the pioneers of MedFT have illustrated in their texts the versatility of MedFT in primary care, particularly in family medicine (Hodgson, Lamson, Mendenhall, & Crane, 2014; McDaniel et al., 1992, 2014). However, regardless of one's amount and quality of training or one's ability to execute MedFT in a particular setting, MedFTs have to respect the workflow, reimbursement, and transformation processes common to integration of behavioral health into a healthcare context (Cohen et al., 2015; Hodgson et al., 2014; McDaniel et al., 1992, 2014). These operational, systemic factors will have an impact on the care provided. This section aims to highlight, using the case example at the beginning of this chapter, the various ways that MedFTs may be assimilated into family medicine settings.

Depending on one's job duties, MedFTs at *Levels 1 and 2* of the continuum may have the ability to function as clinician, researcher, and/or policy advocate who executes components of a relational and BPSS framework (Engel, 1977, 1980; Wright et al., 1996). At these levels, the MedFT may have the skills to practice at a more advanced level but may not have the "green light" of the system to do so.

Table 2.3 MedFTs in Family Medicine: Advanced Knowledge and Skills

MedFT Healthcare Continuum Level	Level 4	Level 5
Knowledge	Consistently applied understanding of the more commonly treated health conditions and BPSS impacts in family medicine. Knowledgeable about benefits and risks of associated treatments of the more commonly seen biological and mental health conditions across the lifespan in family medicine (e.g., diabetes mellitus, hypertension, COPD, asthma, depression, anxiety). Understands how to collaborate with other disciplines to implement evidence-based BPSS and family therapy protocols in traditional and integrated behavioral healthcare contexts. Identifies self as a MedFT. Knowledgeable about designing and advocating for policies that govern BPSS-oriented inpatient and outpatient family medicine care services.	Understands and educates others about treatment and care sequences for unique and/or challenging topics in family medicine practice (e.g., delirium, medication interaction effects, comorbidities); can consult proficiently with professionals about BPSS topics from other fields. Proficient at explaining evidence-based treatments regarding most mental health disorders and their role(s) in the family; has background to provide psychoeducation to patients and families about a variety of symptoms, medications, and behavioral health management. Very knowledgeable about BPSS research designs and execution, policies, and advocacy needs as relevant to family medicine care. Proficient in developing a curriculum on integrated behavioral healthcare, BPSS applications, MedFT, etc. to mental health and other health professionals. Understands leadership and supervision strategies for building integrated behavioral healthcare teams in outpatient and inpatient family medicine settings.

(continued)

Table 2.3 (continued)

MedFT Healthcare Continuum Level	Level 4	Level 5
Skills	Able to deliver seminars and workshops to a variety of professional types (e.g., mental health, biomedical) about the BPSS complexities of a variety of commonly reported health and wellness topics found in family medicine settings.	Proficient in nearly all aspects of commonly seen presenting problems in a family medicine setting; able to synthesize and conduct research and clinical work; engages in community-oriented projects outside of the family medicine.
	Can apply several BPSS interventions in care (including most types of brief interventions); can administer mood- and disease-specific assessment tools as the family medicine context requires.	Goes beyond intervention routine for this population; can integrate specific models of integrated behavioral healthcare into routine practice (e.g., PCBH, Chronic Care Model).
	Consistently collaborates with key family medicine team members (e.g., primary care providers, nurses, medical assistants, behavioral health providers, pharmacists, dieticians); initiates and facilitates team visits with multiple providers when working with patients and families.	Works proficiently as a MedFT and collaborates with other providers from a variety of disciples.
		Leads, supervises, and/or studies success of the implementation and dissemination of BPSS curriculum on integrated behavioral healthcare, BPSS applications, MedFT, etc.
	Can independently and collaboratively construct research and program evaluation studies that study the impact of BPSS interventions with a variety of diagnoses and patient/family units of care.	Leads and explains at a high level of skill evidence-based treatments regarding most commonly seen family medicine presenting problems and their impact(s) on family systems; has background to provide psychoeducation to patients and families about a variety of symptoms, medications, and behavioral health management techniques that facilitate managing chronic illnesses well, returning to optimal health, or managing one's health successfully.

Contemporary MedFTs in family medicine settings are more commonly in roles where they provide both integrated behavioral healthcare (IBHC) services and traditional psychotherapy services, as well as teaching and research. Their expertise is in working relationally and applying the BPSS framework, but at *Levels 1 and 2*, this expertise is often sought after for "special" cases or situations rather than as a routine service. For example, the case example presented at the beginning of this chapter started with how the family medicine resident contacted the MedFT to request that she join her in the patient's next visit (*Levels 1 and 2*). At this point, it is hopeful that Dr. Robbins will continue to work along with the MedFT throughout the duration of the case, but many *Level 1 and 2* engagements end at the initial consult phase with little or no coordination of services or treatment plans, and no BPSS interventions or family therapy provided. Consulting with the MedFT is rare to occasional in its occurrence. Then, when the MedFT incorporated the family into the treatment in a hallway consult during the visit, this began to showcase more of the MedFT's BPSS and relational skills. However, Martha moved beyond *Level 2* when she incorporated the family into the treatment plan versus being strictly in a consulting role.

While MedFTs at *Levels 1 and 2* have a complementary skill set to other members of the team, they should also have a working knowledge of the pharmaceuticals more commonly being prescribed by the team and a familiarity with non-family medicine diagnoses that may exacerbate or be a consequence of treatments for family medicine conditions (e.g., polypharmacy effects due to metabolism changes in aging adults). These skills should be executed more frequently and advanced across the entire continuum as the MedFT becomes more fully integrated. As he or she becomes more integrated, he or she then moves beyond a siloed "mental health or discipline-specific" role into one where he or she is a member of the team where expertise among all members, including the patient and his/her support system member, is shared and respected collectively. Additionally, with regard to research and policy/advocacy, MedFTs operating at *Levels 1 or 2* may rarely to occasionally be asked or inspired to add to a study or policy addendum that taps into BPSS interactional dynamics. They may also advocate or be consulted with on occasion regarding relational and BPSS factors that influence the family medicine setting's clinical, operational, financial, and training/education policies and protocols. One example of this would be the modification of a policy on how information may be documented and exchanged between the healthcare team members and which members of the patient's support system should be routinely invited to visits.

In the case example presented for this chapter, the MedFT functions at a *Level 3* when she applies her MedFT knowledge and skills through BPSS and relational interventions. While not all MedFTs will have relational and BPSS research or policy/advocacy opportunities in family medicine settings, this level of MedFT has skills and experience necessary for participating in opportunities related to each and is able to contribute effectively. In relation to the chapter's case example, something appears to be embedded in the procedures of the system, where providers of different disciplines know about and refer to one another. At a *Level 3*, collaboration usually continues past the referral point and how frequently it occurs may depend upon the complexity of the case and how much the providers value it. The fact that Martha was called in advance of Dr. Robbins meeting with the patient and her family, and not just in response to a crisis, demonstrated a *Level 3* application of MedFT clinical and collaborative knowledge and skills. She also responded to and included the patient's family in treatment, acknowledging that they are important to the success of managing the patient's BPSS health. Those living and interacting with the patient outside of the healthcare context are able to separate out sudden versus gradual changes that may point to different diagnoses. For example, a urinary tract infection in an older adult may rapidly lead to mental status changes and get treated as a purely mental health issue although a biomedical intervention is the critical first step. This is why it is important that providers remain BPSS aware of patient's health and well-being and family/support system members be permitted to participate in treatment and contribute to providers' understanding of the problem.

MedFTs at *Levels 4 and 5* highlight consistent and then proficient application of MedFT knowledge and skills. At these levels, the clinician, like Martha, will identify as a MedFT professionally. She will be seen as part of the healthcare team versus exclusively as a colocated specialty care provider. An example of this advanced level of skill would be when she led the family interventions sessions to help the family plan for future declines in cognitive functioning. The *Level 5* skills were also evident with this case when Martha led the team in developing a treatment plan that would be best for the family unit, not just the patient. It permitted the opportunity for the providers to address the guilt expressed by the family members over needing to consider a care facility at some point in the future. The team also recognized the cultural components of the system and did not exclude the kin from the treatment plan but incorporated them into it. Team members had access to each other's notes, and everyone shared responsibility for encouraging the team's overall goals with the patient and her family versus only the goals aligned for the patient's best interests. Also at their sessions, incorporation of the family's spirituality into the plan was also recognized as a vital need. Martha as a *Level 5* MedFT also displayed skills in alternating between integrated behavioral healthcare and traditional psychotherapy services, being able to blend them well and maintain a BPSS and relational perspective throughout.

Research-Informed Practices

For a MedFT in a primary care setting, there are numerous opportunities for intervening in patient care. Interactions between a MedFT and a patient may occur in the form of a patient introduction, same-day responses to referrals, brief assessments or point of care interventions (i.e., under 30 minutes), short-term psychotherapy (e.g., 4 to 6 sessions; Vogel, Kirkpatrick, Collings, Cederna-Meko, & Grey, 2012), or as interprofessional collaboration with other healthcare providers (McDaniel et al., 2014). Research has emphasized the importance of brevity and cost-effectiveness in these behavioral interventions, recognizing that there are unique limits, focuses, and constraints for this particular kind of work (Polaha, Volkmer, & Valleley, 2007). These interventions are often educational, cognitive- and/or behaviorally based, and solution-focused (Vogel et al., 2012); they are not intended to dig deep into one's past as a professional in a traditional therapy context would. Rather, they are meant to empower and equip a patient to traverse forward in accord with the design set within their treatment team. The following section will review several individual, family, and community research-informed practices commonly used by MedFTs in family medicine.

Individual Approaches

Cognitive behavioral therapy. Cognitive behavioral therapy (CBT) represents a way to help patients restructure their maladaptive preconceptions and corresponding behaviors, which often interfere with or impede successful compliance with treatments. CBT has been found to be effective for treating common concerns in primary care such as chronic fatigue (Meng, Friedberg, & Castora-Binkley, 2014), depression (Kessler et al., 2009; Linde et al., 2015), anxiety and other stress-related problems (Craske et al., 2006; Ejeby et al., 2014), and somatic physical symptoms (Escobar et al., 2007). Beyond primary care, CBT has been shown successful in treating mild to moderate dementia and general mental functioning (Robinson et al., 2010; van Ravesteijn, Lucassen, Bor, van Wheel, & Speckens, 2013) and disordered eating (Agras, Walsh, Fairburn, Wilson, & Kraemer, 2000). Research has demonstrated that helping patients in primary care settings emotionally process their experiences (i.e., integrate their thoughts and feelings) via CBT predicted improved outcomes (Godfrey, Chalder, Ridsdale, Seed, & Ogden, 2007). The effects of CBT have been shown at completion of therapy and at 6-month follow-up (Escobar et al., 2007).

Interpersonal psychotherapy. Interpersonal psychotherapy (IPT) is another well-documented, empirically based clinical intervention commonly used in primary care. IPT is designed to focus on the patient's current interpersonal relationships while addressing primary areas of concern (e.g., grief, role transitions, role disputes, interpersonal deficits; Kindaichi & Mebane, 2011; Markowitz & Weissman, 2004). The goal of this particular approach is to intervene by considering significant life changes that may precipitate negative symptoms (e.g., grief and loss) and addressing identifiable triggers of the patient's health concern(s). In primary care, IPT is an effective approach to treating depression and postpartum depression (van Schaik et al., 2006). Beyond primary care, IPT has been found successful in treating depression and postpartum depression, (Markowitz & Weissman, 2004; O'Hara, Stuart, Gorman, & Wenzel, 2000), disordered eating (Wilfley et al., 2002), posttraumatic stress disorder (Markowitz et al., 2015), multisomatoform disorder (Sattel et al., 2012), and anxiety (Stangier, Schramm, Heidenreich, Berger, & Clark, 2011). IPT has been found to be ineffective in treating dysthymic disorder in primary care (Browne et al., 2002).

Motivational interviewing. Motivational interviewing (MI; Miller, 1983) is a collaborative, patient-centered approach focused on assessing patients' readiness for change and empowering patients to move toward change. This approach reaffirms patients' freedom of choice and self-efficacy and avoids provider-driven treatment plans that often fail to consider patients' ambivalence toward making a change. The overarching goal of MI is behavior change through collaboration between patient and MedFT, supporting patient autonomy and drawing out the patient's concerns and ideas for solutions (Anstiss, 2009).

The original description of MI (Miller, 1983) was based on implicit principles derived from intuitive practices (e.g., alcohol addiction, smoking cessation) and was elaborated upon by Miller and Rollnick (1991). Since then, hundreds of studies, including meta-analyses, have been conducted evaluating the effectiveness of this approach. One meta-analysis by Lundahl et al. (2013) reported MI to have a significant positive impact on cholesterol levels, blood pressure, HIV viral load, weight, physical strength, quality of life (e.g., worrying, pain, adjustment to illnesses), self-monitoring activities (e.g., blood sugar levels), reducing sedentary behavior, and increasing confidence and engagement in treatment. MI has also been found to significantly increase medical adherence for older adults (mean age of 75 years) in primary care when compared to a control group that received an advice approach (Moral et al., 2015). MI is also a good approach when working with problems that are often found to be comorbid in patients (e.g., alcohol dependence, drug abuse, eating disorders; Britt, Hudson, & Blampied, 2004; Vanbuskirk & Wetherell, 2014).

Psychoeducation. The use of psychoeducation in primary care can be a helpful strategy to deliver information about topics like sleep hygiene, smoking cessation, lifestyle habits, medication management, and mental health (Substance Abuse and Mental Health Services Administration, 2009). The main components of psychoeducation include therapeutic interaction, clarification, and enhancing coping competence (Bäuml, Froböse, Kraemer, Rentrop, & Pitschel-Walz, 2006). Psychoeducation may be offered in a one-on-one conversation between a MedFT and patient or via multi-person visits or group classes. In research to date, psychoeducation has been shown to be helpful in patients' positive adjustment to receiving a breast cancer diagnosis (Dastan & Buzlu, 2012). Findings from systematic reviews and meta-analyses have suggested that for adult patients with major depressive disorder, psychoeducation is an effective approach in improving clinical course, treatment adherence, and psychosocial functioning (Donker, Griffiths, Cuijpers, & Christensen, 2009; Tursi, Baes, Camacho, Tofoli, & Juruena, 2013). Research has also shown that a significant percentage of parents who received psychoeducation about nutrition, family meals, and physical activity have reduced the amount of screen time and sugary drinks consumed by their children (Stovitz et al., 2014).

Family Approaches

Families are important for health. Research has consistently linked better family relationships to positive health (e.g., Campbell, 2003; Chesla, 2010; Garcia-Huidobro & Marsalis, 2012; Hartmann, Bzner, Wild, Eisler, & Herzog, 2010; Martire, Lustig, Schulz, Miller, & Helgeson, 2004; Martire, Schulz, Helgeson, Small, & Saghafi, 2010; Shields, Finley, & Chawla, 2012). Interventions that have integrated a family approach can be grouped in two broad types: family therapy and family-based interventions. Family therapy approaches are structured interventions that have focused in improving family relationships and consequentially mental health outcomes including depressive, anxiety, eating, and substance use disorders. Although these approaches require specific training, it is important that MedFTs are familiar with them, as certain communities might not have access to providers who can deliver effective family therapy interventions. Family-based interventions use the relational principles of family therapy and aim at improving physical health outcomes (McDaniel et al., 2005). These have been more commonly implemented in primary care settings, targeting patients with a wide array of physical health conditions. In the following sections, research on these two family-focused approaches is reviewed.

Family therapy approaches. Traditional family therapy approaches, such as structural, strategic, narrative, and systemic family therapy, among others, have focused on relational outcomes. Yet, few of them are supported with empirical research (Sprenkle, 2002). In this section, we review the evidence-based family therapy approaches for mental health problems commonly seen in primary care across the lifespan. As practicing these techniques requires specific training, it is unlikely that MedFTs will use all of these therapy styles; however, it is important to be familiar with them, as some primary care patients might benefit from specific types of interventions.

Frequent mental health problems in *children* are related to problematic behaviors. Parent-child interaction therapy has shown positive effects in preschool- and school-aged children with attention-deficit hyperactivity disorder (Matos, Bauermeister, & Bernal, 2009; Nixon, 2001) and children with oppositional defiant disorder (Nixon, Sweeney, Erickson, & Touyz, 2004). This approach aims to enhance positive parent-child interactions and subsequently improve parent-child relationship quality. For example, MedFTs often provide direct coaching to assist parents in practicing skills while interacting with their children in the therapy session.

Common mental health problems for adolescents that are seen in family medicine settings include depression, anxiety, conduct problems, substance use, and suicide ideation. Multidimensional family therapy, solution-focused family therapy, attachment-based family therapy, functional family therapy, family cognitive behavioral therapy, and Maudsley family therapy are evidence-based approaches to treat adolescent depression, anxiety, bipolar disorder, suicide ideation, substance use, conduct problems, and eating disorders and improve overall family functioning (Ewing, Diamond, & Levy, 2015; Liddle, Dakof, Turner, Henderson, & Greenbaum, 2008; Liddle, Rowe, Dakof, Henderson, & Greenbaum, 2009; Lock, Agras, Bryson, & Kraemer, 2005; Santisteban et al., 2003; Wood, Piacentini, Southam-Gerow, Chu, & Sigman, 2006; Storch et al., 2007; Waldron & Turner, 2008; Wood, Piacentini, Southam-Gerow, Chu, & Sigman, 2006). Multidimensional family therapy is a comprehensive intervention that provides individual and joint care to parents and adolescents. This approach is focused in helping adolescents and their parents develop effective coping and problem-solving skills as a way to improve their relationships as a protective factor for substance abuse. Research studies have provided strong evidence for its effectiveness and cost-effectiveness at improving substance abuse among other significant outcomes (e.g., education, delinquency, and crime; Liddle et al., 2008; Liddle et al., 2009).

Solution-focused family therapy posits that troublesome adolescent behaviors originate in negative family interactions; therefore, improving family functioning will help to improve adolescents' behaviors. Under this approach, MedFTs join the family to diagnose patterns of family interactions and then help restructure their dynamics. After receiving this treatment, youth have reported improved conduct problems, substance use, and family functioning (Gingerich & Peterson, 2013; Santisteban et al., 2003).

Attachment-based family therapy aims to repair attachment injuries that predispose adolescents to experience depression, anxiety, and suicide ideation, by rebuilding secure relationships (Ewing et al., 2015). It assumes that symptoms can be triggered, exacerbated, or reduced by family relations. This approach has shown significant effects reducing all mental health outcomes while also improving family support (Ewing et al., 2015).

Functional family therapy is focused in family adaptation and overall functionality. It is a strength-based model of care that targets family engagement, motivation, relational assessment, behavioral changes, and generalization of the behaviors changed in the family to other contexts. This short-term treatment has shown effectiveness helping families with adolescents overcome depression, substance abuse, HIV risk behaviors, and behavioral problems (Sexton & Turner, 2010; Waldron & Turner, 2008).

Family cognitive behavioral therapy shares the same principles of individual CBT that is focused on thoughts (cognitions), emotions, and behaviors. As a family therapy approach, it extends its strategies to other family members and relationships. Research has shown positive effects at improving multiple anxiety disorders in youth, including generalized anxiety disorder, social phobia, and obsessive-compulsive disorder (Storch et al., 2007; Wood et al., 2006).

Finally, the Maudsley approach was developed to help families with a member experiencing eating disorders. This approach combines multiple family therapy techniques with guidance on healthy eating behaviors and strategies to gain weight. Multiple randomized trials support the effectiveness of this approach to treat anorexia and bulimia nervosa, including short (10 sessions) and long (20 sessions) treatment (Lock et al., 2005), and these were conducted conjoint or separated from the family (Eisler, Simic, Russell, & Dare, 2007; Loeb et al., 2007).

Among *adults*, frequent mental health problems seen in primary care include mood and anxiety disorders and substance use. Emotionally focused therapy (EFT) and cognitive behavioral couples therapy (CBCT) are the family therapy approaches that have been studied the most. EFT aims at helping couples improve their attachment and, thereby, their relationship. It is centered on helping patients develop a secure emotional attachment with their partner. CBCT includes a focus on substance use behaviors and the couple's relationship. Both of these approaches improve relationship satisfaction and dyadic distress (Fals-Stewart, Birchler, & Kelley, 2006). EFT also contributes improving depressive symptoms and distress caused by chronic illnesses (Dessaulles, Johnson, & Denton, 2003; Wiebe &

Johnson, 2016); CBCT has shown robust findings improving mood and substance use disorders (Fischer, Baucom, & Cohen, 2016; Schumm, O'Farrell, Kahler, Murphy, & Muchowski, 2014).

Although parenting interventions are not necessarily family therapy interventions, these types of interventions aim to improve parents' parenting skills and parent-child relationships. These interventions are structured and can be effectively delivered in primary care settings by family educators, social workers, and MedFTs in either individual or group formats. A recent literature review of parenting interventions delivered in primary care identified that Incredible Years and Triple P are the programs with that most evidence supporting feasibility and effectiveness (Cluxton-Keller, Riley, Noazin, & Umoren, 2015; Leslie et al., 2016). Given the longitudinal relationship between primary care providers and parents, MedFTs could have a significant impact in helping parents to raise their children in positive and healthy ways, leading to short- and long- term health and well-being. Children of parents who took part in parenting interventions are less likely to exhibit behavioral, substance use, and other mental health problems and are more likely to be healthier (Svetaz, Garcia-Huidobro, & Allen, 2014).

Family-based approaches. Family-based interventions are grounded in family therapy principles, but oftentimes these are less structured and include components of multiple approaches (Campbell, 2003). These types of interventions include separate or joint sessions, family meetings, home visits, multi-family groups, or a combination of these interventions (McDaniel et al., 2005). These interventions are frequently interdisciplinary, as when Dr. Robbins and Martha met with Mary's family in several family meetings. Even though for research purposes these interventions have structured manuals and protocols, these interventions are flexible and can be adapted according to the circumstances of the environments where they are being implemented. For example, García-Huidobro, Bittner, Brahm, and Puschel (2011) implemented a family-based intervention to improve the metabolic control of patients with type 2 diabetes. This intervention advanced a family approach to diabetes care and included components such as having medical assistants ask how the family were helping them with their condition, pharmacists discussing with patients and their families about the use of the medications, and providers extending family consultations in home visits to discuss in-depth strategies and increase family involvement in the patient's care. These last components were conducted by physicians, nurses, psychologists, or social workers who were trained in principles of family therapy, how to conduct family assessments and support family relationships (but they were not asked to follow a scripted intervention for each meeting). As with this example, many family-based interventions are focused at strengthening family relationships and promoting involvement in patients' care. Training is required for MedFTs to deliver these interventions effectively.

Research in support of family-based interventions, especially those focused on physical health outcomes, is growing. In the last decades, multiple systematic reviews have been published reporting the benefit of including family members in preventive or therapeutic interventions (Campbell, 2003; Chesla, 2010;

Hartmann et al., 2010; Martire et al., 2004, 2010; Shields et al., 2012). In preventive care, family-based interventions are useful at increasing healthy eating and physical activity and preventing overweight/obesity, high blood pressure, dyslipidemia, smoking, and overall cardiovascular risk (Garcia-Huidobro & Marsalis, 2012). In addition to improving relationship outcomes (Martire et al., 2010), family-based interventions are also useful at improving the management of multiple medical conditions such as arthritis and chronic pain (Hartmann et al., 2010; Martire et al., 2010), type 1 and type 2 diabetes control (Baig, Benitez, Quinn, & Burnet, 2015; Torenholt, Schwennesen, & Willaing, 2014), anti-HIV medication management (Hartmann et al., 2010), cardiovascular disease and stroke (Hartmann et al., 2010; Sher et al., 2014), and improved coping with cancer (Hartmann et al., 2010; Shields et al., 2012). Involving spouses only or a diverse group of family members seems to produce similar results (Hartmann et al., 2010). Effects on family members' health have been observed in interventions targeting cardiovascular disease, cancer, and arthritis, but there is less evidence supporting these extended effects (Hartmann et al., 2010; Martire et al., 2010). With all these encouraging results, family medicine clinics are a prime location for the work of MedFTs.

Community Approaches

Integrated primary care services go beyond the clinic or healthcare networks. Integrated behavioral healthcare includes collaborating with community agencies, faith organizations, among other groups that also have an impact in patient health (McDaniel et al., 2014). MedFTs working in primary care settings with the required skills to successfully interact with members of the community can be tremendous assets to collaborate maximizing the resources that would help patients and their local communities become happier and healthier.

Research in this area is also growing and oftentimes has been conducted under the principles of community-based participatory research (CBPR; Minkler & Wallerstein, 2011), which emphasize the participation of the community in all phases of the research projects. Community Partners in Care (CPIC) was the first randomized study that compared "traditional" research methods with CBPR methods (Wells et al., 2013). This study focused on improving mental health in Los Angeles, CA, using community engagement and planning or resources for services. After 6 months of intervention, participants in the community engagement group achieved better outcomes, including better health-related quality of life, reduced behavioral health hospitalizations, and increased depression visits among users of primary care.

Beck et al. (2014) developed a collaborative intervention between primary care clinics and community organizations called Keeping Infants Nourished and Developing [KIND]. In this partnership, pediatricians and community collaborators developed processes to link food-insecure families of infants with supplementary formula, educational materials, and other resources (e.g., community referrals, food a banks, and job training programs). After 14 months, recipients were more likely to have undergone lead testing and developmental screening procedures and to have received well-infant visits. Another example is presented by Ariza et al. (2013), where they linked pediatric primary care with community services focused in obesity via the Promoting Health Project [PHP]. Although this project was centered in processes related to partnership success, authors reported that this coordination required many unanticipated resources that ended up affecting patients' results.

Allen et al. (2013) present how a partnership between academics and community organizations (including primary care clinics) was developed using a paralleling community-academic partnership development with Erikson's stages of human development. As a way to reconcile the research interests of the academic partner in tobacco use prevention, alongside needs within parenting programs for immigrant Latino families, they developed a parenting curriculum using the academic and community expertise that led them to secure funding to conduct a large randomized study over 5 years (Allen et al., 2012). This intervention blended core Latino cultural values such as *respeto* (respect), *familismo* (importance of family relationships), and *personalismo* (importance of individual relationships) with evidence-based parenting education. As a product, the intervention had similar or higher attendance than other parenting programs, while improving parent-child relationships (Allen et al., 2017).

The population health approach, originally developed by the Canadian Institute for Advanced Research in the 1990s, aims to improve the health status of an entire population or subpopulations. This alternate approach was developed to oppose current standard (i.e., individualistic) approaches to care. Its primary focus is to reduce health inequities among population groups by recognizing and addressing factors and conditions that have a strong influence on our health, known as *determinants of health* (Sox, 2013). Examples of determinants of health include employment/working conditions, health services, education, income, and social environments (Richmond & Ross, 2008). This approach is based on the understanding that the health of populations as a whole is correlated with factors that fall outside the health system and which are not routinely addressed (Public Health Agency of Canada [PHAC], 2013). The population health approach calls for innovative and interrelated strategies that recognize the connections between the social, economic, and environmental health determinants. The focus, then, is on developing and implementing policies and actions to improve the health and well-being of those populations. Benefits of a population health approach extend beyond improved population health outcomes but also include a more wholly integrated health system.

Dr. Jeffrey Brenner, founder of the Camden Coalition of Healthcare Providers, has been recognized for his work in the field of population health. He has identified the term, *hotspotting*, as the strategic reallocation of resources to a small subset of high-needs, high-cost patients (Camden Coalition of Healthcare Providers [CCHP], 2016). These patients are known as *super-utilizers*—those that account for much of the cost in the healthcare system. As these patients' chronic conditions worsen over time, they require more complex and expensive treatments. Hotspotting uses data to identify these super-utilizers and focuses efforts on understanding the problem, reallocating resources, and intervening. Multidisciplinary, coordinated care attends to both the medical and nonmedical needs that affect health (e.g., housing, mental health, substance abuse), providing a more holistic approach to patient care (CCHP, 2016). Considering a family medicine practice through the lens of a population health approach—including hotspotting to address the impact of super-utilizers on the health of the larger population—could be an advantageous way for MedFTs to focus in their integrated behavioral healthcare in a culturally relevant way.

In sum, MedFTs can support healthcare integration beyond their work in traditional clinical settings. However, they need to be aware that this work requires additional skills outlined in higher levels of the MedFT healthcare continuum (Table 2.3).

Conclusion

Family medicine has a long-standing relationship with family therapy and has been a place where integrated behavioral healthcare has gotten its footing. Given the exponential opportunities for family therapists to hold positions as administrators, clinicians, researchers, and faculty in family medicine settings, it is imperative that there are working models and resources to help provide the necessary training. When it comes down to it, we are all focused on health. While family therapists do not make diagnoses rooted in the physical body, they understand that all diagnoses, whether mental or medical, have psychosocial implications. There is a place at the table for relationally trained behavioral health providers. There is evidence that supports that approaching health from a relational perspective leads to positive health outcomes. Therefore, as clinical, operational, and financial models for integrated behavioral healthcare are becoming sustainable services in settings like family medicine, there will be an increase in demand for trained MedFT clinicians and researchers.

Reflection Questions
1. If you were given the opportunity to integrate into a family medicine setting, what strengths do you already possess that you believe would be transferable? What areas would be notable ones for future growth—and where could you get this training locally, regionally, and/or nationally?
2. What reimbursement mechanisms exist in your state that permit family therapists to bill for services in a family medicine setting? What reimbursement mechanisms exist but are not available to family therapists currently?
3. What are the top three things you know to recommend for patients who are developing health goals in each of the following areas: (a) sleep hygiene, (b) stress management, (c) physical activity, and (d) healthy eating?

Glossary of Important Terms for Care in Family Medicine

Attending physician In medical residency training, the attending physician is a faculty member responsible for the training of residents and supervision of patient care. At times the term "preceptor" may be used to describe an attending physician who is providing specific teaching and supervision during a focused period of time (such as a clinic session).

Collaborative care A model of healthcare delivery that requires collaborative efforts from people of different disciplines.

Colocated care A model of care where behavioral health providers are working in the same facility as physical health providers, but there is limited collaboration in their care.

Community-based participatory research (CBPR) An approach to research (and accompanying methodologies) that emphasize the co-ownership of the investigative process between professionals and community members; these efforts are carrying out within the contexts and processes of flat professional hierarchies.

Fellowship training Additional years of clinical experience focused on a specific area of interest, such as adolescent medicine, emergency medicine, palliative care, sports medicine, geriatrics, or others.

Healthcare disparities Systematic differences in the provision of healthcare; groups from marginalized populations tend to have less access to care and poorer health outcomes.

Hotspotting An innovative approach to managing healthcare disparities; it involves strategic reallocation of resources to a small subset of high-needs, high-cost patients.

Integrated behavioral healthcare A model of healthcare delivery that embeds behavioral healthcare providers within the traditional healthcare environment. At varying levels of integration, teams of providers share access to patients, electronic records, and physical space, and they collaborate and coordinate on plans for treatment.

Primary care Full-spectrum healthcare; primary care providers often serve as the patient's "medical home" by managing chronic conditions, treating acute concerns, and coordinating treatment from various specialists.

Primary care provider The clinician who provides preventive and medical care for patients over time; this includes physicians, nurses, and physician assistants.

Residency Medical training that takes places after the completion of medical school but before independent practice. Most family medicine residency programs are 3 years long; a few require 4 years of training.

Resident A person who has graduated from medical school and is pursuing further training in a particular specialty area and may be referred to as an "intern" during the first year of training. The resident's year of training is designated as PGY1 (program year 1), PGY2, etc. "Chief resident" is a senior leadership position with varying responsibilities based on the specific program but frequently includes some additional organizational and teaching responsibilities.

Silo A term that refers to the traditional separation between behavioral health and biomedical treatment.
Secondary care Specialist care focusing on a specific body system, disease, or condition (e.g., medical family therapist, endocrinologist, cardiologist, etc.).
Tertiary care Higher-level specialty care within the hospital requiring highly specialized equipment and expertise or complex treatments or procedures (e.g., burn units, neonatal intensive care unit).

Additional Resources

Literature

Blount, A. (2003). Integrated primary care: Organizing the evidence. *Families, Systems, & Health, 21*, 121–133. https://doi.org/10.1037/1091-7527.21.2.121.

Crane, D., & Christenson, J. D. (2014). A summary report of cost-effectiveness: Recognizing the value of family therapy in health care. In J. Hodgson, A. Lamson, T. Mendenhall, and D. Crane (Eds.), *Medical family therapy: Advanced applications* (pp. 419–436). New York, NY: Springer.

Hodgson, J., Lamson, A., Mendenhall, T., & Crane, D. (Eds.). (2014). *Medical family therapy: Advanced applications.* New York, NY: Springer.

Marlowe, D., Hodgson, J., Lamson, J., White, M., & Irons, T. (2012). Medical family therapy in a primary care setting: A framework for integration. *Contemporary Family Therapy, 34*, 244–258. https://doi.org/10.1007/s10591-012-9195-5.

McDaniel, S. H., Doherty, W. J., & Hepworth, J. (2014). *Medical family therapy and integrated care.* Washington, DC: American Psychological Association.

McDaniel, S., Campbell, T. L., Hepworth, J., & Lorenz, A. (2005). *Family-oriented primary care.* New York, NY: Springer.

Peek, C. J. (2008). Planning care in the clinical, operational, and financial worlds. In R. Kessler and D. Stafford (Eds.), *Collaborative medicine case studies* (pp. 25–38). New York, NY: Springer.

Electronic Resources

Collaborative Families and Health Blog. http://www.cfha.net/blogpost/753286/Families-and-Health

Integrated Behavioral Health Project (2007). http://www.ibhp.org/

Society of Teachers of Family Medicine (resource section). http://www.stfm.org/Resources

Substance Abuse and Mental Health Services Administration (2016). *What is Integrated Care?* http://www.integration.samhsa.gov/about-us/what-is-integrated-care

Measures/Instruments

Brief Pain Inventory. https://www.mdanderson.org/education-and-research/departments-programs-and-labs/departments-and-divisions/symptom-research/symptom-assessment-tools/brief-pain-inventory.html
CAGE Assessment. http://www.tobaccofreemaine.org/channels/providers/documents/CAGE.pdf
Edinburgh Postnatal Depression Scale (EPDS). http://www.fresno.ucsf.edu/pediatrics/downloads/edinburghscale.pdf
Generalized Anxiety Disorder 7-item (GAD-7) scale. http://www.integration.samhsa.gov/clinical-practice/GAD708.19.08Cartwright.pdf
Healthy Living Questionnaire. http://www.integration.samhsa.gov/clinical-practice/Healthy_Living_Questionnaire2011.pdf
Kessler 6 Assessment of Mood. http://www.integration.samhsa.gov/images/res/K6%20Questions.pdf
Patient Health Questionnaire (PHQ-9). http://www.cqaimh.org/pdf/tool_phq9.pdf
Patient Satisfaction Questionnaire. http://www.rand.org/health/surveys_tools/psq.html
Patient Stress Questionnaire. http://www.integration.samhsa.gov/Patient_Stress_Questionnaire.pdf
Primary Care-PTSD Screen. http://www.mirecc.va.gov/docs/visn6/2_primary_care_ptsd_screen.pdf
Quality of Life Scale (QOLS). https://www.theacpa.org/uploads/documents/Life_Scale_3.pdf
Suicide Behaviors Questionnaire (SBQ-R). http://www.integration.samhsa.gov/images/res/SBQ.pdf
Vanderbilt Assessment Scale. http://www.nichq.org/childrens-health/adhd/resources/vanderbilt-assessment-scales

Organizations/Associations

American Academy of Family Physicians. www.aafp.org
American Association for Marriage and Family Therapy. www.aamft.org
Collaborative Family Healthcare Association. www.cfha.net
Society of Teachers of Family Medicine. www.stfm.org

References[1]

Agras, W. S., Walsh, B. T., Fairburn, C. G., Wilson, G. T., & Kraemer, H. C. (2000). A multicenter comparison of cognitive-behavioral therapy and interpersonal psychotherapy for bulimia nervosa. *Archives of General Psychiatry, 57*, 459–466. https://doi.org/10.1001/archpsyc.57.5.459

Allen, M., Svetaz, M. V., Hurtado, G. A., Linares, R., Garcia-Huidobro, D., & Hurtado, M. (2013). The developmental stages of a community-university partnership: The experience of padres informados/jovenes preparados. *Progress in Community Health Partnerships: Research, Education, and Action, 7*, 271–279. https://doi.org/10.1353/cpr.2013.0029

Allen, M. L., Garcia-Huidobro, D., Bastian, T., Hurtado, G. A., Linares, R., & Svetaz, M. V. (2017). Reconciling research and community priorities in a multisite participatory trial (mPaT): Application to padres informados/jovenes preparados. *Family Practice, 34*, 347–352.

Allen, M. L., Garcia-Huidobro, D., Hurtado, G. A., Allen, R., Davey, C. S., Forster, J. L., … Trebs, L. (2012). Immigrant family skills-building to prevent tobacco use in Latino youth: Study protocol for a community-based participatory randomized controlled trial. *Trials, 13*, 242–252. https://doi.org/10.1186/1745-6215-13-242

American Academy of Family Physicians (2015). *Member census*. Retrieved from http://www.aafp.org/about/the-aafp/family-medicine-facts/table-13.html

American Diabetes Association. (2015). Classification and diagnosis of diabetes. *Diabetes Care, 38*, S8–S16. https://doi.org/10.2337/dc15-S005

American Diabetes Association. (2016). Standards of medical care in diabetes. *Diabetes Care, 39*, S1–S106. https://doi.org/10.2337/diaclin.34.1.3

Anstiss, T. (2009). Motivational interviewing in primary care. *Journal of Clinical Psychology in Medical Settings, 16*, 87–93. https://doi.org/10.1007/s10880-009-9155-x

Ariza, A. J., Hartman, J., Grodecki, J., Clavier, A., Ghaey, K., Elsner, M., … Binns, H. J. (2013). Linking pediatric primary care obesity management to community programs. *Journal of Health Care for the Poor and Underserved, 24*, 158–167. https://doi.org/10.1353/hpu.2013.0112

Baig, A. A., Benitez, A., Quinn, M. T., & Burnet, D. L. (2015). Family interventions to improve diabetes outcomes for adults. *Annals of the New York Academy of Sciences, 1353*, 89–112. https://doi.org/10.1111/nyas.12844

Bäuml, J., Froböse, T., Kraemer, S., Rentrop, M., & Pitschel-Walz, G. (2006). Psychoeducation: A basic psychotherapeutic intervention for patients with schizophrenia and their families. *Schizophrenia Bulletin, 32*(Suppl 1), s1–s9. https://doi.org/10.1093/schbul/sbl017

Beck, A. F., Henize, A. W., Kahn, R. S., Reiber, K. L., Young, J. J., & Klein, M. D. (2014). Forging a pediatric primary care–community partnership to support food-insecure families. *Pediatrics, 134*, e564–e571. https://doi.org/10.1542/peds.2013-3845

Bitar, G. W., Springer, P., Gee, R., Graff, C., & Schydlower, M. (2009). Barriers and facilitators of adolescent behavioral health in primary care: Perceptions of primary care providers. *Families, Systems, and Health, 27*, 346–361. https://doi.org/10.1037/a0018076

Blair, I. V., Havranek, E. P., Price, D. W., Hanratty, R., Fairclough, D. L., Farley, T., … Steiner, J. F. (2013). An assessment of biases against Latinos and African Americans among primary care providers and community members. *American Journal of Public Health, 103*, 92–98. https://doi.org/10.2105/AJPH.2012.300812

*Blount, A. (2003). Integrated primary care: Organizing the evidence. *Families, Systems, & Health, 21*, 121–133. https://doi.org/10.1037/1091-7527.21.2.121

Bostock, S., & Steptoe, A. (2012). Association between low functional health literacy and mortality in older adults: Longitudinal cohort study. *British Journal of Medicine, 344*, 1–10. https://doi.org/10.1136/bmj.e1602

---

[1] Note: References that are prefaced with an asterisk are recommended readings

Bridges, A. J., Andrews, A. R., Villalobos, B. T., Pastrana, F. A., Cavell, T. A., & Gomez, D. (2014). Does integrated behavioral health care reduce mental health disparities for Latinos? Initial findings. *Journal of Latino/a Psychology, 2*, 37–53. https://doi.org/10.1037/lat0000009

Britt, E., Hudson, S. M., & Blampied, N. M. (2004). Motivational interviewing in health settings: A review. *Patient Education and Counseling, 53*, 147–155. https://doi.org/10.1016/S0738-3991(03)00141-1

Brook, R. D., Appel, L. J., Rubenfire, M., Ogedegbe, G., Bisognano, J. D., Elliot, W. J., ... Rajagopalan, S. (2013). Beyond medications and diet: Alternative approaches to lowering blood pressure: A scientific statement from the American Heart Association. *Hypertension, 61*, 1360–1383. https://doi.org/10.1161/HYP.0b013e318293645f

Browne, G., Steiner, M., Roberts, J., Gafni, A., Byrne, C., Dunn, E., ... Kraemer, J. (2002). Sertraline and/or interpersonal psychotherapy for patients with dysthymic disorder in primary care: 6-month comparison with longitudinal 2-year follow-up of effectiveness and costs. *Journal of Affective Disorders, 68*, 317–330. https://doi.org/10.1016/S0165-0327(01)00343-3

Camden Coalition of Healthcare Providers. (2016). *Healthcare hotspotting: A project of the Camden Coalition of Healthcare Providers.* Retrieved from http://hotspotting.camdenhealth.org/

Campbell, T. L. (2003). The effectiveness of family interventions for physical disorders. *Journal of Marriage and Family Therapy, 29*, 263–281. https://doi.org/10.1111/j.1752-0606.2003.tb01204.x

Caplan, L., Wolfe, F., Michaud, K., Quinzanos, I., & Hirsh, J. M. (2014). Strong association of health literacy with functional status among rheumatoid arthritis patients: A cross-sectional study. *Arthritis Care & Research, 66*, 508–514. https://doi.org/10.1002/acr.22165

Centers for Disease Control & Prevention (CDC). (2016), *Most recent asthma data.* Retrieved from http://www.cdc.gov/asthma/most_recent_data.htm

Centers for Medicare & Medicaid Services (CMS). (2013). *Common codes for family practice.* Retrieved from http://www.roadto10.org/specialty-references/common-codes-family-practice/

Chapman, E. N., Kaatz, A., & Carnes, M. (2013). Physicians and implicit bias: How doctors may unwittingly perpetuate health care disparities. *Journal of General Internal Medicine, 28*, 1504–1510. https://doi.org/10.1007/s11606-013-2441-1

Chesla, C. (2010). Do family interventions improve health? *Journal of Family Nursing, 16*, 355–377. https://doi.org/10.1177/1074840710383145

Cluxton-Keller, F., Riley, A. W., Noazin, S., & Umoren, M. V. (2015). Clinical effectiveness of family therapeutic interventions embedded in general pediatric primary care settings for parental mental health: A systematic review and meta-analysis. *Clinical Child and Family Psychology Review, 18*, 395–412. https://doi.org/10.1007/s10567-015-0190-x

Cohen, D. J., Balasubramanian, B. A., Davis, M., Hall, J., Gunn, R., Stange, K. C., ... Miller, B. F. (2015). Understanding care integration from the ground up: Five organizing constructs that shape integrated practices. *Journal of the American Board of Family Medicine, 28*(Suppl 1), S7–S20. https://doi.org/10.3122/jabfm.2015.S1.150050

Conner, K. O., Copeland, V. C., Grote, N. K., Koeske, G., Rosen, D., Reynolds, C. F., & Brown, C. (2010). Mental health treatment seeking among older adults with depression: The impact of stigma and race. *American Journal of Geriatric Psychiatry, 18*, 531–543. https://doi.org/10.1097/JGP.0b013e3181cc0366

Cook, B. L., Zuvekas, S. H., Carson, N., Wayne, G. F., Vesper, A., & McGuire, T. J. (2014). Assessing racial/ethnic disparities in treatment across episodes of mental health care. *Health Services Research, 49*, 206–229. https://doi.org/10.1111/1475-6773.12095

Crane, D., & Christenson, J. D. (2012). A summary report of the cost-effectiveness of the profession and practice of marriage and family therapy. *Contemporary Family Therapy, 34*, 204–216. https://doi.org/10.1007/s10591-012-9187-5

*Crane, D., & Christenson, J. D. (2014). A summary report of cost-effectiveness: Recognizing the value of family therapy in health care. In J. Hodgson, A. Lamson, T. Mendenhall, and D. Crane. (Eds.), *Medical family therapy: Advanced applications* (pp. 419–436). New York, NY: Springer.

Craske, M. G., Roy-Byrne, P., Stein, M. B., Sullivan, G., Hazlett-Stevens, H., Bystritsky, A., & Sherbourne, C. (2006). CBT intensity and outcome for panic disorder in a primary care setting. *Behavior Therapy, 37*, 112–119. https://doi.org/10.1016/j.beth.2005.05.003

Dastan, N. B., & Buzlu, S. (2012). Psychoeducation intervention to improve adjustment to cancer among Turkish stage I-II breast cancer patients: A randomized controlled trial. *Asian Pacific Journal of Cancer Prevention, 13*, 5313–5318. https://doi.org/10.7314/apjcp.2012.13.10.5313

deGruy, F. (1996). Mental health care in the primary care setting. In M. S. Donaldson, K. D. Yordy, K. N. Lohr, and N. A. Vanselow (Eds.), *Primary care: America's health in a new era* (pp. 285–311). Washington, D.C: Institute of Medicine.

Dessaulles, A., Johnson, S. M., & Denton, W. H. (2003). Emotion-focused therapy for couples in the treatment of depression: A pilot study. *American Journal of Family Therapy, 31*, 345–353. https://doi.org/10.1080/01926180390232266

Doherty, W. J., & Baird, M. A. (1983). *Family therapy and family medicine: Toward the primary care of families*. New York, NY: Guilford Press.

Doherty, W. J., & Baird, M. A. (1987). *Family centered medical care: A clinical casebook*. New York, NY: Guilford Press.

Donker, T., Griffiths, K. M., Cuijpers, P., & Christensen, H. (2009). Psychoeducation for depression, anxiety, and psychological distress: A meta-analysis. *BMC Medicine, 7*, 79–88. https://doi.org/10.1186/1741-7015-7-79

Dowell, D., Haegerich, T. M., & Chou, R. (2016). CDC guideline for prescribing opioids for chronic pain – United States, 2016. *Recommendations and reports, 65*, 1–49. 10.15585/mmwr.rr6501e1er

Druss, B. G., Hwang, I., Petukhova, M., Sampson, N. A., Wang, P. S., & Kessler, R. C. (2009). Impairment in role functioning in mental and chronic medical disorders in the United States: Results from the national comorbidity survey replication. *Molecular Psychiatry, 14*, 728–737. https://doi.org/10.1038/mp.2008.13

Eisler, I., Simic, M., Russell, G. F. M., & Dare, C. (2007). A randomized controlled treatment trial of two forms of family therapy in adolescent anorexia nervosa: A five-year follow-up. *Journal of Child Psychology and Psychiatry, 48*, 552–560. https://doi.org/10.1111/j.1469-7610.2007.01726.x

Ejeby, K., Savitskij, R., Ost, L., Ekbom, A., Brandt, L., Ramnero, J., … Backlund, L. G. (2014). Randomized controlled trial of transdiagnostic group treatments for primary care patients with common mental disorders. *Family Practice, 31*, 273–280. https://doi.org/10.1093/fampra/cmu006

Endevelt, R., Peled, R., Azrad, A., Kowen, G., Valinsky, L., & Heymann, A. D. (2015). Diabetes prevention program in a Mediterranean environment: Individual or group therapy? An effectiveness evaluation. *Primary Care Diabetes, 9*, 89–95. https://doi.org/10.1016/j.pcd.2014.07.005

*Engel, G. L. (1977). The need for a new medical model: A challenge for biomedicine. *Science, 196*, 129–136. https://doi.org/10.1016/b978-0-409-95009-0.50006-1

*Engel, G. L. (1980). The clinical application of the biopsychosocial model. *American Journal of Family Medicine, 137*, 535–544. https://doi.org/10.1176/ajp.137.5.535

Escobar, J. I., Gara, M. A., Diaz-Martinez, A. M., Interian, A., Warman, M., … Rodgers, D. (2007). Effectiveness of a time-limited cognitive behavior therapy-type intervention among primary care patients with medically unexplained symptoms. *Annals of Family Medicine, 5*, 328–335. https://doi.org/10.1370/afm.702

Ewing, E. S. K., Diamond, G., & Levy, S. (2015). Attachment-based family therapy for depressed and suicidal adolescents: Theory, clinical model and empirical support. *Attachment & Human Development, 17*, 136–156. https://doi.org/10.1080/14616734.2015.1006384

Fals-Stewart, W., Birchler, G. R., & Kelley, M. L. (2006). Learning sobriety together: A randomized clinical trial examining behavioral couples therapy with alcoholic female patients. *Journal of Consulting and Clinical Psychology, 74*, 579–591. https://doi.org/10.1037/0022-006x.74.3.579

Felt, B. T., Biermann, B., Christner, J. G., Kochhar, P., & Van Harrison, R. (2014). Diagnosis and management of ADHD in children. *American Family Physician, 90*, 456–464. Retrieved from http://www.aafp.org/journals/afp.html

Fischer, M. S., Baucom, D. H., & Cohen, M. J. (2016). Cognitive-behavioral couple therapies: Review of the evidence for the treatment of relationship distress, psychopathology, and chronic health conditions. *Family Process, 55*, 423–442. https://doi.org/10.1111/famp.12227

Fries, J., Koop, E., Beadle, D., Cooper, P., England, M., Greaves, J., Sokoilov, J., Wright, D., & the Health Project Consortium. (1993). Reducing health care costs by reducing the need and demand for medical services. *New England Journal of Medicine, 329*, 321–325. https://doi.org/10.1056/NEJM199307293290506

Galanti, G. A. (2014). *Caring for patients from different cultures* (2nd ed.). Philadelphia, PA: University of Pennsylvania Press.

García-Huidobro, D., Bittner, M., Brahm, P., & Puschel, K. (2011). Family intervention to control type 2 diabetes: A controlled clinical trial. *Family Practice, 28*, 4–11. https://doi.org/10.1093/fampra/cmq069

Garcia-Huidobro, D., & Marsalis, S. (2012). *Family interventions for the primary prevention of cardiovascular disease.* Presentation at the annual conference for the Collaborative Family Healthcare Association, Austin.

Gardner, W., Murphy, M., Childs, G., Kelleher, K., Pagano, M., Jellinek, M., ... Sturner, R. (1999). The PSC-17: A brief pediatric symptom checklist with psychosocial problem subscales. A report from PROS and ASPN. *Ambulatory Child Health, 5*, 225–236. Retrieved from http://onlinelibrary.wiley.com/journal/10.1111/(ISSN)1467-0658/issues

Gatchel, R., & Oordt, M. (2003). *Clinical health psychology and primary care: Practical advice and clinical guidance for successful collaboration.* Washington, DC, US: American Psychological Association.

George, C. M., Bruijn, L. L., Will, K., & Howard-Thompson, A. (2015). Management of blood glucose with noninsulin therapies in type 2 diabetes. *American Family Physician, 92*, 27–34. Retrieved from http://www.aafp.org/journals/afp.html

Gingerich, W. J., & Peterson, L. T. (2013). Effectiveness of solution-focused brief therapy: A systematic qualitative review of controlled outcome studies. *Research on Social Work Practice, 23*, 266–283. https://doi.org/10.1177/1049731512470859

Godfrey, E., Chalder, T., Ridsdale, L., Seed, P., & Ogden, J. (2007). Investigating the 'active ingredients' of cognitive behaviour therapy and counselling for patients with chronic fatigue in primary care: Developing a new process measure to assess treatment fidelity and predict outcome. *British Journal of Clinical Psychology, 46*, 253–272. ttps://doi.org/10.1348/014466506X147420

Goldstein, D., & Holmes, J. (2011). *Health and wellness survey: 2011 physicians' daily life poll.* Retrieved from http://www.rwjf.org/content/dam/web-assets/2011/11/2011-physicians--daily-life-report

Hartmann, M., Bzner, E., Wild, B., Eisler, I., & Herzog, W. (2010). Effects of interventions involving the family in the treatment of adult patients with chronic physical diseases: A meta-analysis. *Psychotherapy and Psychosomatics, 79*, 136–148. https://doi.org/10.1159/000286958

Hatala, A. R. (2012). The status of the "biopsychosocial" model in health psychology: Towards an integrated approach and a critique of cultural conceptions. *Open Journal of Medical Psychology, 1*, 51–62. https://doi.org/10.4236/ojmp.2012.14009

Hayes, C., Naylor, R., & Egger, G. (2012). Understanding chronic pain in a lifestyle context: The emergence of a whole-person approach. *American Journal of Lifestyle Medicine, 6*, 421–428. https://doi.org/10.1177/1559827612439282

Hodgson, J., Fox, M., & Lamson, A. (2014). Family therapists in primary care settings: Opportunities for integration through advocacy. In J. Hodgson, A. Lamson, T. Mendenhall, and D. Crane (Eds.), *Medical family therapy: Advanced applications* (pp. 357–380). New York, NY: Springer.

*Hodgson, J., Lamson, A., Mendenhall, T., & Crane, D. (Eds.). (2014). *Medical family therapy: Advanced applications.* New York, NY: Springer. https://doi.org/10.1007/978-3-319-03482-9

Hodgson, J., Lamson, A., Mendenhall, T., & Tyndall, L. (2014). Introduction to medical family therapy: Advanced applications. In J. Hodgson, A. Lamson, T. Mendenhall, and D. Crane (Eds.), *Medical family therapy: Advanced applications* (pp. 1–9). New York, NY: Springer.

Huang, L., Yang, L., Shen, X., & Yan, S. (2016). Relationship between glycated hemoglobin A1c and cognitive function in nondemented elderly patients with type 2 diabetes. *Metabolic Brain Disorders, 31,* 347–353. https://doi.org/10.1007/s11011-015-9756-z

Hudon, C., Fortin, M., Haggerty, J., Loignon, C., Lambert, M., & Poitras, M. E. (2012). Patient-centered care in chronic disease management: A thematic analysis of the literature in family medicine. *Patient Education and Counseling, 88,* 170–176. https://doi.org/10.1016/j.pec.2012.01.009

Jackman, R. P., Purvis, J. M., & Mallett, B. S. (2008). Chronic nonmalignant pain in primary care. *American Family Physician, 78,* 1155–1162. Retrieved from http://www.aafp.org/journals/afp.html

Kelly, E. L., Davis, L., & Brekke, J. S. (2015). PBRN findings: Integrated care for individuals with serious mental illness. *Psychiatric Services, 66,* 1253–1253. https://doi.org/10.1176/appi.ps.201500075

Kessler, R., Chiu, W., Demler, O., & Walters, E. (2005). Prevalence, severity, and comorbidity of 12-Month DSM-IV disorders in the National Comorbidity Survey replication. *Archives of General Psychiatry, 62,* 617–627. https://doi.org/10.1001/archpsyc.62.6.617

Kessler, R., & Stafford, D. (2008). Primary care is the de facto mental health system. In In R. Kessler and D. Stafford (Eds.), *Collaborative medicine case studies* (pp. 9-21). New York, NY: Springer.

Kessler, D., Lewis, G., Kaur, S., Wiles, N., King, M., Weich, S., ... Peters, T. J. (2009). Therapist-delivered internet psychotherapy for depression in primary care: A randomised controlled trial. *The Lancet, 374,* 628–634. https://doi.org/10.1016/S0140-6736(09)61257-5

Kindaichi, M. M., & Mebane, S. (2011). Considerations for treating depression in adolescent and college-enrolled females. In P. K. Lundberg-Love, K. L. Nadal, and M. A. Paludi (Eds.), *Women and mental disorders* (pp. 93–109). Santa Barbara, CA: Praeger.

Kozakowski, S. M., Becher, K., Hinkle, T., Blackwelder, R., Knight, C., Bentley, A., & Pugno, P. A. (2016). Responses to medical students' frequently asked questions about family medicine. *American Family Physician, 93,* 1–8. Retrieved from http://www.aafp.org/journals/afp.html

Kroenke, K., & Mangelsdorff, D. (1989). Common symptoms in ambulatory care: Incidence,evaluation, therapy and outcome. *American Journal of Medicine, 86,* 262–266. https://doi.org/10.1016/0002-9343(89)90293-3

Langan, R., & Jones, K. (2015). Common questions about the initial management of hypertension. *American Family Physician, 91,* 172–177. Retrieved from http://www.aafp.org/journals/afp.html

Leslie, L. K., Mehus, C. J., Hawkins, J. D., Boat, T., McCabe, M. A., Barkin, S., ... Beardslee, W. (2016). Primary health care: Potential home for family-focused preventive interventions. *American Journal of Preventive Medicine, 51*(4 Suppl 2), S106–S118.

Liddle, H. A., Dakof, G. A., Turner, R. M., Henderson, C. E., & Greenbaum, P. E. (2008). Treating adolescent drug abuse: A randomized trial comparing multidimensional family therapy and cognitive behavior therapy. *Addiction, 103,* 1660–1670. https://doi.org/10.1111/j.1360-0443.2008.02274.x

Liddle, H. A., Rowe, C. L., Dakof, G. A., Henderson, C. E., & Greenbaum, P. E. (2009). Multidimensional family therapy for young adolescent substance abuse: Twelve-month outcomes of a randomized controlled trial. *Journal of Consulting and Clinical Psychology, 77,* 12–25. https://doi.org/10.1037/a0014160

Linde, K., Rücker, G., Sigterman, K., Jamil, S., Meissner, K., Schneider, A., & Kriston, L. (2015). Comparative effectiveness of psychological treatments for depressive disorders in primary care: Network meta-analysis. *BMC Family Practice, 16,* 1–14. https://doi.org/10.1186/s12875-015-0314-x

Lock, J., Agras, W. S., Bryson, S., & Kraemer, H. C. (2005). A comparison of short- and long term family therapy for adolescent anorexia nervosa. *Journal of the American Academy of Child and Adolescent Psychiatry, 44,* 632–639. https://doi.org/10.1097/01.chi.0000161647.82775.0a

Loeb, K. L., Walsh, T., Lock, J., le Grange, D., Jones, J., Marcus, S., et al. (2007). Open trial of family-based treatment for full and partial anorexia nervosa in adolescence: Evidence of successful dissemination. *Journal of the American Academy of Child and Adolescent Psychiatry, 46,* 792–800. https://doi.org/10.1097/chi.0b013e318058a98e

Lundahl, B., Moleni, T., Burke, B. L., Butters, R., Tollefson, D., Butler, C., & Rollnick, S. (2013). Motivational interviewing in medical care settings: A systematic review and meta-analysis of randomized controlled trials. *Patient Education and Counseling, 93,* 157–168. https://doi.org/10.1016/j.pec.2013.07.012

Makaroff, L. A., Xierali, I. M., Petterson, S. M., Shipman, S. A., Puffer, J. C., & Basexmore, A. W. (2014). Factors influencing family physicians' contribution to the child health care workforce. *Annals of Family Medicine, 12,* 427–431. https://doi.org/10.1370/afm.1689

Markowitz, J. C., Petkova, E., Neria, Y., Van Meter, P. E., Zhao, Y., Hembree, E., ... Marshall, R. D. (2015). Is exposure necessary? A randomized clinical trial of interpersonal psychotherapy for PTSD. *American Journal of Psychiatry, 172,* 430–440. https://doi.org/10.1176/appi.ajp.2014.14070908

Markowitz, J. C., & Weissman, M. M. (2004). Interpersonal psychotherapy: Principles and applications. *World Psychiatry, 3,* 136–139. Retrieved from http://onlinelibrary.wiley.com/journal/10.1002/(ISSN)2051-5545

*Marlowe, D., Hodgson, J., Lamson, J., White, M., & Irons, T. (2012). Medical family therapy in a primary care setting: A framework for integration. *Contemporary Family Therapy, 34,* 244–258. https://doi.org/10.1007/s10591-012-9195-5

Martire, L., Schulz, R., Helgeson, V., Small, B., & Saghafi, E. (2010). Review and meta-analysis of couple-oriented interventions for chronic illness. *Annals of Behavioral Medicine, 40,* 325–342. https://doi.org/10.1007/s12160-010-9216-2

Martire, L. M., Lustig, A. P., Schulz, R., Miller, G. E., & Helgeson, V. S. (2004). Is it beneficial to involve a family member? A meta-analysis of psychosocial interventions for chronic illness. *Health Psychology, 23,* 599–611. https://doi.org/10.1037/0278-6133.23.6.599

Matos, M., Bauermeister, J. J., & Bernal, G. (2009). Parent-child interaction therapy for Puerto Rican preschool children with ADHD and behavior problems: A pilot efficacy study. *Family Process, 48,* 232–252. https://doi.org/10.1111/j.1545-5300.2009.01279.x

McCann, C. M., & le Roux, P. (2006). Individual, family, and group therapy for adolescents. *Adolescent Medicine Clinics, 17,* 217–231. https://doi.org/10.1016/j.admecli.2005.09.003

*McDaniel, S., Campbell, T. L., Hepworth, J., & Lorenz, A. (2005). *Family-oriented primary care.* New York, NY: Springer.

*McDaniel, S. H., Doherty, W. J., & Hepworth, J. (2014). *Medical family therapy and integrated care* (2nd ed.). Washington, DC: American Psychological Association.

McDaniel, S. H., Hepworth, J., & Doherty, W. J. (1992). *Medical family therapy: A biopsychosocial approach to families with health problems.* New York, NY: Basic Books.

Meng, H., Friedberg, F., & Castora-Binkley, M. (2014). Cost-effectiveness of chronic fatigue self-management versus usual care: A pilot randomized controlled trial. *BMC Family Practice, 15,* 184–192. https://doi.org/10.1186/s12875-014-0184-7

Miller, W. R. (1983). Motivational interviewing with problem drinkers. *Behavioural Psychotherapy, 11,* 147–172. https://doi.org/10.1017/S0141347300006583

Miller, W. R., & Rollnick, S. (1991). *Motivational interviewing: Preparing people to change addictive behavior.* New York, NY: Guilford Press.

Minkler, M., & Wallerstein, N. (Eds.). (2011). *Community-based participatory research for health: From process to outcomes.* San Francisco: John Wiley & Sons.

Moral, R. R., de Torres, L., Angel, P., Ortega, L. P., Larumbe, M. C., Villalobos, A. R., ... Rejano, J. M. P. (2015). Effectiveness of motivational interviewing to improve therapeutic adherence in patients over 65 years old with chronic diseases: A cluster randomized clinical trial in primary care. *Patient Education and Counseling, 98,* 977–983. https://doi.org/10.1016/j.pec.2015.03.008

National Institute of Diabetes and Digestive and Kidney Disease. (2012). *Overweight & obesity statistics.* Retrieved from https://www.niddk.nih.gov/health-information/health-statistics/overweight-obesity

Nixon, R. D. V. (2001). Changes in hyperactivity and temperament in behaviourally disturbed preschoolers after Parent-Child Interaction Therapy (PCIT). *Behaviour Change, 18*, 168–176. https://doi.org/10.1375/bech.18.3.168

Nixon, R. D. V., Sweeney, L., Erickson, D. B., & Touyz, S. W. (2004). Parent-child interaction therapy: One- and two- year follow-up of standard and abbreviated treatments for oppositional preschoolers. *Journal of Abnormal Child Psychology, 32*, 263–271. https://doi.org/10.1023/b:jacp.0000026140.60558.05

Nouwen, A., Winkley, K., Twisk, J., Lloyd, C. E., Peyrot, M., Ismail, K., & Pouwer, F. (2010). Type 2 diabetes mellitus as a risk factor for the onset of depression: A systematic review and meta-analysis. *Diabetologia, 53*, 2480–2486. https://doi.org/10.1007/s00125-010-1874-x

O'Hara, M. W., Stuart, S., Gorman, L. L., & Wenzel, A. (2000). Efficacy of interpersonal psychotherapy for postpartum depression. *Archives of General Psychiatry, 57*, 1039–1045. https://doi.org/10.1001/archpsyc.57.11.1039

Oza, R., & Garcellano, M. (2015). Nonpharmacologic management of hypertension: What works? *American Family Physician, 91*, 772–776. Retrieved from http://www.aafp.org/journals/afp.html

*Peek, C. J. (2008). Planning care in the clinical, operational, and financial worlds. In R. Kessler and D. Stafford (Eds.), *Collaborative medicine case studies* (pp. 25–38). New York, NY: Springer.

*Petterson, S., Miller, B. F., Payne-Murphy, J. C., & Phillips, R. L. (2014). Mental health treatment in the primary care setting: Patterns and pathways. *Families, Systems, & Health, 32*, 157–166. https://doi.org/10.1037/fsh0000036.

Petznick, A. (2011). Insulin management of type 2 diabetes mellitus. *American Family Physician, 84*, 183–190. Retrieved from http://www.aafp.org/journals/afp.html

Phillips, R. L., Brungardt, S., Lesko, S. E., Kittle, N., Marker, J. E., Tuggy, M., ... Krug, N. (2014). The future role of the family physician in the United States: A rigorous exercise in definition. *Annals of Family Medicine, 12*, 250–255. https://doi.org/10.1370/afm.1651

Piper, M. A., Evans, C. V., Burda, B. U., et al. (2014). *Screening for high blood pressure in adults: A systematic evidence review for the U.S. preventive services task force, Evidence synthesis no. 121. AHRQ publication no. 13–05194-EF-1*. Rockville: Agency for Healthcare Research and Quality.

Pippitt, K., Li, M., & Gurgle, H. E. (2016). Diabetes mellitus: Screening and diagnosis. *American Family Physician, 93*, 103–109. Retrieved from http://www.aafp.org/journals/afp.html

Polaha, J., Volkmer, A., & Valleley, R. J. (2007). A call-in service to address parent concerns about child behavior in rural primary care. *Families, Systems, & Health, 25*, 333–343. https://doi.org/10.1037/1091-7527.25.3.333

Public Health Agency of Canada. (2013). *What is the population health approach?* Retrieved from http://www.phac-aspc.gc.ca/ph-sp/approach-approche/appr-eng.php

Purnell, T. S., Calhoun, E. A., Golden, S. H., Halladay, J. R., Krok-Schoen, J. L., Appelhans, B. M., & Cooper, L. A. (2016). Achieving health equity: Closing the gaps in health care disparities, interventions, and research. *Health Affairs, 35*, 1410–1415. https://doi.org/10.1377/hlthaff.2016.0158

Ranson, N. E., Terry, D. R., Glenister, K., Adam, B. R., & Wright, J. (2016). Integrated and consumer-directed care: A necessary paradigm shift for rural chronic ill health. *Australian Journal of Primary Health, 22*, 176–180. https://doi.org/10.1071/PY15056

Rao, G. (2008). Childhood obesity: Highlights of AMA expert committee recommendations. *American Family Physician, 78*, 56–63. Retrieved from http://www.aafp.org/journals/afp.html

Regier, D., Goldberg, I., & Taube, C. (1978). The de facto US mental health services system. *Archives of General Psychiatry, 35*, 685–693. https://doi.org/10.1001/archpsyc.1978.01770300027002

Regier, D., Narrow, W., Rae, D., Manderscheid, R., Locke, B., & Goodwin, F. (1993). The de facto US mental and addictive disorders service system: Epidemiologic catchment area prospective 1-year rrevalence rates of disorders and services. *Archives of General Psychiatry, 50*, 85–94. https://doi.org/10.1001/archpsyc.1993.01820140007001

*Reiss-Brennan, B., Brunisholz, K. D., Dredge, C., Briot, P., Grazier, K., Wilcox, A., ... James, B. (2016). Association of integrated team-based care with health care quality, utilization, and cost. *Journal of the American Medical Association, 316*, 826–834. https://doi.org/10.1001/jama.2016.11232

Reitz, R., & Sudano, L. (2014). The medical family therapist as transdisciplinary trainer. In J. Hodgson, A. Lamson, T., Mendenhall, and D. Crane (Eds.), *Medical family therapy: Advanced applications* (pp. 177–195). New York, NY: Springer.

Richmond, C. A. M., & Ross, N. A. (2008). The determinants of first nation and inuit health: A critical population health approach. *Health & Place, 15*, 403–411. https://doi.org/10.1016/j.healthplace.2008.07.004

Robinson, L., Iliffe, S., Brayne, C., Goodman, C., Rait, G., Manthorpe, J., ... Moniz-Cook, E. (2010). Primary care and dementia: 2 long-term care at home: Psychosocial interventions, information provision, career support and case management. *International Journal of Geriatric Psychiatry, 25*, 657–664. https://doi.org/10.1002/gps.2405

Rollnick, S., Miller, W. R., & Butler, C. C. (2008). *Motivational interviewing in health care: Helping patients change behavior.* New York, NY: Guilford.

Sacks, F. M., Svetkey, L. P., Vollmer, W. M., Appel, L. J., Bray, G. A., Harsha, D., ... Cutler, J. A. (2001). Effects on blood pressure of reduced dietary sodium and the Dietary Approaches to Stop Hypertension (DASH) diet. *New England Journal of Medicine, 344*, 3–10. https://doi.org/10.1056/NEJM200101043440101

*Sanchez, K., Ybarra, R., Chapa, T., & Martinez, O. N. (2016). Eliminating behavioral health disparities and improving outcomes for racial and ethnic minority populations. *Psychiatric Services, 67*, 13–15. https://doi.org/10.1176/appi.ps.201400581

Santisteban, D. A., Coatsworth, J. D., Perez-Vidal, A., Kurtines, W. M., Schwartz, S., LaPerriere, A., & Szapocznik, J. (2003). The efficacy of Brief Strategic Family Therapy in modifying Hispanic adolescent behavior problems and substance use. *Journal of Family Psychology, 17*, 121–133. https://doi.org/10.1037/0893-3200.17.1.121

Sattel, H., Lahmann, C., Gundel, H., Guthrie, E., Kruse, J., Noll-Hussong, M., ... Henningsen, P. (2012). Brief psychodynamic interpersonal psychotherapy for patients with multisomatoform disorder: Randomised controlled trial. *British Journal of Psychiatry, 200*, 60–67. https://doi.org/10.1192/bjp.bp.111.093526

Schumm, J. A., O'Farrell, T. J., Kahler, C. W., Murphy, M. M., & Muchowski, P. (2014). A randomized clinical trial of behavioral couples therapy versus individually based treatment for women with alcohol dependence. *Journal of Consulting and Clinical Psychology, 82*, 993–1004. https://doi.org/10.1037/a0037497

Sexton, T., & Turner, C. W. (2010). The effectiveness of functional family therapy for youth with behavioral problems in a community practice setting. *Journal of Family Psychology, 24*, 339–348. https://doi.org/10.1037/a0019406

Sher, T., Braun, L., Domas, A., Bellg, A., Baucom, D. H., & Houle, T. T. (2014). The Partners for Life Program: A couples approach to cardiac risk reduction. *Family Process, 53*, 131–149. https://doi.org/10.1111/famp.12061

*Shields, C. G., Finley, M. A., Chawla, N., & Meadors, P. (2012). Couple and family interventions in health problems. *Journal of Marital and Family Therapy, 38*, 265–280. https://doi.org/10.1111/j.1752-0606.2011.00269.x

Siu, A. L. (2015). Screening for abnormal blood glucose and type 2 diabetes mellitus: U.S. Preventive Services Task Force recommendation statement. *Annals of Intern Medicine, 163*, 861–868. https://doi.org/10.7326/M15-2345

Siu, A. L. (2016). Screening for depression in adults: US Preventive Services Task Force recommendation statement. *Journal of the American Medical Association, 315*, 380–387. https://doi.org/10.1001/jama.2015.18392

Smock, S. A., Trepper, T. S., Wetchler, J. L., McCollum, E. E., Ray, R., & Pierce, K. (2008). Solution-focused group therapy for level 1 substance abusers. *Journal of Marital and Family Therapy, 34*, 107–120. https://doi.org/10.1111/j.1752-0606.2008.00056.x

Sox, H. C. (2013). Resolving the tension between population health and individual health care. *Journal of the American Medical Association, 310*, 1933–1934. https://doi.org/10.1001/jama.2013.281998

Sprenkle, D. H. (2002). *Effectiveness research in marriage and family therapy*. Alexandria, VA: American Association for Marriage and Family Therapy.

Stangier, U., Schramm, E., Heidenreich, T., Berger, M., & Clark, D. M. (2011). Cognitive therapy vs. interpersonal psychotherapy in social anxiety disorder: A randomized controlled trial. *Archives of General Psychiatry, 68*, 692–700. https://doi.org/10.1001/archgenpsychiatry.2011.67

Storch, E. A., Geffken, G. R., Merlo, L. J., Mann, G., Duke, D., Munson, M., ... Goodman, W. K. (2007). Family-based cognitive-behavioral therapy for pediatric obsessive-compulsive disorder: Comparison of intensive and weekly approaches. *Journal of the American Academy of Child and Adolescent Psychiatry, 46*, 469–478. https://doi.org/10.1097/chi.0b013e31803062e7

Stovitz, S. D., Berge, J. M., Wetzsteon, R. J., Sherwood, N. E., Hannan, P. J., & Himes, J. H. (2014). Stage 1 treatment of pediatric overweight and obesity: A pilot and feasibility randomized controlled trial. *Childhood Obesity, 10*, 50–57. https://doi.org/10.1089/chi.2013.0107

Strosahl, K. (1994). New dimensions in behavioral health/primary care integration. *HMO Practice, 8*, 176–179. https://doi.org/10.1016/S1077-7229(05)80084-7

Strosahl, K. (2005). Training behavioral health and primary care providers for integrated care: A core competencies approach. In W. T. O'Donohue, M. R. Byrd, N. A. Cummings, and D. A. Henderson (Eds.), *Behavioral integrative care: Treatments that work in the primary care setting* (pp. 15–52). New York, NY: Brunner-Routledge.

Substance Abuse and Mental Health Services Administration. (2009). *Illness management and recovery: The evidence*. Retrieved from http://store.samhsa.gov/shin/content/SMA09-4463/TheEvidence-IMR.pdf

Svetaz, M. V., Garcia-Huidobro, D., & Allen, M. (2014). Parents and family matter: Strategies for developing family-centered adolescent care within primary care practices. *Primary Care: Clinics in Office Practice, 41*, 489–506. https://doi.org/10.1016/j.pop.2014.05.004

Taylor, R. B. (2006). The promise of family medicine: History, leadership, and the age of aquarius. *Journal of the American Board of Family Medicine, 19*, 183–190. https://doi.org/10.3122/jabfm.19.2.183

Thornton, R. L. J., Glover, C. M., Cene, C. W., Glik, D. C., Henderson, J. A., & Williams, D. R. (2016). Evaluating strategies for reducing health disparities by addressing the social determinants of health. *Health Affairs, 35*, 1416–1423. https://doi.org/10.1377/hlthaff.2015.1357

Torenholt, R., Schwennesen, N., & Willaing, I. (2014). Lost in translation – The role of family in interventions among adults with diabetes: A systematic review. *Diabetic Medicine, 31*, 15–23. https://doi.org/10.1111/dme.12290

Tursi, M. F., Baes, C. V., Camacho, F. R., Tofoli, S. M., & Juruena, M. F. (2013). Effectiveness of psychoeducation for depression: A systematic review. *Australian & New Zealand Journal of Psychiatry, 47*, 1019–1031. https://doi.org/10.1177/0004867413491154

*Tyndall, L., Hodgson, J., Lamson, A., White, M., Knight, S. (2014). Medical family therapy: Charting a course in competencies. In J. Hodgson, A. Lamson, T., Mendenhall, and D. Crane (Eds.), *Medical family therapy: Advanced applications* (pp. 33–53). New York, NY: Springer.

U.S. Centers for Disease Control. (2010). *National ambulatory medical care survey: General/family practice* [fact sheet]. Retrieved from https://www.cdc.gov/nchs/data/ahcd/namcs_2010_factsheet_general_family_practice.pdf

U.S. Preventive Services Task Force. (2016). *About the USPSTF*. Retrieved from http://www.uspreventiveservicestaskforce.org/Page/Name/about-the-uspstf

van Ravesteijn, H., Lucassen, P., Bor, H., van Weel, C., & Speckens, A. (2013). Mindfulness based cognitive therapy for patients with medically unexplained symptoms: A randomized controlled trial. *Psychotherapy and Psychosomatics, 82*, 299–310. https://doi.org/10.1159/000348588

van Schaik, A., van Marwijk, H., Adèr, H., van Dyck, R., de Haan, M., Penninx, B., ... Beekman, A. (2006). Interpersonal psychotherapy for elderly patients in primary care. *American Journal of Geriatric Psychiatry, 14*, 777–786. https://doi.org/10.1097/01.JGP.0000199341.25431.4b

Vanbuskirk, K. A., & Wetherell, J. L. (2014). Motivational interviewing with primary care populations: A systematic review and meta-analysis. *Journal of Behavioral Medicine, 37*, 768–780. https://doi.org/10.1007/s10865-013-9527-4

Vander Wielen, L. M., Gilchrist, E. C., Nowels, M. A., Petterson, S. M., Rust, G., & Miller, B. F. (2015). Not near enough: Racial and ethnic disparities in access to nearby behavioral health care and primary care. *Journal of Health Care for the Poor & Underserved, 26*, 1032–1047. https://doi.org/10.1353/hpu.2015.0083

Visser, S. N., Danielson, M. L., Bitsko, R. H., Holbrook, J. R., Kogan, M. D., Ghandour, R. M., … Blumberg, S. J. (2014). Trends in the parent-report of health care provider-diagnosed and medicated attention-deficit/hyperactivity disorder, United States, 2003-2011. *Journal of the American Academy of Child & Adolescent Psychiatry, 53*, 34–46. https://doi.org/10.1016/j.jaac.2013.09.001

Vogel, M. E., Kirkpatrick, H. A., Collings, A. S., Cederna-Meko, C., & Grey, M. J. (2012). Integrated care: Maturing the relationship between psychology and primary care. *Professional Psychology: Research and Practice, 43*, 271–280. https://doi.org/10.1037/a0029204

Waldron, H. B., & Turner, C. W. (2008). Evidence-based psychosocial treatments for adolescent substance abuse. *Journal of Clinical Child and Adolescent Psychology, 37*, 238–261. https://doi.org/10.1080/15374410701820133

Wells, K. B., Jones, L., Chung, B., Dixon, E. L., Tang, L., Gilmore, J., … Ramos, E. (2013). Community-partnered cluster-randomized comparative effectiveness trial of community engagement and planning or resources for services to address depression disparities. *Journal of General Internal Medicine, 28*, 1268–1278. https://doi.org/10.1007/s11606-013-2484-3

Wiebe, S. A., & Johnson, S. M. (2016). A review of the research in emotionally focused therapy for couples. *Family Process, 55*, 390–407. https://doi.org/10.1111/famp.12229

Wilfley, D. E., Welch, R. R., Stein, R. I., Spurrell, E. B., Cohen, L. R., Saelens, B. E., … Matt, G. E. (2002). A randomized comparison of group cognitive-behavioral therapy and group interpersonal psychotherapy for the treatment of overweight individuals with binge-eating disorder. *Archives of General Psychiatry, 59*, 713–721. https://doi.org/10.1001/archpsyc.59.8.713

Wood, J. J., Piacentini, J. C., Southam-Gerow, M., Chu, B. C., & Sigman, M. (2006). Family cognitive behavioral therapy for child anxiety disorders. *Journal of the American Academy of Child and Adolescent Psychiatry, 45*, 314–321. https://doi.org/10.1097/01.chi.0000196425.88341.b0

Wrenn, G., Kasiah, F., & Syed, I. (2015). Using a self-service kiosk to identify behavioral health needs in a primary care clinic serving an urban, underserved population. *Journal of Innovation in Health Informatics, 22*, 323–328. 10.14236/jhi.v22i3.134

Wright, L. M., Watson, W. L., & Bell, J. M. (1996). *Beliefs: The heart of healing in families and illness*. New York, NY: Basic Books.

Chapter 3
Medical Family Therapy in Pediatrics

Keeley Pratt, Catherine Van Fossen, Katharine Didericksen, Rola Aamar, and Jerica Berge

Pediatric medicine—or "pediatrics" as an umbrella term—promotes the physical, mental, and social well-being of infants, children, adolescents, and young adults (American Academy of Pediatrics, 2011). Pediatric practices are generally situated within primary and specialty care/tertiary care settings. Primary care settings—also called pediatric patient-centered medical homes (PPMH; Ader et al., 2015)—include those where annual well-baby and well-child visits, sick visits, and routine physical exams take place. They are usually led by generalist pediatricians. Specialty/tertiary care settings require additional training tailored to a specific content areas, such as pediatric endocrinology and/or obesity, pediatric pulmonary, pediatric oncology, pediatric hematology, pediatric orthopedics, pediatric intensive care, neonatology, neonatal intensive care, pediatric palliative care, pediatric nephrology, pediatric audiology and speech pathology, pediatric rheumatology, pediatric urology, pediatric gastroenterology, and other health conditions/presentations (see Glossary for term definitions). Healthcare providers—and the roles that they serve—in pediatric specialty care teams are tailored to the specialty itself (e.g., a registered dietician in a pediatric endocrinology and obesity clinic).

Pediatric primary care visits often deal with sickness, infections, injuries, and diseases. This is also the setting where childhood chronic conditions—including asthma, cystic fibrosis, overweight and obesity, malnutrition, and developmental

---

K. Pratt (✉) · C. Van Fossen
Department of Human Sciences, The Ohio State University, Columbus, OH, USA
e-mail: pratt.192@osu.edu

K. Didericksen · R. Aamar
Department of Human Development and Family Science, East Carolina University, Greenville, NC, USA

J. Berge
Department of Family Medicine and Community Health, University of Minnesota Medical School, Minneapolis, MN, USA

© Springer International Publishing AG, part of Springer Nature 2018
T. Mendenhall et al. (eds.), *Clinical Methods in Medical Family Therapy*, Focused Issues in Family Therapy, https://doi.org/10.1007/978-3-319-68834-3_3

disabilities (Torpy, Campbell, & Glass, 2010)—are diagnosed and treated. Pediatric primary care teams also assess for psychosocial stressors that children and adolescents may encounter which could potentially develop into mental and behavioral health conditions (e.g., depression, anxiety). Given the long-term relationships that pediatric primary care providers and care teams have with children and their families (i.e., from birth to 21 years; American Academy of Pediatrics, 2011), they are often the first place that people go to when they have a question about their child's well-being. Further, the relationships between children and their healthcare team, and those relationships that are modeled by their parent(s) and their healthcare team, set the foundation for children to take active roles in their own healthcare as they age.

Medical Family Therapists (MedFTs), often referred to as "behavioral health providers" in pediatric settings, can work fluidly in pediatric settings to promote child and family self-efficacy (or "agency," as previously referred to in MedFT texts). They can also facilitate communication and support around healthcare issues such as assessment, diagnosis, and treatment of mental, behavioral, and social health issues. Additionally, MedFTs can collaborate with pediatric treatment teams to ensure that children and families are receiving comprehensive family-based care. MedFTs bring a unique family systems lens that can help promote understandings of child illnesses or conditions within the family system. They can help facilitate role definition and boundaries/limits for families and healthcare providers in pediatric settings.

There have been increases in childhood chronic illness diagnoses in the past few decades (Van Cleave, Gortmaker, & Perrin, 2010). There is a significant association between childhood obesity and other childhood chronic illnesses (Pulgaron, 2013). The vignette below details the healthcare and coordination of a family and highlights the challenges in assessing family dynamics and mental health and coordinating patient care in pediatrics as a MedFT.

> **Clinical Vignette**
> [Note: This vignette is a compilation of cases that represent treatment in pediatrics. All patients' names and/or identifying information have been changed to maintain confidentiality.]
>
> *Janelle's pediatric primary care physician has been coordinating her medical care since she was 4 years old. The last time that she visited her pediatrician, Janelle, now aged 12, was identified as overweight (85th–94th percentile for her age). Janelle also started showing signs of becoming insulin resistant, as her fasting blood sugar and A1c levels were high. The pediatrician also noticed signs of acanthosis nigricans on Janelle's neck, an early warning sign of insulin changes. The pediatrician prescribed Metformin® and discussed dietary recommendations with Janelle and her mother. These included decreasing consumption of sugar-sweetened beverages and increasing intake*

of lean proteins, low-fat dairy, complex carbohydrates (e.g., whole-grain bread), and vegetables. He sent Janelle and her mother home with educational pamphlets discussing the current dietary recommendations (via MyPlate®) in further detail. A referral was also made in the electronic medical record (EMR) to a pediatric endocrinologist at a nearby pediatric specialty care clinic.

The treatment team at the pediatric endocrinology office consisted of a pediatric endocrinologist, pediatric diabetologist, nurse practitioner, dietician, and behavioral health provider (i.e., MedFT). On Janelle's first visit, she was accompanied by her grandmother. At intake, Janelle completed a PHQ-9A to assess her depressive symptoms. Upon seeing Janelle's high scores, the pediatric endocrinologist introduced Janelle to the MedFT. During the brief therapy session, the MedFT worked to build a strong connection and communication channel with Janelle so that she and her grandmother would feel supported by the healthcare team and others in their community. Additionally, she worked to increase self-efficacy in Janelle so she would feel empowered to address her health concerns and questions. Janelle shared with the MedFT that she had been feeling sad and angry, since she is now in the care of her grandmother and no longer has contact with her mother. Before concluding the consultation, the MedFT spoke with Janelle about how she would like her family members included in her treatment going forward. They also discussed what information Janelle is comfortable with the MedFT sharing with various members of the treatment team and her own family.

The MedFT scheduled follow-up visits with Janelle and her grandmother. Janelle agreed that she was comfortable with the MedFT sharing her family history with the other members of the treatment team, so that the MedFT was able to recommend incorporating Janelle's grandmother into treatment plans, rather than her mother. The MedFT also worked to facilitate communication amongst the treatment team members, which now included Janelle's grandmother, the pediatrician, and the pediatric endocrinology treatment team. It was decided that Janelle would continue to see her pediatrician for general medical care and that her pediatrician would communicate with the specialty team about her endocrine issues. The MedFT also agreed to work on communicating with Janelle's school about any important information regarding Janelle's medications and potential need for blood sugar checks. Finally, the MedFT continued to work with Janelle and her grandmother on Janelle's depressive symptoms and the family's strengths and challenges with adopting necessary behavioral health goals (e.g., medication adherence, dietary changes, and increasing physical activity) related to her healthcare needs.

The MedFT in this vignette was able to provide direct therapeutic care for Janelle and communicate Janelle's wishes with the treatment team about her care going forward. The initial behavioral health consultation with the MedFT is a time to begin planting the seeds of promoting connection, communication, and self-efficacy among patients and families, as well as keeping the patient and family at the center of the treatment plan—which can often be challenging when coordinating school, pediatric primary care, and pediatric specialty care settings.

What Is Pediatrics?

Pediatric care is focused on prevention, detection, and management of physical, behavioral, developmental, and social challenges that affect children and adolescents (American Academy of Pediatrics, 2011). Given the family focus and interdisciplinary nature of pediatrics, MedFTs are well trained to provide patient and family care and collaborate in these settings. In both primary and specialty care, treatment teams focus on early intervention, child-centered and family-based care, and delivery of developmentally appropriate anticipatory guidance in their clinical encounters.

The field of pediatrics promotes *early intervention* in an effort to prevent undue harm to children and families long term and to further connect families to needed services. Early intervention screenings at well-baby and well-child visits are done to ensure that children are meeting developmental milestones and to identify if a child is at risk for a developmental or other disorder (American Academy of Pediatrics, 2016). These screenings are advanced when critical developmental and motor milestones are expected, such as when children are 0–3 years old (American Academy of Pediatrics, 2016). Identifying infants and toddlers with developmental delays or complex chronic conditions early facilitates connecting them with intervention services in a timely manner—ideally setting up the family to successfully work through their child's needs. Specific early intervention efforts are aimed at identifying children who may be at risk for child developmental disorders, such as autism spectrum disorder. MedFTs can be particularly helpful in early intervention when caregivers are faced with the uncertainty of diagnosis, lengthy waiting periods for further assessment and testing, and helping caregivers and family members process their potential feelings of guilt or blame, or fears about not having a "typically" developing child.

The child-centered medical home (CCMH) is a comprehensive model of medical care that integrates multiple providers to deliver care across the continuum of pediatric needs (Stille et al., 2010). According to the American Academy of Pediatrics (AAP), a CCMH should provide a comprehensive and high-quality primary care experience for children and their families. Specifically, it should encompass the following attributes: (a) accessible, so that the care is easy for the child and family to obtain; (b) family-centered, where the healthcare team partners with the family to make decisions and care plans; (c) continuous, so that the same provider cares for the child from birth to young adulthood; (d) coordinated, so that families, healthcare teams, and any relevant community agencies and organizations work together in the care of the child; (e) compassionate, so that genuine concern for the child and family is emphasized; and (f) culturally effective, where the family's culture, language, beliefs, and traditions are valued and respected (AAP, 2016). The training that MedFTs have in family systems theory and family-based models of care situates them well to facilitate putting the family at the center of prevention and treatment, while also honoring the child and family's own contextual background (including culture, religion/spirituality) and family structure (e.g., single parent, blended families, fictive kin).

Children reside in families; therefore, care should involve the family members and caregivers who maintain responsibility for children's day-to-day care. *Family involvement* in pediatric care has been described as family-centered, family-focused, and family-based. Family-centered care, then, is an approach to the planning, delivery, and evaluation of care that is grounded in mutually beneficial partnerships between pediatric treatment teams and families (Institute for Patient- and Family-Centered Care, 2016). *Family-centered care* is a true partnership wherein the needs and wishes of families are respected and valued by the pediatric team. The AAP enforces family-centered care as one critical component of a CCMH. *Family-focused care* includes pediatric providers providing care from the position of an "expert" in the assessment and treatment of the patient. The family is seen as the "unit" of intervention in family-focused care; however, the relationship tends to be more hierarchical (Institute for Patient- and Family-Centered Care, 2010). Lastly, *family-based care* is used to describe care that targets the child and at least one family member (often caregiver) in treatment or intervention of a health condition (e.g., obesity). Family-based care is extensively used in research studies when intervening via the parent-child dyad to effect health behavior change in the child (Berge & Everts, 2011). It is important to note that these terms are not mutually exclusive. For example, treatment teams can be both family-focused and family-based in their care.

Anticipatory guidance is a developmentally based counseling technique that focuses on the needs of children at different stages (Reisinger & Bires, 1980). It is delivered by healthcare providers to assist caregivers in understanding their child's growth and development and to offer age-specific guidance to promote health and decrease risk (AAP, 2016). Often these messages are tailored to child mental health and healthy lifestyles. For example, the AAP's Bright Futures™ guidelines for anticipatory guidance are extensively used to assist pediatric providers in their care of infants, children, adolescents, and their families to promote child mental health and healthy weight. The Bright Futures™ guidelines instruct providers to use open-ended questions and other motivational interviewing techniques (Britt, Hudson, & Blampied, 2004; Emmons & Rollnick, 2001; Irby, Kaplan, Garner-Edwards, Kolbash, & Skelton, 2010; Miller & Rollnick, 2013; Resnicow et al., 2002) to encourage open and supportive communication in the family, using affirming questions to highlight strengths in the family, provide ample time for families to respond to questions, use active listening to identify concerns, recognize teachable moments to give personalized advice and seek feedback, and to conduct developmental observations on the parent-child interaction, developmental milestones, and social competence (Hagan, Shaw, & Duncan, 2008).

Although pediatric providers recognize the importance of anticipatory guidance, time limitations and resources are frequently challenges to care delivery. Anticipatory guidance can be delivered in different formats, such as handouts, video screenings, and in-person consultation between providers and families. Often these messages are tailored to the treatment setting (primary or specialty care), condition (obesity, diabetes, etc.), and children's age/development. During healthcare visits, pediatric providers should observe which family members are responsive to questions (and verbal/nonverbal behaviors and communication) in order to understand more about family dynamics, structure, and family decision-making to provide better care. MedFTs can also assist in providing anticipatory feedback by observing families during the pediatric visits. For example, MedFTs can stay after the pediatrician is done with his/her visit to make sure the family understands, or can repeat back/apply, information that has been provided to them. MedFTs can help to simplify pediatricians' messages to families by selecting one goal that is measurable and specific that the pediatrician will work on with the family, to increase the likelihood of success.

The ways that providers and treatment teams interact with children and families should be both developmentally and age appropriate. For example, some pediatric specialty care clinics have detailed developmental and age-appropriate care based on specific conditions, such as pediatric obesity (see Barlow, 2007). Additionally, parental involvement in clinical visits varies across child developmental age and stage. For example, caregivers are involved more in clinical visits when children are younger. The focus of the medical encounter evens-out between caregivers and children when children are of school age and becomes more one-on-one during adolescence.

Young children (ages 0–5 years) are dependent on their caregiver(s) to meet basic needs and do not have the cognitive capacity to make decisions about care or health behaviors. Given these factors, providers should focus on anticipatory guidance on the caregiver to increase his or her knowledge and address parenting behaviors that may be amendable to change. Although the discussion should be focused on the caregiver(s) role in facilitating the provider's directives, MedFTs can still find ways to involve young children in the clinical encounter by having developmentally appropriate books, toys, and activities available. Additionally, MedFTs can be versed in play therapy techniques (Phillips, 2010; Reddy, Files-Hall, & Schaefer, 2005) often used in hospital-based settings to make children feel more comfortable with new medical procedures and environments.

As youth age and reach various developmental milestones (e.g., reading, speaking in sentences), the focus of the clinical encounter shifts to equally target the child and caregiver. Focusing on both children and caregivers is typical between 6 and 11 years old (Barlow, 2007). These children are depending on their caregivers to provide them with basic needs (e.g., food, shelter, transportation). They are largely still influenced by the structure that caregivers put in place and the parenting behaviors established. Ideally, parents are engaging in authoritative parenting practices that provide both support/nurturance and promote independence and structure when appropriate (Darling & Steinberg, 1993). MedFTs can work with parents to encourage authoritative parenting practices and with parents and children on communication strategies around developmentally appropriate challenges such as chores, curfews, etc.

In adolescence, the clinical encounter shifts to focus more on the youth's thoughts and behaviors. Caregivers may still be present in the exam room, but they are primarily involved to make the home environment healthy and supportive of their adolescent to promote indicated behavior or health changes. Given that adolescents are growing in autonomy and independence, often caregivers and adolescents may not agree on healthcare goals, treatments, or behaviors to change. Providers may wish to collaborate with additional providers (e.g., MedFTs) when these dynamics get particularly tense and/or difficult (see below).

Pediatric providers should be well acquainted with internal and external referrals and resources for collaboration in order to meet patient and family needs. Common collaborators in pediatric care include teachers, social service professionals, specialty providers, behavioral health providers, and dietary and/or nutrition services. MedFTs are highly trained in the integrated behavioral healthcare model, which often makes them leaders of collaborative care within the sites that they are employed. Pediatric settings are ripe with opportunities for collaboration, both inside and outside of healthcare (e.g., schools, religious settings, childcare).

Treatment Teams in Pediatrics

Pediatric healthcare teams are as diverse as the conditions and challenges they treat. The providers listed below represent the most common team members. Often in pediatric specialty settings, treatment teams are tailored to the specialty or diagnoses being treated (which is beyond the scope of this chapter).

Primary care pediatricians. These physicians collaborate with other healthcare providers and specialists in the treatment of childhood diseases and disorders. They manage serious and life-threatening illness; diagnose and treat acute and chronic disorders; conduct developmental screenings; track physical and psychosocial development; provide anticipatory guidance, referrals, and consultations; and engage in a variety of community-based activities.

Pediatric subspecialists. These pediatricians focused their residency training or fellowship (after residency) on a specific aspect of child health (e.g., endocrinologists, rheumatologists). Subspecialists are more likely to work in academic settings conducting research, teaching, and providing direct patient care.

Pediatric nurses. These nurses specialize in pediatrics by obtaining advanced training post-degree. They conduct physical examinations, assess child vitals, take biological specimens and samples, and order diagnostic tests. Pediatric nurses with advanced training also interpret test results to make diagnoses and subsequent treatment plans. They also spend time providing families with education relevant to pediatric healthcare prevention and treatment.

Pediatric dietician and/or nutritionists. These registered dieticians (RDs) are trained to teach about, and coordinate care involving, healthy food choices for children from infancy until early adulthood.

Child and adolescent psychiatrists. These physicians diagnose, treat, and focus on the prevention of mental disorders in children and adolescents by assessing the biopsychosocial-spiritual factors in the development of mental health disorders and responsiveness to intervention and treatment.

Child psychologists. These providers apply psychological principles in the contexts of pediatric health to promote the well-being and development of children, adolescents, and their families using evidence-based methods. They also may specialize in different areas of child health.

Pediatric behavioral health providers. These providers conduct behavioral assessments, brief therapy, family therapy, and consultation to children and families experiencing acute and chronic conditions. Examples of pediatric behavioral health providers include medical family therapists, marriage and family therapists, counselors, and health coaches. The main aim of the behavioral health provider is to facilitate integrated behavioral healthcare across healthcare providers to increase biopsychosocial-spiritual holistic care for patients and families.

Pediatric social workers. These providers work in inpatient and outpatient settings to facilitate the care of children who are experiencing chronic or severe medical conditions. They also provide support to families with children to provide emotional support, coordinate care, connect families to resources, and aid them in navigating the healthcare system.

Fundamentals of Care in Pediatrics

The landscape of pediatric healthcare is changing with increasing demands to meet serious chronic conditions for the youngest of patients and their families. The disciplines of pediatric healthcare providers and their various professional roles continue to change and increase (Katz & Faridi, 2008; Mastro, Mastro, Mastro, Flynn, & Preuster, 2014). This transformation in pediatric treatment teams may in part be due to the evolving needs of pediatric patients and their families. In pediatric settings, it is important for MedFTs to have a strong foundation in the knowledge of common pediatric ailments and conditions, resources, and referrals available to children and families internally and externally; knowledge and skills in promoting integrated behavioral healthcare; skills in brief behavioral, psychological, and relational screeners; and solid understanding of the challenges and pitfalls MedFTs may experience in pediatric care and collaboration.

Common Chronic Pediatric Conditions

MedFTs working in pediatric settings should be competent in the assessment and treatment of common child and adolescent chronic conditions (e.g., pediatric asthma, obesity, and diabetes). These conditions are often diagnosed in primary care with referrals made to specialty care after initial diagnosis. When a pediatric chronic illness diagnosis is made, families may be distressed and worried about the future health and quality of life for their child. Parents and caregivers also may have to rearrange their schedules to provide oversight of their child's treatment (e.g., blood sugar monitoring, dietary planning, inhaler management). Details regarding pediatric obesity are provided below as an example for the type of knowledge MedFTs should have.

Pediatric obesity. MedFTs working with children and adolescents with overweight and obesity should be familiar with measures of height and weight used to obtain body mass index (BMI), BMI percentile, and BMI z-scores. In addition, MedFTs need to be knowledgeable about dietary guidelines for children, physical activity recommendations, and screen time guidelines. In 2005, the American Medical Association (AMA), Health Resources and Services Administration (HRSA), and Centers for Disease Control and Prevention (CDC) brought together an expert committee including representatives from the areas of medicine, mental health, and epidemiology to develop recommendations for the care of overweight and obese children (Barlow, 2007). The report entitled *Expert Committee Recommendations Regarding the Prevention, Assessment, and Treatment of Child and Adolescent Overweight and Obesity* summarizes the findings of the expert committee of currently accepted practices for pediatric obesity prevention, assessment, intervention, and treatment. A concurrent publication by the National Initiative for Children's Healthcare Quality (NICHQ, 2007), entitled *An Implementation Guide from the Childhood Obesity Action Network*, offers a combination of important aspects of the expert recommendations with real-world practice tools identified from primary care groups who have developed obesity care strategies. Thus, the implementation guide offers suggestions and tools for practical application of the expert recommendations. The expert committee recommendations describe prevention and treatment strategies that are applicable for children of all weight statuses (Barlow, 2007), including (a) prevention plus; (b) structured weight management; (c) comprehensive, multidisciplinary intervention; and (d) tertiary care intervention.

A prevention or stage one "prevention plus" visit most commonly takes place at a child's primary care office during an annual well-care visit. At this time, the following should be assessed by the healthcare provider: plot a body mass index (BMI), identify a weight category (e.g., underweight <5%, healthy weight 5–84%, overweight 85–94%, obese 95–98%, and ≥99%), measure blood pressure, take a family-focused medical history, take a focused review of systems (e.g., review different body systems, such as endocrine, that may be impacted by obesity), perform a thorough medical physical examination, order appropriate laboratory tests, and give consistent evidence-based messages for physical activity and nutrition. For stage one, MedFTs can assess the child's attitude including self-perceptions or concerns about weight, readiness to change, successes, barriers, and challenges (Barlow, 2007; NICHQ, 2007; Spear et al., 2007). Finally, it is recommended that the primary care physician follows certain communication strategies (e.g., empathize, elicit, and provide) to improve the effectiveness of counseling.

In stage two, structured weight management visits take place at a primary care office (i.e., the medical care children receive at first contact before being referred to a specialist) with the added support of a healthcare provider who has specific training in weight control. Visits provide an increase in structure and support, specifically toward setting physical activity and nutritional goals and creating rewards. During stage two encounters, MedFTs can monitor goals, aid in barrier removals relevant to setting goals, and make sure that support is provided for both the patient and his/her parent. Stage two visits ideally occur on a monthly basis, either with the child seen individually or as part of a group visit.

Stage three—comprehensive, multidisciplinary intervention—goes beyond stage two by employing interdisciplinary childhood obesity treatment and a structured behavioral program (e.g., negotiating and reinforcing positive healthy behaviors). Ideally, families are seen weekly for 8–12 weeks with additional follow-up services. Stage four, tertiary care intervention, is aimed at severely obese youth by utilizing treatments such as medications (e.g., sibutramine or orlistat), very low calorie diets, and/or weight control surgery (e.g., gastric bypass or lap-band) alongside behavioral treatment. In stage three and four settings, MedFTs are often included as behavioral health partners on the team, consistently seeing all patients for both consultations and when needed traditional individual or family therapy. Obesity treatment can occur in traditional one-on-one medical encounters in a primary care context but also can evolve to interdisciplinary and integrated behavioral healthcare. The history and evolution of these diverse treatment modalities are described below.

It is clear that pediatric settings demand different levels of collaboration, and for some settings, integrated behavioral healthcare may not be feasible. However, in order to explore if such care may be feasible, the healthcare setting needs to be assessed according to the MedFT Healthcare Continuum (Hodgson, Lamson, Mendenhall, & Tyndall, 2014). The next section of this paper describes pediatric care across this continuum for clinical methods and outcomes relevant to pediatrics.

Pediatric Care Across the MedFT Healthcare Continuum

Regardless of the level of integration and therapeutic approach, MedFTs should have a basic knowledge and training in the biopsychosocial-systemic approach (McDaniel, Doherty, & Hepworth, 2014). Hodgson, Lamson, Mendenhall, and Tyndall (2014) introduced the MedFT Healthcare Continuum based on five levels of integration and suggested that MedFTs may work in any of these levels depending on their experience and training. Each level of integration highlights differing skills and training needs for providers and clinics. While the main focus of the MedFT

Healthcare Continuum initially was intended for the general healthcare population, it can easily be applied to pediatric healthcare.

Hodgson et al. (2014) described *Level 1* integration as MedFTs who may have experience, training, and/or biopsychosocial-spiritual (Engel, 1977, 1980; Wright, Watson, & Bell, 1996) and relational approaches; however, guidance regarding application of these approaches in professional settings (e.g., clinical, research, advocacy, and policy) is absent. Clinically, consultation may happen as it is needed or in crisis situations—but collaborative work is not typical. For example, in pediatric care, the MedFT may be asked by a provider for consultation only when the provider is finding a family challenging to work with, such as parent-child conflict, rather than having it be a part of the healthcare routine. Providers in *Level 1* settings should have a basic understanding of the most common pediatric chronic conditions (e.g., asthma, cystic fibrosis, overweight, and obesity) and evidence-based approaches for treatment of these conditions, including national prevention and health promotion strategies (e.g., ChooseMyPlate.gov; Healthy People 2020). Janelle's primary care physician provided the family with general guidance for dietary modifications based on MyPlate recommendations.

At *Level 2* care, collaboration happens occasionally, where BPSS is a portion of what a MedFT does at this level—but it happens less than 50% of the time. Collaboration may consist of intermittent work with other healthcare providers, spiritual advisers, and people in the patient's support system (e.g., family and friends) when BPSS and relational concerns are explicitly present. However, MedFTs at this level may not actively seek to understand BPSS and relational concerns that are more implicit or to collaborate with others regarding these challenges. In pediatrics, this "occasional" collaboration is often seen with the involvement of schools or childcare centers, often with more severe conditions and/or patients with more challenges, wherein these settings and individuals within them may be involved, but not consistently. This is evidenced within the vignette when Janelle's primary care provider makes a referral in the electronic health record to a pediatric endocrinologist at a nearby specialty care clinic so that Janelle and her family can receive more specialized care. MedFTs working in *Level 2* care are familiar with the kinds of family lifestyle behavioral changes necessary to treat the child's chronic conditions (e.g., asthma, cystic fibrosis), and are mostly determining goals relevant to the care they are providing, with outside collaboration on an as needed basis. Finally, because providers working in at this level have more continuity, they can tailor the implementation of national prevention and health promotion strategies (e.g., ChooseMyPlate.gov in public schools) to the settings their patients commonly encounter (see Table 3.1).

Level 3 care consists of collaboration happening "usually," where providers may have more formalized training in their approaches, such as specialty training in weight management, resulting in more collaboration and attention to BPSS and relational needs. The treatment team within the pediatric endocrinologist clinic that Janelle's family was referred to is an example of a specialty care clinic. Hodgson et al. (2014) estimate that MedFTs at this level provide integrated behavioral healthcare up to 75% of the time and collaborate with patients and their support

Table 3.1 MedFTs in Pediatrics: Basic Knowledge and Skills

MedFT Healthcare Continuum Level	Level 1	Level 2	Level 3
Knowledge	Basic training and knowledge about BPSS approaches to pediatrics. Basic understanding regarding most common pediatric chronic conditions (e.g., asthma, cystic fibrosis, overweight and obesity) and recommended treatment strategies. Familiar with national prevention and health promotion strategies targeted toward youth (e.g., child-centered medical homes; healthy people 2020; ChooseMyPlate.gov).	Proficient training and knowledge about BPSS approaches to pediatrics. Familiar with family lifestyle behavior changes necessary to treat common chronic conditions (e.g., asthma, cystic fibrosis, overweight, and obesity). Familiar with implementation of national prevention and health promotion strategies targeted toward youth in specific settings (e.g., ChooseMyPlate.gov in public schools).	Familiar with strategies for inclusion of caregivers and other family members in treatment planning. Trained in disease-specific treatment and collaboration strategies (e.g., weight management, diabetes, asthma). Familiar with specialty providers and multidisciplinary treatment teams. Disease-specific knowledge prioritized above general prevention and health promotion strategies.
Skills	Provides psychoeducation to families related to BPSS principles. Minimal collaborative skills with pediatrician and specialist providers. Consultation may happen as needed or in crisis situations; MedFTs likely to be consulted when the provider is finding a family challenging to work with, such as parent-child conflict.	Collaborates when BPSS and relational concerns are explicitly present; however, collaboration is most likely with schools and childcare centers and is an inconsistent practice. Goals are likely still determined independently from other providers.	Adept at inclusion of caregivers and other family members in treatment planning. Integrates respective team members' perspectives and advice into treatment planning in tertiary care clinics. Assesses family dynamics around disease-specific challenges. Familiar with pediatric specialty providers and able to aid primary care pediatricians in making referrals to specialty mental and behavioral health providers.

system and various providers. In the case of pediatric care, a MedFT in this group would include the child's caregivers and potentially additional family (e.g., siblings, grandparents) and support members in treatment planning (e.g., teachers, spiritual/religious leaders, childcare providers, specialty healthcare providers, and additional extended family or fictive kin who are noted supports). MedFTs at this level would be collaborating within multidisciplinary teams (e.g., pediatric providers, dieticians) to attend to BPSS, systemic, and family variables with similar frequency. MedFTs can assess family strengths and skills for management of their child's diagnosis. Finally, MedFTs should be familiar with pediatric specialty providers and clinics to aid primary care pediatricians to make relevant referrals.

Level 4 care represents another step leading toward full integration of operationalizing skill and identity as a MedFT. Providers at this level have a working knowledge of evidence-based treatments for the most common chronic pediatric conditions. MedFTs in *Level 4* care attend to integration in almost all of their professional work, collaborate consistently with each patient and encounter, and utilize BPSS and systemic intervention in both traditional and integrated behavioral healthcare visits. Integration and collaboration take on additional skills now (e.g., attending to each member of the healthcare team for collaboration and wellness, treatment planning with all members of the patient's healthcare and personal support system, and implementing systemic interventions in working toward the treatment goals). In the vignette, the MedFT works with Janelle's grandmother to illuminate problematic family dynamics that may be impeding the adoption of the behavior changes and goals made by other providers. The MedFT also gains consent from the family to share relevant information with the treatment team, enabling more thorough and inclusive treatment planning. In pediatrics, this level of treatment integration may mean that systems beyond the immediate family need to be involved, like the aforementioned settings of school, childcare, and extracurricular leaders and coaches.

MedFTs in *Level 5* settings have additional training and skills to serve in administration and supervisory contexts that help others to learn integrated behavioral healthcare skills. This may include care provided in various types of healthcare contexts and may be applied in both traditional and integrated settings. Collaboration happens routinely and proficiently with patients, providers, and members of the patient's support system. MedFTs at this level are able to work at an even higher level of integration than the previous level and train other providers and researchers to do so also. *Level 5* MedFTs are able to contribute and create models of integration to enable other providers to increase their levels of collaboration and integration. In pediatrics, a MedFT would be interested in examining the patient, parent, and provider relationships and assessing each relationship from each person's point of view (e.g., the patient's view of his/her relationship with the parent and provider, the provider's view of his/her relationship with the parent and patient, and the parent's view of his/her relationship with the patient and provider). Regarding provider's knowledge, MedFTs working at this level are proficient in all aspects of general pediatric care (i.e., child medical homes and specialty care). They are conversant with evidence-based treatment for the most common pediatric chronic conditions and family responses to these conditions. Providers are also able to give education to patients about a variety of symptoms, medications, and diet management for common chronic conditions. Finally, these MedFTs are able to assess and intervene on relational dynamics between multiple parties responsible for day-to-day child healthcare (e.g., providers, family members, patients, and childcare providers). The MedFT working with Janelle attends to both the needs of Janelle's family and helps

Table 3.2 MedFTs in Pediatrics: Advanced Knowledge and Skills

MedFT Healthcare Continuum Level	Level 4	Level 5
Knowledge	Highly trained and collaborate consistently with each patient and encounter and utilizes BPSS and systemic intervention in both traditional and integrated behavioral healthcare visits. Working knowledge of evidence-based treatments regarding most common chronic pediatric conditions.	Extensive knowledge of integrated behavioral health care and collaboration; able to help others to learn integrated behavioral healthcare skills. Conversant with evidence-based treatments regarding most common pediatric chronic conditions and their role(s) in the family. Extensive knowledge of evidence-based treatments for specific condition if located in tertiary care (e.g., extensive pediatric obesity knowledge in weight management setting).
Skills	Integrates systems beyond the immediate family (e.g., school, childcare, and extracurricular). Integration and collaboration take-on additional skills (e.g., attending to each member of the healthcare team for collaboration and wellness, treatment planning with all members of the patient's healthcare and personal support system, and implementing systemic interventions in working toward the treatment goals).	Training and skills to serve in administration and supervisory contexts that help others to learn integrated behavioral healthcare skills. Collaborates routinely and proficiently with patients, providers, and members of the patient's support system. Proficient in all aspects of general pediatric care (e.g., child medical homes and specialty care). Provides education to patients about a variety of symptoms, medications, and dietary guidance for common chronic conditions. Assesses and intervenes on relational dynamics between providers, families, patients, and childcare providers (e.g., day care, school).

to coordinate the endocrinology treatment team and Janelle's school to ensure that Janelle and her family receive consistent and comprehensive care (see Table 3.2).

As stated previously, each level of integration requires the MedFT to have a certain level of skill and training to perform the given tasks. The level of integration is positively correlated with the amount of skill and training a MedFT must have to implement the required tasks. Hodgson et al. (2014) encourage MedFTs to examine their own skills and training and then decide which level best fits their skill level and training. In pediatric care, much like other types of healthcare populations, higher levels of integration are often preferable to enable better engagement of the patients, providers, family, and support system members.

Research-Informed Practices

Pediatricians are encouraged to focus on preventative efforts because childhood is an ideal time to reduce risk factors. Secondly, providers should make efforts to include caregivers and other family members in treatment planning due to the dependence of children upon caregivers for support. Finally, school personnel can be an important resource for the integrated behavioral healthcare team, as a large majority of the pediatric population is involved in some form of a formal education system (Ader et al., 2015).

Child-Centered and Pediatric Primary Care Medical Home (PCMH)

While researchers continue to refine investigative questions and study designs, preliminary evidence shows that PCMHs show promise in servicing the health needs of children and their families (Ader et al., 2015; Stille et al., 2010). A review of studies examining various aspects of the PCMH indicated that there was a positive relationship between PCMHs and increases in behaviors associated with child wellness, as well as child and family health outcomes (e.g., health status, timeliness of care, family centeredness, and improved family functioning; Homer et al., 2008). PCMH utilization has been shown to lower rates of hospitalization and lower emergency department use (Cooley, McAllister, Sherrieb, & Kuhlthau, 2009). Finally, integrated behavioral healthcare services in primary care have also been found to be effective in treating child behavioral challenges (e.g., oppositional defiant disorder; Kolko, Campo, Kilbourne, & Kelleher, 2012).

Providers should develop competencies for serving unique patient populations. In order to address the lower rates of PCMH utilization in African American, Latino, and non-English speaking families, Coker, Rodriguez, and Flores (2010) recommend that providers spend more time with patients and develop cultural competencies related to learning more about diverse families and their value systems. Providers expecting to work in integrated behavioral healthcare should also receive training specific to working on care teams such as learning how to negotiate and define team roles, sharing decision-making responsibilities, and debriefing in a team setting (McDaniel et al., 2014).

Family Involvement in Care

Caregiver and family involvement are essential for the effective treatment of multiple health conditions. Pediatric patient-centered medical homes encourage the involvement of caregivers and other family members in prevention, intervention, and treatment (Stille et al., 2010). Furthermore, several reviews have demonstrated the effectiveness of family involvement in the treatment of multiple chronic pediatric health conditions (e.g., Morgan et al., 2017; Nichols, Newman, Nemeth, & Magwood, 2015; Raber et al., 2016; Wiebe & Johnson, 2016).

Pediatric diabetes. Family-based behavioral treatments (e.g., goal setting and behavioral contracts) have demonstrated efficacy in increasing glycemic control and regimen adherence (Delamater, de Wit, McDarby, Malik, & Acerini, 2014). Family support increases child adherence to diabetes regimens; however, older children are less likely to receive support from their parents than younger children, placing adolescents at higher risk for nonadherence (Delamater et al., 2014). Additionally, when families noted improvements in family functioning, children also had better glycemic control, further indicating that MedFTs have the potential to promote positive health outcomes through family involvement. During the transition from pediatric to adult care, patients are more likely to experience poorer glycemic control (Lotstein et al., 2013), possibly indicating that patients need support throughout this transition process. Behavioral health providers and PCPs should find ways to solicit family support in developing behavioral treatment plans. Care teams should be sensitive to the risks of this transition and work to engage family supports while increasing patient autonomy.

Pediatric asthma. There is evidence that integrated behavioral healthcare improves outcomes for the treatment of pediatric asthma. Cunningham et al. (2008) found that integrated behavioral healthcare was effective in improving parent education and decreased duration of hospital stays in the treatment of children who had been admitted to the emergency room for an acute asthmatic episode. Children with better asthma control were more likely to be treated in care resembling a PCMH than children presenting with any other chronic illness (Brachlow, Ness, McPheeters, & Gurney, 2007); this suggests that interventions offered through the PCMH are most likely to reach families of children with asthma. Additionally, in a recent randomized control trial, researchers saw increases in symptom-free days and reductions in emergency department visits and hospitalizations (Garbutt, Yan, Highstein, & Strunk, 2015). Components of this intervention included a telephone-based peer training module, which connected parents to peer educators, and an educational component for pediatricians about effective asthma management.

Pediatric obesity. Expert recommendations for the prevention and treatment of childhood obesity endorse the inclusion of families (Barlow, 2007). Randomized control trials have demonstrated the efficacy of a variety of family-based treatments in treating children who are overweight or obese; however, the majority of family-based interventions utilize family-based behavioral therapy to target child and/or parent behaviors relevant for weight loss (Epstein, Paluch, Roemmich, & Beecher, 2007; Sung-Chan, Sung, Zhao, & Brownson, 2013). Other strategies that demonstrate promise for preventing and intervening upon obesity include parental support and home activities. These strategies encourage children to engage in weight management behaviors like increased consumption of nutritious foods, less screen time, and more physical activity (Waters et al., 2011), further highlighting the need for pediatricians and behavioral health providers to include families in treatment efforts.

While models of pediatric care are still being explored, evidence suggests that the PCMHs provide children with consistent and effective medical care. The discussion above highlights the necessity of integrated behavioral healthcare medical teams that provide consistent care to children. Family involvement in treatment planning and implementation is essential for effective treatment of chronic pediatric health conditions. Providers working with pediatric populations should make every effort to understand the unique aspects of working with children and their families in integrated behavioral healthcare systems.

Conclusion

This chapter highlighted the role of MedFTs in pediatric healthcare settings. There are several types of pediatric settings that MedFTs may work in, ranging from pediatric primary care to specialty and tertiary care. They may also work with multidisciplinary providers, including pediatricians, pediatric psychiatrists, pediatric dietitians, and/or pediatric endocrinologists. MedFTs may work with children and families targeting multiple pediatric conditions, including asthma, diabetes, and childhood obesity. Overall, pediatric healthcare settings provide an excellent opportunity for MedFTs to be involved with family-centered care. Given their training in family systems theory and integrated behavioral healthcare practice(s), MedFTs are able to facilitate family-centered care that can promote biopsychosocial-spiritual holistic care within pediatric settings.

Reflection Questions

1. How could you use your knowledge of family systems as a MedFT to work collaboratively with a pediatric healthcare provider to implement family-centered care practices?
2. How might your role as part of the healthcare team be different in a pediatric primary care setting versus a specialty care setting?
3. How can you use anticipatory guidance practices as a way to engage diverse families in the treatment process? In what ways can you use the family's expertise about the patient to frame the dialogue about the child's current and future growth and development?

Glossary of Important Terms for Care in Pediatrics

Anticipatory guidance The practice of educating parents about what they can expect for their child's development over the next few months or years. Education and recommendations are delivered at each visit and are specific to the child's age.

Asthma A chronic inflammatory condition that involves constriction of the airway resulting in symptoms such as coughing, wheezing, and shortness of breath. This is likely to occur when the child is engaging physical activity behaviors. Asthma can have multiple triggers (e.g., smoke, strong odors, pollen, dust mites, pet dander) that need to be identified and is most commonly treated using medication management and environmental/behavioral changes.

Cerebral Palsy The most commonly diagnosed motor disability in children resulting in problems with movement and posture. It can be caused by either abnormal brain development or brain damage in utero. CP has no cure, but early intervention can improve quality of life.

Child-centered medical home An approach to pediatric healthcare endorsed by the American Academy of Pediatrics that encourages a long-term, collaborative relationship between the child's family and a primary medical provider that is aware of the child's health history and can serve as base for all the child's healthcare needs.

Developmentally and age-appropriate care Healthcare that is tailored to the needs of the child based on his/her level of physical, social, emotional, and cognitive development. This practice involves the provider shifting their focus from the parent to the child as the child becomes older, more independent, and capable of engaging in their visits.

Diabetes Type 1 diabetes is a disease characterized by the body's inability to make insulin, the hormone that is responsible for breaking down and storing energy from food. It needs to be treated with insulin injections, often through the use of a pump. Type 1 diabetes is typically diagnosed during childhood; it is the most common form of diabetes present in children. Type 2 diabetes is a chronic condition caused by insulin resistance, wherein the body can make insulin but does not use it effectively. Type 2 diabetes is now being diagnosed in children because of the rise in childhood obesity. It is most commonly treated with the use of medications and lifestyle changes, such as increased physical activity and improved nutrition intake.

Early intervention A system of services that promotes helping children with developmental delays or disabilities as soon as they are discovered. Early intervention typically takes place in the first 3 years of life.

Family-based care Healthcare practice where the intervention or treatment focuses on the child patient and at least one other family member, typically the caregiver.

Family-centered care A collaborative approach to healthcare where the patient, the family, and the healthcare team are equally involved in the assessment of needs and development of a treatment plan.

Family-focused care An approach where the healthcare provider assumes the role of the expert when assessing and treating. The patient and family are considered the unit of intervention, and the provider does the intervening by creating a treatment plan.

General pediatrician A primary care physician with specialty training in pediatric care. A qualified general pediatrician, in the United States, will be board certified by the American Association of Pediatrics.

Malnutrition A condition that occurs as a result of poor nutrition, which can include either undernutrition and overnutrition. It can lead to other conditions, including changes in weight status, behavioral and mental health problems, and inadequate immune system functioning.

Neonatal intensive care An inpatient unit that specializes in caring for premature or severely ill newborn infants.

Neonatology A subspecialty that focuses on providing medical care to newborn infants, especially premature and medically ill newborns.

Overweight/obesity The most commonly diagnosed chronic childhood illness; it is diagnosed when a child weighs too much for their height, based on their age and sex, and is often characterized by excessive adipose (fat) tissue. It is often related to comorbidities such as insulin resistance and diabetes, high blood pressure, sleep apnea, and musculoskeletal pain.

Pediatric audiology and speech pathology Evaluation, diagnosis, and treatment specialty care for children with hearing and communication disorders. These providers encourage early screening and intervention practices.

Pediatric endocrinology The management and treatment of disorders associated with the endocrine glands, including growth disorders, puberty, sex differentiation, glucose metabolism, bone and mineral metabolism, as well as problems with the adrenal, thyroid, and pituitary glands. The most common disease treated by pediatric endocrinology is type 1 diabetes.

Pediatric gastroenterology A specialization in the treatment of digestive system diseases, including bowel syndromes, constipation, diarrhea, vomiting, food allergies and intolerances, nutritional problems, gastroesophageal reflux disease, and liver disease.

Pediatric hematology The study and treatment of blood disorders, which often include bleeding disorders, blood cell disorders, anemia, blood transfusions, and bone marrow and stem cell transplant. Specialists in hematology work closely with pediatric oncology.

Pediatric intensive care An inpatient unit that specializes in caring for critically ill infants, children, and teenagers by providing continuous monitoring of symptoms.

Pediatric nephrology A subspecialty of pediatric care responsible for the management of kidney function and kidney problems, including dialysis and transplants. The most common disease treated by pediatric nephrology is high blood pressure.

Pediatric obesity Pediatricians who offer evidenced-based treatment on lifestyle changes aimed at reducing a child's weight, while also managing and treating weight-related illnesses such as high blood pressure and insulin resistance.

Pediatric oncology The treatment of research of childhood cancers, commonly including leukemia, lymphoma, brain tumors, and bone tumors. Often closely associated with hematology, and both specialties may be available in the same practice.

Pediatric orthopedics Specialists in the musculoskeletal system. They most commonly treat limb and spine deformations, gait abnormalities, broken bones, and bone or joint diseases, infections, and tumors.

Pediatric palliative care Healthcare focused on improving the quality of life for a child and family with serious illness. It focuses on symptom relief from and easing stressors associated with the illness. It should not be confused with end-of-life care or hospice.

Pediatric pulmonary Specialty care in the management and treatment of breathing and lung diseases. The most common diseases treated by pediatric pulmonologists include asthma, cystic fibrosis, and apnea.

Pediatric rheumatology Specialists in musculoskeletal and autoimmune conditions, including arthritis, chronic musculoskeletal pain or weakness, and lupus.

Pediatric urology A surgical subspecialty in the evaluation, diagnosis, and treatment of diseases in the urinary tract and genitals. The most common diseases treated include urination and reproductive organ disorders.

Sleep apnea A sleep disorder characterized by heavy, loud snoring, typically associated with pauses, gasps, and snorts during sleep. A child with sleep apnea may experience restless sleep, bedwetting, fatigue, and sleepiness when woken up/during the day and behavioral problems. This disorder is commonly found in children with severe obesity.

Additional Resources

Literature

Briggs, R. D. (2016). *Integrated early childhood behavioral health in primary care: A guide to implementation and evaluation.* Switzerland: Springer International Publishing.

Durand, V. M. (2008). *When children don't sleep well: Interventions for pediatric sleep disorders therapist guide.* New York, NY: Oxford University Press.

Hassink, S. G. (2014). *Pediatric obesity: Prevention, intervention, and treatment strategies for primary care* (2nd ed.). Elk Grove, IL. American Academy of Pediatrics.

Jenkins, R., & World Health Organization. (2004). *WHO guide to mental and neurological health in primary care: A guide to mental and neurological ill health in adults, adolescents, and children.* London, U.K.: Royal Society of Medicine Press.

Reiff, M. I. (2011). *ADHD: What every parent needs to know. Expert guidance from the American Academy of Pediatrics.* Elk Grove Village, IL: American Academy of Pediatrics.

Roemer, J. B. (2011). *American Diabetes Association guide to raising a child with diabetes*. Alexandria, VA: American Diabetes Association.

Simmonds, J. (2014). *Seeing red: An anger management and anti-bullying curriculum for kids*. Gabriola Island, B.C., Canada: New Society Publishers.

Welch, M. J. & American Academy of Pediatrics. (2000). *American Academy of Pediatrics guide to your child's allergies and asthma: Breathing easy and bringing up healthy, active children*. Elk Grove Village, IL: American Academy of Pediatrics.

Electronic Resources

A Family Guide: Integrating Mental Health and Pediatric Primary Care. http://www.integration.samhsa.gov/integrated-care-models/FG-Integrating,_12.22.pdf

Childhood Asthma. https://www.aaaai.org/conditions-and-treatments/library/at-a-glance/childhood-asthma

Healthy Children/Healthychildren.org. https://www.healthychildren.org/English/Pages/default.aspx

Kids Health. www.kidshealth.org

Strategies to Support the Integration of Mental Health into Pediatric Primary Care. http://www.nihcm.org/pdf/PediatricMH-FINAL.pdf

Measures/Instruments

Motivation for Youth Treatment Scale. http://peabody.vanderbilt.edu/docs/pdf/cepi/ptpb_2nd_ed/PTPB_2010_AppendixB_MYTS_031212.pdf

Patient Health Questionnaire (modified for adolescents). http://www.integration.samhsa.gov/images/res/8.3.4%20Patient%20Health%20Questionnaire%20(PHQ-9)%20Adolescents.pdf

Pediatric Intake Form. https://www.brightfutures.org/mentalhealth/pdf/professionals/ped_intake_form.pdf

Pediatric Symptom Checklist. http://www.massgeneral.org/psychiatry/assets/PSC-35.pdf

Screening for Child Anxiety Related Disorders (SCARED). http://psychiatry.pitt.edu/sites/default/files/Documents/assessments/SCARED%20Child.pdf

Vanderbilt ADHD Diagnostic Parent Rating Scale. http://www.childrenshospital.vanderbilt.org/uploads/documents/DIAGNOSTIC_PARENT_RATING_SCALE(1).pdf

Organizations/Associations

American Academy of Pediatrics/Family-Centered Care. https://brightfutures.aap.org/
American Diabetes Association. http://www.diabetes.org/living-with-diabetes/parents-and-kids/
Academy of Nutrition and Dietetics. www.eatright.org
Obesity Action Coalition. www.obesityaction.org

References[1]

Ader, J., Stille, C. J., Keller, D., Miller, B. F., Barr, M. S., & Perrin, J. M. (2015). The medical home and integrated behavioral health: Advancing the policy agenda. *Pediatrics, 135*, 909–917. https://doi.org/10.1542/peds.2014-3941

American Academy of Pediatrics. (2011). *Pediatrics 101: A resource guide from the American Academy of Pediatrics* (2nd ed.). Washington, DC: Author.

American Academy of Pediatrics. (2016). *HealthyChildren.Org*. Retrieved from https://www.healthychildren.org/English/Pages/default.aspx

*Barlow, S.E. (2007). Expert committee recommendations regarding the prevention, assessment, and treatment of child and adolescent overweight and obesity: Summary report. *Pediatrics, 120*, 164–92. https://doi.org/10.1542/peds.2007-2329C

*Berge, J. M., & Everts, J. C. (2011). Family-based interventions targeting childhood obesity: A meta-analysis. *Childhood Obesity, 7*, 110–121. https://doi.org/10.1089/chi.2011.07.02.1004.berge

*Brachlow, A. E., Ness, K. K., McPheeters, M. L., & Gurney, J. G. (2007). Comparison of indicators for a primary care medical home between children with autism or asthma and other special health care needs: National Survey of Children's Health. *Archives of Pediatrics & Adolescent Medicine, 161*, 399–405. https://doi.org/10.1001/archpedi.161.4.399

*Briggs, R. D. (2016). *Integrated early childhood behavioral health in primary care: A guide to implementation and evaluation*. Switzerland: Springer International Publishing.

Britt, E., Hudson, S. M., & Blampied, N. M. (2004). Motivational interviewing in health settings: A review. *Patient Education and Counseling, 53*, 147–155. https://doi.org/10.1016/S0738-3991(03)00141-1

Coker, T. R., Rodriguez, M. A., & Flores, G. (2010). Family-centered care for US children with special health care needs: Who gets it and why? *Pediatrics, 125*, 1159–1167. https://doi.org/10.1542/peds.2009-1994

Cooley, W. C., McAllister, J. W., Sherrieb, K., & Kuhlthau, K. (2009). Improved outcomes associated with medical home implementation in pediatric primary care. *Pediatrics, 124*, 358–364. https://doi.org/10.1542/peds.2008-2600

Cunningham, S., Logan, C., Lockerbie, L., Dunn, M. J., McMurray, A., & Prescott, R. J. (2008). Effect of an integrated care pathway on acute asthma/wheeze in children attending hospital: Cluster randomized trial. *Journal of Pediatrics, 152*, 315–320. https://doi.org/10.1016/j.jpeds.2007.09.033

Darling, N., & Steinberg, L. (1993). Parenting style as context: An integrative model. *Psychological Bulletin, 113*, 487–496. Retrieved from http://www.apa.org/pubs/journals/bul/

---

[1] Note: References that are prefaced with an asterisk are recommended readings.

Delamater, A. M., de Wit, M., McDarby, V., Malik, J., & Acerini, C. L. (2014). Psychological care of children and adolescents with type 1 diabetes. *Pediatric Diabetes, 15*, 232–244. https://doi.org/10.1111/pedi.12191

*Durand, V. M. (2008). *When children don't sleep well: Interventions for pediatric sleep disorders therapist guide*. New York, NY: Oxford University Press.

Emmons, K. M., & Rollnick, S. (2001). Motivational interviewing in health care settings: Opportunities and limitations. *American Journal of Preventive Medicine, 20*, 68–74. Retrived from http://www.ajpmonline.org/

Engel, G. L. (1977). The need for a new medical model: A challenge for biomedicine. *Science, 196*, 129–136. https://doi.org/10.1016/b978-0-409-95009-0.50006-1

Engel, G. L. (1980). The clinical application of the biopsychosocial model. *American Journal of Family Medicine, 137*, 535–544. https://doi.org/10.1176/ajp.137.5.535

Epstein, L. H., Paluch, R. A., Roemmich, J. N., & Beecher, M. D. (2007). Family-based obesity treatment, then and now: Twenty-five years of pediatric obesity treatment. *Health Psychology, 26*, 381–391. https://doi.org/10.1037/0278-6133.26.4.381

Garbutt, J. M., Yan, Y., Highstein, G., & Strunk, R. C. (2015). A cluster-randomized trial shows telephone peer coaching for parents reduces children's asthma morbidity. *Journal of Allergy and Clinical Immunology, 135*, 1163–1170. https://doi.org/10.1016/j.jaci.2014.09.03

Hagan, J. F., Shaw, J. S., & Duncan, P. M. (2008). *Bright futures: Guidelines for health supervision of infants, children, and adolescents*. Elks Grove Village: American Academy of Pediatrics.

*Hassink, S. G. (2014). *Pediatric obesity: Prevention, intervention, and treatment strategies for primary care* (2nd ed.). Elk Grove: American Academy of Pediatrics.

Hodgson, J., Lamson, A., Mendenhall, T., & Tyndall, L. (2014). Introduction to medical family therapy: Advanced applications. In J. Hodgson, A. Lamson, T. Mendenhall, and D. Crane (Eds.), *Medical family therapy: Advanced applications* (pp. 1–9). New York, NY: Springer.

Homer, C. J., Klatka, K., Romm, D., Kuhlthau, K., Bloom, S., Newacheck, P., ... Perrin, J. M. (2008). A review of the evidence for the medical home for children with special health care needs. *Pediatrics, 122*, e922–e937. https://doi.org/10.1542/peds.2007-3762

Institute for Patient- and Family-Centered Care. (2010). *Frequently asked questions*. Retrieved from http://www.ipfcc.org/faq.html

Institute for Patient- and Family-Centered Care. (2016). *Patient- and family-centered care is working "with" patients and families, rather than just doing "to" or "for" them*. Retrieved from http://www.ipfcc.org/about/pfcc.html

Irby, M., Kaplan, S., Garner-Edwards, D., Kolbash, S., & Skelton, J. A. (2010). Motivational interviewing in a family-based pediatric obesity program: A case study. *Families, Systems, & Health, 28*, 236–245. https://doi.org/10.1037/a0020101

*Jenkins, R., & World Health Organization. (2004). *WHO guide to mental and neurological health in primary care: A guide to mental and neurological ill health in adults, adolescents, and children*. London: Royal Society of Medicine Press.

Katz, D., & Faridi, Z. (2008). Public health approaches to the control of pediatric and adolescent obesity. In W. O'Donoghue, B. Moore, and B. Scott (Eds.), *Handbook of pediatric and adolescent obesity treatment* (pp. 251–271). New York, NY: Taylor and Francis.

*Kolko, D. J., Campo, J. V., Kilbourne, A. M., & Kelleher, K. (2012). Doctor-office collaborative care for pediatric behavioral problems: A preliminary clinical trial. *Archives of Pediatrics & Adolescent Medicine, 166*, 224–31. https://doi.org/10.1001/archpediatrics.2011.201

Lotstein, D. S., Seid, M., Klingensmith, G., Case, D., Lawrence, J. M., Pihoker, C., ... Imperatore, G. (2013). Transition from pediatric to adult care for youth diagnosed with type 1 diabetes in adolescence. *Pediatrics, 131*, 1062–1070. https://doi.org/10.1542/peds.2012-1450

Mastro, K. A., Mastro, K. A., Mastro, K. A., Flynn, L., & Preuster, C. (2014). Patient- and family-centered care: A call to action for new knowledge and innovation. *Journal of Nursing Administration, 44*, 446–451. https://doi.org/10.1097/NNA.0000000000000099

McDaniel, S. H., Doherty, W. J., & Hepworth, J. (2014). *Medical family therapy and integrated care* (2nd ed.). Washington, DC: American Psychological Association.

Miller, W. R., & Rollnick, S. (2013). *Motivational interviewing: Helping people change.* New York, NY: Guilford Press.

Morgan, P. J., Young, M. D., Lloyd, A. B., Wang, M. L., Eather, N., Miller, A., ... Pagoto, S. L. (2017). Involvement of fathers in pediatric obesity treatment and prevention trials: A systematic review. *Pediatrics, 139,* 1–11. https://doi.org/10.1542/peds.2016-2635

National Initiative for Children's Health Care Quality. (2007). *Implementation guide for expert committee recommendations on the assessment, prevention and treatment of child and adolescent overweight and obesity.* Retrieved from www.ihs.gov/nonmedicalprograms/dirinitiatives/documents/coan%20implementation%20guide%20dr.%20scott%20gee.doc

Nichols, M., Newman, S., Nemeth, L. S., & Magwood, G. (2015). The influence of parental participation on obesity interventions in African American adolescent females: An integrative review. *Journal of Pediatric Nursing, 30,* 485–493. https://doi.org/10.1016/j.pedn.2014.12.004

Phillips, R. D. (2010). How firm is our foundation? Current play therapy research. *International Journal of Play Therapy, 19,* 13–25. https://doi.org/10.1037/a0017340

Pulgaron, E. R. (2013). Childhood obesity: A review of increased risk for physical and psychological comorbidities. *Clinical Therapeutics, 35,* A18–A32. https://doi.org/10.1016/j.clinthera.2012.12.014

Raber, M., Swartz, M. C., Santa Maria, D., O'Connor, T., Baranowski, T., Li, R., & Chandra, J. (2016). Parental involvement in exercise and diet interventions for childhood cancer survivors: A systematic review. *Pediatric Research, 80,* 338–346. Retrieved from http://txcercit.org/Files/publications/27064243_Raber.pdf

Reddy, L. A., Files-Hall, T. M., & Schaefer, C. E. (2005). *Empirically based play interventions for children.* Washington, DC: American Psychological Association.

*Reiff, M. I. (2011). *ADHD: What every parent needs to know. Expert guidance from the American Academy of Pediatrics.* Elk Grove Village: American Academy of Pediatrics.

Reisinger, K. S., & Bires, J. A. (1980). Anticipatory guidance in pediatric practice. *Pediatrics, 66,* 889–892. Retrieved from http://pediatrics.aappublications.org/content/139/5?current-issue=y

Resnicow, K., DiIorio, C., Soet, J. E., Borrelli, B., Hecht, J., & Ernst, D. (2002). Motivational interviewing in health promotion: It sounds like something is changing. *Health Psychology, 21,* 444–3351. Retrieved from http://www.apa.org/pubs/journals/hea/

*Roemer, J. B. (2011). *American Diabetes Association guide to raising a child with diabetes.* Alexandria, VA: American Diabetes Association.

*Simmonds, J. (2014). *Seeing red: An anger management and anti-bullying curriculum for kids.* Gabriola Island: New Society Publishers.

Spear, B. A., Barlow, S. E., Ervin, C., Ludwig, D. S., Saelens, B. E., Schetzina, K. E., & Taveras, E. M. (2007). Recommendations for treatment of child and adolescent overweight and obesity. *Pediatrics, 120,* 254–288. https://doi.org/10.1542/peds.2007-2329F

Stille, C., Turchi, R. M., Antonelli, R., Cabana, M. D., Cheng, T. L., Laraque, D., & Perrin, J. (2010). The family-centered medical home: Specific considerations for child health research and policy. *Academic Pediatrics, 10,* 211–217. https://doi.org/10.1016/j.acap.2010.05.002

Sung-Chan, P., Sung, Y. W., Zhao, X., & Brownson, R. C. (2013). Family-based models for childhood-obesity intervention: A systematic review of randomized controlled trials. *Obesity Reviews, 14,* 265–278. https://doi.org/10.1111/obr.12000

Torpy, J. M., Campbell, A., & Glass, R. M. (2010). Chronic diseases of children. *JAMA, 303,* 682. https://doi.org/10.1001/jama.303.7.682

Van Cleave, J., Gortmaker, S. L., & Perrin, J. M. (2010). Dynamics of obesity and chronic health conditions among children and youth. *JAMA, 303,* 623–630. https://doi.org/10.1001/jama.2010.104

Waters, E., de Silva-Sanigorski, A., Hall, B. J., Brown, T., Campbell, K. J., Gao, Y., ... Summerbell, C. D. (2011). Interventions for preventing obesity in children. *Cochrane Database of Systematic Reviews, 12,* 1–224. https://doi.org/10.1002/14651858.CD001871.pub3

*Welch, M. J. and the American Academy of Pediatrics. (2000). *American Academy of Pediatrics guide to your child's allergies and asthma: Breathing easy and bringing up healthy, active children*. Elk Grove Village: American Academy of Pediatrics.

Wiebe, S. A., & Johnson, S. M. (2016). A review of the research in emotionally focused therapy for couples. *Family Process, 55*, 390–407. https://doi.org/10.1111/famp.12229

Wright, L. M., Watson, W. L., & Bell, J. M. (1996). *Beliefs: The heart of healing in families and illness*. New York, NY: Basic Books.

Chapter 4
Medical Family Therapy in Internal Medicine

Jennifer Harsh and Rachel Bonnema

Whether a puzzling diagnostic dilemma or multiple severe chronic illnesses, Internal Medicine providers are trained to manage both simple and complex medical conditions. They are equipped to handle the broad and comprehensive spectrum of illnesses that affect adults, and are experts in diagnosis, treatment of chronic illness, and health promotion and disease prevention. They are not limited to one type of medical problem or organ system. This includes care across the continuum of outpatient (community-based) to inpatient (hospital) facilities, with particular attention paid to times of transition when risk for adverse outcomes from chronic medical conditions increases. Nearly one-fifth of Medicare patients discharged from a hospital have an acute medical problem within the subsequent 30 days that necessitates another hospitalization, and the majority of the time, it is for a different medical condition than the original hospitalization (Jencks, Williams, & Coleman, 2009). The transition from hospital to home is a high-risk time for most patients but particularly for patients who are elderly or those with more chronic medical conditions. Internists, by nature of their training in balancing multiple medical conditions in adults, are well-equipped to provide care to patients at any inpatient or outpatient site.

Managing complex conditions, including acute and chronic illness, has many behavioral and psychosocial implications for patients and families. People with serious physical health problems often have comorbid behavioral health difficulties (Kessler, Chiu, Demler, & Walters, 2005). For example, depression and anxiety are two psychosocial difficulties that commonly accompany serious medical illness (Murri et al., 2017; Vancampfort, Koyanagi, Hallgren, Probst, & Stubbs, 2017). Research suggests that there is a bidirectional relationship between anxiety and depression and serious medical illness (Chauvet-Gelinier & Bonin, 2017). That is,

---

J. Harsh (✉) · R. Bonnema
Department of Internal Medicine, University of Nebraska Medical Center, Omaha, NE, USA
e-mail: jennifer.harsh@unmc.edu

© Springer International Publishing AG, part of Springer Nature 2018
T. Mendenhall et al. (eds.), *Clinical Methods in Medical Family Therapy*, Focused Issues in Family Therapy, https://doi.org/10.1007/978-3-319-68834-3_4

anxious and depressive symptoms can stem from difficult-to-manage physical symptoms, and anxiety and depression may contribute to participation in health behaviors that exacerbate physical symptoms, such as smoking, nonadherence to medication regimens, and poor diet (Chauvet-Gelinier & Bonin, 2017; Katon, 2003). Also, medical conditions such as chronic pain, diabetes, and cardiovascular disease, which are commonly treated by Internal Medicine providers, are highly comorbid with sleep difficulties (Dikeos & Georgantopoulos, 2011). Sleep is very important for overall function. Sleep difficulties are associated with psychological distress (Morin, LeBlanc, Daley, Gregoire, & Merette, 2006), decreased quality of life (Katz & McHorney, 2002), and medical difficulties (e.g., diabetes; Vgontzas et al., 2009). Furthermore, sleep problems adversely impact health outcomes and patients' ability to manage disease (Dikeos & Georgantopoulos, 2011).

Because patients do not generally exist in isolation, families and friends of patients with complex and difficult-to-manage health problems can be greatly impacted as well. Caring for a family member can be rewarding. Family members may learn new skills and feel good about themselves. Conversely, caregiving family members often experience increased rates of chronic stress, depression, and decreased physical and psychological health (Schultz & Sherwood, 2008).

The aforementioned difficulties are just a handful of the complex acute and chronic medical conditions experienced by patients and families who receive care in Internal Medicine settings. The need for whole person and whole family care, which simultaneously includes assessment and treatment of biomedical and psychosocial challenges, is evident. The following case example highlights the experience of Maria and her family as they transition from acute hospital care to chronic illness management in an Internal Medicine primary care clinic.

Clinical Vignette
[Note: This vignette is a compilation of cases that represent treatment in Internal Medicine. All patients' names and/or identifying information have been changed to maintain confidentiality.]

Maria, 45, has poorly controlled Type 2 diabetes mellitus and is being discharged from the hospital today after an amputation of her left foot. She was in and out of the hospital battling infections in her foot prior to the amputation. In addition to diabetes, Maria has been managing hypertension, chronic kidney disease, obesity, and obstructive sleep apnea. She was just prescribed four new medications, bringing her total medication regimen to 40 pills per day. Dr. Rachel Bonnema, her attending (primary) physician during her hospital stay, met Maria during her hospital stay. As Maria and Dr. Bonnema discussed the impact of Maria's health on her quality of life, Maria reported that she has felt "sad" and "lonely" over the past few years as her medical conditions have become increasingly difficult to manage.

> *Upon hearing this, Dr. Bonnema contacted Dr. Jennifer Harsh, a medical family therapist, via electronic medical record message, and provided an overview of Maria's medical history and psychosocial difficulties.*
>
> *Shortly after this, Dr. Harsh met Maria, her husband Ronaldo, and their son Richard, 28, during Maria's hospital follow-up appointment with her primary care provider. During a 20-minute discussion, Maria spoke about feeling overwhelmed by all of the medications she has been asked to take, the dietary changes she has been asked to make, and the new limitations she is experiencing following her amputation. She and her husband expressed concern that they would be unable to meet all of Maria's healthcare needs. Richard also expressed concern that his mother and father were "stressed out" and "depressed." Because of these emotional difficulties and feelings of being overwhelmed, Maria reported that she has not been taking her medications as prescribed. In fact, she hasn't taken her insulin since leaving the hospital.*
>
> *Dr. Harsh initiated a discussion in which the family was asked to talk about their goals. Each reported that they wanted to travel to visit family and wanted to start "living life again," which they felt they had not been doing since Maria's medical conditions began to worsen. Additionally, Maria mentioned that she wanted to "be around" to meet her grandchildren someday. Dr. Harsh then asked the family to think about how Maria's health and caring for her health might fit into these goals. Maria felt that "taking medications the doctors prescribe" and "eating differently" may help her to attain these goals. Maria's husband mentioned that he would like to help Maria by cooking "healthier food" when Maria does not feel up to the task. Richard mentioned that he felt his parents didn't really know how to care for Maria's many medical conditions and was (is) concerned about his parents' ability to afford the prescribed medications.*
>
> *Dr. Harsh provided a summary of the discussion including goals and strategies developed to meet these goals to the family. She then asked the family if they would be interested in meeting with a diabetes educator to create a specific diabetes care plan, including healthier food options, and a social worker who could assist them in finding resources for procuring medication at a reduced cost. The family agreed and met with each provider before leaving the clinic. Dr. Harsh also relayed patient and family difficulties, family goals, and strategies for achieving the goals to the patient's primary care physician.*

This case example showcases some of the many ways in which medical family therapists (MedFTs) collaborate with Internal Medicine care teams. The remainder of this chapter will provide an in-depth look at the practice of Internal Medicine and practice settings. It will highlight the role of Internal Medicine care team members, with special attention paid to the role of the MedFT. Additionally, this chapter will outline important skills and concepts that allow MedFTs to effectively function as part of an Internal Medicine team.

What Is Internal Medicine?

Internal Medicine providers are specialists who apply scientific knowledge and clinical expertise to the diagnosis, treatment, and compassionate care of adults across the spectrum from health to complex illness. General internists (or simply, internists) handle a broad spectrum of illnesses that affect adults; they are recognized as experts in the treatment of chronic illness, often managing several different illnesses that affect patients concurrently. They are competent in solving diagnostic problems and are trained in health promotion and disease prevention. Because internists often care for patients over the duration of their adult lives in primary care clinics, during hospitalization, and in nursing homes, internists have an opportunity to establish long and oftentimes rewarding relationships with their patients.

There has been an important evolution in the field of Internal Medicine that has separated outpatient care from inpatient care over the last 15 years. Often, patients have an identified internist as an outpatient provider and a separate internist as a primary hospital provider, should hospital care be needed. This creates an important transition point for a care plan to be continued between settings. For example, a patient may have been hospitalized for a heart arrhythmia and can quickly be stabilized in a matter of 1–2 days to no longer need intensive monitoring or hospital care. However, that patient may have testing or studies that still need to occur, still need medication adjustment to control the arrhythmia, and possibly need further work-up regarding the underlying cause of the heart arrhythmia. Outpatient internists may be referred to as primary care providers (PCPs); inpatient internists are called hospitalists. They both function to manage multiple conditions and coordinate care in their respective environments, and they may each have different care team members.

As of 2012, about half of all adults in the United States—117 million people—had one or more chronic health conditions, and one in four adults had two or more chronic health conditions (Ward, Schiller, & Goodman, 2014). Frequent diagnoses include type 2 diabetes mellitus, hypertension, chronic obstructive pulmonary disease (COPD), heart disease, and congestive heart failure. Internists also manage chronic pain syndromes such as fibromyalgia, headache, and back pain. As primary care practitioners, they are also first-line providers for depression and anxiety (Ansseau et al., 2004).

Internal Medicine care teams manage a number of complicated medical conditions and, as a result, manage an abundance of medications. According to the Centers for Disease Control and Prevention (CDC, 2014a), about half of all people over the age of 18 used a prescription medication in the last 30 days; 30% over the age of 45 used three different prescription medications in the last 30 days. Managing these medications, and the potential interactions between various medications, is an important aspect of Internal Medicine.

Because of the complexities within—and interactions between—biomedical and psychosocial difficulties inherent to chronic and complex illness, patients and their families oftentimes must adapt to a great deal of change. Maria and her family in our clinical vignette are no exception. She and her husband are trying their best to care for Maria's many health difficulties and will now have to make further adaptations secondary to Maria's foot amputation. With the variety of patient conditions and biopsychosocial (BPS; Engel, 1977) needs, team-based care and collaboration between medical and psychosocial providers are of utmost importance if the myriad of patient and family needs are to be met effectively.

Treatment Teams in Internal Medicine

There are many different types of collaborative relationships between medical and behavioral health professionals in Internal Medicine. Coordinated, co-located, and integrated behavioral healthcare models of collaboration represent three types of relationships (e.g., Blount, 2003; Substance Abuse and Mental Health Services Administration-Health Resources and Services Administration Center for Integrated Health Solutions [SAMHSA-HRSA], 2013). Coordinated care involves two or more professionals from different settings working together by sharing information about a common patient. These relationships, which often begin with a referral, provide the opportunity for important medical and behavioral health information to travel between providers (Blount, 2003). Co-located care is very similar to coordinated care in that information is shared between colleagues. However, with colocated care, behavioral health and medical providers share the same facilities. Integrated behavioral health care describes patient care that focuses on both mental and physical health simultaneously. Care is provided by *one* team of medical and behavioral health professionals with *one* treatment plan that focuses simultaneously on behavioral and physical components of health (Blount, 2003; Doherty, McDaniel, & Baird, 1996).

In addition to different models of collaboration, there are multiple members of Internal Medicine care teams that differ depending on the setting and type of care that patients and families need. Because Internal Medicine providers care for patients in both hospital and primary care outpatient settings, this chapter will provide an overview of healthcare professionals in both settings who collaborate with MedFTs to provide optimal team-based treatment. Most hospital Internal Medicine care teams have each of the team members outlined below:

Primary care physicians (PCPs). Primary care physicians are providers who see patients in an outpatient clinic for regular appointments to care for a multitude of physical conditions, follow labs and related studies, manage medications, and coordinate care plans.

Hospitalists. Hospitalists are physician providers who see hospitalized patients daily to monitor and treat physical conditions, follow labs and related studies, manage medications, and make decisions about the conduct of care plans.

Advanced practice providers (APPs). Advanced practice providers are either physician assistants or nurse practitioners. They have particular advanced medical training (beyond that of a nurse) and assist the primary care provider (PCP or hospitalist) with care provision. Depending on state requirements, APPs can evaluate and manage the care of a patient under the indirect supervision of a primary care provider, including prescribing medications.

Nurses. Nursing care can be provided by a registered nurse (RN) or a licensed practical nurse (LPN) who maintains responsibility for assisting with care delivery, monitoring and educating patients, and triaging patient needs. RNs often serve as case managers, assisting with population health, coordinating care for the sickest or more complex patients, and coordinating next steps in care, including discharge planning.

Medical assistants/patient care technicians. Medical assistants and patient care technicians have completed some post-high school training in assessing patients and providing care. They typically assist with rooming patients, checking vital signs, administering vaccinations, and assisting with the flow of patients through a primary care clinic.

Medical receptionists. Medical receptionists are trained to complete a wide variety of tasks that allow a healthcare setting to function properly. They typically complete patient appointment scheduling, manage and appropriately transfer incoming phone calls and faxes, greet and check patients in for appointments, update patient demographic and insurance information, and collect insurance co-pays. Medical receptionists are very important members of the healthcare team, and they often set the tone for the patient experience in a given healthcare environment since they are the first people with whom the patient typically interacts.

Pharmacists. Pharmacists are trained in the advanced management of medications. They assist with patient education and provide recommendations regarding safe dosing regimens, medication interactions, and dose adjustments in common medications for common diseases (e.g., hypertension, hyperlipidemia).

Diabetes educators. Diabetes educators teach patients and families about the complexities of diabetes management, including dietary and lifestyle needs, medications, and side effects. They often provide care in hospital and primary care Internal Medicine settings.

Physical and occupational therapists. Physical therapists are trained in physical medicine and rehabilitation used to remediate physical impairments and promote mobility, function, and quality of life. Similarly, occupational therapists work to develop or maintain the daily living and work skills of patients and focus much of their effort on identifying and eliminating environmental barriers to independence and participation in daily activities.

Dieticians. Dieticians have specific training in assessing patients' nutritional needs; they work with patients and families to design a diet that minimizes negative health effects from chronic medical conditions (e.g., outlining a renal diet for patients with kidney disease).

Social workers. Social workers provide care for patients and families in both hospital and primary care Internal Medicine settings. Their roles look different in each setting, depending on setting type, patient needs, and unique/respective training and skill sets. Responsibilities may include case management skills to help resolve social and financial difficulties for patients and families, helping patients and families adjust to an extended hospital stay, educating patients about the roles of the healthcare treatment team, and coordinating hospital discharge planning, including continuity of care with community resources (National Association of Social Workers [NASW], 2011). Social workers with clinical training may also conduct comprehensive psychosocial assessments and deliver psychological interventions to assist patients in coping with emotional and behavioral difficulties related to their health condition/s.

Behavioral health providers. Behavioral health providers are responsible for attending to patients' psychosocial needs through the provision of brief psychosocial interventions and/or psychotherapy sessions. They may be trained as psychologists, clinical social workers, marriage and family therapists, professional counselors, or MedFTs. There can be overlap in the duties and responsibilities of practitioners in the social worker and behavioral health provider roles. Specific functions of each are generally practice site-specific.

Fundamentals of Care in Internal Medicine

MedFTs working in an Internal Medicine setting would benefit from gaining an understanding of the Internal Medicine culture, including norms and language. The following is an overview of aspects of the Internal Medicine culture that we believe are instrumental to successful integration into the Internal Medicine environment. Remember, too, that even after gaining insight into Internal Medicine culture and practice, MedFTs can benefit from maintaining a learner's role, in which they continue to search for new information and insight.

Brevity

Because both hospital and primary care Internal Medicine settings are fast-paced environments, MedFTs should focus on keeping interactions with collaborators and patients and families no longer than clinically necessary. For example, no more time should be spent than is needed when talking about patient care recommendations with a physician or physician extender, assessing for patient depression, providing an intervention for anxiety, or documenting a patient encounter. Also, through using brief psychosocial assessment and intervention, MedFTs have the ability to provide care for more patients and families. Intervention specifics will be discussed in the following section.

Health Behavior Change

In Internal Medicine settings, patients' illnesses are complex and impacted, either negatively or positively, by their health behaviors (e.g., diet and exercise). MedFTs in Internal Medicine frequently assist patients and families with health behavior change and, more specifically, with finding motivation for change and developing change strategies. For example, 69% of the U.S. population is overweight or obese (Ogden, Carroll, Kit, & Flegal, 2014). MedFTs help patients with weight-related issues to determine reasons for losing weight and to develop specific and attainable strategies for reaching weight loss goals.

Isolation

Extant literature and our personal experiences with patients highlight the social isolation that often accompanies the common chronic illnesses seen in Internal Medicine (Glozier et al., 2013; Wong et al., 2014). Patients with limited functional ability and/or limited resources (e.g., transportation, money) may find themselves with low levels of social interaction. Not surprisingly, social isolation is correlated with an array of unwanted health outcomes, including negative effects on blood pressure, depression, pain, and fatigue (Hawkley, Thisted, Masi, & Cacioppo, 2010; Jaremka et al., 2012). In fact, loneliness is associated with immune system dysregulation, which means that people who are lonely have a higher chance of becoming ill (Cohen, Doyle, Turner, Alper, & Skoner, 2003). MedFTs can assist this group of patients in identifying barriers that impede social connection and developing strategies for initiating connection with others.

Common Illnesses in Internal Medicine

Gaining an understanding of the common illnesses and associated symptoms seen by Internal Medicine care teams can assist the MedFT in developing appropriate BPS assessment and intervention strategies. The following are six such illnesses:

Diabetes mellitus (DM). Diabetes mellitus is an endocrine disorder resulting in elevated blood sugar. Chronically elevated blood sugar can have negative effects on essentially all organ systems. This leads to medical conditions such as chronic kidney disease, heart attacks, strokes, and vascular disease. The most common type of DM in the Internal Medicine population is type 2, which is often linked with obesity and physical inactivity. Common lab tests for DM are blood sugar tests and hemoglobin A1c. MedFTs assist patients with DM in developing strategies for adapting to the array of daily changes (e.g., taking insulin, eating a diabetes-friendly diet) that medical providers ask them to make.

Heart disease. Heart disease is a term often used by the public to denote any heart problem; however, to a primary care provider, the term typically refers to a syndrome of high cholesterol and disease in the blood vessels that supply blood to the heart, which can ultimately lead to a heart attack. If patients suffer from heart disease, they are often encouraged to regulate diet, physical activity, cholesterol, and blood pressure. The MedFT role can vary greatly with patients with heart disease, depending on the severity of illness. For example, MedFTs may assist patients at risk of serious heart problems with developing motivation and a plan for prevention. Following a heart attack, patients may experience both functional and psychosocial difficulties. MedFTs can work with this group of patients and their caregivers to normalize and validate accompanying emotional distress. MedFTs may also assist these families in adapting to role changes that result from patients' functional limitations.

Congestive heart failure (CHF). Congestive heart failure refers to dysfunction of the heart muscle causing it to pump inefficiently. This often occurs after a heart attack with resultant poor heart function (due to dead heart muscle tissue). CHF can also result from high blood pressure or drug/alcohol use. One measure of heart failure is the "ejection fraction" (EF), which is evaluated by performing an ultrasound of the heart (echocardiogram). Because of the drastic life changes that often accompany CHF, MedFTs can help patients and families develop strategies to practically and emotionally adjust to a new level of daily functioning.

Chronic obstructive pulmonary disease (COPD). Chronic obstructive pulmonary disease, often referred to as emphysema, can have significant effects on patients' quality of life and activity levels. It is most commonly linked to tobacco use but can also be due to occupational exposures. Severe COPD can result in patients needing supplemental oxygen therapy, which can further limit activity. Since COPD often results from patient behavior (e.g., smoking), patients may experience guilt or remorse about the behavior that caused functional limitations. MedFTs can assist patients with processing this guilt and can use motivational interviewing strategies to assist patients with any desired behavior changes.

Medically unexplained symptoms (MUS). Medically unexplained symptoms are often chronic, lack a definitive biological basis, and account for between 25 and 50% of patients seen in primary care (Dumit, 2005; Rosendal, Carlsen, Rask, & Moth, 2015). This makes MUS the most common set of complaints seen by primary care providers (Edwards, Stern, Clarke, Ivbijaro, & Kasney, 2010). Coping with MUS is multifaceted and can contribute to many difficulties in patients' and families' lives, such as lifestyle changes due to symptoms, dealing with perceived lack of legitimacy from the medical system, and living with uncertainty (Dumit, 2005; Nettleton, 2006). In addition to patient difficulties, medical providers experience challenges when working with this group of patients. For example, providers can experience frustration and a lack of confidence with diagnostic strategies and treatment planning (Harsh, Hodgson, White, Lamson, & Irons, 2015). MedFTs can assist both patients and providers experiencing stress and frustration surrounding

MUS. For example, MedFTs can work with patients and families to develop coping strategies and validate frustration stemming from difficult interactions with the medical system. MedFTs can also validate provider frustration and can normalize the array of feelings that stem from not knowing exactly how to effectively treat a patient's symptoms.

Chronic pain. Chronic pain often leads to functional impairment and emotional difficulties; it impacts the lives of over 76 million Americans (National Institutes for Health [NIH], 2013). The prevalence of patients consulting healthcare providers due to chronic pain has dramatically increased in recent years. Prescriptions for opioid pain medications have quadrupled in the past 17 years, and approximately 44 people die each day in the United States of a prescription opioid overdose (CDC, 2015). Chronic pain is often a challenging clinical disorder for Internal Medicine providers to treat and, as such, often leaves both providers and patients frustrated. MedFTs can be instrumental in assisting patients and providers in decreasing frustration and developing helpful care strategies. MedFTs may teach providers about evidence-based psychosocial chronic pain treatment strategies that can be used in lieu of or in conjunction with medication therapy. MedFTs can also work directly with patients and their families to provide education about the biopsychosocial experience(s) of pain. Pain education can help to normalize the physical, emotional, and social impacts that pain has on patients' lives. Additionally, MedFTs may teach management strategies for coping with pain, such as relaxation techniques, scheduling pleasurable activities, and tracking pain to discover activities and/or interventions that are associated with decreased levels of pain.

Medical Collaborator Knowledge Base

Collaboration between MedFTs, patients, and medical providers is one of the most instrumental aspects of providing successful, effective care that attends to biomedical and psychosocial aspects of the patient and family experience (McDaniel, Doherty, & Hepworth, 2014). In Internal Medicine settings, facilitating communication between patients and providers is an instrumental aspect of a MedFT's role. Ideally, for collaborative efforts between professionals on the healthcare team to yield positive results, medical and behavioral health providers should communicate with one another on a consistent basis about patient care (McDaniel et al., 2014). Understanding differences in training, professional goals, and ways of thinking can help medical and behavioral health providers work together in a way that invites effective communication and, ultimately, effective patient care. Recognizing the educational background, the hierarchical relationships between Internal Medicine providers (e.g., attending physicians supervise resident physicians), vocabulary, and treatment goals of team members can improve collaborative relationships.

Sensitivity to Diversity

Many patients cared for in Internal Medicine settings experience unemployment, poverty, lack of access to transportation needed to procure healthy food options and needed medication, and lack of health insurance. MedFTs and other members of the Internal Medicine healthcare team must take these determinants of health into account when developing effective assessment and intervention strategies with patients and families. For example, if a patient decides they would like to increase exercise, asking that they join a gym and drive to the gym each day would not be an effective intervention if the patient does not have access to reliable transportation (to get to the gym) or money (to pay for membership fees).

Clinical Evaluation

While not the focus of this chapter, learning how to design and carry out research projects to evaluate the impact of clinical work is needed. It is important for MedFTs to know how clinical care enhances both the system in which they work (e.g., financial impact, medical provider well-being) and the lives of patients and families for whom they provide care (e.g., improved metabolic control (A1C), improved quality of life). Through evaluation, MedFTs can continually modify existing clinical programs or create new programs that effectively and efficiently meet patient, family, and medical system needs.

Internal Medicine Across the MedFT Healthcare Continuum

The Medical Family Therapy Healthcare Continuum, developed by Hodgson, Lamson, Mendenhall, and Tyndall (2014), provides a helpful framework that can be used to highlight necessary skills and knowledge for MedFT providers in Internal Medicine settings. Tables 4.1 and 4.2 contain overviews of the skills and knowledge that MedFTs providing clinical care in Internal Medicine should possess at each level of the continuum.

At *Level 1*, MedFTs know about the interplay between the most common health conditions seen in Internal Medicine primary care clinics (e.g., heart disease, hypertension) and psychosocial difficulties (e.g., anxiety and depression). They are versed in the ways in which patients' family members and friends impact and are impacted by patients' illness and resulting lifestyle changes. MedFTs at this level can name some of the Internal Medicine team members in both hospital and primary care settings but may have a limited understanding of the role each member plays on the healthcare team. They can collaborate with an Internal Medicine healthcare team member when deemed absolutely necessary for patient care. In Maria's case, a

Table 4.1 MedFTs in Internal Medicine: Basic Knowledge and Skills

MedFT Healthcare Continuum Level	Level 1	Level 2	Level 3
Knowledge	Can name the common medical difficulties treated in Internal Medicine settings. Has a basic knowledge of the biopsychosocial and systemic impact of common health difficulties (e.g., diabetes mellitus, heart disease) but does not generally apply this knowledge to clinical work with patients. Minimal understanding of the roles held by members of an Internal Medicine team of providers.	Holds a general knowledge of the physical limitations and lifestyle changes that often accompany common medical difficulties treated in Internal Medicine settings. Knows about the impact lifestyle (e.g., diet and exercise) has on health and illness. Some understanding of the roles held by members of an Internal Medicine team of providers, but limited interaction or collaboration. Basic understanding of the role brief psychosocial interventions can play in promoting patient and family well-being in Internal Medicine settings.	Understands the roles and responsibilities of each member on the Internal Medicine care team. Recognizes the reciprocal relationship between family function and patients' experienced common medical difficulties. Can articulate the positive impact health behavior change may have for patients with the most common diagnoses treated in Internal Medicine settings.
Skills	Can collaborate with Internal Medicine team members when deemed absolutely necessary, but does not participate in routine collaboration.	Able to provide individual psychotherapy with patients diagnosed with acute or chronic medical difficulty, using a biopsychosocial lens.	Can provide effective couple and family psychotherapy with patients and families with acute or chronic illness, using a biopsychosocial and systemic lens, and can also provide effective, brief psychosocial interventions. Adept at collaborating with Internal Medicine providers regarding patient care and providing referrals to specialists (e.g., substance abuse, dietetics) as determined by patient need.

Table 4.2 MedFTs in Internal Medicine: Advanced Knowledge and Skills

MedFT Healthcare Continuum Level	Level 4	Level 5
Knowledge	Can articulate the types of physical symptoms, medication regimens, tests, and general treatment associated with medical difficulties treated in Internal Medicine settings.	Understands many of the complexities associated with comorbid health conditions and how theses complexities impact patient and family well-being.
	Holds a basic knowledge of Internal Medicine team member perspectives on patient care and reasons behind choosing specific treatment plans.	Remains cognizant of medical provider perspectives.
	Has a working knowledge of types of medical treatment that takes place in hospital and primary care settings.	
Skills	Attends to the well-being of the healthcare system and members of the healthcare team.	Generates collaborative treatment plans with members of the healthcare team.
	Practices evidence-based integrated behavioral health care that includes brief psychosocial interventions during patient medical encounters and brief biopsychosocial and systemic psychotherapy that attends to the interplay between the patient, family, medical system, and illness.	Able to participate in facilitating transitions of psychosocial care from hospital to primary care settings. Measures the effectiveness of psychosocial interventions and is able to modify how or which type of care is provided based on outcomes.
	Consistently collaborates with each medical provider on the Internal Medicine care team (e.g., primary care provider, nurse case manager, diabetes educator).	

MedFT practicing at this level would have a base of knowledge about the ways in which Maria's ability to care for her diabetes may be impacted by her feelings of being overwhelmed and down. They would also know that Maria's husband's adjustment to her illness and his psychosocial well-being would impact Maria's own psychosocial adjustment and illness management.

MedFTs practicing at *Level 2* hold a basic understanding about the physical difficulties and limitations that stem from specific medical illnesses treated in Internal Medicine inpatient and outpatient healthcare settings. They know that patients' health behaviors impact illness. MedFTs at this level hold a basic understanding of the functions of many members on the healthcare team. They are able to provide individual psychotherapy with patients diagnosed with acute or chronic illness and maintain a basic understanding of the benefits of brief psychosocial interventions. A MedFT at *Level 2* would be readily able to assist Maria and her family by providing brief psychosocial assessment and intervention for Maria during her medical visits. They would also be able to provide follow-up psychotherapy for Maria to help her adjust to her illness and promote health behavior change.

At *Level 3*, MedFTs understand the roles and responsibilities of each member of the Internal Medicine care team. They can discuss the impacts that health behaviors have on illness and health for many of the illnesses treated in Internal Medicine settings. *Level 3* MedFTs provide effective psychotherapy with patient and families, taking into consideration BPS and systemic components of patient and family experience. These MedFTs are adept at collaborating with Internal Medicine providers regarding patient care, and they are able to provide appropriate referrals to specialists (e.g., substance abuse counselors, dieticians). In our clinical vignette example, a MedFT at this level could work with Maria and her family to help them discover ways in which current health behaviors may be impacting Maria's physical symptoms. They could discern and collaborate with appropriate members of the healthcare team regarding the specific barriers to care Maria and her family are experiencing (e.g., financial barriers, lack of health-related knowledge).

MedFTs practicing at *Level 4*, which is the beginning of advanced practice, are able to articulate the physical symptoms, medication regimens, diagnostic tests, and treatment regimens associated with the most common medical difficulties treated in Internal Medicine settings. These MedFTs have a working knowledge of the perspectives on patient care that members of the healthcare team hold. They attend to patient and family needs and recognize and promote the well-being of the medical team within which they function. A MedFT at this level practices evidence-based behavioral health care and is able to facilitate individual, couple, and family psychotherapy, in addition to brief psychosocial interventions during patients' medical visits. These MedFTs also collaborate frequently with each member of the healthcare team. In Maria's case, a *Level 4* MedFT would assess and intervene with Maria, her husband, and her son to promote optimal systemic function. They would also use their understanding of Maria's various disease processes to help create appropriate interventions. For example, because Maria has been managing diabetes and obesity, evidence-based interventions such as motivational interviewing may be employed to assist the family with health behavior change that could promote management of multiple comorbid conditions.

At *Level 5*, MedFTs understand many complexities associated with comorbid and complex health conditions and recognize the ways in which these complexities impact patient and family well-being. MedFTs at this level remain aware of the perspectives of team members and collaborate consistently regarding patient care, including generating collaborative treatment plans with members of the healthcare team. These MedFTs can facilitate psychosocial care transitions between Internal Medicine settings. They are also adept at measuring the effectiveness of clinical interventions and modifying treatment based on outcomes. A MedFT practicing at this level could provide education for Maria and her family on the ways in which

Maria's health complexities may be impacting her emotional well-being and family functioning. This MedFT could also work with the PCP, hospitalist, diabetes educator, and social worker involved in Maria's care to develop a BPS treatment plan that attends to each aspect of Maria and her family's illness experience. As part of ongoing care, this MedFT could also utilize assessment tools to measure improvements in family functioning across time.

Research-Informed Practices

There are many approaches to psychosocial care that could be used in Internal Medicine settings. Examples of brief research-informed approaches and interventions that are well suited for use in Internal Medicine are highlighted below. The common themes between all of the chosen approaches are that they can be carried out in a short period of time and can be used to address systemic components of the patient and family experience. The following approaches can be applied systemically, regardless of how many people are in the room:

Individual, Couple, and Family Approaches

Fast-paced Internal Medicine settings are conducive to brief psychosocial interventions, delivered in 5–20-minute brief encounters during patients' medical visits and brief, goal-oriented psychotherapy sessions. Research suggests that brief interventions are effective in working with people with multiple health difficulties such as diabetes (Osborn et al., 2010) and substance use/abuse (Kaner et al., 2009), which are commonly seen in Internal Medicine. Furthermore, expanding brief interventions to include patients' family systems can lead to better overall BPS outcomes for patients and their families because systemic interventions can target adjustment and coping at both the individual and family system levels (Campbell, 2003; Chesla, 2010; Lister, Fox, & Wilson, 2013; Yorgason et al., 2010). For example, brief systemic interventions can lower anxiety and depressive symptoms among patients and their family members (Chesla, 2010) and can increase individual and family involvement in chronic illness management (Campbell, 2003).

Therapeutic relationship. The therapeutic relationship is largely responsible for the outcome of psychosocial interventions and is a significant contributor to creating positive change (Blow, Sprenkle, & Davis, 2007). Thus, the most important part of working with patients and families in Internal Medicine is that MedFTs are able to rapidly build rapport, regardless of therapeutic approach. MedFTs who are positive, convey warmth and affirmation, refrain from attacking and blaming, and stay away from critical and rejecting actions are generally the most successful in building relationships.

Motivational interviewing. Motivational interviewing (MI) is a collaborative clinical approach that focuses on resolving patient ambivalence and eliciting patients' motivations for making health-promoting behavior change. MI techniques include providing empathy, asking open-ended questions, giving positive affirmations, using reflective listening, and summarizing patient remarks, including the patient's motivations for change (Rollnick, Miller, & Butler, 2008). Research has found that MI can be used effectively in patient encounters as brief as 15 minutes (Rubak, Sandaek, Lauritzen, & Christiansen, 2005), making it an ideal intervention for Internal Medicine settings. MI is an effective intervention for many presenting patient difficulties commonly seen in Internal Medicine settings, including substance abuse/use (Bernstein et al., 2005), medication adherence difficulties (Palacio et al., 2016), and weight-related problems (Rubak et al., 2005). Engaging the patient's family using MI can be done by asking a present family member directly about his/her own ideas and insights into potentially beneficial changes that the patient and family can make to improve well-being. If family members are not present, the MedFT can ask the patient questions about how the family can be involved in change plans and how the patient's relationships can either facilitate or hinder progress toward desired goals.

Solution-focused therapy. Solution-focused therapy (SFT) helps patients and families to use strengths and resources to move away from problems and toward identified solutions. Basic principles of SFT include: the patient is the expert; if it isn't broken, don't fix it; if something works, continue doing it; and if something doesn't work, do something else (de Shazer, 1985). Using SFT, MedFTs can help patients and families with eliciting solutions to problems and developing strategies to move away from problems and toward identified solutions and future possibilities. Multiple groups of researchers have found that using SFT is an effective strategy for helping people with medical issues such as diabetes (Viner, Christie, Taylor, & Hey, 2003), pain (Simm, Iddon, & Barker, 2014), and the difficult impacts of addictions (Smock et al., 2008)—all of which are frequently the foci of care provided in Internal Medicine. Patients and families can take part in discussing possible strategies for movement away from problems and toward solutions. With Maria and her family, MedFTs can discuss how each family member can be included in strategies to improve Maria's well-being and strategies to help the family reach their goal of traveling. The MedFT may also task the family with having a conversation about developed goals with medical professionals with whom they interact during future appointments.

Relaxation strategies. Relaxation strategies are commonly used for reducing symptoms associated with depression, anxiety, and pain (Finlay & Rogers, 2015; Klainin-Yobas, Oo, & Lau, 2015). Progressive muscle relaxation (PMR) is a particularly effective strategy that is easy to teach to patients and families in a short period of time. PMR involves the purposeful, systematic tensing and relaxing of each large muscle group in the body (Bernstein & Borkovec, 1973). Patients learn the exercise in the clinical setting, practice at home, and follow-up on success or barriers to success with members of the healthcare team at subsequent appointments. If family members or friends are present, they can be included in learning the exercise. If they are not present, the MedFT can ask the patient to name at least one person with whom they can practice this skill before their next medical visit.

Guided imagery is a relaxation technique in which patients visualize pleasant images while focusing on associated physical experiences in their bodies (Abdoli, Rahzani, Safaie, & Sattari, 2012). Guided imagery can lead to decreases in anxiety and pain symptoms, alongside improving sleep and overall life quality (Chen & Francis, 2010). Patients can learn guided imagery during the medical encounter, with instructions to practice it on a regular schedule. As with PMR, the MedFT can ask the patient to think about one person with whom they can practice guided imagery and develop a plan for meeting with this person to practice this skill together.

Screening, brief intervention, and referral to treatment approach (SBIRT). SBIRT is a public health approach that is used to identify, prevent, and reduce risky substance use and abuse. Following this protocol, patients are asked to complete brief assessments about substance use habits and participate in a brief motivational interviewing intervention and are provided with a referral to specialty substance use treatment as needed. SBIRT can reduce risky drinking, reduce dangerous behaviors associated with substance use, and improve health outcomes (CDC, 2014b). MedFTs can include the patient's family members in a discussion about possible reasons for cutting down on drinking or drug use. If a family member is not present during the patient's medical encounter, MedFTs can discuss with the patient the possible impacts that substance use has on important relationships.

Goal setting/action plans. Goal setting and creating action plans with patients and families is one of the hallmarks of psychosocial interventions in Internal Medicine settings. Action plans with specific patient goals can help patients in their quest to create behavior change (Handley et al., 2006). Assisting patients with creating small, specific goals can be accomplished in a short period of time (5–10 minutes) and can provide patients with a clear framework for steps they can take to improve well-being. Using a systemic lens to develop an action plan, MedFTs can assist patients in developing useful goals that include family members and friends. For example, if a patient wishes to increase exercise, the MedFT can ask the patient if a family member or friend might be interested in exercising with them. The MedFT can also request that the patient chooses a family member with whom s/he can discuss healthcare goals and plans for achieving set goals. Documenting action plans in the patient's electronic medical record allows each member of the healthcare team to remain aware of patient's goals. This also gives team members the ability to check in with patients on progress toward goal achievement and facilitators and barriers to reaching goals at each subsequent visit.

The aforementioned are examples and may be employed as stand-alone interventions or in tandem. For example, although listed separately, solution-focused therapy and motivational interviewing interventions and objectives have a lot in common and can be used together effectively (Sterminsky & Brown, 2014).

Community Approaches

The community in which patients and families reside holds many resources that, when utilized to their full potential, can provide a variety of helpful support opportunities. Support groups, in person or online, exist for people with specific medical conditions, behavioral health and substance use difficulties, and for caregivers. These group experiences can provide much-needed outlets to discuss multifaceted and complex illness experiences. Many hospital systems provide support groups on different topics that patients and their families can attend. Also, religious communities, get-togethers for people with shared interests (e.g., hiking, painting), and other social gatherings can increase social interaction. As previously mentioned, these experiences can enhance both emotional well-being and physical well-being (Hawkley et al., 2010; Jaremka et al., 2012). Maria may benefit, for example, from an online support group in which she is able to connect with other people who have experienced an amputation. She could share the grief she feels regarding the loss of her foot and ask the group for suggestions of practical strategies she might use to participate in activities she enjoys.

Conclusion

MedFTs greatly enhance patient and family care as members of a multidisciplinary Internal Medicine care team. Because MedFTs focus on BPS and systemic components of health and illness experiences (McDaniel et al., 2014), they are uniquely positioned to provide critical components of care for the complex patient and family needs that present in Internal Medicine settings. Through purposefully assimilating into the Internal Medicine culture, MedFTs play an important role in providing psychosocial assessment and intervention for patients and families and facilitating and enhancing communication between patients and families and members of the healthcare team.

Reflection Questions
1. How might you retain positive regard for patients and families (and manage your own potential feelings of frustration) when patients continue to participate in behaviors that lead to poor health?
2. As you begin to practice in an Internal Medicine setting, how can you learn to effectively provide brief psychosocial interventions and brief therapy? How will you choose which models of care and specific interventions are the best fit for the patient populations with whom you work?
3. Think about a specific patient and family with whom you have provided clinical care that would likely be seen in an Internal Medicine setting. With the com-

plexities of illness and subsequent patient and family experiences, how can you attend to the large array of patient and family needs? Which resources do you need to include when providing care for this family system?

Glossary of Important Terms for Care in Internal Medicine

Acute An acute complaint occurs for less than 2 weeks (e.g., cough or cold symptoms); acute visits are typically for a new, quickly arising problem that cannot wait until the next scheduled visit.

Adherence The extent to which medications and healthcare regimens prescribed by healthcare providers are followed by patients. For example, providers ask patients to adhere to taking medications, following diet plans, and increasing exercise.

Attending physician A physician who has completed all medical training and serves as the provider of record. Attending physicians supervise residents and medical students; they are ultimately responsible for the patient care residents and medical students provide.

Chronic A complaint occurring for 3–4 weeks or more. This may be a disease that patients still have, thought it may be managed with medication (e.g., hypertension), or may be a complaint that has persisted over time (e.g., cough for 2 months); chronic visits are typically for management of ongoing medical conditions.

Differential diagnosis A short list of possible diagnoses. As internists are working through potential diagnoses to consider, they may discuss the differential diagnosis for a patient. This can occur during an H&P or with a new problem presented by a patient. This term is generally used while diagnostic labs or studies are still pending.

History and Physical (H&P) Evaluation that is completed by medical doctors, including internists, and serves as the complete evaluation of a patient, including the patient's story of events and physical exam findings.

Progress/Encounter note Typical documentation done by a member of the care team after the patient visit, highlighting which issues were discussed, physical exam or lab findings, and assessment and care plan moving forward.

Resident physician A physician who has completed an undergraduate college degree and 4 years of medical school and is essentially in an apprenticeship position. They work semi-independently, depending on skill level. An attending physician either directly observes, is available to join, or is available via telephone to provide supervision and instruction. Internal medicine residency is 3 years.

Vital signs Physical exam/data that include temperature, heart rate, respiratory rate, and blood pressure. At times, other objective measures may be added, including weight or pulse oximetry (measure of oxygen level in the blood).

Additional Resources

Literature

Galanti, G. (2014). *Caring for patients from different cultures.* Philadelphia, PA: University of Pennsylvania Press.
McDaniel, S. H., Campbell, T. L., Hepworth, J., & Lorenz, A. (2005). *Family-oriented primary care.* New York, NY. Springer.
Miller, W. R. & Rollnick, S. (2013). *Motivational interviewing: Helping people change* (3rd ed.). New York, NY: Guilford Press.
Oyama, O., & Burg, M. A. (2016). *The behavioral health specialist in primary care: Skills for integrated practice.* New York, NY: Springer.
Peek, C. & National Integration Academy Council. (2013). *Lexicon for behavioral health and primary care integration: Concepts and definitions developed by expert consensus.* (AHRQ Publication No.13-IP001-EF). Retrieved from http://integrationacademy.ahrq.gov/sites/default/files/Lexicon.pdf
Rollnick, S., Miller, W. R., & Butler, C. C. (2008). *Motivational interviewing in health care: Helping patients change behavior.* New York, NY: Guilford Press.

Measures/Instruments

Alcohol Use Disorders Identification Test (AUDIT). http://www.talkingalcohol.com/files/pdfs/WHO_audit.pdf
Drug Abuse Screening Test (DAST-7). https://www.drugabuse.gov/sites/default/files/files/DAST-10.pdf
Generalized Anxiety Disorder 7-Item Scale (GAD-7). http://www.integration.samhsa.gov/clinical-practice/GAD708.19.08Cartwright.pdf
Patient Health Questionnaire-9 (PHQ-9). http://www.phqscreeners.com/

Organizations/Associations

American College of Physicians. https://www.acponline.org/
Collaborative Family Healthcare Association. http://www.cfha.net/
Society of General Internal Medicine. http://www.sgim.org/

References[1]

Abdoli, S. A., Rahzani, K., Safaie, M., & Sattari, A. (2012). A randomized control trial: The effect of guided imagery with tape and perceived happy memory on chronic tension type headache. *Scandinavian Journal of Caring Sciences, 26*, 254–226. https://doi.org/10.1111/j.1471-6712.2011.00926.x

Ansseau, M., Dierick, M., Buntinkx, F., Cnockaert, P., De Smedt, J., Van Den Haute, M., & Mijnsbrugge, D. (2004). High prevalence of mental disorders in primary care. *Journal of Affective Disorders, 78*, 49–55. https://doi.org/10.1016/SO165-0327(02)00219-7

Bernstein, E. A., & Borkovec, T. D. (1973). *Progressive relaxation training: A manual for the helping professions*. Champaign, IL: Research Press.

Bernstein, J., Bernstein, E., Tassiopoulos, K., Herren, T., Levenson, S., & Hingson, R. (2005). Brief motivational intervention at a clinic visit reduces cocaine and heroin use. *Journal of Drug and Alcohol Dependency, 7*, 49–59. https://doi.org/10.1016/j.drugalcdep.2004.07.006

Blount, A. (2003). Integrated primary care: Organizing the evidence. *Families, Systems & Health, 21*, 121–134. https://doi.org/10.1037/1091-7527.21.2.121

Blow, A. J., Sprenkle, D. H., & Davis, S. D. (2007). Is who delivers the treatment more important than the treatment itself? The role of the therapist in common factors. *Journal of Marital and Family Therapy, 33*, 298–317. https://doi.org/10.1111/j.1752-0606.2007.00029.x

Campbell, T. (2003). The effectiveness of family interventions for physical disorders. *Journal of Marital and Family Therapy, 29*, 263–281. https://doi.org/10.1111/j.1752-0606.2003.tb01204.x

Centers for Disease Control and Prevention. (2014a). *Health, United States, 2014- individual charts and tables: Spreadsheets, PDF, and PowerPoint files*. Retrieved from http://www.cdc.gov/nchs.hus/contents2014.htm#085

Centers for Disease Control and Prevention. (2014b). *Alcohol screening and counseling: An effective but underused health service*. Retrieved from http://www.cdc.gov/vitalsigns/www.cdc.gov/vitalsigns/

Centers for Disease Control and Prevention. (2015). *Understanding the epidemic*. Retrieved from http://www.cdc.gov/drugoverdose/epidemic/index.html

Chauvet-Gelinier, J. C., & Bonin, B. (2017). Stress, anxiety and depression in heart disease patients: A major challenge for cardiac rehabilitation. *Annals of Physical and Rehabilitation Medicine, 60*, 6–12. https://doi.org/10.1016/j.rebah.2016.09.002

Chen, Y. L., & Francis, A. J. P. (2010). Relaxation and imagery for chronic, nonmalignant pain: Effects on pain symptoms, quality of life and mental health. *Pain Management Nursing, 11*, 159–168. https://doi.org/10.1016/j.pmn.2009.05.005

Chesla, C. A. (2010). Do family interventions improve health? *Journal of Family Nursing, 16*, 355–377. https://doi.org/10.1177/1074840710383145

Cohen, S., Doyle, W. J., Turner, R., Alper, C. M., & Skoner, D. P. (2003). Sociability and susceptibility to the common cold. *Psychological Science, 14*, 389–395. https://doi.org/10.1111/1467-9280.01452

de Shazer, S. (1985). *Keys to solution in brief therapy*. New York, NY: Norton.

Dikeos, D., & Georgantopoulos, G. (2011). Medical comorbidity of sleep disorders. *Current Opinion in Psychiatry, 24*, 346–354. https://doi.org/10.1097/yco.0b013e3283473375

Doherty, W. J., McDaniel, S. H., & Baird, M. A. (1996). Five levels of primary care/behavioral healthcare collaboration. *Behavioral Healthcare Tomorrow*, October Edition, 25–28. Retrieved from http://in.bgu.ac.il/en/fohs/communityhealth/Family/Documents/ShlavB/physician%20involvement%20with%20families.pdf

Dumit, J. (2005). Illnesses you have to fight to get: Facts as forces in uncertain, emergent illness. *Social Science & Medicine, 62*, 577–590. https://doi.org/10.1016/j.socscimed.2005.06.018

---

[1] Note: References that are prefaced with an asterisk are recommended readings.

Edwards, T. M., Stern, A., Clarke, D. D., Ivbijaro, G., & Kasney, L. M. (2010). The treatment of patients with medically unexplained symptoms in primary care: A review of the literature. *Mental Health in Family Medicine, 7,* 209–221. Retrieved from http://eds.a.ebscohost.com/eds/pdfviewer/pdfviewer?sid=641e1740-5f4a-4786-a0ab-0eea6f11c28a%40sessionmgr4010&vid=2&hid=4210

Engel, G. L. (1977). The need for a new medical model: A challenge for biomedicine. *Science, 196,* 129–136. https://doi.org/10.1016/b978-0-409-95009-0.50006-1

Finlay, K. A., & Rogers, J. (2015). Maximizing self-care through familiarity: The role of practice effects in enhancing music listening and progressive muscle relaxation for pain management. *Psychology of Music, 43,* 511–529. https://doi.org/10.1177/0305735613513311

*Galanti, G. (2014). *Caring for patients from different cultures.* Philadelphia, PA: University of Pennsylvania Press.

Glozier, N., Tofler, G. H., Colquhoun, D. M., Bunker, S. J., Clarke, D. M., Hare, D. L., ... Branagan, M. G. (2013). Psychosocial risk factors for coronary heart disease. *Medical Journal of Australia, 199,* 179–180. https://doi.org/10.5694/mja13.10440

*Handley, M., MacGregor, K., Schillinger, D., Sharifi, C., Wong, S., & Bodenheimer, T. (2006). Using action plans to help primary care patients adopt healthy behaviors: A descriptive study. *Journal of the American Board of Family Medicine, 19,* 224–231. https://doi.org/10.3122/jabfm.19.3.224.

*Harsh, J., Hodgson, J., White, M. B., Lamson, A. L., & Irons, T. G. (2015). Medical residents' experiences with medically unexplained illness and medically unexplained symptoms. *Qualitative Health Research, 26,* 1091–1101. https://doi.org/10.1177/1049732315578400.

Hawkley, L. C., Thisted, R. A., Masi, C. M., & Cacioppo, J. T. (2010). Loneliness predicts increased blood pressure: Five-year cross-lagged analyses in middle-aged and older adults. *Psychology and Aging, 25,* 132–141. https://doi.org/10.1037/a0017805

*Hodgson, J., Lamson, A., Mendenhall, T., & Tyndall, L. (2014). Introduction to medical family therapy: Advanced applications. In J. Hodgson, A. Lamson, T. Mendenhall., and D. Crane (Eds.). *Medical family therapy: Advanced applications* (pp. 1–9). New York, NY: Springer.

Jaremka, L. M., Fagundes, C. P., Glaser, R., Bennett, J. M., Malarkey, W. B., & Kiecolt-Glaser, J. K. (2012). Loneliness predicts pain, depression, and fatigue: Understanding the role of immune dysregulation. *Psychoneuroendocrinology, 38,* 1310–1317. https://doi.org/10.1016/j.psyneuen.2012.11.016

Jencks, S. F., Williams, M. V., & Coleman, E. A. (2009). Rehospitalizations among patients in the Medicare fee-for-service program. *New England Journal of Medicine, 360,* 1418–1428. https://doi.org/10.1056/NEJMsa0803563

Kaner, E. N., Dickinson, H. O., Beyer, F., Pienaar, E., Schlesinger, C., Campbell, F., ... Heather, N. (2009). The effectiveness of brief alcohol interventions in primary care settings: A systematic review. *Drug & Alcohol Review, 28,* 301–323. https://doi.org/10.1111/j.1465-3362.2009.00071.x

*Katon, W. J. (2003). Clinical and health services relationships between major depression, depressive symptoms, and general medical illness. *Biological Psychiatry, 54,* 216–226. https://doi.org/10.1016/s0006-3223(03)00273-7.

*Katz, D., & McHorney, C. A. (2002). The relationship between insomnia and health-related quality of life in patients with chronic illness. *Journal of Family Practice, 51,* 229–235. Retrieved from http://pmmp.cnki.net/Resources/CDDPdf/evd%5Cbase%5CJournal%20of%20Family%20Practice%5C%E6%A8%AA%E6%96%AD%E9%9D%A2%E7%A0%94%E7%A9%B6%5Cjfp20025103229.pdf

Kessler, R., Chiu, W., Demler, O., & Walters, E. (2005). Prevalence, severity, and comorbidity of twelve-month DSM-IV disorders in the National Comorbidity Survey Replication. *Archives of General Psychiatry, 62,* 617–627. https://doi.org/10.1001/archpsyc.62.6.617

Klainin-Yobas, P., Oo, W. N., & Lau, Y. (2015). Effects of relaxation interventions on depression and anxiety among older adults: A systematic review. *Aging and Mental Health, 19,* 1043–1055. https://doi.org/10.1080/13607863.2014.997191

*Lister, Z. C., Fox, C., & Wilson, C.M. (2013). Couples and diabetes: A 30-year narrative review of dyadic relational research. *Contemporary Family Therapy: An International Journal, 35*, 613–638. https://doi.org/10.1007/s10591-013-9250-x.
*McDaniel, S. H., Campbell, T. L., Hepworth, J., & Lorenz, A. (2005). *Family-oriented primary care*. New York, NY: Springer.
*McDaniel, S. H., Doherty, W. J., & Hepworth. (2014). *Medical family therapy and integrated care* (2nd ed.). Washington, DC: American Psychological Association.
*Miller, W. R. & Rollnick, S. (2013). *Motivational interviewing: Helping people change* (3rd ed.). New York, NY: Guilford Press.
Morin, C., LeBlanc, M., Daley, M., Gregoire, J. P., & Merette, C. (2006). Epidemiology of insomnia: Prevalence, self-help treatments, consultations and determinants of help-seeking behaviors. *Sleep Medicine, 7*, 123–130. https://doi.org/10.1016/j.sleep.2005.08.008
Murri, B. M., Mamberto, S., Briatore, L., Mazzucchelli, C., Amore, M., & Cordera, R. (2017). The interplay between diabetes, depression and affective temperaments: A structural equation model. *Journal of Affective Disorders, 219*, 64–71. https://doi.org/10.1016/j.jad.2017.05.018
National Association of Social Workers (2011). *Social workers in hospital & medical settings*. Retrieved from http://workforce.socialworkers.org/studies/profiles/Hospitals.pdf
National Institutes of Health. (2013). *Chronic pain*. Retrieved from https://report.nih.gov/nihfactsheets/ViewFactSheet.aspx?csid=57
Nettleton, S. (2006). 'I just want permission to be ill': Towards a sociology of medically unexplained symptoms. *Social Science & Medicine, 62*, 1167–1178. https://doi.org/10.1016/j.socscimed.2005.07.030
Ogden, C. L., Carroll, M. D., Kit, B. K., & Flegal, K. M. (2014). Prevalence of childhood and adult obesity in the United States, 2011-2012. *Journal of the American Medical Association, 311*, 806–814. https://doi.org/10.1097/01.sa.0000451505.72517.a5
Osborn, C. Y., Amico, K. R., Cruz, N., O'Connell, A. A., Perez-Escamilla, R., Kalichman, S. C., … Fisher, J. D. (2010). A brief culturally tailored intervention for Puerto Ricans with Type 2 Diabetes. *Health Education and Behavior, 37*, 849–862. https://doi.org/10.1177/1090198110366004
*Oyama, O., & Burg, M. A. (2016). *The behavioral health specialist in primary care: Skills for integrated practice*. New York, NY: Springer.
*Palacio, A., Garay, D., Langer, B., Taylor, J., Wood, B. A., & Tamariz, L. (2016). Motivational interviewing improves medication adherence: A systematic review and meta-analysis. *Journal of General Internal Medicine, 31*, 929–940. https://doi.org/10.1007/s11606-016-3685-3.
*Peek, C. & National Integration Academy Council. (2013). *Lexicon for behavioral health and primary care integration: Concepts and definitions developed by expert consensus*. (AHRQ Publication No.13-IP001-EF). Retrieved from http://integrationacademy.ahrq.gov/sites/default/files/Lexicon.pdf
*Rollnick, S., Miller, W. R., & Butler, C. C. (2008). *Motivational interviewing in health care: Helping patients change behavior*. New York, NY: Guilford Publications.
Rosendal, M., Carlsen, A. H., Rask, M. T., & Moth, G. (2015). Symptoms as the main problem in primary care: A cross-sectional study of the frequency and characteristics. *Scandinavian Journal of Primary Health Care, 33*, 91–99. https://doi.org/10.3109/02813432.2015.1030166
Rubak, S., Sandaek, A., Lauritzen, T., & Christiansen, B. (2005). Motivational interviewing. A systematic review and meta-analysis. *British Journal of General Practice, 55*, 305–312. Retrieved from https://www.ncbi.nlm.nih.gov/pmc/articles/PMC1463134/
*Schultz, R., Sherwood, P. R. (2008). Physical and mental health effects of family caregiving. *American Journal of Nursing, 108*, 23–27. https://doi.org/10.1097/01.NAJ.0000336406.45248.4c.
Simm, R., Iddon, J., & Barker, C. (2014). A community pain service solution-focused pain management programme: Delivery and preliminary outcome data. *British Journal of Pain, 8*, 49–56. https://doi.org/10.1177/2049463713507910

Smock, S. A., Trepper, T. S., Wetchler, J. L., McCollum, E. E., Ray, R., & Pierce, K. (2008). Solution-focused group therapy for level 1 substance abusers. *Journal of Marital and Family Therapy, 34*, 107–120. https://doi.org/10.1111/j.1752-0606.2008.00056.x

*Sterminsky, G., & Brown, K. S. (2014). The perfect marriage: Solution-focused therapy and motivational interviewing in medical family therapy. *Journal of Family Medicine and Primary Care, 3*, 383–387. https://doi.org/10.4103/2249-4863.148117.

Substance Abuse and Mental Health Services Administration-Health Resources and Services Administration Center for Integrated Health Solutions. (2013). *A review and proposed standard framework for levels of integrated healthcare*. Retrieved from http://www.integration.samhsa.gov/integrated-care-models/A_Standard_Framework_for_Levels_of_Integrated_Healthcare.pdf

Vancampfort, D., Koyanagi, A., Hallgren, M., Probst, M., & Stubbs, B. (2017). The relationship between chronic physical conditions, multimorbidity and anxiety in the general population: A global perspective across 42 countries. *General Hospital Psychiatry, 45*, 1–6. https://doi.org/10.1016/j.genhosppsych.2016.11.002

Vgontzas, A. N., Liao, D., Pejovic, S., Calhoun, S., Karataraki, M., & Bixler, E. O. (2009). Insomnia with objective short sleep duration is associated with type 2 diabetes: *A population-based study. Diabetes Care, 32*, 1980–1985. https://doi.org/10.2337/dc09-0284

Viner, R. M., Christie, D., Taylor, V., & Hey, S. (2003). Motivational/solution-focused intervention improves HbA1c in adolescents with type 1 diabetes: A pilot study. *Diabetic Medicine, 20*, 739–742. https://doi.org/10.1046/j.1464-5491.2003.00995.x

Ward, B. W., Schiller, J. S., Goodman, R. A. (2014). *Multiple chronic conditions among US adults: A 2012 update (130389)*. Retrieved from https://www.cdc.gov/pcd/issues/2014/13_0389.htm

Wong, S. S., Abdullah, N., Abdullah, A., Liew, S. M., Ching, S. M., Khoo, E. M., ... Chia, Y. C. (2014). Unmet needs of patients with chronic obstructive pulmonary disease (COPD): A qualitative study on patients and doctors. *BMC Family Practice, 15*, 67–74. https://doi.org/10.1186/1471-2296-15-67

Yorgason, J. B., Roper, S. O., Wheeler, B., Crane, K., Byron, R., Carpenter, L., ... Higley, D. (2010). Older couples' management of multiple-chronic illnesses: Individual and shared perceptions and coping in type 2 diabetes and osteoarthritis. *Families, Systems, & Health, 28*, 30–47. https://doi.org/10.1037/a0019396

Part II
Medical Family Therapy in Secondary Care

Chapter 5
Medical Family Therapy in Intensive Care

Angela Lamson and Jessica Goodman

The history of intensive care units and critical care dates back to the early to mid-1900s. Critical care is commonly described as a form of medical care for patients who have an acute, life-threatening, or medically complex condition or illness which requires a close, constant watch by specialized providers (Fulbrook, 2010; Lakanmaa, Suominenb, Perttila, Puukkae, & Leino-Kilpi, 2012). Most critical care services take place in an environment known as an intensive care unit (ICU).

Critical care exists in a multitude of intensive care specializations, across both pediatric and adult populations. To name a few, neonatal ICUs (NICUs) provide extensive specialized care for newborn babies postdelivery. Once a child is discharged from a healthcare context after delivery and must return for critical care services, he or she would most likely be cared for in a pediatric ICU (PICU). For adults, critical care units include coronary care (CCU), medical–surgical (MSICU), surgical (SICU), neurosurgical (NCC for neurocritical care or NSICU for neurosurgical intensive care), and trauma (TICU) units. Furthermore, there are a number of forms of progressive care units (PACUs) that are aligned with critical care units, including telemetry, step-down, intermediate, and progressive care.

With years of work in attempting to solidify the competencies needed to care for patients in critical care units, as well as controversy over the patient–nurse or provider ratio needed in critical care units, is also a growing focus on the importance and role of family as part of the patient's care team. The inclusion of family and psychosocial support in ICUs is not surprising to most medical family therapists (MedFTs), especially since one of George Engel's earliest publications was in relation to Monica—an infant patient with esophageal atresia who was fed by gastrostomy and

---

A. Lamson (✉) · J. Goodman
Department of Human Development and Family Science, East Carolina University, Greenville, NC, USA
e-mail: lamsona@ecu.edu

whose feeding intake was especially influenced by psychosocial interactions with one happy and one somber medical provider (Engel & Reichsman, 1956).

This chapter includes information for MedFTs that may cut across or be useful within a variety of critical care units (i.e., due to the multitude and levels of critical care services, specific attention is not given to the function of MedFTs in every type of intensive care unit). Details are provided regarding typical treatment team members in critical care, knowledge and skills necessary to work in critical care environments, and research-informed practices in caring for patients, including ways to maximize family involvement. The following segment is a MedFT clinical example from a real case that occurred in a children's hospital.

Clinical Vignette
[Note: This vignette is a compilation of cases representative of treatment in intensive care. All patients' names and/or identifying information have been changed to maintain confidentiality.]

More than a decade ago, a MedFT received a call from a nurse who served as a nurse educator and leader for her unit within a children's hospital. She described a unique need within the hospital; she sensed that the healthcare team was struggling with grief associated with the loss of a long-time pediatric patient. Based on that call, she and the MedFT met in person and discussed some of the interactions she had witnessed between providers and patients as well as among the providers and staff. From this discussion, the MedFT shared with her a curiosity about the role that grief was having in the NICU, PICU, and pediatric units and providers. In particular, the MedFT began to wonder with her about the presence of grief, secondary traumatic stress, burnout, and compassion fatigue.

*Over the next few weeks, that nurse educator pulled together a multidisciplinary team that included nurses, nurse managers, nurse educators, a pharmacist, a chaplain, and a MedFT. They discussed ways to develop education and support for providers when a need was determined, following a trauma or death on the unit. From the biweekly meetings, a doctoral student and MedFT faculty member developed a seminar that would be provided to all interested physician and extenders, mental health, and spiritual providers on the topics of grief, compassion fatigue, and burnout (*Meadors, Lamson, & Sira, 2010*). Nearly 300 providers attended the large psychoeducation sessions. Following these initial seminars, small group sessions were provided as a part of the orientation for the children's hospital. These orientation sessions proved immediately meaningful as some of the newest staff and providers at the hospital stated that they had never experienced death in their professional or personal lives and were most concerned about how to handle the loss of a patient.*

In addition, a program was developed called the HUGS (Hearts United Giving Strength) team. Any provider or staff member within the children's hospital could go to a person on their unit's leadership team and request a HUGS team; these requests typically followed the death of a patient (or series of patient deaths) on a unit. The HUGS team included a team of MedFTs who would come onto the unit, food catered in, and a series of mindfulness practices (soft music, journals, messages for self-care) that were all provided in a designated room on the pediatric intensive care unit (PICU), neonatal intensive care unit (NICU), or pediatric (PEDS) unit. Throughout these sessions, the MedFT would offer a time for a group reflection and rejoicing of a patient(s) who had died or experienced a trauma. Traditional MedFT sessions were made available for any provider who requested support, as well as a way to honor the patient who had passed away (e.g., commonly quilt squares were available in the room so that each provider could draw or write a message to the family of the patient who had died).

The MedFTs were called many times at the start or end of a shift or on weekends to come and provide a HUGS team for providers on the NICU, PICU, or PEDS unit. These experiences were a unique addition; beyond providing MedFT to patients on the units, the MedFTs also cared for the hidden grievers (e.g., providers and staff on these units). The MedFT faculty member had distinctly remembered one experience when she was out of state and received a telephone call that there had been multiple deaths in the NICU within a very short amount of time. Upon her return, the HUGS team came together on the NICU and talked about what these providers were able to do for their own self-care while also extending rituals that were meaningful to the families during an incredible time of loss. In the NICU, pictures were taken of babies with the parents (upon parents' consent) and sent home with the parents, spiritual rituals were offered, and baby blankets were made for each family.

Another vivid experience was the loss of young boy who had struggled with cancer. His death was a reminder to the hospital and larger community of how experiences of grief and voices of collaboration can and do make a difference in honoring the family and the providers who interface with each patient. To this day, an event is celebrated each fall in honor of this child's life. The event that celebrates his life is not isolated; the medical and larger community offer many events throughout the year that celebrate the lives lost in our youngest warriors.

Many of the chapters in this text include examples of how MedFTs interface with providers in direct patient care. In the clinical example above, it is hoped that MedFTs can also learn how to care for the carers. It is important to highlight that the HUGS team, the psychoeducation seminars, and the push to incorporate information about death, grief, compassion fatigue, and burnout into orientation could not have been possible without the vision and passion of a diverse multidisciplinary team.

What Is Intensive Care?

In this section, we define the designations given to intensive care units, describe the types of providers and expertise needed at different levels of ICU care, and provide examples of patient conditions and interventions that MedFTs may encounter. ICUs are located in hospitals that have appropriate resources to ensure that the multifaceted needs of ICU medicine are met (Ramnarayan et al., 2010, Valentin, Ferdinande, & ESICM, 2011). ICUs, or critical care centers, are designated in each of three areas, including by level of care, "academic" or nonacademic," and "open" or "closed" (Haupt et al., 2003). Factors including disorders treated, availability of sophisticated equipment, level of provider specialization, and availability of support services determine which of the three levels critical care centers are designated as, and these factors determine the level of patient acuity that the ICU can serve. ICUs should accommodate at least six beds; however, 8 to 12 beds are considered the optimum number (Valentin et al., 2011). Larger ICUs can be subdivided into separate, specialized subunits of 6 to 8 beds but share geographic, administrative, and facility resources.

Levels of Care

Level 1 critical care centers deliver comprehensive care to critically ill patients experiencing a range of disorders that require hourly and likely invasive monitoring (Nates et al., 2016; Sarode & Hawker, 2014). In level 1 ICUs' sophisticated equipment, specialized nurses and physicians, nurse practitioners, or physician assistants with critical care training must be available at all times. Level 1 centers also provide support services including pharmaceutical, respiratory, nutritional, pastoral care, and social services. The nurse-to-patient ratio in these centers is greater than, or equal to, one nurse for every one or more patients (Nates et al., 2016; Valentin et al., 2011). Examples of interventions that can be provided in a Level 1 center include cerebrospinal fluid drainage for elevated intracranial pressure management, invasive mechanical ventilation, vasopressors, extracorporeal membrane oxygenation, intra-aortic balloon pump, left ventricular assist device, and continuous renal replacement therapy.

Level 2 critical care centers are able to serve unstable patients in need of nursing interventions, laboratory workups, and monitoring every 2–4 hours (Nates et al., 2016). Level 2 centers may be able to deliver comprehensive, high quality care to most critically ill patients (Nates et al., 2016; Sarode & Hawker, 2014). Level 2 centers may have a dearth of specialty care services such as neurosurgical, cardiac surgical, or a trauma program, for example. As a result, Level 2 centers are obliged to have transfer agreements established in advance for patients with specific problems (Warren et al., 2004). The nurse-to-patient ratio in these centers is greater than, or equal to, one nurse for every three or more patients (Nates et al., 2016; Valentin et al., 2011). Examples of interventions that can be provided in a Level 2 center include noninvasive ventilation, IV infusions, and titration of vasodilators or antiarrhythmic substances.

Level 3 centers primarily provide monitoring, initial stabilization of critically ill patients (Nates et al., 2016), or close monitoring of stable patients. Such centers have written policies to address the transfer of critically ill patients to critical care centers that can provide necessary comprehensive critical care (Level 1 or Level 2; Sarode & Hawker, 2014). Level 3 centers care for patients whose conditions are stable but require close monitoring (Nates et al., 2016). The nurse-to-patient ratio in these centers is one nurse for every four or more patients (Nates et al., 2016; Valentin et al., 2011). Examples of interventions that can be provided in a Level 3 center include IV infusions and titration of medications such as vasodilators or antiarrhythmics or necessary laboratory workups that must occur on a regular basis (e.g., every 2–4 hours).

Academic or Nonacademic Categorizations

In addition to levels, critical care centers are given the categorization of academic or nonacademic (Haupt et al., 2003). Level 1 and 2 centers can be classified as having an academic mission through affiliation with a medical, nursing, or other health service school or educational program. In academic facilities, physicians and extenders, nurses, pharmacists, and respiratory therapists have required times whereby they must participate in scholarly pursuits, including clinical and basic research, care reports, and critical thinking. These professionals also need to possess extensive knowledge and teaching skills that enable them to provide education to critical care nursing staff, physicians in training, and staff physicians in the ICU. Nonacademic centers also keep current with changes in the field of critical care through participation in continuing education and maintaining current certification in applicable areas of expertise; however, they are not mandated to attend to scholarly pursuits.

Open or Closed System

Some critical care centers use an added designation of "open," "closed," or a combination of both to define their ICUs (Haupt et al., 2003). Open-system ICUs have committed nursing, pharmacy, and respiratory therapy staff resources, but the physicians and extenders directing the care of ICU patients may have roles and responsibilities outside of the ICU, for example, in other outpatient and inpatient contexts or in the operating room (Chawla & Todi, 2012). In some centers, providers are able to choose whether to consult an intensivist to support patient management, while in others critical care consultation is required for all patients (Haupt et al., 2003). An

ICU is also considered open when any attending physician with the correct hospital admitting privileges can be the patient's physician of record and has definitive responsibility for care quality and coordination (Brilli et al., 2001).

In a closed ICU system, critical care physicians, nurses, pharmacists, respiratory therapists, and other healthcare professionals work together as an ICU-based team (Chawla & Todi, 2012). Intensivists are the attending physician of record for all patients admitted into a closed-system ICU (Skinner, Warrillow, & Denehy, 2015). All other physicians are considered consultants in this system.

Although the 2001 Society of Critical Care Medicine (SCCM) suggested that closed ICU systems produce better ICU outcomes (Brilli et al., 2001), results of an updated study found that closed ICUs were not associated with better outcomes compared to open systems (Weled et al., 2015). Regardless of the type of system, the SCCM recommends that the intensivist and the ICU patient's primary care provider and consultants proactively collaborate in the care of all patients. Both open and closed systems should have an intensivist with authority to intervene and directly care for the critically ill patient in urgent and emergent situations, and all orders regarding ICU patients' care should be channeled through an ICU-based intensivist and his or her extender team (Skinner, Warrillow, & Denehy, 2015). The differences between open and closed ICUs fade when these principles are followed.

Regardless of the level of care, academic or nonacademic, or open or closed systems across ICUs, MedFTs are uniquely positioned for success given their biopsychosocial–spiritual and systemic approach to care (Engel, 1977, 1980; Wright, Watson & Bell, 1996). This is especially important when considering the large, diverse, and often fluctuating composition and size of ICU treatment teams (Baggs, 1993; Baggs, Ryan, Phelps, Richeson, & Johnson, 1992; Baggs, Schmitt, Mushlin, Eldredge, Oaks, & Huston, 1997; Baggs, Schmittm, Mushlin, Mitchell, Eldrege, & Oakes, 1999). MedFTs have the training to support care coordination and deliver a wide range of BPSS-grounded assessments and interventions in tandem with interdisciplinary teams in the ICU. MedFTs are committed to supporting the diverse needs and concerns faced by ICU patients and their families.

Treatment Teams in Intensive Care

A critical care team is specially trained to work in an ICU (Despins, 2009). Delivery of care in ICUs has required an even greater team effort over the past several decades. A critical care team must be self-organizing and able to expand and contract based on sometimes competing needs at any given time (Hawryluck, Espin, Garwood, Evans, & Lingard, 2002). The ICU team typically is comprised of a bedside nurse, respiratory therapist, and physician and can grow to include other disciplines like MedFTs, dietitians, and physical therapists based on the needs of each patient. Levels of collaboration and conflict can fluctuate within the team, not unlike the size and composition of the team.

Optimal patient care requires a collaborative team approach to care delivery among many groups of professionals utilizing a diverse range of interventions, treatments, and procedures (Rose, 2011; Valentin et al., 2011). Collaboration among team members supports joint decision-making, focused on the needs of the patient while at the same time valuing and acknowledging individual members' respective contributions that lead to improved care quality, patient safety, and outcomes (Herbert, 2005; Manojlovich, Antonakos, & Ronis, 2009; Rose, 2011; Zwarenstein & Reeves, 2006). Below, the roles of specific team members often engaged in critical care units are described.

Care and case managers. Care management has been defined as a general concept covering assessment, care planning, coordination, and reviewing of services (Haupt et al., 2003). This is commonly a very patient-centered approach and is distinguished from case management (an activity of advocacy and coordination of services for patients who needs a designated level of support). Upon discharge, case managers typically meet with patients and/or healthcare proxies to talk about medications, oxygen therapy, home care, physical therapy, and/or post-discharge transition to home and follow up care with a primary care provider.

Chaplains. Chaplains are nondenominational clergy members who talk with patients, families, and staff in the hospital. In the ICU, chaplains provide spiritual support and may help find a clergy member of the patient's faith to better support the patient's spiritual needs (Society of Critical Care Medicine, 2016). Chaplains commonly play an important role in end-of-life care. Involving clergy or spiritual leaders during the last 24 hours of a patient's life in the ICU can contribute to greater family satisfaction with spiritual care (Wall, Engelberg, Gries, Glavan, and Curtis, 2007). Additionally, there is a strong association between satisfaction with spiritual care and satisfaction with the total ICU experience.

Child life specialists. Child life specialists may be found in a variety of ICUs but most particularly in NICUs or PICUs. Child life specialists are experts in child development who typically collaborate with other providers to support ill children in the PICU or work with children visiting adult family members or siblings in an ICU, PICU, and NICU (Child Life Council, 2010; Society of Critical Care Medicine, 2016). In their work they often provide theory-based play therapy. Having families and children visit critically ill family members in the ICU has been shown to have wide-ranging positive impacts, including decreased patient anxiety (Sims & Miracle, 2006), decreased intracranial pressure (Bell, 2012), better coping and integration of experiences in the ICU by patients (Clarke & Harrison, 2001), and improved patient and family satisfaction (Khaleghparast et al., 2016). The unhampered presence of supportive loved ones can also improve communication between the patient, family, and providers, understanding of the patient and their condition, patient- and family-centered care, and enhance staff satisfaction (Bell, 2012; Thompson, 2009).

Successful visitation can be supported through such things as supporting staff and families in discussion about their concerns with children visiting the ICU (Hanley & Piazza, 2012); identification of tools that will support visitation, such as educational books for children preparing to visit the ICU; overview of developmental goals; and guidance on appropriate language and explanations to use with children based on their stage of development. A comprehensive plan for introducing children and adolescents to the ICU should include an overview of what the environment is like, the sights and sounds they will experience; changes their family may experience; normalizing responses to visitation; identification of hospital support people available before, during, and after the child or adolescent visit; discussion of why it is important for the child or adolescent to share their feelings about the hospital experience in order to receive needed care and support; and identification of language to describe things, as well as words that they might encounter during their family member's hospitalization.

Critical care nurses. Critical care nurses provide many facets of care to patients in the ICU (Society of Critical Care Medicine, 2016). They are formally trained in intensive care medicine and emergency medicine (Valentin et al., 2011). The critical care nursing staff led by a head nurse, who is responsible for the function and quality of nursing care in the ICU, as well as education and evaluation of the nursing staff's competencies. Critical care nurses are an important part of decision-making processes with the patient, family, and care team (SCCM, 2016). They facilitate dialogue and collaboration among those involved in care, maintain close contact with the patient and family, and work to uphold the patient's wishes.

Critical care nursing practice is focused on a number of areas, including patient assessment, physical care, and oversight of the plan of care (Brilli et al., 2001). This occurs in collaboration with the ICU attending physician. In the ICU, the ratio of patients to bedside nurses is usually 2:1 (Hinds & Watson, 2008). This allows the critical care nursing staff to spend several hours per patient, per shift collecting and integrating information into meaningful patient care (Brilli et al., 2001). Critical care nurses use their experience and critical thinking skills to identify clinical changes and prevent further deterioration in patient health conditions. Critical care nurses possess expertise in organizational leadership and have the ability to implement unit-based protocols, quality improvement, and outcome data based on staff and patient satisfaction (Hillman & Bishop, 2004).

Intensivists. The ICU has a director who is a medical doctor responsible for the administrative and medical management of the ICU (Valentin et al., 2011). Between 75 and 100% of the director's time should be dedicated to the ICU, and they cannot hold other top-level positions within the hospital. Typical prior degree specialties include anesthesiology, internal medicine, or surgery. The director of the ICU is supported by medical doctors qualified in intensive care medicine called intensivists.

Intensivists have academic and clinical training as well as credentials focused on caring for very ill patients (Hinds & Watson, 2008; SCCM, 2016). Intensivists coordinate and lead multidisciplinary, multispecialty critical care teams; act as coordinators of management activities for safe, efficient, timely, and consistent delivery of care in the ICU; delegate authority and responsibilities; and provide resources and administrative leadership for the team (Valentin et al., 2011; Wheelan, Burchill, & Tilin, 2003; Yoo, Edwards, Dean, & Dudley, 2016). Examples of an intensivist's responsibilities may include patient triage based on admission and discharge criteria, discharge planning, development and enforcement of clinical and administrative protocols for the purpose of improving the safe and efficient delivery of clinical care, meeting regulatory requirements in collaboration with other ICU team disciplines, and coordination and support of the implementation of quality improvement activities within the ICU (Brilli et al., 2001).

Intensivists also take on roles in offering emotional support and information to families during patient admissions to the ICU (Brilli et al., 2001). They facilitate and collaborate with other team members including nurses, chaplain services, and social service team members who provide counseling to families. Collaboration with diverse providers is also essential given the likelihood that together they must attend to ethical care issues and decisions. Across all levels of ICU, difficult decisions pertaining to healthcare delivery or life and death alterations are common; thus, intensivists must be prepared to offer information and support to families and other providers in order to assist in making informed decisions regarding the patient's care.

Occupational therapists. Occupational therapists work collaboratively with the treatment team to support the goals for each patient (Kwiecinska, 2008). Interventions may focus on the prevention of problems secondary to the illness, psychological and physiological impacts of treatment in the ICU, or modification of functional capacity or occupational performance. Examples of goals that occupational therapists may set with patients in the ICU include relearning activities of daily skills (such as grooming, feeding, dressing) or instrumental activities of daily living skills (such as balancing a checkbook), rebuilding muscle strength and endurance, or attending to ways to maximize body function in context of the diagnosis or condition (Kwiecinska, 2008). Through these interventions, occupational therapists help patients live as independently as possible (Society of Critical Care Medicine, 2016).

Pharmacists. Pharmacists are experts in a multitude of medicines, their side effects, and potential interactions with daily vitamins, alcohol (or other substances), and environmental factors (e.g., sun exposure) and in counseling needs pertaining to their use. Pharmacists work with the critical care team on prescribed treatments and check on the progress of patients' pharmacotherapy needs during their stay in the ICU (Hinds & Watson, 2008; Society of Critical Care Medicine, 2016). They also help manage pain and discomfort, agitation and sedation, and delirium (Gagnon & Fraser, 2013).

Physical therapists. Physical therapists in the ICU focus on restoring body functionality and maximizing health and wellness involving muscles, bones, tissues, and nerves (Society of Critical Care Medicine, 2016). Physical therapists help patients improve mobility in daily life, for example, walking and going up and down the stairs, by using techniques like stretching and applying heat to reduce pain and swelling. Such assistance is also aimed at preventing permanent physical disability.

Physical therapy interventions commonly utilized in the ICU include therapeutic exercises and functional mobility retraining (Hodgin, Nordon-Craft, McFann, Mealer, & Moss, 2009).

Registered dieticians. Registered dieticians working in the ICU are trained and licensed in nutrition in context of diverse illnesses (Society of Critical Care Medicine, 2016). Registered dieticians collaborate with the care team and the family to help improve the patient's health, particularly when they lack nutrients. Registered dieticians in the ICU direct or perform feedings by the mouth, tube, or vein.

Respiratory therapists. Respiratory therapists in the ICU have special knowledge and experience in healing patients with breathing problems (Society of Critical Care Medicine, 2016). Respiratory therapists focus primarily on management of the patient/ventilator system, airway care, delivery of bronchodilators, monitoring of hemodynamics and blood gases, and the delivery of protocol-regulated respiratory care (Brilli et al., 2001).

Fundamentals of Intensive Care

The following section includes fundamental knowledge and skills that are helpful for MedFTs who work in neonatal intensive care units, pediatric intensive care units, and a variety of critical care units. The majority of content in this section focuses on most common diagnoses in ICU contexts, so that MedFTs are aware of the complexity and prognosis of conditions as they collaborate with patients, families, and diverse healthcare providers.

Neonatal Intensive Care Unit (NICU)

MedFTs' primary work in NICU environments may be in facilitating and modelling integrated behavioral healthcare that connects the biopsychosocial–spiritual needs of a parent/guardian with the child. This work may also include building a model that strengthens efficient and quality interactions between a parent/guardian and the variety of providers and staff. While the MedFT will have very limited direct engagement with the patient in this context, researchers have found extraordinary benefits of integrated behavioral healthcare on babies in the NICU. O'Brien et al. (2013), for example, tested a family integrated care (FIC) model involving parents in the care of their NICU infants (and allows them to participate in the care team) against a control group; they found a 25% increase in weight gain in the FIC babies, an 80% increase in the rate of breastfeeding, a 25% decrease in parental stress, and a significant reduction in nosocomial infection and critical incident reports. In particular, MedFT skills may include assisting parents with building confidence in attending to the nonmedical needs of their baby (e.g., diaper changes, feeding, cleaning/bathing), attending to parents' concerns related to developmental questions about having a new baby with any unexpected health needs, and facilitating integrated behavioral healthcare models. For those who experience the death of a child or patient, skills can also include offering brief therapy for families and/or providers.

In addition to the skills described above, MedFTs should have knowledge of a number of diagnoses that are most prevalent among babies who are cared for in NICUs (e.g., apnea, jaundice, intraventricular hemorrhage, necrotizing enterocolitis, respiratory distress syndrome, and sepsis). MedFTs must be knowledgeable enough about these diagnoses in order to help families process both acute and long-term familial and systemic changes that may occur. MedFTs are also great ambassadors for hope and can help to facilitate solution-based conversations between families and healthcare providers in relation to projected treatments and optimal health.

Researchers have also investigated leading causes of death in NICUs (e.g., congenital malformations (28%), diseases closely associated with perinatal disorders (25%), disorders of the cardiovascular system (18%), and infections (15%)) that MedFTs must be prepared to discuss with bereaving family members and the patient's healthcare team (Widmann et al., 2017). MedFTs are an integral partner with palliative care teams, when needed. MedFTs have taken an important stance to suggest that all patients, regardless of age or severity of diagnoses, deserve the attention received from palliative care services (Williams-Reade et al., 2013a, 2013b).

Apnea. Apnea is a common occurrence with neonatal patients (March of Dimes, 2014; Sleep Education, 2017). Apnea is a pause in breathing that lasts 15–20 (or more) seconds. The most common form of apnea occurs due to disruptions in the central nervous system (Gardner, Carter, Enzman-Hines, & Hernandez, 2011). It is most highly correlated with being born too early (i.e., prior to 34 weeks) or from maintaining a low birth weight. Apnea occurs in approximately 85% of all babies born under two pounds and in 25% of babies born less than 5.5 pounds. It typically appears between the second and seventh day after birth (American Academy of Sleep Medicine, 2017). Interestingly, apnea has not been correlated as a risk factor with sudden infant death syndrome.

Intraventricular hemorrhage (IVH). IVH is the most common type of neonatal intracranial hemorrhage and typically develops within 3 days after delivery. This diagnosis may be reflected through seizures, decreased motor activity, hypotension, and/or bradycardia.

Jaundice. This condition is when babies have a yellowish color to their eyes or skin. Jaundice occurs when the baby's liver is not functioning well due to a form of waste that is not being effectively eliminated from the blood. This is more likely to occur when the baby has a different blood type from his or her mother. Babies may be placed under a special form of lighting to help break down and eliminate the toxin.

Necrotizing enterocolitis (NEC). NEC is a disease of the bowels. Unfortunately, NEC has a very high mortality rate within the NICU (Gregory, DeForge, Natale, Phillips, & Van Marter, 2011). Risk factors that may result in NEC include perinatal stress, prematurity, and hypothermia.

Respiratory distress syndrome (RDS). Distress primarily happens shortly after birth and is particularly prone to those born prematurely. Signs of RDS include shallow respiration, apnea, and grunting noises in attempts to breathe.

Sepsis. While sepsis also occurs in adults, in newborns it differs in types and origins of symptoms. Sepsis in newborns is a toxic condition (bacterial, fungal, parasitic, or viral) that spreads throughout the bloodstream or body tissues. In newborns it can occur because of intergenerational risk factors (e.g., substance use, malnutrition, fever, current urinary tract infection of mother) or neonatal risks (e.g., meconium aspiration, low birth weight, or prematurity) (Gardner, Carter, Enzman-Hines & Hernandez, 2011).

Pediatric Intensive Care Unit (PICU)

According to researchers, essential skills necessary in PICU care include communication and professionalism with families and healthcare professionals (Turner et al., 2013). While this research was written for pediatric critical care medical fellows, it is likely that these skills are just as important for MedFTs, including the ability to

> communicate effectively with patients, families and the public across a broad range of socioeconomic and cultural backgrounds; communicate effectively with physicians, or other health professionals, and health related agencies; work effectively as a member or leader of a health care team or other professional group; maintain comprehensive, timely, and legible records; extend compassion, integrity, and respect for others; responsiveness to patient needs that supersedes self-interest; respect for patient privacy and autonomy, accountability to patients, society, and the profession; and sensitivity and responsiveness to diverse patient populations, including but not limited to diversity in gender, age, culture, race, religion, disabilities, and sexual orientation. (p. 456)

Beyond recognizing the importance of communication and professionalism in pediatric intensive care, an essential element that was punctuated by Turner et al. (2013) is that many residency and fellowship programs have no mechanism to teach fellows about the impact(s) of grief and loss on themselves. As such, MedFTs should be leaders in PICUs in establishing training and retreats for providers as well as for the primary caregivers of children. Topics, such as compassion fatigue and burnout, should be addressed in order to keep these carers as emotionally healthy as possible.

A widespread number of conditions are treated in PICUs, spanning the ages from the time a newborn is discharged from a healthcare context after delivery (or directly after delivery if at-home birth) through 21 years of age. It is not possible to list every condition treated in a PICU context. However, MedFTs in PICUs should be knowledgeable about issues recognized as most prevalent and complex, including severe breathing problems from asthma (respiratory illness are the most common diagnoses treated in PICUs), serious infections (including poisoning), complications of diabetes, childhood cancer, and trauma (e.g., those associated with automobile accidents, near-drowning incidents, and other crises), and childhood-onset chronic conditions like congenital heart abnormalities, cerebral palsy, and chromosomal abnormities (Edwards et al., 2012).

Childhood cancer. Each year approximately 16,000 children aged 0–19 years are diagnosed with cancer (Ward, DeSantis, Robbins, Kohler, & Jemal, 2014). There are numerous types and complexities of cancer that a child and his or her family may face. There are a myriad of experiences that can be encountered by the family throughout treatments, including complex decision-making, engaging with extended family, managing side effects from treatments, and dealing with potential psychosocial challenges associated with care (e.g., long-term care in the hospital, parental/guardian absence from work to be present with child, having to split time between children at home and child at the hospital). Biopsychosocial–spiritual care is necessary with cancer patients and their families in order to reduce the likelihood for depression and post-traumatic stress in relation to the child's experience with the diagnosis, support healthy communication between family members related to systemic changes, and facilitate family involvement through integrated behavioral healthcare throughout the treatment process in the PICU.

Congenital heart abnormalities/diseases (CHDs). About 1 out of every 120 children is born with a congenital hearth abnormality (Hoffman & Kaplan, 2002). There are many types of CHDs that may influence a newborn's life. CHDs occur because too little or too much blood passes through the lungs or too little blood passes through the body. These abnormalities are typically diagnosed during pregnancy or shortly after delivery and commonly last throughout one's life. However, there are some abnormalities that will wane as the child ages. Children with CHDs should be followed by a pediatric cardiologist as indicated.

Endocrine disorders. While Type 1 and Type 2 diabetes are likely the most recognized names aligned with endocrine disorders (Mayer-Davis et al., 2017), there are other diagnoses associated with endocrinology among pediatric populations as well. These including thyroid and pituitary disorders, congenital hypothyroidism, Hashimoto's thyroiditis, isolated growth hormone deficiency (GHD), Graves' disease, polycystic ovarian syndrome, adrenal gland disorders, and hypoglycemia (Neary & Nieman, 2010). The endocrine system affects growth and development, metabolism, and mood.

Respiratory diseases. Respiratory diseases include several conditions; those most commonly treated in the PICU include bronchiolitis, bronchitis, asthma, and acute respiratory distress syndrome. Asthma is the most common of the respiratory diagnoses for youth. However, pneumonia and its associated complications lead to the most deaths, particularly in those aged five and younger (Zar & Ferkol, 2014). Still too common of a diagnosis is tuberculosis (TB); nearly one-fifth of all persons diagnosed with TB are youth. Many respiratory diseases can be better managed by reducing toxins in youths' living and school environments (e.g., minimizing exposure to smoke, dust, pesticides, vermin feces, stress).

Unintentional injury. Unintentional injuries are considered any incident that was not done deliberately. Of all of the presenting concerns addressed in the PICU context, unintentional injury is the leading cause of death among children under the age of 14 years old. It is estimated that more than one million children die each year due to unintentional injuries. Leading causes of accidental injury for children and youth typically occur in the home; the most common include burns, drowning, suffocation, choking, poisonings, falls, and injury from firearms (Acar et al., 2015).

Adult Intensive Care Unit (AICU)

About 20% of acute care admissions and approximately 58% of emergency department admissions in the United States result in an ICU admission (Wunsch, Angus, Harrison, Linde-Zwirble, & Rowan, 2011). The most common reasons to be admitted in AICU units include acute myocardial infarction, intracranial hemorrhage (or cerebral infarction), percutaneous cardiovascular procedure with drug-eluting stent, respiratory system diagnosis with ventilator support, and septicemia or severe sepsis without mechanical ventilation. While ICUs are still considered in many contexts as part of a hospital's geography, critical care patients may be treated in diverse units throughout most any hospital context. However, when on a unit, healthcare providers must be adept at the management of catheters, surgical outcomes, and central lines. They must also be prepared to best attend to the 20% of all AICU patients who meet criteria for palliative care services (Lamas, Owens, Bernacki, & Block, 2014).

Medical family therapists can be of great assistance in meeting families where they are at in ensuring that there is transparent and beneficial communication between family members and healthcare provider teams in relation to the loved one's progress and health-related decisions. It is also important that MedFTs be skilled at working with families who have difficult biopsychosocial–spiritual decisions to make in collaboration with or on behalf of a loved one. Addressing psychosocial well-being in the context of critical care conditions is particularly important, given that ICU survivors commonly experience symptoms of post-traumatic stress and depression that then negatively influence their health-related quality of life (Bienvenu, & Neufeld, 2011; Davydow, Gifford, Desai, Needham, & Bienvenu, 2008). Below are descriptions of common concerns experienced by critical care patients that should be cared for by interdisciplinary healthcare teams that include MedFTs.

Acute myocardial infarction. Cardiac diagnoses make up the most common reason for entry into an ICU in the United States (44.6%), with almost one-tenth of those admitted due to coronary artery disease or acute myocardial infarction (Wunsch et al., 2011). Unfortunately, as is the case with many chronic physical health conditions, it does not exist in isolation. Smolderen et al. (2017), for example, conducted a longitudinal study that enforced the need to attend to psychological diagnoses, particularly focusing on depression comorbid to acute myocardial infarction and its associated adverse outcomes.

Cardiovascular illnesses. It is estimated that 38% of patients admitted to ICUs have a primary cardiovascular diagnosis and that another 33% are experiencing a cardiovascular complication in relation to their presenting illness (van Diepen et al., 2015). Cardiovascular illnesses rarely emerge without being accompanied by other chronic conditions, such as diabetes mellitus, hypertension, renal dysfunction, and obstructive lung disease. As such, patients with cardiovascular disease may be deemed critically ill due to the likelihood toward major systemic complications, including those that may occur or be exacerbated while in an ICU (e.g., bleeding, catheter-related infections, ventilator-acquired pneumonia, and multi-organ dysfunction).

Intracranial hemorrhage/cerebral infarction. These serious conditions result from airway or respiratory compromise, large cerebral swelling, and—sometimes—seizures. As cerebral swelling increases, the likelihood to maintain consciousness decreases. Oftentimes, neuroimaging and neurological monitoring are needed to best care for patients experiencing these conditions. In particular, most serious cases are recommended to be served in intensive care or stroke units so that they are treated by neurointensivists. In the ICU, complex medical care often includes airway management and mechanical ventilation, blood pressure control, fluid management, and glucose and temperature control (Wijdicks et al., 2014).

Respiratory system diseases. Respiratory and pulmonary diseases include diagnoses such as influenza, pneumonia, chronic obstructive pulmonary disease, asthma, cystic fibrosis, and pulmonary hypertension. While many of these conditions may worsen without much awareness from the patient, attention to self-management is essential. Cognitive behavioral therapy has been used to bring attention to self-management, while also treating the distress that often accompanies respiratory diseases (Baraniak & Sheffield, 2011). More recently, internet-based self-management systems have been created that attend to both physical and psychosocial symptom regulation. One example of such a system is EDGE (sElf-management anD support proGrammE). The EDGE was designed to help patients identify exacerbations of physical and psychosocial symptoms while also providing them with psychoeducation about ways to maximize compliance to treatments and overall well-being (Farmer et al., 2017). The results from EDGE research show clinical significance toward reducing depression, but not statistical significance. Still, long-term findings should be tracked given that these comorbid diagnoses typically span many years without improved outcomes.

Septicemia/sepsis. Sepsis is an inflammatory response to infection (Kaukonen, Bailey, Suzuki, Pilcher, & Bellomo, 2014; Prescott, Osterholzer, Langa, Angus & Iwashyna, 2016). It has the capacity to influence multiple systems and organs in the body that can, and typically does, lead to impairments on both physical and mental abilities during and after discharge from the ICU (Winters, Eberlein, Leung, Needham, Pronovost, & Sevransky, 2010).

Toxicity from drugs/substances. Common substances resulting in toxicity or overdose include recreational stimulants, tricyclic antidepressants, monoamine oxidase inhibitors, and opioids. Growth in opioid abuse, as well as other prescription and illicit drugs, has led to a growth in concerns related to treatment of these patients in ICUs. One serious concern is serotonin syndrome, which can lead to hyperthermia, tachycardia, and rhabdomyolysis (Altman & Jahangiri, 2010). The likelihood for this syndrome increases when selective serotonin reuptake inhibitors (SSRIs) or serotonin and norepinephrine reuptake inhibitors (SNRIs) are administered alongside other serotonergic medications (Kelly, Rubenfeld, Masson, Min, & Adhikari, 2017). Patients who arrive at a hospital with cognitive impairment, or who have overdosed, typically are unable to report their drug of choice or last substance used. This can present additional treatment challenges as it can influence their treatment process.

Intensive Care Across the MedFT Healthcare Continuum

Medical family therapy on critical care or intensive care units is not likely occurring in smaller healthcare contexts (i.e., MedFTs are more likely in larger trauma-1 hospitals) and as such may be more likely to be practiced off-site or in central mental health arenas of a healthcare context. MedFT is more likely to take place on location in larger trauma or critical care complexes. Skills and knowledge of MedFTs range from a primary focus on the psychosocial needs of a family member who has a loved one in a critical care context toward more advanced relational and BPSS skills and knowledge of MedFTs who function as a part of collaborative teams within NICU, PICU, and AICU contexts. Tables 5.1 and 5.2 highlight specific knowledge and skills that characterize MedFTs' involvement in ICU contexts across Hodgson, Lamson, Mendenhall, and Tyndall's (2014) MedFT Healthcare Continuum.

Medical family therapists functioning at *Levels 1* and *2* are likely to be either off-site or in a behavioral health hub in a particular part of a hospital where there is minimal collaboration or opportunity to directly collaborate with ICU providers or staff. While they may be aware of BPSS health and relational well-being as a researcher and/or clinician, these MedFTs only rarely or occasionally address the interface of the physical complications into the psychosocial assessments or care. MedFTs at these levels will not likely recognize the idiosyncrasies of a medical diagnosis, but rather attend to the criticality. That is, they are more likely to extend services to a family member who has a loved one in an ICU than the patient himself or herself. As such, MedFTs at these levels may be maintaining a systemic lens (considering the loved one who is in ICU), but attention is primarily given to the psychosocial concerns of the family member. In relation to the vignette at the start of this chapter, a MedFT at these levels would likely provide services for ICU families once a family member has been discharged, treating relational dynamics that have shifted after an ICU experience, for example, or grief after the death of a loved one.

Table 5.1 MedFTs in Intensive Care: Basic Knowledge and Skills

MedFT Healthcare Continuum Level	Level 1	Level 2	Level 3
Knowledge	MedFTs at this level are more likely to extend services to a family member who has a loved one in an ICU than the patient himself or herself; thus, knowledge would be focused on coping or grief pertaining to a loved one's condition. Minimal awareness of potential for collaboration or how to access diverse treatment team members.	MedFT may be aware of BPSS health and relational well-being as a researcher and/or clinician, but he/she only occasionally addresses the interface of the physical complications into the psychosocial assessments or care.	Has a working knowledge of specific team members and medical terminology within the ICU. Is aware of family therapy interventions appropriate for siblings, couples, and families who have a loved one in the ICU.
Skills	Incorporates family systems or BPSS assessments into sessions on an irregular, rare occasion. May request discharge documents to better understand complexity of condition. Able to conceptualize behavioral health concerns with families associated with a loss that occurred in an ICU.	Facilitates conversations with family members about questions that they could ask of the healthcare team on the ICU in relation to BPSS or systemic questions of concern. Attends to relational changes that may occur after discharge of a family member from the ICU.	Attending to multiple family members' needs, including crisis response pertaining to an ICU admission or death on a unit. Recognizes BPSS and systemic health outcomes associated with having a family member admitted to or die in the ICU. Deliver research-informed and culturally aware family therapy and BPSS interventions to family members in ICU contexts. Can identify ways in which psychosocial and spiritual health can exacerbate or support health complications.

Table 5.2 MedFTs in Intensive Care: Advanced Knowledge and Skills

MedFT Healthcare Continuum Level	Level 4	Level 5
Knowledge	Biopsychosocial–spiritual (BPSS) implications for the patient and family members during stay in ICU and any related trauma on patient, family, and provider systems. Systemic and relational concerns unique to the patient and family experiences in the ICU and with related trauma.	Proficient in theories, assessments, and interventions that capture BPSS and systemic healthcare in ICU contexts for families and in collaboration with diverse healthcare providers. Systemic and relational concerns unique to patient and family experiences in the ICU, including death of a loved one/death of a patient. Design, implement, lead, and evaluate integrated behavioral healthcare teams in the ICU.
Skills	Consistently engages as part of the ICU team. Assesses for BPSS factors unique to ICU patients and intervenes with families and providers accordingly. Delivers systemic and family therapy and BPSS interventions to support patient, family, and provider systems. Encourages interprofessional collaboration to maximize care.	Administers, supervises, conducts program evaluations and policy formation in the ICU. Trains healthcare professionals in family therapy and MedFT practice, research, policy, and/or administration in ICU contexts. Advocates and analyzes healthcare policy effectively to maximize patient care and ethical research in ICUs.

MedFTs at *Level 3* must be highly adaptable, attending to multiple family members' needs, including attention to crisis responses in family members who have encountered acute trauma or critical health concerns in a loved one. MedFT can be complicated at this level because of the acuteness of the presenting concern. MedFTs who are trained in family therapy and BPSS interventions can assist family members in recognizing their immediate needs. At this level, too, MedFTs are informed about the most common diagnoses encountered in an intensive care unit and can identify ways in which psychosocial and spiritual health can exacerbate or support health complications in order to share these types of challenges with family members. In relation to the vignette at the start of this chapter, interventions at this level included ways that the MedFT worked to integrate rituals into the ICU that fit with the beliefs and needs of the family members. The MedFT works to interact with families to minimize stressful interactions among family members during ICU treatments or a loss experience and also assists families with ways to maximize communication between family members and their loved one's healthcare team.

MedFT research may include research on ways in which families are influenced by critical care encounters and experiences. Examples of this at *Level 3* could include attention to family communication following child or partner treatment for sepsis. This work may focus on ways in which communication and BPSS health are altered following a critical care encounter with sepsis.

At *Level 4*, MedFT clinicians and/or researchers are trusted as reputable and consistent healthcare team members; they offer family therapy interventions and expertise through a biopsychosocial–spiritual lens for families engaged in an ICU. As described in the vignette at the start of the chapter, some families may be awaiting happy news from the healthcare team (e.g., that the patient will be released to go home in a stable medical condition); others may also be expecting a release from the hospital but recognize that a chronic healthcare battle will lie ahead for their family member; others still may find the ICU as a final resting place. MedFTs at *Level 4* must be able to weave in and out of the emotional tapestry that exists in the ICU for families, as well as in the healthcare team. MedFTs' systemic training allows them to interface with patients at the clinical level in an ICU room, recognize the processes and procedures that can positively influence care (e.g., discussing procedures for rituals and healthcare logistics that can take place to honor the loss of a loved one in an ICU unit), and identify ways to reduce provider burnout and compassion fatigue given the high level of empathy and energy given to each patient. At *Level 4*, the MedFT would encourage interprofessional collaboration in order to maximize quality care; this may be done through clinical, operational, and larger system processing groups, research groups, or grand round/national presentations.

At *Level 5*, MedFTs are experienced at administration, supervision, program evaluation, and policy formation in the ICU. They are also experienced in training healthcare professionals in family therapy and MedFT practice, research, policy, and/or administration. Examples of this through the vignette were that the MedFT faculty member had mentored a doctoral student in developing a research-based educational seminar focused on grief, trauma, reduction of burnout, and compassion fatigue that was administered to over 300 NICU and PICU providers and staff (Meadors et al., 2010). She and the student collaborated on a pre- and posttest for the seminars (approved through the institutional review board [IRB] processes to be used for program evaluation and research purposes). Content from the pre- and posttest outcomes led to an increase in clinical service debriefings with providers across the children's hospital. These outcomes also further resulted in a number of publications and sparked additional research and practice requests from diverse medical disciplines who wanted to better attend to infant loss, palliative care processes, and family-centered care practices in ICU contexts.

In relation to policies that influence ICUs, MedFTs advocate for healthcare policy, particularly in relation to the inclusion of family-centered care in ICU contexts, including the removal/restrictions of visitation hours for family members. MedFTs at *Level 5* should analyze existing policies in their local healthcare system with particular attention toward operational processes and procedures that are linked to health disparities and barriers to treatment. Given the research presented throughout this chapter, involvement of *Level 5* MedFTs may help (through their systemic lens

Table 5.3 Critical Care ICU Research by Role

Role	Responsibilities	Interprofessional Research that Informs Practice
Care/case manager	Deliver home health services. Determine if assisted living or other transitional care is needed. Help to coordinate the transition from the inpatient to outpatient setting.	Researchers have highlighted the role of care management for outpatient health care services particularly to ensure reductions in mortality post-discharge and attention to aging patient populations (Katz et al., 2010). *This research may benefit a MedFT who can assist by collaborating with family members on ways in which these decisions align with the family's health beliefs and also how they may influence the family's role in the care of their loved one.*
Chaplain	Provide spiritual support to patient and family.	Research has been limited yet positive about the role of chaplains in addressing patients' spiritual concerns in ICUs (Johnson et al., 2014); much more exists in relation to chaplains' presence in patient and family end-of-life decision-making (Shinall, Ehrenfeld, & Guillamondegui, 2014). *MedFTs are often close collaborators with chaplains, because of their shared attention to meaning making in relation biopsychosocial–spiritual health.* *MedFTs recognize the important role that chaplains and spiritual beliefs bring to decision-making processes, the need for more research on spirituality and religion in relation to health, and as such are likely to build strong bonds in practice and research with chaplaincy teams.*
Child life specialist	Deliver various types of family-centered supportive care for infants and children. Support staff and families in preparation for child visitation in ICU.	By 2022, all child life specialists will be required to have a graduate degree in order to be clinically active. Researchers have reported that child life specialists have a role in understanding developmental care tasks developed in the ICU, providing sibling support, and assisting with nonpharmacologic pain management support (Smith, Desai, Sira, & Engelke, 2014). *MedFTs and child life specialists are often trained in child and family development departments and thus typically share a systemically oriented foundation to care, making them a logical partnership in practice, research, and advocacy for children and families.*

(continued)

Table 5.3 (continued)

Role	Responsibilities	Interprofessional Research that Informs Practice
Critical care nurse/nurse practitioner	Assessment. Oversight of plan of care. Care delivery. Organizational leadership. Implementation of unit-based protocols. Quality improvement. Outcomes data analysis. Staff and patient satisfaction.	Researchers have found that specified training for nurses and nurse practitioners in ICU care following degree completion maximizes unit-based protocols and care delivery outcomes (Simone, Mccomiskey, & Andersen, 2016); training options that maximize patient outcomes may include orientation to ICU daily routines, rounding processes, competencies in ICU knowledge and systems, unit level work models, and rotations through a series of ICU/trauma units (Weled et al., 2015). *This research may benefit MedFTs by encouraging Level 5 leaders to develop cite-based protocol, trainings, and metrics that can maximize operational outcomes that benefit the patient, patient's family, and interprofessional team practices.*
Intensivist	Team leader. Assessment and treatment. Coordinate and delegate. Administrative. Regulatory. Quality improvement. Support patients and families. Discharge.	Consistently, researchers have found over the past decade that between 30% and 50% fewer patients would die if an intensivist rounded daily with critically ill patients (Durbin, 2006; Wilcox et al., 2013). High-intensity staffing is consistently tied to better patient outcomes and lower patient mortality; however still in question is whether 24-hours intensivist staffing is needed, given contradictory outcomes in full-day versus daytime-only coverage (Kerlin & Halpern, 2016; Wilcox et al., 2013). *MedFTs may benefit from this research by conducting a cost–benefit analysis on provider type, time spent with each patient, interprofessional processes, and patient outcomes in order to develop a time and cost-effective model of care.*
Pharmacist	Medication monitoring. Medication delivery. Pharmacotherapy evaluation.	A quarter of ICUs have no dedicated clinical pharmacists, despite studies demonstrating a reduction in medication errors and increase in benefits to patient outcomes (Beardsley, Jones, Williamson, Chou, Currie-Coyoy, & Jackson, 2016). Advanced practice training is recommended for pharmacists who work on ICUs, particularly because preventable adverse drug events are at least twice as likely to occur on an ICU than on an acute unit (Durbin, 2006). *From this research, MedFTs can raise awareness on the unit about the importance of pharmacists in patient care, the role of medication adherence, recognition of a family history with substance use, and barriers to long-term medication management.*

(continued)

Table 5.3 (continued)

Role	Responsibilities	Interprofessional Research that Informs Practice
Physical therapist	Develop treatment plan. Utilize stretching, movement, and heat to reduce disability. Focus on early mobility of patients.	Emerging evidence suggests the safety and efficacy of physical therapist-guided ambulation to promote recovery postsurgery and improve patient mobility in the ICU (Fields, Trotsky, Fernandex & Smith, 2015). *MedFTs are able to collaborate with PTs and learn about the role of pain in tandem with in-unit physical therapy. MedFTs can provide pre- and post-PT interventions that may assist pain management.*
Registered dietician	Plan diet based on patient needs. Direct or perform feedings.	Given the complex chronic health and illness conditions presented in the ICU, nutritional assessments are essential in order to determine the unique nutritional needs for each patient; the prevalence of malnutrition among critically ill patients is estimated to exceed 50%, again supporting the need for registered dieticians or nutritionists as part of the ICU team (Fontes, Generoso, & Correia, 2014). *MedFTs can take away many lessons when collaborating with registered dieticians, particularly addressing the meaning associated with eating and the roles in the family (e.g., who does the grocery shopping; who cooks the food); psychoeducation is also important in that nutrition influences most chronic conditions and thus requires family meal planning and goals that support better biopsychosocial health.*
Respiratory therapist	Manage delivery of protocol-regulated respiratory care. Patient/ventilator system. Airway care. Deliver bronchodilators. Monitor hemodynamics and blood gases.	With increasing percentages of ICU patients who are mechanically ventilated, respiratory therapists have become an integral part of the ICU team, particularly in improving adherence to weaning protocols, decreasing ventilator days, and reducing ICU costs (Bourke, 2016). *MedFTs and RTs may deliver a most unique collaboration both for the patient and their family, after all struggles with breathing often heighten anxiety for patients and for loved ones; evidence-based interventions can be taught to providers, to families, and in best-case scenarios to patients in order to best regulate breathing that maximizes their biopsychosocial health.*

of practice, research, and policy) to reduce the mortality rates within the ICU and improve biopsychosocial health of the patient and family within the year after discharge.

Research-Informed Practices

All of these forms of ICU performance can be further enhanced by MedFT contributions to clinical practice, research, and policy efforts, as seen in Table 5.3 (which describes critical care ICU teams by role, responsibilities, and interprofessional research in tandem with MedFT). Collectively, these efforts serve to better inform integrated behavioral healthcare practice and research.

Intensive care unit performance can be assessed using a number of measures focused on medical, economic, psychological, and institutional outcomes (Ko et al., 2017; Kohn et al., 2017). Medical outcomes are tied to variables including patient survival, complication rates, adverse events, and symptom control (Rose, 2011). Economic outcomes involve analysis examining resource consumption and cost-effectiveness of care, in particular, related to specified treatment plans (e.g., antimicrobial stewardship (Reader, Reddy & Brett, 2017; Rose, 2011; Ruiz-Ramos et al., 2017). Psychological outcomes, as presented earlier in the chapter, are largely missing from the research. Yet these are necessary to examine, not just in relation to patients who survive the ICU, but also for parents of critically ill children (Stremler, Haddad, Pullenayegum, & Parshuram, 2017). Institutional and operational outcomes are essential to the patient flow and quality of perceived outcome for patient/family and providers, including the importance of patient/family–provider communication as a key indicator toward quality care (Kohn et al., 2017). Institutional outcomes have also been measured by staff satisfaction and turnover, ICU bed utilization, efficiency of ICU services, and satisfaction of other hospital departments with these services (Garland, 2005).

Family Approaches

According to researchers, only one-quarter of ICUs include patients and family members in their daily rounds and even less have protocols that promote a family meeting as part of care or treatment planning (Cypress, 2012). While research about family involvement in ICU care is limited, it is clear that there are some essential elements that are regarded as important in family-centered care and influence patient outcomes. These elements include transparent and genuine interpersonal communication between patients/patients' families and providers (including communication about the roles of parents and professional caregivers) and empathy through challenging decision-making processes.

Transparent and genuine interpersonal communication. In a study conducted with neonatal–perinatal medicine fellows by Boss, Hutton, Donohue, and Arnold (2009), researchers found that 41% of respondents had no formal training on communication skills and 75% had never even participated in role-plays or simulated trainings for clinical encounters with families. These skills are critical for providers to have, given that communication affects parental stress, satisfaction, care, treatment, decision-making, and health outcomes for the child, parent, and family (Curtis, Engelberg, Wenrich, Shannon, Treece, & Rubenfeld, 2005; Curtis & Rubenfeld, 2005; Foster, Whitehead, and Maybee, 2015).

Family-centered care research may more naturally bend toward the involvement of families in the care for young children. However, family-centered care is just as important when engaging in care of a spouse, partner, or parent. Curtis et al. (2001) developed five objectives that can help guide providers when engaging in conversations with families throughout the lifespan. These objectives are summarized by the mnemonic VALUE; researchers have adapted this to strengthening providers' ability to value family statements, acknowledge family emotions, listen to the family, understand the patient as a person, and elicit family questions (Lautrette et al., 2007). While family-centered care, and thus level of interpersonal communication, lies on a continuum from more provider-directed conversations at times to times when the conversation is more family led, the important element is that providers and family feel as though they are collaborators toward the best care for the patient (Lilly et al., 2000; Lilly, Sonna, Haley, & Massaro, 2003; Stapleton, Engelberg, Wenrich, Goss, & Curtis, 2006).

Family-centered care becomes even more interesting when considering the diverse nature of patients served in ICUs. In a study done with Latino families (Walker-Vischer, Hill, & Mendez, 2015), participants stated that they felt as though there was greater trust with the healthcare team when they were involved in decision-making processes on behalf of their loved one and that this comfort grew even stronger when providers on the healthcare team were fluent in Spanish. Walker-Vischer et al. (2015) also supported the importance of transparent and genuine communication from providers when considering concepts such as *respecto* and *simpatía* (i.e., honoring those in authority without questioning decisions by those higher in the hierarchy and respecting the value of relationships, particularly by avoiding conflict). Thus, providers will need to continue to strengthen their skill set in growing transparent and genuine communication with families as well as their cultural awareness. These skills will likely transpire into more empathetic exchanges between families and providers regardless of the patient's health outcome.

Empathy. Foster et al. (2015) extended multiple recommendations that can enhance empathy through family and provider communication and decision-making processes. Through their systematic review, they encouraged parent involvement and connection in the ICU via

> parental presence during life-threatening events and procedures; regular health care professional, parent, and child meetings; development of PICU parental support groups; access to interactive web-based communication systems; and integration of research into clinical practice where health care providers, parents, and children are active participants. (p. 59)

Again, these recommendations were put forth for family-centered care when the child was the identified patient. However, empathy is needed throughout the lifespan and may be most noticed in times of difficult decision-making. Empathic statements exchanged with the ICU team have been found to be associated with higher overall family satisfaction (Selph, Shiang, Engelberg, Curtis, & White, 2008). Empathic statements made by physicians and physician extenders may include the way in which one discusses the difficulty of having a critically ill loved one, the difficulty of surrogate decision-making related to determining the patient's wishes, and statements about the difficulty of confronting death related to the process of accepting the impending loss of a loved one (Selph et al., 2008). When a loved one is dying in the ICU, families report higher levels of satisfaction when providers spend more time listening (Heyland, Rocker, O'Callaghan, Dodek, & Cook, 2003; Keenan, Mawdsley, Plotkin, Webster, & Priestap, 2000; Malacrida et al., 1998; McDonagh et al., 2004). More recently, researchers are finding that placing a family support coordinator (e.g., a MedFT) into the ICU may enhance family-focused empathy, increase the possibility for family-provider consensus on decision-making, and reduce conflict and thus symptoms of post-traumatic stress for the patient and family (Azoulay et al., 2005; Moore et al., 2012).

Overall, MedFTs have a great deal to offer in neonatal, pediatric, and adult ICUs. There is still much to learn about the role of psychosocial health for patients and families during and post their ICU stays. Furthermore, MedFTs have the opportunity to contribute as clinicians and researchers to understanding what happens for patients and families after discharge that leads to better longevity and quality of life. In particular, integrated behavioral healthcare teams are well suited to assess best practices while on the unit that can result in evidence-based practice and evidence-based research for these patient populations.

Conclusion

One of the most challenging elements of working in a critical care unit is that any given day is filled with a multitude of unexpected events. Providers may have the opportunity to go into one patient room and deliver good news and then walk into the next to deliver bad news about a poor prognosis or loss of life. MedFTs' value is added to these contexts is extensive, particularly in their ability to assist in the reorganization of a family's life in the face of the event that led to the ICU experience. Furthermore, MedFTs have the ability to use their relational training to strengthen the quality of work and personal life for providers who extend care in ICU contexts. These contributions are further strengthened when their relational and BPSS expertise is integrated into research and policy that can maximize family-based care for patients and their providers.

Reflection Questions
1. How might you prepare yourself and promote self-care among the healthcare team when going from best-case scenario situations to worst-case scenario situations (or vice versa) within the ICU?
2. What knowledge, skills, and outcome research will assist you in providing best practice to families receiving care in ICU contexts?
3. What are the biopsychosocial–spiritual implications for a medical procedure that occurs on any given ICU unit, and how might these implications influence the family system while on the ICU and at time of discharge?

Glossary of Important Terms in Intensive Care[1]

Arterial catheterization A thin, hollow tube that is placed into an artery (large blood vessel) in the wrist, groin, or other location to measure blood pressure. This is often called an "art line" in the intensive care unit (ICU).

Bubble CPAP Devices that apply pressure to the neonatal respiratory system via nasal prongs placed into the nostrils, forming a tight seal to minimize leak.

Central venous catheter (central line) A long, soft, thin hollow tube that is placed into a largevein. Also known as a central line or CVC.

Chest tube thoracostomy Chest tubes are inserted between ribs into one's chest in order to drain blood, fluid, or air and allow full expansion of the lungs. The tube may be connected to a suction machine to help with drainage.

High-frequency oscillation A type of high frequency ventilation characterized by the use of active expiration.

Intensive care unit-acquired weakness Clinically detected weakness in critically ill patients when there is no other explanation for the weakness other than critical illness.

Intubation The introduction of a tube into a hollow organ (such as the trachea).

Mechanical ventilation The technique through which gas is moved toward and from the lungs through an external device connected directly to the patient.

Neuromuscular blockers A group of drugs that prevent motor nerve endings from exciting skeletal muscle. They may be used during surgery to produce paralysis and facilitate manipulation of muscles.

Tracheostomy This procedure involves surgically constructing a hole that goes through the front of the neck into the trachea or windpipe. A breathing tube is placed through the hole and directly into the windpipe to facilitate breathing.

Additional Resources

Literature

Davidson, J. E., Powers, K., Hedayat, K. M., Tieszen, M., Kon, A. A., Shepard, E., … Armstrong, D. (2007). Clinical practice guidelines for support of the family in the patient-centered intensive care unit: American College of Critical Care Medicine Task Force 2004–2005. *Critical Care Medicine, 35,* 605–622. https://doi.org/10.1097/01.ccm.0000254067.14607.eb

---

[1] Note: Due to diversity of diagnoses across neonatal, pediatric, and adult intensive care units, terms are defined within the "Fundamentals of Intensive Care" section of this chapter. Below are key terms related to intervention in ICUs that are important for MedFTs to know regardless of a patient's age.

Foster, M., Whitehead, L., & Maybee, P. (2015). The parents', hospitalized child's, and health care providers' perceptions and experiences of family-centered care within a pediatric critical care setting: A synthesis of quantitative research. *Journal of Family Nursing, 22*, 6–73. https://doi.org/10.1177/1074840715618193

Johnson, J. R., Engelberg, R. A., Nielsen, E. L., Kross, E. K., Smith, N. L., Hanada, J. C., ... Curtis, J. R. (2014). The association of spiritual care providers' activities with family members' satisfaction with care after a death in the ICU. *Critical Care Medicine, 42*, 1991–2000. https://doi.org/10.1097/ccm.0000000000000412

Wall, R.J., Engelberg, R.A., Gries, C.J., Glavan, B., & Curtis, J.R. (2007). Spiritual care of families in the intensive care unit. *Critical Care Medicine, 35*, 1084–1090. https://doi.org/10.1097/01.CCM.0000259382.36414.06

Electronic Resources

Critical Care Reviews (free, full access, peer reviewed articles related to critical care). http://www.criticalcarereviews.com/

iCritical Care Podcasts (produced by the Society of Critical Care Medicine; free to download). https://itunes.apple.com/nz/podcast/sccm-podcast-icritical-care/id76207297/

Learn ICU.org (offered by the Society of Critical Care Medicine; provides a variety of journal articles and presentations about different ICU topics). http://www.learnicu.org/Pages/default.aspx

Organizations/Associations

American Thoracic Society. http://www.thoracic.org/default.asp
National Association of Neonatal Nurses. http://nann.org/
Society of Critical Care Medicine. http://www.sccm.org/index.asp
World Federation of Societies of Intensive and Critical Care Medicine. http://www.world-critical-care.org/index.php?option=com_content&view=article&id=278&Itemid=47

References[2]

Acar, E., Dursun, O. B., Esin, İ. S., Öğütlü, H., Özcan, H., & Mutlu, M. (2015). Unintentional injuries in preschool age children: Is there a correlation with parenting style and parental attention deficit and hyperactivity symptoms. *Medicine, 94*, e1378-e1382. https://doi.org/10.1097/MD.0000000000001378

Altman, C. S., & Jahangiri, M. F. (2010). Serotonin syndrome in the perioperative period. *Anesthesia & Analgesia, 110*, 526–528. https://doi.org/10.1213/ane.0b013e3181c76be9

American Academy of Sleep Medicine. (2017). *Infant sleep apnea—Symptoms & risk factors*. Retrieved May 18, 2017, from http://www.sleepeducation.org/sleep-disorders-by-category/sleep-breathing-disorders/infant-sleep-apnea/symptoms-risk-factors

Azoulay, E., Pochard, F., Kentish-Barnes, N., Chevret, S., Aboab, J., Adrie, C., ... Fassier, T. (2005). Risk of post-traumatic stress symptoms in family members of intensive care unit patients. *American Journal of Respiratory and Critical Care Medicine, 171*, 987–994. https://doi.org/10.1164/rccm.200409-1295OC

Baggs, J., Ryan, S., Phelps, C., Richeson, J., & Johnson, J. (1992). The association between interdisciplinary collaboration and patient outcomes in a medical intensive care unit. *Heart & Lung, 21*, 18–24.

Baggs, J. (1993). Collaborative interdisciplinary bioethics decision making in intensive care units. *Nursing Outlook, 41*, 108–112.

Baggs, J., Schmitt, M., Mushlin, A., Eldredge, D., Oakes, D., & Hutson, A. (1997). Nurses and resident physicians' perceptions of the process of collaboration in an MICU. *Research in Nursing Health, 20*, 71–80. https://doi.org/10.1002/(SICI)1098-240X(199702)20:1<71::AID-NUR8>3.0.CO;2-R

Baggs, J., Schmitt, M., Mushlin, A., Mitchell, P., Eldrege, D., & Oakes, D. (1999). Association between nurse-physician collaboration and patient outcomes in three intensive care units. *Critical Care Medicine, 27*, 1991–1998. Retrieved from https://www.ncbi.nlm.nih.gov/pubmed/10507630

Baraniak, A., & Sheffield, D. (2011). The efficacy of psychologically based interventions to improve anxiety, depression and quality of life in COPD: A systematic review and meta-analysis. *Patient Education and Counseling, 83*, 29–36. https://doi.org/10.1016/j.pec.2010.04.010

Beardsley, J. R., Jones, C. M., Williamson, J., Chou, J., Currie-Coyoy, M., & Jackson, T. (2016). Pharmacist involvement in a multidisciplinary initiative to reduce sepsis-related mortality. *American Journal of Health-System Pharmacy, 73*, 143–149. https://doi.org/10.2146/ajhp150186

*Bell, L. (2012). Family presence: visitation in the adult ICU. *Critical Care Nurse, 32*, 76–78.

Bienvenu, O. J., & Neufeld, K. J. (2011). Post-traumatic stress disorder in medical settings: Focus on the critically ill. *Current Psychiatry Reports, 13*, 3–9. https://doi.org/10.1007/s11920-010-0166-y

Boss, R. D., Hutton, N., Donohue, P. K., & Arnold, R. M. (2009). Neonatologist training to guide family decision making for critically ill infants. *Archives of Pediatrics & Adolescent Medicine, 163*, 783–788. https://doi.org/10.1001/archpediatrics.2009.155

Bourke, M. E. (2016). Coronary care unit to cardiac intensive care unit: Acute medical cardiac care—Adapting with the times. *Canadian Journal of Cardiology, 32*, 1197–1199. https://doi.org/10.1016/j.cjca.2016.02.001

Brilli, R. J., Spevetz, A., Branson, R. D., Campbell, G. M., Cohen, H., Dasta, J. F., ... Andre, A. C. S. (2001). Critical care delivery in the intensive care unit: Defining clinical roles and the best practice model. *Critical Care Medicine, 29*, 2007–2019. https://doi.org/10.1097/00003246-200110000-00026

---

[2] Note: References that are prefaced with an asterisk are recommended readings.

Chawla, R., & Todi, S. (Eds.). (2012). *ICU protocols: A stepwise approach*. New Delhi, IN: Springer.
Child Life Council, Inc. (2010). *Vision statement*. Retrieved from http://www.childlife.org
Clarke, C., & Harrison, D. (2001). The needs of children visiting on adult intensive care units: A review of the literature and recommendations for practice. *Journal of Advanced Nursing, 34*, 61–68. https://doi.org/10.1046/j.1365-2648.2001.3411733.x
Curtis, J. R., Patrick, D. L., Shannon, S. E., Treece, P. D., Engelberg, R. A., & Rubenfeld, G. D. (2001). The family conference as a focus to improve communication about end-of-life care in the intensive care unit: Opportunities for improvement. *Critical Care Medicine, 29*, N26–N33. https://doi.org/10.1097/00003246-200102001-00006
Curtis, J. R., Engelberg, R. A., Wenrich, M. D., Shannon, S. E., Treece, P. D., & Rubenfeld, G. D. (2005). Missed opportunities during family conferences about end-of-life care in the intensive care unit. *American Journal of Respiratory and Critical Care Medicine, 171*, 844–849. https://doi.org/10.1164/rccm.200409-1267OC
Curtis, J. R., & Rubenfeld, G. D. (2005). Improving palliative care for patients in the intensive care unit. *Journal of Palliative Medicine, 8*, 840–854. https://doi.org/10.1089/jpm.2005.8.840
*Cypress, B. S. (2012). Family presence on rounds: A systematic review of literature. *Dimensions of Critical Care Nursing, 31*, 53–64. https://doi.org/10.1097/dcc.0b013e31824246dd.
*Davidson, J. E., Powers, K., Hedayat, K. M., Tieszen, M., Kon, A. A., Shepard, E., ... Armstrong, D. (2007). Clinical practice guidelines for support of the family in the patient-centered intensive care unit: American College of Critical Care Medicine Task Force 2004–2005. *Critical Care Medicine, 35*, 605–622. https://doi.org/10.1097/01.ccm.0000254067.14607.eb.
Davydow, D. S., Gifford, J. M., Desai, S. V., Needham, D. M., & Bienvenu, O. J. (2008). Posttraumatic stress disorder in general intensive care unit survivors: A systematic review. *General Hospital Psychiatry, 30*, 421–434. https://doi.org/10.1016/j.genhosppsych.2008.05.006
Despins, L. A. (2009). Patient safety and collaboration of the intensive care unit team. *Critical Care Nurse, 29*, 85–91. https://doi.org/10.4037/ccn2009281
Durbin, C. (2006). Team model: advocating for the optimal method of care delivery in the intensive care unit. *Critical Care Medicine, 34*, S12–S17. https://doi.org/10.1097/01.CCM.0000199985.72497.D1
Edwards, J. D., Houtrow, A. J., Vasilevskis, E. E., Rehm, R. S., Markovitz, B. P., Graham, R. J., & Dudley, R. A. (2012). Chronic conditions among children admitted to U.S. pediatric intensive care units. *Critical Care Medicine, 40*, 2196–2203. https://doi.org/10.1097/ccm.0b013e31824e68cf
Engel, G. L. (1977). The need for a new medical model: A challenge for biomedicine. *Science, 196*, 129–136. https://doi.org/10.1016/b978-0-409-95009-0.50006-1
Engel, G. L. (1980). The clinical application of the biopsychosocial model. *American Journal of Family Medicine, 137*, 535–544. https://doi.org/10.1176/ajp.137.5.535
Engel, G. L., & Reichsman, F. (1956). Spontaneous and experimentally induced depressions in an infant with a gastric fistula. *Journal of American Psychoanalytic Association, 4*, 428–452. https://doi.org/10.1177/000306515600400302
Farmer, A., Williams, V., Velardo, C., Shah, S. A., Yu, L., Rutter, H., ... Tarassenko, L. (2017). Self-management support using a digital health system compared with usual care for chronic obstructive pulmonary disease: Randomized controlled trial. *Journal of Medical Internet Research, 19*, e144. https://doi.org/10.2196/jmir.7116
Fields, C., Trotsky, A., Fernandez, N., & Smith, B. A. (2015). Mobility and ambulation for patients with pulmonary artery catheters. *Journal of Acute Care Physical Therapy, 6*, 64–70. https://doi.org/10.1097/jat.0000000000000012
Fontes, D., Generoso, S. D., & Correia, M. I. (2014). Subjective global assessment: A reliable nutritional assessment tool to predict outcomes in critically ill patients. *Clinical Nutrition, 33*, 291–295. https://doi.org/10.1016/j.clnu.2013.05.004
*Foster, M., Whitehead, L., & Maybee, P. (2015). The parents', hospitalized child's, and health care providers' perceptions and experiences of family-centered care within a pediatric critical

care setting: A synthesis of quantitative research. *Journal of Family Nursing, 22,* 6–73. https://doi.org/10.1177/1074840715618193.

Fulbrook, P. (2010). Critical care or intensive care? *Connect: The World of Critical Care Nurses, 7,* 107. Retrieved from http://en.connectpublishing.org/issues.php?author_id=144

Gagnon, D. J., & Fraser, G. L. (2013). Pain, sedation, and delirium in the ICU: The pharmacist's role. *Pharmacy Practice News,* 1–8. Retrieved from http://c.ymcdn.com/sites/www.kphanet.org/resource/resmgr/KYP_Provider/PainMedSedation.pdf

Garland, A. (2005). Improving the ICU. *Chest, 127,* 2151–2164. https://doi.org/10.1378/chest.127.6.2151

Gardner, S. L., Carter, B. S., Enzman-Hines, M., & Hernandez, J. (2011). *Merenstein & Gardner's handbook of neonatal intensive care* (7th ed.). St. Louis, MO: Mosby Elsevier.

Gregory, K. E., Deforge, C. E., Natale, K. M., Phillips, M., & Marter, L. J. (2011). Necrotizing enterocolitis in the premature infant. *Advances in Neonatal Care, 11,* 155–164. https://doi.org/10.1097/anc.0b013e31821baaf4

Hanley, J. B., & Piazza, J. (2012). A visit to the intensive cares unit. *Critical Care Nursing Quarterly, 35,* 113–122. https://doi.org/10.1097/cnq.0b013e31823b1ecd

Haupt, M. T., Bekes, C. E., Brilli, R. J., Carl, L. C., Gray, A. W., Jastremski, M. S., ... Horst, M. (2003). Guidelines on critical care services and personnel: Recommendations based on a system of categorization of three levels of care. *Critical Care Medicine, 31,* 2677–2683. https://doi.org/10.1097/01.CCM.0000094227.89800.93

Hawryluck, L. A., Espin, S. L., Garwood, K. C., Evans, C. A., & Lingard, L. A. (2002). Pulling together and pushing apart: Tides of tension in the ICU team. *Academic Medicine, 77,* S73–S76. https://doi.org/10.1097/00001888-200210001-00024

Herbert, C. (2005). Changing the culture: Interprofessional education for collaborative patient centered practice in Canada. *Journal of Interprofessional Care, 19,* 1–4. https://doi.org/10.1080/13561820500081539

Heyland, D. K., Rocker, G. M., O'Callaghan, C. J., Dodek, P. M., & Cook, D. J. (2003). Dying in the ICU: Perspectives of family members. *Chest, 124,* 392–397. https://doi.org/10.1378/chest.124.1.392

Hillman, K., & Bishop, G. (2004). Organisation of an intensive care unit. In K. Hillman and G. Bishop (Eds.), *Clinical intensive care and acute medicine* (pp. 7–14). Cambridge, GB: Cambridge University Press.

Hinds, C. J., & Watson, D. (2008). Planning, organization and management. In C. Hinds and D. Watson (Eds.), *Intensive care: A concise textbook.* New York, NY: Saunders/Elsevier.

Hodgin, K. E., Nordon-Craft, A., McFann, K. K., Mealer, M. L., & Moss, M. (2009). Physical therapy utilization in intensive care units: Results from a national survey. *Critical Care Medicine, 37,* 561–568. https://doi.org/10.1097/CCM.0b013e3181957449

Hodgson, J., Lamson, A., Mendenhall, T., & Tyndall, L. (2014). Introduction to medical family therapy: Advanced applications. In J. Hodgson, A. Lamson, T., Mendenhall, and D. Crane (Eds.), *Medical family therapy: Advanced applications* (pp. 1-9). New York, NY: Springer.

Hoffman, J. I., & Kaplan, S. (2002). The incidence of congenital heart disease. *Journal of the American College of Cardiology, 39*(12), 1890–1900. https://doi.org/10.1016/S0735-1097(02)01886-7

*Johnson, J. R., Engelberg, R. A., Nielsen, E. L., Kross, E. K., Smith, N. L., Hanada, J. C., ... Curtis, J. R. (2014). The association of spiritual care providers' activities with family members' satisfaction with care after a death in the ICU. *Critical Care Medicine, 42,* 1991–2000. https://doi.org/10.1097/ccm.0000000000000412.

Katz, J. N., Shah, B. R., Volz, E. M., Horton, J. R., Shaw, L. K., Newby, L. K., ... Becker, R. C. (2010). Evolution of the coronary care unit: Clinical characteristics and temporal trends in healthcare delivery and outcomes. *Critical Care Medicine, 38,* 375–381. https://doi.org/10.1097/ccm.0b013e3181cb0a63

Kaukonen, K., Bailey, M., Suzuki, S., Pilcher, D., & Bellomo, R. (2014). Mortality related to severe sepsis and septic shock among critically ill patients in Australia and New Zealand, 2000-

2012. *Journal of the American Medical Association, 311*, 1308–1316. https://doi.org/10.1001/jama.2014.2637

Keenan, S. P., Mawdsley, C., Plotkin, D., Webster, G. K., & Priestap, F. (2000). Withdrawal of life support: How the family feels, and why. *Journal of Palliative Care, 16*, S40–S44. Retrieved from http://search.proquest.com/openview/988a67ed6b2d1637108697f84233ca4c/1?pq-origsite=gscholar&cbl=31334

Kelly, J. M., Rubenfeld, G. D., Masson, N., Min, A., & Adhikari, N. K. (2017). Using selective serotonin reuptake inhibitors and serotonin-norepinephrine reuptake inhibitors in critical care. *Critical Care Medicine, 45*, e607–e616. https://doi.org/10.1097/ccm.0000000000002308

Kerlin, M. P., & Halpern, S. D. (2016). Nighttime physician staffing improves patient outcomes: No. *Intensive Care Medicine, 42*, 1469–1471. https://doi.org/10.1007/s00134-016-4367-7

Khaleghparast, S., Joolaee, S., Ghanbari, B., Maleki, M., Peyrovi, H., & Bahrani, N. (2016). A review of visiting policies in intensive care units. *Global Journal of Health Science, 8*, 267–276. https://doi.org/10.5539/gjhs.v8n6p267

Ko, A., Harada, M. Y., Dhillon, N. K., Patel, K. A., Kirillova, L. R., Kolus, R. C., ... Ley, E. J. (2017). Decreased transport time to the surgical intensive care unit. *International Journal of Surgery, 42*, 54–57. https://doi.org/10.1016/j.ijsu.2017.04.030

Kohn, R., Madden, V., Kahn, J. M., Asch, D. A., Barnato, A. E., Halpern, S. D., & Kerlin, M. P. (2017). Diffusion of evidence-based intensive care unit organizational practices. A state-wide analysis. *Annals of the American Thoracic Society, 14*, 254–261. https://doi.org/10.1513/AnnalsATS.201607-579OC

Kwiecinska, K. M. (2008). *Investigating occupational therapists' perceived role in the ICU*. Retrieved from http://search.proquest.com.jproxy.lib.ecu.edu/docview/304329354?accountid=10639

Lakanmaa, R., Suominen, T., Perttilä, J., Puukka, P., & Leino-Kilpi, H. (2012). Competence requirements in intensive and critical care nursing—Still in need of definition? A Delphi study. *Intensive and Critical Care Nursing, 28*, 329–336. https://doi.org/10.1016/j.iccn.2012.03.002

*Lamas, D. J., Owens, R. L., Bernacki, R. E., & Block, S. D. (2014). Palliative care: A core competency for intensive care unit doctors. *American Journal of Respiratory and Critical Care Medicine, 189*, 1569–1569. https://doi.org/10.1164/rccm.201403-0467le.

Lautrette, A., Darmon, M., Megarbane, B., Joly, L. M., Chevret, S., Adrie, C., ... Curtis, J. R. (2007). A communication strategy and brochure for relatives of patients dying in the ICU. *New England Journal of Medicine, 356*, 469–478. https://doi.org/10.1056/NEJMoa063446

Lilly, C. M., De Meo, D. L., Sonna, L. A., Haley, K. J., Massaro, A. F., Wallace, R. F., & Cody, S. (2000). An intensive communication intervention for the critically ill. *American Journal of Medicine, 109*, 469–475. https://doi.org/10.1016/S0002-9343(00)00524-6

Lilly, C. M., Sonna, L. A., Haley, K. J., & Massaro, A. F. (2003). Intensive communication: Four-year follow-up from a clinical practice study. *Critical Care Medicine, 31*, S394–S399. https://doi.org/10.1097/01.CCM.0000065279.77449.B4

Malacrida, R., Bettelini, C. M., Degrate, A., Martinez, M., Badia, F., Piazza, J., ... Rapin, C. H. (1998). Reasons for dissatisfaction: A survey of relatives of intensive care patients who died. *Critical Care Medicine, 26*, 1187–1193. Retrieved from http://journals.lww.com/ccmjournal/Abstract/1998/07000/Reasons_for_dissatisfaction__A_survey_of_relatives.18.aspx

Manojlovich, M., Antonakos, C. L., & Ronis, D. L. (2009). Intensive care units, communication between nurses and physicians, and patients' outcomes. *American Journal of Critical Care, 18*, 21–30. https://doi.org/10.4037/ajcc2009353

March of Dimes. (2014). *Common conditions treated in the NICU*. Retrieved May 18, 2017, from http://www.marchofdimes.org/baby/common-conditions-treated-in-the-nicu.aspx

Mayer-Davis, E. J., Lawrence, J. M., Dabelea, D., Divers, J., Isom, S., Dolan, L., ... Wagenknecht, L. (2017). Incidence trends of type 1 and type 2 diabetes among youths, 2002–2012. *New England Journal of Medicine, 376*, 1419–1429. https://doi.org/10.1056/nejmoa1610187

McDonagh, J. R., Elliott, T. B., Engelberg, R. A., Treece, P. D., Shannon, S. E., Rubenfeld, G. D., ... Curtis, J. R. (2004). Family satisfaction with family conferences about end-of-life care in the intensive care unit: Increased proportion of family speech is associated with increased satisfaction. *Critical Care Medicine, 32*, 1484–1488. https://doi.org/10.1097/01.CCM.0000127262.16690.65

Meadors, P., Lamson, A., & Sira, N. (2010). Development of an educational module on provider self-care. *Journal for Nurses in Staff Development, 26*, 152–158. https://doi.org/10.1097/NND.0b013e3181b1b9e4

Moore, C. D., Bernardini, G. L., Hinerman, R., Sigond, K., Dowling, J., Wang, D. B., & Shelton, W. (2012). The effect of a family support intervention on physician, nurse, and family perceptions of care in the surgical, neurological, and medical intensive care units. *Critical Care Nursing Quarterly, 35*, 378–387. https://doi.org/10.1097/cnq.0b013e318268fde3

Nates, J. L., Nunnally, M., Kleinpell, R., Blosser, S., Goldner, J., Birriel, B., ... Sprung, C. L. (2016). ICU admissions, discharge, and triage guidelines: A framework to enhance clinical operations, development of institutional policies and further research. *Critical Care Medicine, 44*, 1553–1602. https://doi.org/10.1097/CCM.0000000000001856

Neary, N., & Nieman, L. (2010). Adrenal insufficiency: Etiology, diagnosis and treatment. *Current Opinion in Endocrinology, Diabetes and Obesity, 17*, 217–223. https://doi.org/10.1097/med.0b013e328338f608

O'Brien, K., Bracht, M., Macdonell, K., Mcbride, T., Robson, K., O'Leary, L., ... Lee, S. K. (2013). A pilot cohort analytic study of family integrated Care in a Canadian neonatal intensive care unit. *BioMed Central Pregnancy and Childbirth, 13*, S12. https://doi.org/10.1186/1471-2393-13-s1-s12

Prescott, H. C., Osterholzer, J. J., Langa, K. M., Angus, D. C., & Iwashyna, T. J. (2016). Late mortality after sepsis: Propensity matched cohort study. *British Medical Journal, 353*, i2375. https://doi.org/10.1136/bmj.i2375

Ramnarayan, P., Thiru, K., Parslow, R. C., Harrison, D. A., Draper, E. S., & Rowan, K. M. (2010). Effect of specialist retrieval teams on outcomes in children admitted to paediatric intensive care units in England and Wales: A retrospective cohort study. *Lancet, 376*, 698–704. https://doi.org/10.1016/S0140-6736(10)61113-0

Reader, T. W., Reddy, G., & Brett, S. J. (2017). Impossible decision? An investigation of risk trade-offs in the intensive care unit. *Ergonomics*, 1–12. https://doi.org/10.1080/00140139.2017.1301573

Rose, L. (2011). Interprofessional collaboration in the ICU: How to define? *Nursing in Critical Care, 16*, 5–10. https://doi.org/10.1111/j.1478-5153.2010.00398.x

Ruiz-Ramos, J., Frasquet, J., Romá, E., Poveda-Andres, J. L., Salavert-Leti, M., Castellanos, A., & Ramirez, P. (2017). Cost-effectiveness analysis of implementing an antimicrobial stewardship program in critical care units. *Journal of Medical Economics, 20*, 652–659. https://doi.org/10.1080/13696998.2017.1311903

Sarode, V. V., & Hawker, F. H. (2014). Design and organisation of intensive care units. In A. Bernsten and N. Soni (Eds.), *Oh's intensive care manual* (7th ed., pp. 3–9). China: Elsevier.

Selph, R. B., Shiang, J., Engelberg, R., Curtis, J. R., & White, D. B. (2008). Empathy and life support decisions in intensive care units. *Journal of General Internal Medicine, 23*, 1311–1317. https://doi.org/10.1007/s11606-008-0643-8

Simone, S., Mccomiskey, C. A., & Andersen, B. (2016). Integrating nurse practitioners into intensive care units. *Critical Care Nurse, 36*, 59–69. https://doi.org/10.4037/ccn2016360

Sims, J. M., & Miracle, V. A. (2006). A look at critical care visitation: The case for flexible visitation. *Dimensions of Critical Care Nursing, 25*, 175–180. https://doi.org/10.1097/00003465-200607000-00011

Shinall, M. C., Ehrenfeld, J. M., & Guillamondegui, O. D. (2014). Religiously affiliated intensive care unit patients receive more aggressive end-of-life care. *Journal of Surgical Research, 190*, 623–627. https://doi.org/10.1016/j.jss.2014.05.074

Skinner, E., Warrillow, S., & Denehy, L. (2015). Organisation and resource management in the intensive care unit: A critical review. *International Journal of Therapy & Rehabilitation, 22*, 187–196. https://doi.org/10.12968/ijtr.2015.22.4.187

Sleep Education. (2017). *Infant sleep apnea: Symptoms & risk factors*. Retrieved from http://www.sleepeducation.org/sleep-disorders-by-category/sleep-breathing-disorders/infant-sleep-apnea/symptoms-risk-factors

Smith, J. G., Desai, P. P., Sira, N., & Engelke, S. C. (2014). Family-centered developmentally supportive care in the neonatal intensive care unit: Exploring the role and training of child life specialists. *Children's Health Care, 43*, 345–368. https://doi.org/10.1080/02739615.2014.880917

Smolderen, K. G., Spertus, J. A., Gosch, K., Dreyer, R. P., D'Onofrio, G., Lichtman, J. H., ... Krumholz, H. M. (2017). Depression treatment and health status outcomes in young patients with acute myocardial infarction. *Circulation, 135*, 1762–1764. https://doi.org/10.1161/circulationaha.116.027042

Society of Critical Care Medicine. (2016). *Team*. Retrieved from http://www.myicucare.org/About-Critical-Care/Pages/Team.aspx

Stapleton, R. D., Engelberg, R. A., Wenrich, M. D., Goss, C. H., & Curtis, J. R. (2006). Clinician statements and family satisfaction with family conferences in the intensive care unit. *Critical Care Medicine, 34*, 1679–1685. https://doi.org/10.1097/01.CCM.0000218409.58256.AA

*Stremler, R., Haddad, S., Pullenayegum, E., & Parshuram, C. (2017). Psychological outcomes in parents of critically ill hospitalized children. *Journal of Pediatric Nursing, 34*, 36–43. https://doi.org/10.1016/j.pedn.2017.01.012.

Thompson, R. (Ed.). (2009). *The handbook of child life: A guide for psychosocial care*. Springfield, IL: Charles C. Thomas.

Turner, D. A., Mink, R. B., Lee, K. J., Winkler, M. K., Ross, S. L., Hornik, C. P., ... Goodman, D. M. (2013). Are pediatric critical care medicine fellowships teaching and evaluating communication and professionalism? *Pediatric Critical Care Medicine, 14*, 454–461. https://doi.org/10.1097/pcc.0b013e31828a746c

van Diepen, S., Granger, C. B., Jacka, M., Gilchrist, I. C., Morrow, D. A., & Katz, J. N. (2015). The unmet need for addressing cardiac issues in intensive care research. *Critical Care Medicine, 43*, 128–134. https://doi.org/10.1097/ccm.0000000000000609

Valentin, A., Ferdinande, P., & ESICM Working Group on Quality Improvement. (2011). Recommendations on basic requirements for intensive care units: Structural and organizational aspects. *Intensive Care Medicine, 37*, 1575–1587. https://doi.org/10.1007/s00134-011-2300-7

*Walker-Vischer, L., Hill, C., & Mendez, S. S. (2015). The experience of Latino parents of hospitalized children during family-centered rounds. *Journal of Nursing Administration, 45*, 152–157. https://doi.org/10.1097/nna.0000000000000175.

*Wall, R.J., Engelberg, R.A., Gries, C.J., Glavan, B., & Curtis, J.R. (2007). Spiritual care of families in the intensive care unit. *Critical Care Medicine, 35*, 1084–1090. https://doi.org/10.1097/01.CCM.0000259382.36414.06.

Ward, E., Desantis, C., Robbins, A., Kohler, B., & Jemal, A. (2014). Childhood and adolescent cancer statistics, 2014. *CA: A Cancer Journal for Clinicians, 64*, 83–103. https://doi.org/10.3322/caac.21219

Warren, J., Fromm, R. E., Jr., Orr, R. A., Rotello, L. C., Horst, H. M., & American College of Critical Care Medicine. (2004). Guidelines for the inter- and intra- hospital transport of critically ill patients. *Critical Care Medicine, 32*, 256–262. https://doi.org/10.1097/01.CCM.0000104917.39204.0A

Weled, B. J., Adzhigirey, L. A., Hodgman, T. M., Brilli, R. J., Spevetz, A., Kline, A. M., ... Wheeler, D. S. (2015). Critical care delivery: The importance of process of care and ICU structure to improved outcomes. *Critical Care Medicine, 1*, 1520–1525. https://doi.org/10.1097/CCM.0000000000000978

Wheelan, S., Burchill, C., & Tilin, F. (2003). The link between teamwork and patients' outcomes in intensive care units. *American Journal of Critical Care, 12*, 527–534. Retrieved from http://ajcc.aacnjournals.org/content/12/6/527.full

Widmann, R., Caduff, R., Giudici, L., Zhong, Q., Vogetseder, A., Arlettaz, R., ... Bode, P. K. (2017). Value of postmortem studies in decreased neonatal and pediatric intensive care unit patients. *Virchows Archive, 470*, 217–223. https://doi.org/10.1007/s00428-016-2056-0

Wijdicks, E. F., Sheth, K. N., Carter, B. S., Greer, D. M., Kasner, S. E., Kimberly, W. T., … Wintermark, M. (2014). Recommendations for the management of cerebral and cerebellar infarction with swelling: A statement for healthcare professionals from the American Heart Association/American Stroke Association. *Stroke, 45*, 1222–1238. https://doi.org/10.1161/01.str.0000441965.15164.d6

Wilcox, M. E., Chong, C. A., Niven, D. J., Rubenfeld, G. D., Rowan, K. M., Wunsch, H., & Fan, E. (2013). Do intensivist staffing patterns influence hospital mortality following ICU admission? A systematic review and meta-analyses. *Critical Care Medicine, 41*, 2253–2274. https://doi.org/10.1097/ccm.0b013e318292313a

Williams-Reade, J., Lamson, A. L., Knight, S. M., White, M. B., Ballard, S. M., & Desai, P. P. (2013a). The clinical, operational, and financial worlds of neonatal palliative care: A focused ethnography. *Palliative and Supportive Care, 13*, 179–186. https://doi.org/10.1017/s1478951513000916

Williams-Reade, J., Lamson, A. L., Knight, S. M., White, M. B., Ballard, S. M., & Desai, P. P. (2013b). Pediatric palliative care: A review of needs, obstacles and the future. *Journal of Nursing Management, 23*, 4–14. https://doi.org/10.1111/jonm.12095

Winters, B. D., Eberlein, M., Leung, J., Needham, D. M., Pronovost, P. J., & Sevransky, J. E. (2010). Long-term mortality and quality of life in sepsis: A systematic review. *Critical Care Medicine, 38*, 1276–1283. https://doi.org/10.1097/ccm.0b013e3181d8cc1d

Wright, L. M., Watson, W. L., & Bell, J. M. (1996). *Beliefs: The heart of healing in families and illness.* New York, NY: Basic Books.

Wunsch, H., Angus, D. C., Harrison, D. A., Linde-Zwirble, W. T., & Rowan, K. M. (2011). Comparison of medical admissions to intensive care units in the United States and United Kingdom. *American Journal of Respiratory and Critical Care Medicine, 183*, 1666–1673. https://doi.org/10.1164/rccm.201012-1961oc

Yoo, E. J., Edwards, J. D., Dean, M. L., & Dudley, R. A. (2016). Multidisciplinary critical care and intensivist staffing. *Journal of Intensive Care Medicine, 31*, 325–332. https://doi.org/10.1177/0885066614534605

Zar, H. J., & Ferkol, T. W. (2014). The global burden of respiratory disease: Impact on child health. *Pediatric Pulmonology, 49*, 430–434. https://doi.org/10.1002/ppul.23030

Zwarenstein, M., & Reeves, S. (2006). Knowledge translation and interprofessional collaboration: Where the rubber of evidence-based care hits the road of teamwork. *Journal of Continuing Education in the Health Professions, 26*, 46–54. https://doi.org/10.1002/chp.50

Chapter 6
Medical Family Therapy in Obstetrics and Gynecology

Angela Lamson, Kenneth Phelps, Ashley Jones, and Rebecca Bagley

The combined disciplines of obstetrics and gynecology (Ob-Gyn) are committed to the reproductive physiology of women's health throughout the lifespan and include an integration of medical and surgical care. Ob-Gyn providers attend to the social, physiological, environmental, and genetic factors that influence or exacerbate health conditions in women. As such, Ob-Gyns' expertise in and attention to diverse factors that influence the physical health of women makes medical family therapists (MedFTs) a logical partner for integrated behavioral healthcare (IBHC). Both disciplines train providers to recognize and care for the unique biopsychosocial-spiritual (BPSS) health needs (Engel, 1977, 1980; Wright, Watson & Bell, 1996) of each patient over the lifespan and in the context of her family system. Furthermore, both disciplines include training in their respective areas across prevention, health education, assessment, diagnostics, and intervention.

When collaborating, MedFTs and Ob-Gyns may resemble (at times) an IBHC team that delivers services in primary care, because Ob-Gyns oftentimes serve as a primary care provider for many women. However, there are many diagnoses and health factors that call for specialized care or surgery that are beyond what typically occurs in primary care (e.g., cesarean sections, labor, and/or delivery). Furthermore, there are unique complications that MedFTs are more likely to encounter when

---

A. Lamson (✉)
Department of Human Development and Family Science, East Carolina University, Greenville, NC, USA
e-mail: lamsona@ecu.edu

K. Phelps · A. Jones
Department of Neuropsychiatry and Behavioral Science, University of South Carolina, Columbia, SC, USA

R. Bagley
Department of Advanced Nursing Practice and Education, East Carolina University, Greenville, NC, USA

working within departments of obstetrics or gynecology (e.g., endometriosis, pelvic pain, stillbirths) than would typically be encountered in a primary care office setting. Below is just one example of how gynecology, obstetrics, and MedFT have interfaced in one family's life.

Clinical Vignette
[Note: This vignette is a compilation of cases that represent treatment in obstetrics and gynecology. All patients' names and/or identifying information have been changed to maintain confidentiality.]

Jill was referred to a MedFT (known to have worked with several families who had experienced fetal loss) after the loss of her twins at 20 weeks' gestation, one boy and one girl. She shared her story with the MedFT about how she believed that the difficulties in this delivery had led to complications with her fertility and her concern for future pregnancies. Jill's husband was devastated at the loss of the twins. Jill mentioned that she, too, was upset—but that her first loss was much more difficult. She said, "When we lost Isa it was harder on me; when we lost the twins that was harder on my husband, Robert."

Jill and Robert experienced their first loss experience the year before; their baby Isa was stillborn. Jill had just been to her Ob visit the week before Isa's death, and everything seemed okay. She shared with the MedFT how she was told that the baby had died, whereupon she actually left the hospital and drove home alone (overwhelmed and in shock) to get her "delivery suitcase" and then returned to the hospital to deliver Isa. She expressed rage and confusion about having to deliver the baby vaginally knowing that the baby was no longer alive. She explained how she had begged for a cesarean and struggled with every push to deliver this child. During the first MedFT session, Jill shared pictures of her beautiful baby girl. She did not have pictures of her twins but had equal care and detail in her narrative regarding her love for them. It was always an honor to this MedFT to be invited to see these pictures and to hear about the naming of couples' children. Jill and the MedFT met about twice a month over a 10-month time frame.

The MedFT did not have the opportunity to meet Robert until the next spring, during a ceremony that is held each year for children who have died prior to or shortly after their birth. Both Jill and Robert were overcome by emotion during the ceremony as they read Isa's name and the names their twins, Jackson and Jenna. It was through the time together in MedFT sessions that Jill and Robert decided to memorialize their twins by giving them each a unique first name. They had not been able to take this step immediately after the twins' death.

Shortly after the naming ceremony, Jill and Robert were determined that they would try to seek fertility treatments to assist in their future pregnancy. Jill described for the MedFT how she visited a new provider who did not review her chart prior to the medical visit; this provider came in with questions that were painful after experiencing the loss of two children to miscarriage and one to stillbirth (e.g., "Do you have any children?"). Following that experience, the MedFT reached out to the team of providers and recommended that a special flagging system on the medical chart be implemented so that providers and team members who worked with similar patients would be aware that a child's death had occurred. This collaborative action helped to reduce Jill's frustration and sadness as she faced the next provider who was more informed about her medical history.

At this point, the MedFT began working even more closely with Jill's new Ob-Gyn. Over the next few years, Jill and Robert tried multiple times to get pregnant and, at one point, faced an ectopic pregnancy that nearly ended Jill's life. Jill lost a lot of blood prior to hospitalization, and Robert began to worry about the well-being of his wife if they chose to continue with fertility treatments.

After this experience, Jill, Robert, the Ob-Gyn, and the MedFT met to discuss the couple's plans for proceeding since the scare of the last pregnancy. Together, the team continued to reflect on Jill's biopsychosocial-spiritual well-being, Jill's and Robert's relationship as a couple, and the collaborative work needed among all of Jill's personal and professional healthcare team. Jill had made it clear to the MedFT many times in the past that all she wanted in the world was the one thing that she could not seem to have: to give birth to a live baby. Jill understood her husband's concerns about not wanting to continue with their attempts, but she wanted so desperately to share the experience of childbearing and rearing with Robert.

Throughout the following months, Jill and Robert worked with their Ob-Gyn and a well-respected perinatologist with a final hope for pregnancy. Jill was not far into her pregnancy when it was determined that she should be on bed rest. Her status eventually became so high risk that she was transferred to a local hospital, where she would stay until the birth of their baby. During the 3 months that Jill was on hospitalized bed rest, there were a number of collaborators who worked together to ensure a safe and successful delivery. Providers included the perinatologist, women's health care teams, a number and variety of nursing professionals, the MedFT, and nearly a dozen other types of providers/staff. The MedFT would call Jill, or stop by to see her, to hear how she and Robert were doing, and to provide as much support as possible for the two of them. She and the MedFT had a number of conversations about the "What if?" questions that invaded her thoughts every day. Jill and the MedFT also talked about how she could strengthen her attachment to the unborn child and what she would want this baby to know about the brother and sisters who had come before her.

Finally, after years of struggling, Jill and Robert had a beautiful baby boy. To this day, that little boy is called a "miracle baby." Following multiple losses, Jill and Robert had an incredible experience to share with the world.

The role of the MedFT in the life of this family was so small compared to what that family had contributed to the healthcare system (e.g., better ways to identify fetal loss in the electronic health record and feedback regarding what was most helpful during the stay in the hospital following such losses). However, there were some skills implemented by the MedFT that were essential to working with this family. It was critical for the MedFT to know:

1. What a stillbirth is
2. The significance of memorializing a baby who has died (e.g., offering a naming ritual, sharing pictures)
3. What parents who have had a miscarriage or stillbirth encounter via biopsychosocial-spiritual conversations with friends, family, and providers who may or may not be helpful
4. The unique biopsychological-spiritual strains felt by mothers compared to those experienced by fathers
5. How to collaborate with Ob-Gyn providers and families when they consider or plan for future pregnancies following a loss experience

Jill has since collaborated with MedFTs on some state level presentations for providers (mostly labor and delivery, women's health, psychiatry, marriage/couple and family therapy, and MedFT) to teach others more about the biopsychosocial-spiritual influence of miscarriage and stillbirth experiences in a parent's life. Together, they (Jill and the MedFTs) have discussed the systemic challenges of such circumstances, the collaborators that were (are) necessary in Jill's life or those like her, things that were helpful and not helpful in care, and resources for medical and behavioral health providers to consider when caring for families who experience a miscarriage or stillbirth. The remainder of this chapter provides more details into the roles that Ob-Gyn teams and MedFTs extend to a diverse range of issues and patients encountered in an Ob-Gyn practice.

What Are Obstetrics and Gynecology?

Ob-Gyn practices have become a healthcare home for many women across the United States. This is not surprising, given that women meet with their Ob-Gyn provider throughout the life cycle. Some young women may first come to an Ob-Gyn at the onset of menarche to ensure that all biological systems are healthy. With the heightened attention to some vaccinations (e.g., Gardasil) and potential health consequences for human papilloma virus, some young women may arrive at an Ob-Gyn even before menarche to learn about sexual health and the prevention of a number of health conditions beyond those that directly relate to sexual activity.

Ob-Gyns are continuously using research to inform their practice, which also helps to ensure that care is cost-effective for patients. For example, young women do not commonly receive a Pap smear now until the age of 21, and then the exam may only be done every 3 years unless the results are abnormal. Women who are of a reproductive age may receive exams annually in order to request or maintain birth control, be screened for sexually transmitted diseases, and/or ensure that there have been no changes in their health (Osborne, 2017). While many visits to Ob-Gyns may be for preventative care, some appointments are prompted by changes to women's biopsychosocial systems including heavy, prolonged, or irregular menstruation, chronic pelvic pain, typical or atypical changes due to pregnancy, and/or challenges associated with mental health—perhaps in association with developmental shifts such as menarche, pregnancy, post-pregnancy, and menopause.

As stated above, one common concern for women is related to menorrhagia or heavy bleeding, which often leads to the discovery of hormonal imbalances, ovarian dysfunction, polycystic ovary syndrome, uterine fibroids, or polyps (Ahuja & Hertweck, 2010). During an initial or follow-up evaluation, concurrent discussions about mood may arise for some adolescent or adult women. Inquiry into mood states can identify premenstrual dysphoric disorder for up to 5.8% of menstruating women, which is characterized by impaired affective lability, irritability, low mood, and anxiety during the final week before the onset of menses (American Psychiatric Association, 2013). Undoubtedly, these mood changes reverberate through the family system, prompting relational tension for parents, partners, or other family members. Unfortunately, challenges with menorrhagia can exacerbate or be exacerbated by psychosocial challenges that can result in or exist in tandem with chronic pelvic pain (Shin & Howard, 2011; Stein, 2013).

Chronic pelvic pain, commonly defined as noncyclical pain that lasts greater than 6 months, is estimated to occur in 5.7–26.6% of women (Ahangari, 2014). The development and course of genito-pelvic pain remains unclear, particularly because there are commonly reported delays in seeking care and, as such, the initial source of pain may have grown or evolved in uncertain ways. Peaks of reported pain are commonly seen in early adulthood (related to onset of sexual activity) and during perimenopause due to physiologic changes (American Psychiatric Association, 2013). Similar to most pain conditions, the existing literature supports the best practice of treating pelvic pain by using a biopsychosocial stance whereby disease activity, physical condition, self-efficacy, cognitive experience, social support, and relational adjustment can be conceptualized concurrently (Tripp & Nickel, 2013). The assortment of services (e.g., medical, surgical, physical, and psychological treatments) needed by patients to manage pain can all be provided via an IBHC or collaborative care model whereby Ob-Gyn and MedFT providers can work in tandem to extend both BPSS and relationally based interventions as part of acute and complex chronic care (Al-Abbadey, Liossi, Curran, Schoth, & Graham, 2016).

Alongside onset and abnormalities in menarche as an initial foray into gynecologic care, many young women seek care from an Ob-Gyn provider with the desire to start or consider contraception based on their sexual health needs (Osborne, 2017). Of course, contraceptive counseling is not confined to early life, as many women remain on some form of contraception for decades (Murphy, Hewitt, & BeLew, 2017). Best practices exist to ensure that contraceptive counseling incorporates relational- and task-oriented communication grounded in a close, trusting patient-provider relationship (Dehlendorf, Krajewski, & Borrero, 2014). Visits addressing contraceptives often include valuable psychoeducation about anatomy and sexual response, as well as discussions regarding safe sex practices throughout the life cycle (Berishaj, 2017; Cason, 2017). The American College of Obstetricians and Gynecologists (2011) recommends screening for prior sexual abuse, rape trauma histories, and current or past intimate partner violence for every patient. Detection of an assault history during contraceptive counseling can ensure timely referral to psychotherapeutic services to advance psychological healing and combat post-traumatic stress symptomatology. Identification of sexual dysfunction (e.g., low desire, genito-pelvic pain, anorgasmia) during annual examinations is another common topic of concern that activates involvement of a behavioral health provider. These opportunities lend themselves to MedFTs using their systemic lens to analyze the interplay of medical, psychological, and relational factors associated with intimacy and/or intercourse.

Perhaps the most widely seen and known presentations within Ob-Gyn offices relate to women during pregnancy and postpartum periods; these encompass a variety of positive and concerning BPSS stressors. With nearly four million babies born each year in the United States (Martin et al., 2011), there is an abundance of healthcare visits that take place to ensure the safest health measures possible for mother and child throughout and following the pregnancy. At times, women and their partners bear the burden of infertility, characterized by financial duress, lowered moods, and mounting anxieties (Luk & Loke, 2015). The experience of infertility has also been linked to relational problems, including communication difficulties and/or sexual dysfunction (Monga, Alexandrescu, Katz, Stein, & Ganiats, 2004). While most women do not have difficulty becoming pregnant, the role of expected versus unexpected pregnancy may influence mental wellness. In fact, nearly half of pregnancies in the United States are unintended (Finer & Zolna, 2011). This unexpected life event can cue difficult decision points regarding parenthood, abortion, or adoption wherein the safe spaces provided by an Ob-Gyn provider and/or MedFT could be both welcomed and warranted.

For women who continue in their pregnancies, the hormonal fluctuations during the perinatal experience coupled with the demands of this transition into a new role can cue new relational distress or postpartum symptomatology (Wenzel & Kleiman, 2015). The nature of perinatal psychological distress is detailed later in this chapter given the prevalence of this concern within the inpatient and outpatient contexts, including more information pertaining to pregnancy loss via miscarriage and stillbirth. Relational distress is also to be expected in light of the fact that pregnancy and birth are relational experiences; relational factors are described throughout this chapter.

MedFTs, given their systemic stance and focus on life cycle issues, are ideal practitioners for integrated Ob-Gyn contexts. Concerns can range from those outlined above to the discovery of congenital abnormalities on ultrasound, attachment difficulties with a new baby, co-occurring urological problems (e.g., incontinence, interstitial cystitis), vasomotor symptoms of menopause, and intimate partner violence. Regardless of the chief complaint, the psychological and relational nature of

Ob-Gyn practice is evident. While systemically oriented behavioral health providers are a vital part of the treatment team, an array of service providers are needed to assess and treat the complex issues within women's healthcare.

Treatment Teams in Obstetrics and Gynecology

There are many possible members of a treatment team that play an integral role in patient care across an Ob-Gyn practice. The key participants will likely depend on the setting (outpatient versus inpatient), life stage of the patient (adolescent, reproductive years, menopause, postmenopause), and the resources of the office or facility. If there is a physician or physician extender on the treatment team, he or she will typically serve as a medical director of the practice or unit, though all members of the team have distinct and important roles to play in caring for women on the Ob-Gyn service. The goal of the team should be to provide comprehensive and evidence-based care for each patient (including relevant family/social support).

Advanced practice registered nurses (APRN): Nurse practitioners, nurse anesthetists, clinical nurse specialists, and nurse midwives. APRNs have a wide variety of duties within the healthcare setting, including taking histories, performing physicals, counseling patients, making diagnoses, performing procedures, ordering tests, and—in most states—prescribing medications. They are registered nurses with advanced training in a specific field of study. APRNs have a minimum of a master's degree and some have a doctorate in nursing practice. Depending on the state, they may practice independently (consulting with physicians, nurse practitioners, and physician assistants as needed). Certified nurse midwives (CNMs) are trained to provide care for women from adolescence through postmenopause with a focus on labor and birth. They are also trained in the care of the "well" newborn for the first 28 days of life.

Behavioral health providers (BHPs). Behavioral health providers are represented by a number of mental health disciplines within Ob-Gyn settings, including MedFTs, psychologists, social workers, counselors, and psychiatric nurses. These mental health professionals work collaboratively with other healthcare professionals to ensure the delivery of comprehensive, biopsychosocial-spiritual care. BHPs commonly use brief screening, assessment, and treatment models to address adherence, psychological distress, coping difficulties, and relational tension associated with biological or physical wellness, illness, or life-changing experiences (e.g., pregnancy). Diagnosing and intervening at the individual, couple, or family level, providing group therapy, and referral to specialty care for more in depth psychological treatment are also typical functions for BHPs. MedFTs who serve as the BHP will especially focus on assessments, diagnoses, and interventions that are BPSS and relational in nature. Chaplains, religious counselors, and clergy are often consulted in the event of a maternal or fetal death.

Doulas. A doula is a nonmedical person who provides physical, emotional, and informational support during prenatal care and during childbirth. Additionally, postpartum doulas are trained or experienced in providing postpartum care, including care for the mother and newborn, breastfeeding support, cooking, child care, errands, and/or light cleaning. While there are no specific licensing requirements for being a doula, many have completed a seminar and course or have extensive hands on training in maternal and infant care, leading to certification for some.

Genetic counselors. Genetic counselors inform patients and healthcare providers about the risks of inherited conditions before, during, and after pregnancy. These counselors perform detailed histories and often include genograms in their assessments to determine familial patterns of illness or medical conditions. As part of the counseling, options for genetic testing are frequently discussed with a hybrid of information and support offered throughout. Genetic counselors usually hold master's degrees or have completed certificate programs in genetic counseling and are called upon in prenatal settings to discuss abnormal ultrasound findings or when prenatal tests reflect abnormalities.

Lactation consultants. Lactation consultants are members of the healthcare team who provide patients with lactation and breastfeeding care and support often in inpatient settings and during the postpartum period. Typically, lactation consultants have become certified after education in other fields, such as nursing or midwifery. Lactation consultants must have demonstrated education in health sciences before taking the examination to be certified by the International Board of Lactation Consultant Examiners.

Medical assistants (MA). Medical assistants perform clinical and administrative work in various healthcare settings. They take vital signs, schedule appointments, enter patient history or information into the medical record, handle laboratory samples, and in some states can administer medications or injections as ordered by the primary care provider. MAs have completed high school, and many complete a certificate program, while others begin working and learning through clinical experience.

Neonatologists. Neonatologists are medical doctors (M.D. or D.O.) who specialize in treating critically ill infants in the neonatal intensive care unit (NICU). Neonatologists have completed undergraduate school, 4 years of medical school, 3 years of pediatrics residency, and an additional 3 years of a Neonatal-Perinatal Medicine Fellowship.

Obstetrician-gynecologists (Ob-Gyn). Ob-Gyns are medical doctors (MD or DO) who specialize in the medical and surgical care of women. According to the American Congress of Obstetricians and Gynecologists (2005), Ob-Gyns are "dedicated to the broad, integrated medical and surgical care of women's health throughout their lifespan" (para 1). Ob-Gyn physicians and extenders have completed undergraduate school, 4 years of medical school, and 4 years of obstetrics-gynecology residency training. They are licensed to practice medicine and can prescribe medication and perform surgical procedures that are within their scope of practice. Resident physicians start with a limited medical license to practice medicine but can apply during residency for a permanent medical license. Some Ob-Gyn physicians and extenders further specialize after completing residency by doing a fellowship in fields like gynecologic oncology, maternal-fetal medicine, female pelvis medicine and reconstructive surgery, and reproductive endocrinology and infertility.

Palliative care coordinators. This coordinator is typically a nursing professional who provides for patients with life-threatening illnesses and their families with continuity of care through the loss experience. The coordinator often receives referrals, provides or arranges for anticipatory grief counseling, and coordinates bereavement programs.

Physician assistants (PA). Physician assistants are members of the healthcare team who work closely with physicians. The level of supervision from a physician required for PAs varies by state. PAs take patient histories, diagnose and treat illnesses, prescribe medications, and order tests. PAs typically complete 4 years of undergraduate school and then 2 years of a master's degree.

Perinatologists. Perinatologists are medical doctors (MD or DO) who specialize in the care of the fetus and complicated, high-risk pregnancies. This subspecialty is also known as maternal-fetal medicine (MFM). In addition to medical school and 4 years of Ob-Gyn residency training, the MFM specialist receives 2 to 3 years of education in the diagnosis and management of high-risk pregnancies. The MFM physician typically works in close consultation with the obstetrician.

Psychiatrists. Psychiatrists are medical doctors (MD or DO) who specialize in diagnosing, treating and preventing mental disorders, and assessing both physical and mental aspects of psychological illnesses. Psychiatrists have completed undergraduate school, 4 years of medical school, and 4 years of psychiatry residency training. They are licensed to practice medicine and can prescribe medication. Psychiatrists also receive training in psychotherapy, so they may choose to utilize psychotherapy in addition to medications for treatment of patients. Some psychiatrists further specialize after residency by doing fellowships in child and adolescent psychiatry, forensic psychiatry, geriatric psychiatry, addiction psychiatry, sleep medicine, pain medicine, or psychosomatic medicine. Some psychiatrists choose to specialize in reproductive psychiatry, which focuses on the diagnosis and treatment of psychiatric disorders related to a woman's reproductive cycle, pregnancy, and menopause.

Registered nurses (RN). Registered nurses provide patient care and education in a wide variety of patient care settings. They take medical histories, administer medications, provide instructions to patients and families about illnesses and treatments, observe patients, and help with care planning. RNs may have an associate's degree in nursing, a bachelor of science degree in nursing, or graduate from an approved program. RNs have a nursing license.

Fundamentals of Care in Obstetrics and Gynecology

At first glance, one may assume the proficiencies required of a MedFT in the treatment of women in an Ob-Gyn context may be no different than in a traditional mental health setting or primary care environment. However, women seek care during some of the most anxiety provoking and sensitive times of their lives (e.g., deciding to become sexually active, attempting to become pregnant, and transitioning into midlife). Thus, while common disorders (e.g., depression, anxiety) and relational woes may be superficially similar, the amplitude of these struggles may be higher or uniquely presented in Ob-Gyn practices given the BPSS factors at play. The physiological fluctuations and role shifts that occur during pregnancy and postpartum warrant specific mention, too. Diseases and dysfunctions that accompany sexual activity often carry substantial shame or guilt, requiring a MedFT to have as much empathy as information when joining and extending care. When working as a MedFT provider in Ob-Gyn practice, specialized content knowledge and skill sets are essential. The following represent those that are most important to this effort.

Perinatal Distress

Throughout the reproductive years, women may experience different types of mental, behavioral, or emotional issues. Given the importance of optimizing mental well-being, MedFTs should explore the time course of symptom presentation to delineate between an exacerbation and new onset of a mental illness. A pregnant or postpartum woman may experience worsening symptoms of a preexisting mental health condition, like someone who already has obsessive-compulsive disorder, and it worsens during pregnancy or in the postpartum period. Other women may have a new onset of a mental illness during pregnancy or in the postpartum period, since many mental illnesses first present during the reproductive years (e.g., young women are almost three times as likely as young men to develop depression at the onset of puberty (National Institute of Mental Health [NIMH], 2015).

The skill of determining onset of illness is best paired with an appreciation for the relational climate, specifically whether social factors precipitated, exacerbated, or could remediate a current struggle. For many women and their partners, it is not uncommon during pregnancy to have a series of complex conversations that result in partners feeling as though what may have once felt like a healthy relationship is now a relationship filled with conflict or—even worse—is one that is unhealthy or unwanted. MedFTs in Ob-Gyn practices need to have both knowledge and skills in understanding common BPSS challenges associated with pregnancy to facilitate conversations with patients and their partners or other family members and engage in healthy exchanges about complex issues. Some of the common topics that should be addressed include (a) expectations about what it is to be parent (e.g., has the parent(s) discussed parenting styles?), (b) expectations about the baby (e.g., does the parent(s) know about normal developmental stages and engage in discussions about any special needs their infant may have?), (c) financial shifts (e.g., cost of daycare, diapers), and (d) roles of partners (e.g., if a single parent, is there adequate social support?; if partnered, have the parents each talked about how their role within the home will change and have partners talked about how to maintain their couple relationship while also maintaining their role as parents?). An incredible skill set that many MedFTs have is to assist the parent(s) with how life will change upon their child's appearance into the world. Furthermore, parents can be most successful when expectations are right sized and clearly communicated with other support systems. These conversations, when supportive, can also be essential in reducing the likelihood for perinatal distress.

Skills of a family therapist working in labor and delivery were previously outlined in a 2011 Clinical Update for the American Association for Marriage and Family Therapy. Those focused on the relational unit and treatment team include the following (Lamson & Phelps, 2011, p. 122):

1. Utilize theories to recognize and normalize family life changes amongst healthy and/or complex pregnancies and deliveries
2. Recognize that there may be unmet needs by one or both parents or disappointment with regard to expectations associated with prepared birth plans that had to change during the delivery process or complications with breastfeeding, etc.
3. Assess psychosocial trends (e.g. guilt, blame, depression) amongst families navigating complications
4. Explore ways to assist parents so that they may make difficult choices by facilitating discussions using effective communication techniques
5. Collaborate with chaplains, pastors, or priests for families with a strong religious or spiritual faith
6. Conduct small process groups to reduce compassion fatigue among providers

Healthy conversations and support are important for any patient to remediate perinatal or relational distress but may be especially central for women who are identified as lesbian, gay, bisexual, and transgender (LGBT). Discrimination may aggravate psychological health for these patients and/or serve as a barrier to receiving physical and psychosocial health services. Increasingly, LGBT couples are presenting to healthcare providers with a desire for parenthood. Unless the couple is both a transman and transwoman with intact reproductive organs, the only options for LGBT couples are adoption, surrogate pregnancy, or pregnancy with insemination. When both partners identify as lesbian, the decision about which partner is going to attempt the pregnancy and carry the child is necessary. For those who select surrogacy or adoption, there may be additional concerns beyond those experienced by heterosexual couples due to biases or discrimination against LGBT parents. Concerns for the transman—a person born with a female reproductive system who identifies and expresses himself as male (Fenway Health, 2017)—carry other important questions to consider, including decisions to stop hormone therapy so as to conceive. This decision has the potential for the return of female characteristics (Ellis, Wojnar & Pettinato, 2014).

MedFTs are ideally trained to explore these complex decisions within the patient and family's distinct social location. MedFTs working therapeutically with these families should understand the immense subjugation faced by many of these patients. Unfortunately, much of this discrimination originated in the mental health professions with conversion therapy and pathologizing of sexual or gender identities as commonplace in our histories (i.e., diagnostic codes for homosexuality in early version of the Diagnostic and Statistical Manual of Mental Disorders). However, a new generation of thought has risen, where the therapy room can offer a safe place to affirm the identities and attractions of LGBT couples who are seeking Ob-Gyn care. Offering this supportive, nonjudgmental stance for patients and their partners should be common practice, and providers should be particularly attuned to the various presentations of psychological distress during the perinatal period.

Psychological Distress During Pregnancy

Anxiety and depressive disorders have been found in up to 20% of women during pregnancy (Massachusetts General Hospital Center for Women's Mental Health, 2017). As mentioned previously, symptoms may represent challenges associated with a preexisting or a new-onset illness. In women being evaluated for postpartum depression, at least 11% had symptoms of depression during the pregnancy (Newport, Fernandez, Juric, & Stowe, 2009). Given the preponderance of mood and anxiety complaints, screening for mental health symptoms during pregnancy is important not just for the quality of life of the expectant mother but also for the family and fetus. While the assessment of mood and anxiety symptoms might be comfortable for some Ob-Gyn providers, more complex presentations that involve other mental health comorbidities, polypharmacy, or relational conflict would warrant the inclusion of the broader team, including a MedFT and/or reproductive psychiatrist. There is published literature that examines the potential developmental and obstetrical outcomes of untreated maternal mental illness on the fetus (Newport et al., 2009; Suri, Lin, Cohen, & Altshuler, 2014). Though a comprehensive discussion about the risks of untreated illness versus risks of pharmacological treatments in pregnancy is beyond this chapter's scope, it is important to highlight that not recognizing these illnesses in pregnancy can potentially have detrimental effects on the fetus and the mother.

Psychological Distress During Postpartum

In the postpartum period, it is important for MedFTs to understand several different psychiatric illnesses that may occur. In fact, estimates are as high as 85% of women who experience some type of postpartum mood change. The most common of these is called the "postpartum blues" (or the "baby blues"). This is not usually considered a disorder because it is very common and does not typically impair a woman's functioning. Postpartum blues typically occur within the first few weeks after delivery. Women can have mood changes and become more tearful, irritable, and anxious. These struggles peak at approximately day four or five postpartum and typically remit within 2 weeks. Monitoring symptoms of postpartum depression is important, but intensive therapy or pharmacologic intervention is not usually necessary. MedFTs can utilize normalization, openly discuss recent role changes with women and their partners, and provide an outlet to ponder the delicate balance of personal time for self-care and bonding with the new baby (Massachusetts General Hospital Center for Women's Mental Health, 2017).

Postpartum depression. About 15% of patients will experience postpartum depression (PPD) (Postpartum Support International, 2016). Higher rates of depression have been found in teens and in women of lower socioeconomic status (Postpartum Support International, 2016; Postpartum Progress, 2016). Again, this highlights the understanding that the biopsychosocial-spiritual assessment of a patient is crucial in creating the most effective treatment plan. PPD can cause significant dysfunction for a new mother and often the family unit. PPD appears similar to other types of depression. Persistent symptoms may include depressed mood, sadness, little interest in activities (including the baby), feeling guilty, sleep disturbance, appetite changes, low energy, poor concentration, feeling hopeless and/or worthless, and suicidal thoughts (American Psychiatric Association, 2013). One helpful assessment for PPD is the Edinburgh Postnatal Depression Scale (EPDS); it is a validated ten-item screening tool (Cox, Holden, & Sagovsky, 1987).

It is important to recognize and treat PPD, as it potentially impacts maternal-infant bonding, infant and child development, quality of life for the mother, and stabilization of the family unit (Newport et al., 2009). Concerns regarding prenatal and postpartum depression may also extend to fathers. Paulson and Bazemore (2010) documented that approximately 10% of fathers experienced perinatal depression, which was moderately correlated to maternal depression in their meta-analysis. Thus, concerns regarding screening for these symptoms should extend to fathers and partners in LGBT relationships. The MedFT's systemic lens adds an important element to the IBHC team, as tracking the interrelationships between mood, relational cohesion, and familial conflict seems prudent. Moreover, intervention aimed at improving depressive symptoms alongside attachment bonds may hold distinctive benefits as both members of the couple are navigating this transition.

Postpartum anxiety. Postpartum anxiety is not as widely discussed as PPD but is certainly experienced by many new mothers. Women may experience excessive worry and anxious behaviors centered around their baby. Symptoms include restlessness, irritability, muscle tension, and/or insomnia. To classify these symptoms, the MedFT should be familiar with the presentations of generalized anxiety disorder, panic disorder (and/or panic attacks), and post-traumatic stress disorder (American Psychiatric Association, 2013). Many new mothers also experience distressing thoughts (e.g., unwanted, thoughts that involve harm coming to the baby) common with anxiety and, specifically, obsessive-compulsive disorder (OCD) (Uguz & Ayhan, 2011). Data show that a vast majority of new parents have "scary thoughts," but whether they are interpreted as alarming or significant is what morphs these thoughts into obsessions that drive compulsions (Wenzel & Kleiman, 2015). These thoughts can include accidental harm or thoughts of intentional harm to the infant (Fairbrother & Woody, 2008). Intrusive thoughts of harm are different from homicidal ideation or delusions related to postpartum psychosis, as they are ego-dystonic (i.e., not aligned with one's sense of self or wishes), rather than ego-syntonic (i.e., aligned with one's current self, desires, or wishes). Noteworthy risk factors for development of postpartum-onset OCD include an obsessive-compulsive or avoidant personality, as well as a history of major depression (Uguz & Ayhan, 2011).

MedFTs should be aware of the various psychotherapeutic treatments for anxiety disorders, most notably cognitive-behavioral and mindfulness approaches, that have been shown to reduce distress for new parents (Wenzel & Kleiman, 2015). Reassurance giving should be avoided for the patient with OCD, as this is contraindicated because it tends to worsen symptomatology. Instead, exposure and response prevention (E/RP) or systematically approaching the feared stimulus without engaging in rituals or compulsions (Wheaton et al., 2016) is recommended.

Postpartum psychosis. The rarest but most serious postpartum mental illness is postpartum psychosis. Postpartum psychosis occurs in about 1–2 out of 1000 postpartum women (American Psychiatric Association, 2013). This disorder has a high risk of infanticide and suicide; it is thereby considered a psychiatric emergency that usually requires hospitalization. After delivery, women may rapidly develop symptoms (e.g., within 2 weeks). Though it is termed postpartum psychosis, the initial symptoms appear similar to bipolar disorder, including irritability, sleep disturbance, mood shifts, and restlessness. Women also may develop confusion, disorganization, auditory hallucinations, and delusions (American Psychiatric Association, 2013). It is important to ask about the baby when discussing symptoms, as the hallucinations or delusions may involve the baby (Bergink et al., 2015). An overview of the various presentations of perinatal distress along with treatment approaches is presented in the research-informed practices of this chapter (Massachusetts General Hospital Center for Women's Mental Health, 2017).

Additional Difficulties Associated with Pregnancy

While perinatal distress and concurrent relational difficulties into parenthood may be some of the most common presenting concerns for a MedFT to attend to (perhaps even more so when caring for infants who have physical health concerns or diagnoses), MedFTs may also help women (and partners) face a number of other difficulties, such as infertility, miscarriage, and stillbirth that require grieving hopes and dreams for an idealized birth or growing family. These losses may occur in the context of serious health complications during pregnancy, including ectopic pregnancy, placenta previa, placental abruption, preeclampsia, and thromboembolic disease, among others. It is also not uncommon for some women to grieve the loss of a normal spontaneous vaginal delivery when they end up with a cesarean birth, even when mother and baby are both healthy. Below are descriptions of ways in which loss may occur throughout pregnancy.

A pregnancy loss can occur during any trimester. A pregnancy loss prior to 20 weeks' gestation is called an early pregnancy loss or a spontaneous, elective, or medical abortion. Spontaneous abortion (SAB), also known as a miscarriage, occurs in at least 10% of all diagnosed pregnancies, with 80% of these losses occurring in the first trimester (American Congress of Obstetricians and Gynecologists, 2015). This is why many pregnant women wait until they hear the fetal heartbeat at 12 weeks' gestation to announce their pregnancy. An elective abortion (EAB) is a voluntary termination of the pregnancy for nonmedical reasons. A medical reason for an EAB is called a medical abortion; it may be recommended by a healthcare provider because of the mother's poor health or a fetus with an anomaly incompatible with life. After 20 weeks' gestation, a loss of pregnancy is called a stillbirth or intrauterine fetal demise (IUFD). If the gestational age of the pregnancy is not known, a birth weight of 350 grams is used to differentiate an IUFD from a SAB (Cunningham et al., 2014).

There are numerous risk factors for a spontaneous early pregnancy loss, with 50% due to chromosomal abnormalities (Alijotas-Reig & Garrido-Gimenez, 2013; Stephenson, Awartani, & Robinson, 2002). Maternal factors for pregnancy loss may also be due to infection, medical disorders including hypertension (HTN), diabetes mellitus (DM), thyroid disorders, medications, radiation, extremes of nutrition (severe deficiency and morbid obesity), lifestyle choices (smoking, excessive caffeine, illicit drugs), occupational or environmental factors, immunological factors, inherited thrombophilias, or uterine defects (Cunningham et al., 2014).

Causes of a pregnancy loss after the first trimester may be associated with the placenta such as an abruption, fetal growth restriction with a decreased blood flow through the placenta, infections, chronic health conditions in the mother (e.g., hypertension, diabetes, or clotting disorders), and umbilical cord accidents such as a true knot or a tight nuchal cord (Jordan, 2014). Sometimes the pregnancy ends secondary to preterm labor or cervical insufficiency, during which the baby dies due to being previable (or because of complications from being born too early).

An IUFD is generally suspected during a pregnancy when there is an absence of fetal movement after it has been felt by the mother or the inability to auscultate the fetal heartbeat after it had been documented as audible. A diagnosis is not made until confirmed with ultrasonography which visualizes the absence of cardiac motion in the fetus. Once the diagnosis of an IUFD is made, the mother or couple is given options about how to proceed. Depending on the gestation of the pregnancy, these may include a medical induction or surgically evacuation. Some mothers or couples want to end the pregnancy immediately; others need time to accept the diagnosis prior to scheduling the termination. At times, women must labor for an extended length of time after a known loss. An important area of consideration for the MedFT is possible post-traumatic stress disorder (PTSD), especially for those couples experiencing repeated losses or traumatic deliveries. Many women and their families need a safe space to process their options regarding timing and/or method of termination. MedFTs should function as a process consultant in these scenarios, providing a safe space for such considerations.

Additional Difficulties Not Necessarily Associated with Pregnancy

In addition to a variety of challenges that are associated with pregnancies, are a variety of concerns that may or may not coincide with pregnancy. Two examples of these common presenting concerns include (a) sexually transmitted infections or disease and (b) changes due to menopause.

Ob-Gyns have a significant role in screening, preventing, diagnosing, and treating *sexually transmitted infections* (STIs). Some STIs can have significant neurological implications if they are contracted during early pregnancy. STIs are infections that spread through sexual contact in both males and females. Herpes, gonorrhea, chlamydia, human immunodeficiency virus (HIV), and syphilis are a few examples of such infections. In a recent press release, the Centers for Disease Control and Prevention (CDC) reported a concern about the significant increase (and highest combined number) of chlamydia, gonorrhea, and syphilis infections (CDC, 2016). Half of the new STIs have been found in people aged 15–24 (Office of Women's Health, 2017). STIs may not be noticeable upon visual inspection and/or may not present initially with significant symptoms, but they can lead to serious health effects if not treated. Medications are used to treat STIs and may be given to both the patient and his or her partner. Some STIs can be cured with treatment; others require ongoing symptom management (Office of Women's Health, 2017). Patients who complain of vaginal or penile discharge, painful urination, genital sores, or have unprotected sexual encounters, should be examined by their health professional.

The CDC reports that the only way to avoid getting an STI is to not have oral, anal, or vaginal sex. Patients who are sexually active can decrease their risk by correctly using condoms, getting vaccinated (available for human papilloma virus and hepatitis B), or maintaining a monogamous relationship where both partners have negative tests for STIs (CDC, 2016). Education by MedFTs about STI risk, prevention, and screening is an important part of caring for women. It is imperative that MedFTs and medical professionals provide accurate and appropriate information about STIs and sexual practices, especially since the specific content of sexual education in schools (where young women are most likely to first learn about reproduction and sexual health) is variable.

Menopause is the cessation of menstrual cycles, caused by either the ovaries no longer producing estrogen (natural) or removal of the ovaries (surgical). This is considered the transition from being reproductive to nonreproductive. A fact sheet associated with menopause, related terms, and hormone therapies was created by the American College of Obstetrics and Gynecologists [ACOG] (2015). Menopause can last 4–8 years, and in the United States, the average age of menopause is 51 years old. Symptoms initially include changes in frequency and length of menstrual cycles (sometimes called perimenopause), followed by vaginal dryness and vasomotor symptoms (hot flashes and night sweats) that continue after menstrual cycles stop. Women can experience insomnia, urinary changes, and sexual dysfunction throughout menopause. Risks for osteoporosis and heart disease are increased as well. It is essential that MedFTs be aware of changes associated with menses from adolescence through menopause.

Obstetrics and Gynecology Across the MedFT Healthcare Continuum

Medical family therapists may function differently in each Ob-Gyn context based on the needs of the context, collaborative team involved, and relevance of BPSS or relational health to the environment. In some instances, MedFTs may function in one of the five levels of the MedFT Healthcare Continuum (Hodgson, Lamson, Mendenhall, & Tyndall, 2014), ranging from rarely using the BPSS framework or a relational lens with patients or providers in the Ob-Gyn system or up through the highest level of proficiency, by integrating systemic and BPSS practice, research, and policy collaboratives alongside of Ob-Gyn patients and providers. Tables 6.1 and 6.2 highlight specific knowledge and skills that characterize MedFTs' involvement in Ob-Gyn contexts across this continuum.

At *Levels 1 and 2*, MedFTs are likely to be in a context where there is minimal collaboration or opportunity to directly collaborate with Ob-Gyn providers or staff. While the MedFT may be aware of biopsychosocial-spiritual health and relational well-being as a researcher and/or clinician, he or she only rarely or occasionally applies all of these health dimensions into practice. MedFTs at these levels are going to have some of the basic knowledge about the BPSS challenges associated with women's physical health but rarely introduce opportunities to consider biological, psychosocial, and spiritual dimensions of health into care delivery. They are likely to share pertinent information with other providers only as needed. In the vignette at the start of the chapter, a *Level 1 or 2* MedFT may have provided services to Jill, but may not have thought to expand the treatment to include Jill's partner. He or she may, too, have focused more specifically on Jill's emotional health rather than engaging in her BPSS well-being.

At *Level 3*, MedFTs are trained to apply a broad range of family therapy and BPSS interventions and conduct therapy in relation to a variety of women's health

Table 6.1 MedFTs in Obstetrics and Gynecology: Basic Knowledge and Skills

MedFT Healthcare Continuum Level	Level 1	Level 2	Level 3
Knowledge	Basic knowledge about BPSS approaches to obstetrical and gynecological services with an awareness of how physical, mental, and relational health interrelate. Familiar with Ob-Gyn as a profession, demonstrating an understanding of commonly seen diagnoses and treatments. Minimal awareness of treatment team members.	Some specific knowledge of how hormonal changes and medical conditions can influence both mental and relational health with ability to cite data about perinatal distress, infertility, pregnancy loss, pelvic pain, and interpersonal trauma. Knowledge of how to use electronic record to efficiently collaborate with colleagues from a distance. Awareness of treatment team members and their respective roles.	Working knowledge of specific team members and medical terminology (preeclampsia, gestational diabetes, etc.). Broad range of knowledge of research-informed individual, couple/family, and community approaches to care; incorporation of BPSS factors into treatment plans. When able, conducts research and policy/advocacy initiatives to advocate for BPSS-oriented care and inclusion of relational factors into Ob-Gyn settings.
Skills	Able to complete a BPSS conceptualization for patients and families experiencing miscarriage, stillbirth, preterm birth, pelvic pain, and various gynecologic conditions. Uses validation, empathy, and normalization with patients and families navigating life transitions (e.g., onset of menarche, pregnancy, menopause). Applies IPT and CBT techniques to individuals experiencing perinatal distress but within a broader systemic framework. Demonstrates minimal collaborative skills with professionals working in Ob-Gyn contexts; prefers to work as an individual practitioner model but able to refer as needed.	Systemic interventions are used alongside individually oriented modalities of psychotherapy to assist with management of psychological and relational distress, as well as medical compliance and agency in most cases. Facilitates communication between providers via written letters or electronic medical record messages to ensure providers are abreast to the patient or families treatment goals. Conducts a separate treatment plan from other providers with some related goals or interventions (i.e., "reduce subjective reports of pain" or "lower experiences of anxiety and increase social support postpartum").	Includes other treatment team members when conceptualizing and forming treatment plans, engaging in mutual learning. Implements systemic assessments via observational data, subjective reports, and use of enactments. Regularly integrates evidence-based measures to assess mental health among multiple family members (e.g., Edinburgh). Attends and contributes to team meetings to create a BPSS treatment plan for families seen in the Ob-Gyn context.

Table 6.2 MedFTs in Obstetrics and Gynecology: Advanced Knowledge and Skills

MedFT Healthcare Continuum Level	Level 4	Level 5
Knowledge	More advanced knowledge of common presenting problems, diagnoses, and treatments encountered in Ob-Gyn settings. Identifies self as a MedFT. Aware of advocacy needs for patients and families in Ob-Gyn settings. Attends to indicators of compassion fatigue among clinical team members.	Demonstrates command of evidence-based literature and research interprofessional collaboration and integrated behavioral healthcare models in treating Ob-Gyn-related diagnoses. Conveys clinical/research expertise with a variety of psychosocial, behavioral, and relational health diagnoses and interventions to Ob-Gyn patients, families, healthcare teams, community partners, administrators, researchers, policy makers, legislators, trainees, and/or supervisees.
Skills	Ability to design assessment guides or template for patient portals, electronic health records.	Supervises MedFTs or other health team members in integrated and traditional sessions with ability to recognize BPSS health factors that may not be known to the supervisee. Influences local, community, or state policies in relation to women's health disparities or necessary interventions that can maximize health and well-being.

experiences and concerns. They usually collaborate with providers, patients, and patients' support system members in order to ensure that treatment plans are systemically constructed and implemented. At *Level 3*, the MedFT (as described in the vignette) is working to collaborate on a variety of complex issues that may enter into an Ob-Gyn practice (such as a couple's loss via stillbirth). MedFTs at this level will also collaborate on other concerns using research-informed interventions on issues including intimate partner violence, depression, PPD, pain, and common psychosocial experiences that coincide with developmental changes across the lifespan.

MedFT research at this level may include intervention studies with women or dyads based on health experiences or conditions encountered in an Ob-Gyn practice. An example of such inquiry could include assessing for ways in which infertility influences both partners of a dyad or biopsychosocial-spiritual differences in PPD for mothers in comparison to fathers. In policy work, the *Level 3* MedFT advocates for healthcare policy that is inclusive of individuals, couples, families, and diverse populations and cultures across a wide range of BPSS issues pertaining to women's health. Practice recommendations from a MedFT may include requests for inclusion of relational interventions when attending prenatal visits or promoting policies pertaining to assessment and intervention when intimate partner violence is flagged as present.

In this level, the MedFT is implementing research-informed practices with couples and families all the while maintaining an inclusion of BPSS questions that interface with the couple's or family's presenting concern. The MedFT is also likely attending conferences or community forums that attend to the policy needs of women.

At *Level 4*, MedFT clinicians and/or researchers integrate into healthcare contexts with diverse professionals. They are trained to apply a broad range of family therapy and BPSS interventions across both traditional and IBHC formats. They are confident with acute and chronic conditions, including treatment for patients struggling with substance use, past sexual trauma, and/or how expecting mothers manage gestational diabetes. These MedFTs consistently collaborate at each encounter with providers (colocated or integrated), patients, and patients' support system members, including brief assessments for depression, PPD, intimate partner violence, anxiety, and trauma. MedFTs at *Level 4* are skilled in using diverse family therapy and health-based theories, models, and interventions during each traditional and integrated behavioral healthcare visit. They are adept in managing biopsychosocial-spiritual concerns via once per year visits, as well as for patients who require multi-visit continuity of care. Given the volume of patients seen with diverse presenting concerns, these MedFTs are also aware of the ways in which demographics (e.g., ethnicity, religious affiliation, socioeconomics) may influence health disparities and indicated treatment options.

Researchers at *Level 4* consistently form interdisciplinary teams to study the reciprocal relationships between women's BPSS health status and couple/family support systems and the impact(s) of a MedFT or family therapy intervention(s) in traditional and integrated behavioral healthcare practice contexts. MedFT researchers would also work in tandem with medical researchers in Ob-Gyn contexts to further treatment options for health concerns such as pelvic pain, military sexual trauma (further discussed in the *Chapter 18*), or postpartum depression. Furthermore, MedFTs at this level commonly engage in cross-disciplinary collaborations such as with genetic counselors for women concerned about hereditary diseases, substance abuse counselors who assist in detox or treatment options for pregnant women who struggle with addiction, and/or with case managers who may need to investigate the safety of a newly born baby due to a mother's severe PPD with suicidal or homicidal ideation.

At *Level 5*, MedFTs are experienced at administrating and supervising other behavioral health providers in both traditional and integrated care models. In a clinical role, MedFTs collaborate routinely with providers, patients, and patients' support system members and have influence on templates that should be accessible in the electronic health record to account for psychosocial concerns (as described in the vignette at the start of the chapter), including social determinants. These MedFTs are proficient at family therapy and health-based theories, models, and interventions in treating the primary concerns described throughout the chapter. They may develop and lead curriculum for providers on the team in relation to current research in biopsychosocial women's health, common trends in women's health literature, or research-informed ways to improve relational health between patient and her family system, patient-provider dyads, and provider-staff dynamics. These researchers routinely construct interdisciplinary teams to study the relationships between women's BPSS health status and couple/family support systems and/or the impact(s) of MedFT or family therapy intervention(s), including outcome studies for patients and their families/support systems receiving brief and traditional family therapy in both IBHC and conventional mental health settings on women's health issues.

Unique to *Level 5* are the abilities to serve as a supervisor and ambassador for women's health. MedFTs who serve in these roles are not only proficient at extending practice; they are aware that not all women have the same needs and thus advocate for best practices for lesbian and transwomen, racial and ethnic differences, and diverse age groups, recognizing the continuum of ability while honoring spiritual health differences in decision-making. Furthermore, research reflects an awareness of ethics, particularly with the complex circumstances of knowing how to best interface with women, given that so many of the physical exams require that the patient disrobe. With consideration for these elements, MedFTs at *Level 5* have learned—and constructed ways to maximize—patient flow and encounters in order to promote healthy BPSS care, research, and policies.

Research-Informed Practices

Ob-Gyn settings serve as a pivotal healthcare home for millions of women as they encounter diverse and complex transitions throughout the life cycle. Undoubtedly, intrapersonal, interpersonal, and cultural research must be examined when developing a comprehensive treatment plan or policies that promote women's health or reduce health disparities in IBHC contexts (El-Mohandes, Kiely, Gantz, & El-Khorazaty, 2011; Joseph et al., 2009). For MedFTs in IBHC settings, evidence-based research on brief relational and BPSS therapeutic techniques, such as interpersonal therapy, cognitive-behavioral therapy, or interpersonal psychoeducation communication strategies, hold utility in lessening psychological distress. These evidence-based approaches offer a focused way of conceptualizing and treating common symptoms (e.g., sleep disturbance, mood lability, negative thoughts of self or others, social isolation). Common concerns in Ob-Gyn contexts (e.g., pregnancy loss, transition to parenthood or menopause, and sexual difficulties) require research-informed skills and ability in detecting systemic patterns at the individual, family, and community levels.

Individual Approaches

Individual therapeutic skills hold value for many presenting problems encountered in Ob-Gyn contexts, such as preparation for or adjustment to a clinical procedure, sexual desire or pelvic pain issues, and—most notably—depression or anxiety among peri- or postnatal women. Core skills of validating or empathizing with patients remain crucial in both building rapport and ensuring a patient feels understood. Furthermore, psychoeducation regarding the overlay between biological, psychological, social, and spiritual factors can assist women in identifying strengths and concerns associated with their experiences. Psychoeducation that is grounded in a BPSS foundation also offers providers and the patient a multifactorial explanation for any current difficulties and, as such, guides appropriate treatment options. MedFTs in an Ob-Gyn practice should be aware of prevalence for common conditions, as well as evidence-based assessments and interventions. Table 6.3 provides examples of psychosocial symptoms that may be associated with having a baby, alongside treatment recommendations.

The two individual approaches most frequently cited in the remediation of perinatal distress include brief interpersonal therapy (IPT) and cognitive-behavioral therapy (CBT). IPT has been shown to be effective for perinatal depression, including PPD (O'Hara, Stuart, Gorman, & Wenzel, 2000; Weissman, Markowitz, & Klerman, 2000). Though IPT is typically completed in a therapist-patient relationship without involvement of a partner or spouse, IPT focuses primarily on interpersonal relationships as an avenue for change. IPT is the most efficacious therapy for depression, even more so than CBT (Cuijpers et al., 2008), holding particular value in circumstances of (a) grief and loss, (b) interpersonal disputes, and (c) role transitions (Stuart, 2012). The IPT clinician identifies relational conflict and limited social networks as key determinants of depressive symptomatology.

MedFTs can easily integrate common IPT tools of interpersonal inventory (e.g., description of key relationships), interpersonal circle (e.g., bullseye picture where relationships are visually depicted), and interpersonal formulation (e.g., graphing interface between BPSS) into an IBHC context (Stuart, 2012). To some degree, this approach can be thought of as systemic therapy with an individual, as treatment techniques involve a detailed account of interpersonal incidents followed by a communication analysis and role-playing techniques to change relational patterns. For postpartum women, this might involve identifying instrumental or emotional needs, exploring how to best communicate these needs to identified support persons, and problem-solving strategies to avoid criticism and defensiveness. It is not surprising that IPT provides particular benefits for women transitioning to motherhood or adjusting to loss, given that the chances for miscommunications as systemic homeostasis are disrupted.

Cognitive behavior therapy—an active, problem-focused approach—is another individual therapy commonly used in the treatment of perinatal distress (as well as non-perinatal mood and anxiety complaints). CBT is thought to have advantages over IPT in the treatment of anxiety, obsessive-compulsive disorder, and trauma- or

Table 6.3 Treatment Recommendations for Common Psychosocial Symptoms that may be Associated with having a Baby

Illness	Prevalence	Course of Illness	Clinical Symptoms	Treatment
Baby blues	50%–85%	Peak postpartum day 4–5 and typically remits within 2 weeks	• Irritability • Moodiness • Anxiety • Tearfulness • No functional impairment	No intervention usually necessary. Normalization and encourage self-care. Monitor for potential to progress to PPD.
Postpartum depression (PPD)	15%	Typically in the first 3 months after delivery but can be anytime in the postpartum period (up to 12 months)	• Depressed mood, sadness • Tearfulness • Loss of interest • Appetite change • Sleep disturbance • Feeling guilty, hopeless, or worthless • Trouble concentrating • Low energy • Suicidal thoughts	Dependent upon severity of the illness – Work-up for medical illnesses that present with psychiatric symptoms – Pharmacotherapy – Psychotherapy (IPT or CBT)
Postpartum anxiety	10%	Similar to PPD; can be anytime in the postpartum period (up to 12 months)	• Persistent, excessive worrying • Racing thoughts • Sleep disturbance • Appetite change • Inability to relax • Panic attacks • Fear that something bad will happen/is going to happen • Obsessions and/or compulsions	Dependent upon severity of the illness – Work-up for medical illnesses that present with psychiatric symptoms – Pharmacotherapy – Psychotherapy (CBT or ERP)
Postpartum psychosis	1–2/1000	Typically develops 48 hours –2 weeks after delivery	• Early symptoms include: – Sleep disturbance – Restlessness – Irritability • Progress to: – Rapid mood changes – Confusion – Disorganization – Auditory hallucinations – Delusions (usually associated with infant)	– Psychiatric emergency – Partial or full hospitalization – Risk for suicide and infanticide, thus conduct thorough safety assessment – Pharmacotherapy – Family psychoeducation

(Source: MGH Women's Mental Health Center, Postpartum Support International, Postpartum Progress, 2016)

stress-related disorders for perinatal women (Wenzel & Kleiman, 2015). In their detailed account of this approach for perinatal distress, Wenzel and Kleiman presented a biopsychosocial model for perinatal distress (similar to IPT's conceptualization with more focus on cognitions and psychological factors), highlighting how interactions of genetic vulnerability, neurochemical variability, and psychological vulnerability mediated through life stress (including relational factors) cue distress. According to these leading clinicians, CBT for perinatal distress works by evaluating unhelpful automatic thoughts, restructuring core beliefs, developing affective coping skills, and engaging in problem-solving or communication skills training. Some examples of clinical techniques include a patient challenging her thought of being a "terrible mother" or taking graded steps toward being close to her baby even if/when intrusive, ego-dystonic thoughts associated with OCD enter her mind. Of note, this would also be considered a subset of behavioral therapy, E/RP, referenced earlier in this chapter. It is recommended that a MedFT includes psychoeducation about the interplays between triggering stressors, automatic thoughts, emotional dysregulation, and behavioral responses, especially since cognitive distortions often pertain to relational content or worldviews.

CBT's utility extends beyond perinatal distress to many other mental health conditions that are outlined in other chapters within this text. One area that deserves particular mention is the role of cognitions in pelvic pain. Understanding the interplays between psychological appraisal of pain and ongoing symptomatology is a necessary step for the treatment team. The Pain Catastrophizing Scale (Sullivan, Bishop, & Pivik, 1995) outlines three core factors related to pain-related catastrophizing: (a) rumination, (b) magnification, and (c) helplessness. Assessing the cognitive stance toward pain seems to be a valuable first step prior to implementation of individual and relational treatment protocols. Furthermore, inquiry into the following individual psychological factors is important: somatic hypervigilance, fear of pain, negative attitudes about sexuality, distraction from sexual cues, anxiety, negative causal attributions for the pain, feelings of low self-efficacy in coping with pain, and depressive symptoms (Desrochers, Bergeron, Landry, & Jodoin, 2008; Meana, 2012). A recent randomized control trial (RCT) tested the efficacy of cognitive-behavioral couple therapy compared to topical lidocaine for provoked vestibulodynia (PVD), a frequent source of chronic genital pain (Corsini-Munt et al., 2014). While current theories and best practices guide MedFT clinicians toward application of CBT to pelvic or genital pain conditions, future relational research, such as the RCT referenced, will undoubtedly inform the specifics of how to involve partners in treatment of these debilitating conditions. Clinicians interested in learning more about the current treatments for female sexual pain disorders can turn to a recently published systematic review by Al-Abbadey et al. (2016).

While IPT and CBT have provided MedFTs with a roadmap to addressing psychological distress in practice, other clinical researchers have discussed the value of a strengths-based approach to bereavement or other adversity. Calhoun and Tedeschi (2014) have written extensively about the concept of posttraumatic growth (PTG), which is positive psychosocial-spiritual change resulting from adversity. Emerging research over the last several years underscore the importance of assessing PTG and coping strategies in cases of unexpected perinatal loss and pregnancy termination for fetal abnormality (Black & Wright, 2012; LaFarge, Mitchell, & Fox, 2017). Using their model, MedFTs can assess, punctuate, and amplify personal strengths, improved relationships, spiritual changes, and experiences of gratitude as a result of significant and complex circumstances. As MedFTs tend to operate from both a relational and strengths-based stance, attention to the resilience and growth aspects of the transitionary experiences of Ob-Gyn patients seems crucial.

Family Approaches

Emerging science is exploring the utility of including partners and families in a variety of interventional studies (Corsini-Munt et al., 2014). Considerable research has emerged citing the role of partner responses (e.g., solicitousness, negative, facilitative) and societal/cultural factors of religiosity and stigma in genito-pelvic pain (Meana, Maykut, & Fertel, 2015). Existing knowledge guides clinicians to enact facilitative patterns among partners where flexible sexual scripts can build intimate cohesion, for instance, helping a partner know how to verbally or nonverbally adapt to painful sexual scenarios (e.g., "It seems like this is difficult for us; what if we touch in this way instead?") rather than halting all touch or responding critically to a situation. Healthy communication about wants and needs are vital for treatment success. Additional relational and research-informed practices for genito-pelvic pain and other sexual dysfunctions can be found in Hertlein, Weeks, and Gambescia's (2015) recently updated comprehensive guide to sexual health, entitled *Systemic Sex Therapy*. Using this text or a similar resource, MedFTs should familiarize themselves with information about the female sexual response cycle, notably how desire, arousal, and orgasm interact with couple, intergenerational, and societal/cultural factors. Psychoeducation, goal setting, behavioral techniques (e.g., graded exposure, sensate focus), and empathetic attunement are common goals across relationally focused sex therapy (Hertlein et al., 2015).

While there is a growing literature on the relational implications of various Ob-Gyn concerns (e.g. bereavement, STIs, menopause), the efficacy of marital/couple and family therapy interventions for couples dealing with infertility also deserves specific mention. As far back as 2001, Deborah Gerrity published a biopsychosocial theory of infertility. In her paper, treatment suggestions for couples included noting differences in coping styles, exploring dissimilarities in boundary wishes (sustaining privacy versus seeking support), and uniting couples around decision-making about things that they can control. As time has progressed, clinicians have applied evidence-based couple therapy as a way to improve sexual satisfaction, marital adjustment, and emotional distress for those dealing with infertility (Soleimani et al., 2015; Soltani, Shairi, Roshan, & Rahimi, 2014). These investigators found that when emotionally focused couple therapy (EFT) protocols were applied to infertile couples, significant improvements were found in relation to couples' satisfaction, cohesion, and affectional expression (Soleimani et al., 2015).

EFT also reduced rates of depression, anxiety, and stress for men and women who were coping with infertility (Soltani et al., 2014). Advantages of relational therapy are not limited to EFT, either; a recent meta-analysis of 39 studies documented that couple interventions, including cognitive-behavioral couples therapy and mindfulness-based interventions, appear to be efficacious at both lowering mental health concerns and improving pregnancy rates (Frederiksen, Farver-Vestergaard, Skovgard, Ingerslev, & Zachariae, 2015).

Community Approaches

Recognizing the need for communion, manifested through contact, openness, and union (Bakan, 1966), during profound life transitions can help to promote efforts that connect women to community resources as they are navigating the new role of motherhood. Centering Pregnancy is a form of group prenatal care that was first described in the literature the late 1990s (Rising, 1998). A group of 8–12 pregnant women met together for interactive learning and community building (Alliman, Jolles, & Summers, 2015); below are the essential elements required for the program:

1. Health assessment occurs within the group space
2. Women are involved in self-care activities
3. A facilitative leadership style is used
4. Each session has an overall plan
5. Attention is given to the core content; emphasis may vary
6. There is stability of group leadership
7. Group conduct honors the contribution of each member
8. The group is conducted in a circle
9. Group composition is stable, but not rigid
10. Group size is optimal to promote the process
11. Involvement of family support people is optional
12. Opportunity for socialization within the group is provided
13. There is ongoing evaluation of outcomes

Centering Pregnancy groups also provide individual abdominal assessments (performed behind a curtain). Contexts are selected so that pelvic exams and/or MedFT sessions that include sensitive topics can be performed in confidential rooms away from the group. Sessions are longer than traditional models of prenatal care—and the relationships that are formed during these sessions may become an essential part of an expecting mother's support system. These groups may be even more important for women who have been raised in or align with communal societies rather than intra-individually focused societies. Collectively, research has found that those participating in such care show a decrease in the number of preterm births and evidence both positive individual- and community-level outcomes (Magant & Dodgson, 2011).

Freestanding birth centers are another model of maternity care where women receive prenatal care, labor, and give birth in the same facility with midwives. These prenatal visits are also longer than traditional models of care, allowing for education and relationship building between pregnant women and midwives. Freestanding birth centers maintain standards set up by the American Association of Birth Centers (AABC) and have shown "improved health outcomes, cost savings, and increased patient satisfaction" (Alliman et al., 2015, p. 244).

Conclusion

Opportunities for IBHC in Ob-Gyn contexts via the inclusion of MedFT support endless pathways to improve BPSS health for women and their families. The realm of care provided in Ob-Gyn practices reaches from the prevention of unhealthy behaviors and unintended pregnancies to interventions that can increase the likelihood for healthy relationships between partners, between parent(s) and child, and in patients' BPSS well-being. MedFTs are able to contribute their knowledge and skills in tandem with Ob-Gyn providers to improve psychosocial factors associated with diverse medical and mental illnesses, complex relational issues, and trauma. Evidence through research-informed practices and clinical research outcomes continue to support the urgency of having this field integrated into Ob-Gyn practices for the betterment of women's BPSS health.

Reflection Questions
1. How will you prepare yourself to begin a collaborative relationship with patients and/or providers in an Ob-Gyn context?
2. What beliefs do you have about sexual health, common birthing practices, congenital abnormalities, adoption, abortion, and death of a fetus or parent during pregnancy or delivery?
3. What parenting or intergenerational issues could arise that would be a strength or impede MedFT services or IBHC? Consulting your standard of ethics, federal regulations pertaining to privacy, and/or ongoing meetings with supervisors is a great way to stay in-check regarding this question.
4. What evidence-based or outcome research are you familiar with that may be of assistance to clinical services with families receiving care in Ob-Gyn contexts?

Glossary of Important Terms for Care in Obstetrics and Gynecology

Breech presentation When the fetus is positioned inside the uterus in a manner whereby its feet or buttocks would—without intervention—deliver first (instead of the head).

C-section (Cesarean birth) A surgical delivery of a baby through incisions made in the abdomen and uterus.

Cervix The opening to the uterus, located at the top of the vagina.

D&C (dilation and curettage) A surgical procedure for removal of tissue from inside the uterus by opening the cervix and inserting an instrument into the uterus.

Ectopic pregnancy Also known as a mislocated pregnancy; symptoms include unexpected vaginal bleeding and cramping. The fetus may grow enough to rupture the fallopian tube (typically after about 6–8 weeks), whereby a woman usually feels severe pain in her lower abdomen. If the tube ruptures later (after about 12–16 weeks), the risk of death for the woman is increased because the fetus and placenta are larger and lead to an increased loss of blood. In most women, the fetus and placenta from an ectopic pregnancy must be surgically removed.

Hysterectomy A surgery for removal of the uterus. It is termed a "total hysterectomy" if the cervix is removed with the uterus.

Placenta previa A condition that occurs in about one in every 200 deliveries; it refers to when the placenta is mostly or completely covering the cervix, in the lower (rather than upper) part of the uterus. Placenta previa can cause painless bleeding from the vagina that suddenly begins late in pregnancy necessitating emergent delivery. It is a risk for maternal and fetal death due to blood loss.

Preeclampsia An illness that occurs in pregnancy or after delivery where a woman has high blood pressure and symptoms of organ injury or dysfunction. Some of these symptoms include an abnormal amount of protein found in the urine, abnormal liver or kidney function, vision changes, decreased number of platelets, upper abdominal pain, fluid found in the lungs, and severe headache. (note: Eclampsia is an extension of preeclampsia, resulting in maternal seizures.)

Preterm delivery When a baby is born before week 37 of the pregnancy.

Preterm labor Also called premature labor; it refers to when uterine contractions occur before 37 weeks of pregnancy.

Previable delivery A delivery prior to 23 weeks (22 weeks in some facilities).

Sexually transmitted infections/diseases (STI/D) Some women may not know that they are carrying an STI/D; this becomes an even more of complicated issue during pregnancy or at the time of delivery. Some STI/Ds are more dangerous for the fetus than others, especially when considering vaginal deliveries. Some hospitals are using rapid human immunodeficiency virus (HIV) testing during labor and delivery for pregnant women who were not tested previously during pregnancy. If a woman is found to be HIV-infected, providers are then able to begin antiretroviral therapy immediately to prevent perinatal transmission.

Thromboembolic disease In the United States, thromboembolic disease is the leading cause of death in pregnant women. It occurs when blood clots form in blood vessels that travel through the woman's bloodstream and block an artery. This disease most commonly occurs 6–8 weeks after delivery. The risk is much greater after a cesarean section than after vaginal delivery.

Additional Resources

Literature

Coady, D., & Fish, N. (2011). *Healing painful sex: A woman's guide to confronting, diagnosis, and treating sexual pain.* Berkley, CA: Seal Press.
Murkoff, H. & Mazel, S. (2016). *What to expect when you are expecting* (5th ed.). New York, NY: Workman Publishing Company. (note: This text is also available in Spanish).
Wenzel, A. (2014). *Coping with infertility, miscarriage, and neonatal loss: Finding perspective and creating meaning.* Washington, DC: American Psychological Association.

Measures/Instruments

Edinburgh Postnatal Depression Scale (EPDS). http://www.fresno.ucsf.edu/pediatrics/downloads/edinburghscale.pdf
Pain Catastrophizing Scale. http://sullivan-painresearch.mcgill.ca/pcs.php
Perinatal Anxiety Screening Scale (PASS). http://www.kemh.health.wa.gov.au/services/pmcls/docs/PASSAdministrationandScoringGuidelines.pdf
Postpartum Bonding Questionnaire (PBQ). https://www.scribd.com/document/284790115/Postpartum-Bonding-Questionnaire
Postpartum Depression Screening Scale (PDSS). http://www.wpspublish.com/store/p/2902/postpartum-depression-screening-scale-pdss
Postpartum Distress Measure (PDM). http://postpartumstress.com/for-professionals/assessments/

Organizations/Associations

American College of Nurse-Midwives. www.midwife.org
American Congress of Obstetricians and Gynecologists. www.acog.org
American Gynecological and Obstetrical Society. www.agosonline.org
Association of Women's Health, Obstetric and Neonatal Nurses. www.awhoon.org
Compendium of Centering. https://www.centeringhealthcare.org/why-centering/evaluation-research/
International Lactation Consultant Association. www.ilca.org
Massachusetts General Hospital Center for Women's Mental Health. www.womensmentalhealth.org

Office of Women's Health, U.S. Department of Health and Human Services. www.womenshealth.gov
Postpartum Progress. www.postpartumprogress.com
Postpartum Support International. www.postpartum.net
Share: Pregnancy & Infant Loss Support. http://nationalshare.org/

References[1]

Ahangari, A. (2014). Prevalence of chronic pelvic pain among women: An updated review. *Pain Physician, 17,* 141–147. http://www.diva-portal.org/smash/get/diva2:770659/FULLTEXT01.pdf

Ahuja, S. P., & Hertweck, S. P. (2010). Overview of bleeding disorders in adolescent females with menorrhagia. *Journal of Pediatric Adolescent Gynecology, 23,* S15–S21. https://doi.org/10.1016/j.jpag.2010.08.006

*Al-Abbadey, M., Liossi, C., Curran, N., Schoth, D. E., & Graham, C. A. (2016). Treatment of female sexual pain disorders: A systematic review. *Journal of Sex & Marital Therapy, 42,* 99–142. https://doi.org/10.1080/0092623X.2015.1053023.

Alijotas-Reig, J., & Garrido-Gimenez, C. (2013). Current concepts and new trends in the diagnosis and management of recurrent miscarriage. *Obstetrical & Gynecological Survey, 68,* 445–466. https://doi.org/10.1097/OGX.0b013e31828aca19

Alliman, J., Jolles, D., & Summers, L. (2015). The innovation imperative: Scaling freestanding birth centers, centering pregnancy, and midwifery-led maternity health homes. *Journal of Midwifery & Women's Health, 60,* 244–249. https://doi.org/10.1111/jmwh.12320

American Congress of Obstetricians and Gynecologists. (2005). *The scope of practice of obstetrics and gynecology.* Retrieved from https://www.acog.org/About-ACOG/Scope-of-Practice

American Congress of Obstetricians and Gynecologists. (2015). *Frequently asked questions.* Retrieved from https://www.acog.org/Patients/FAQs/Early-Pregnancy-Loss#how

*American Congress of Obstetrics and Gynecology (2015). Practice bulletin number 150: Early pregnancy loss. *Obstetrics & Gynecology, 125,* 1258–1267. https://doi.org/10.1097/01.AOG.0000465191.27155.25

American College of Obstetrics and Gynecologists. (2015). *The menopause years.* http://www.acog.org/Patients/FAQs/The-Menopause-Years

American Psychiatric Association. (2013). *Diagnostic and statistical manual of mental disorders: DSM 5.* Washington, D.C: American Psychiatric Association.

Bakan, D. (1966). *The duality of human existence: Isolation and communion in western man.* Boston, MA: Beacon.

Bergink, V., Burgerhout, K. M., Koorengevel, K. M., et al. (2015). Treatment of psychosis and mania in the postpartum period. *American Journal of Psychiatry, 172,* 115–123. https://doi.org/10.1176/appi.ajp.2014.13121652

Berishaj, K. (2017). Sexual assault. In K. Schuiling and F. Likis (Eds.), *Women's gynecologic health* (3rd ed., pp. 327–356). Burlington, MA: Jones & Bartlett Learning.

Black, B. P., & Wright, P. (2012). Posttraumatic growth and transformation as outcomes of perinatal loss. *Illness, Crisis, & Loss, 20,* 225–237. https://doi.org/10.2190/IL.20.3.b

*Calhoun, L. G., & Tedeschi, R. G. (2014). *Handbook of posttraumatic growth: Research and practice.* New York, NY: Psychology Press.

Cason, P. (2017). Sexuality and sexual health. In K. Schuiling and F. Likis (Eds.), *Women's gynecologic health* (3rd ed., pp. 191–208). Burlington, MA: Jones & Bartlett Learning.

---

[1] Note: References that are prefaced with an asterisk are recommended readings.

Centers for Disease Control and Prevention (2016). *Sexually transmitted disease surveillance 2015.* https://www.cdc.gov/nchhstp/newsroom/2016/std-surveillance-report-2015-press-release.html
*Coady, D., & Fish, N. (2011). *Healing painful sex: A woman's guide to confronting, diagnosis, and treating sexual pain.* Berkley, CA: Seal Press.
Corsini-Munt, S., Bergeron, S., Rosen, N. O., Steben, M., Mayrand, M. H., Delisle, I., ... Santerre-Baillargeon, M. (2014). A comparison of cognitive-behavioral couple therapy and lidocaine in the treatment of provoked vestibulodynia: Study protocol for a randomized control trial. *Trials, 15,* 506–517. https://doi.org/10.1186/1745-6215-15-506
Cox, J. L., Holden, J. M., & Sagovsky, R. (1987). Detection of postnatal depression. Development of the 10-item Edinburgh postnatal depression scale. *British Journal of Psychiatry, 150,* 782–786. https://doi.org/10.1192/bjp.150.6.782
Cuijpers, P., van Straten, A., Andersson, G., & Van Oppen, P. (2008). Psychotherapy for depression in adults: A meta-analysis of comparative outcome studies. *Journal of Consulting Clinical Psychology, 76,* 909–922. https://doi.org/10.1037/a0013075
Cunningham, G., Leveno, K., Bloom, S., Spong, C., Sashe, J., Hoffman, B., ... Sheffield, J. (2014). Stillbirth. In F. Cunningham, K. Leveno, S. Bloom, C. Spong, J. Dashe, B. Hoffman, B. Casey, & J. Sheffield (Eds.), *Williams obstetrics* (24th ed., pp. 661–667). New York, NY: McGraw Hill Education.
Dehlendorf, C., Krajewski, C., & Borrero, S. (2014). Contraceptive counseling: Best practices to ensure quality communication and enable effective contraceptive use. *Clinical Obstetrics and Gynecology, 57,* 659–673. https://www.ncbi.nlm.nih.gov/pmc/articles/PMC4216627/
Desrochers, G., Bergeron, S., Landry, T., & Jodoin, M. (2008). Do psychosexual factors play a role in the etiology of provoked vestibulodynia? A critical review. *Journal of Sex and Marital Therapy, 34,* 198–226. https://doi.org/10.1080/00926230701866083
Ellis, S. A., Wojnar, D. M., & Pettinato, M. (2014). Conception, pregnancy, and birth experiences of male and gender variant gestational parents: It's how we could have a family. *Journal of Midwifery & Women's Health, 60,* 62–69. https://doi.org/10.1111/jmwh.12213
El-Mohandes, A. A., Kiely, M., Gantz, M. G., & El-Khorazaty, M. N. (2011). Very preterm birth is reduced in women receiving an integrated behavioral intervention: A randomized controlled trial. *Maternal and Child Health Journal, 15,* 19–28. https://doi.org/10.1007/s10995-009-0557-z
Engel, G. L. (1977). The need for a new medical model: A challenge for biomedicine. *Science, 196,* 129–136. https://doi.org/10.1016/b978-0-409-95009-0.50006-1
Engel, G. L. (1980). The clinical application of the biopsychosocial model. *American Journal of Family Medicine, 137,* 535–544. https://doi.org/10.1176/ajp.137.5.535
Fairbrother, N., & Woody, S. R. (2008). New mothers' thoughts of harm related to the newborn. *Archives of Women's Mental Health, 11,* 221–229. https://doi.org/10.1007/s00737-008-0016-7
Finer, L. B., & Zolna, M. R. (2011). Unintended pregnancy in the United States: Incidence and disparities, 2006. *Contraception, 84,* 478–485. https://doi.org/10.1016/j.contraception.2011.07.013
*Hertlein, K. M., Weeks, G. R., & Gambescia, N. (2015). *Systemic sex therapy (2nd ed.).* New York, NY: Routledge.
Hodgson, J., Lamson, A., Mendenhall, T., & Tyndall, L. (2014). Introduction to medical family therapy: Advanced applications. In J. Hodgson, A. Lamson, T. Mendenhall, and D. Crane (Eds.), *Medical family therapy: Advanced applications* (pp. 1–9). New York, NY: Springer.
Jordan, R. (2014). Perinatal loss and grief. In R. Jordan, J. Engstrom, J. Marfell, and C. Farley (Eds.), *Prenatal and postnatal care: A woman-centered approach* (pp. 409–415). Iowa: John Wiley & Sons.
Joseph, J. G., El-Mohandes, A. A., Kiely, M., El-Khorazaty, M. N., Gantz, M. G., Johnson, A. A., ... Subramanian, S. (2009). Reducing psychosocial and behavioral pregnancy risk factors: Results of a randomized clinical trial among high-risk pregnant African American women. *American Journal of Public Health, 99,* 1053–1062. https://doi.org/10.2105/AJPH.2007.131425
*Frederiksen, Y., Farver-Vestergaard, I., Skovgard, N. G., Ingerslev, H. J., & Zachariae, R. (2015). Efficacy of psychosocial interventions for psychological and pregnancy outcomes in infer-

tile women and men: A systematic review and meta-analysis. *BMJ Open, 5*, 1–18. https://doi.org/10.1136/bmjopen-2014-006592

Lafarge, C., Mitchell, K., & Fox, P. (2017). Posttraumatic growth following pregnancy termination for fetal abnormality: The predictive role of coping strategies and perinatal grief. *Anxiety, Stress, & Coping*, 1–15. https://doi.org/10.1080/10615806.2016.1278433

Lamson, A., & Phelps, K. (2011). Labor and delivery. In *Clinical updates for family therapists: Research and treatment approaches for issues affection today's families (Volume 4)*. Alexandria, VA: American Association for Marriage and Family Therapy.

*Luk, B. H. K., & Loke, A. Y. (2015). The impact of infertility on the psychological well-being, marital relationships, sexual relationships, and quality of life of couples: A systematic review. *Journal of Sex and Marital Therapy, 41*, 610–625. https://doi.org/10.1080/0092623X.2014.958789

Magant, A., & Dodgson, J. E. (2011). Centering pregnancy: An integrative literature review. *Journal of Midwifery & Women's Health, 56*, 94–102. https://doi.org/10.1111/j.1542-2011.2010.00021.x

Martin, J. A., Hamilton, B. E., Ventura, S. J., Osterman, M. J., Wilson, E. C., Mathews, T. J., et al. (2011). Births: Final data for 2010. *National Vital Statistics Reports, 61*, 1–72. http://waterbirthsolutions.com/Downloadables/1.pdf

Massachusetts General Hospital Center for Women's Mental Health. (2017). *Homepage*. https://womensmentalhealth.org/?doing_wp_cron=1511581621.1843678951263427734375

Meana, M. (2012). *Sexual dysfunction in women*. Cambridge, MA: Hogrefe Press.

Meana, M., Maykut, C., & Fertel, E. (2015). Painful intercourse: Genito-pelvic pain/penetrative disorder. In K. M. Hertlein, G. R. Weeks, and N. Gambescia (Eds.), *Systemic sex therapy* (2nd ed., pp. 191–209). New York, NY: Routledge.

Monga, M., Alexandrescu, B., Katz, S. E., Stein, M., & Ganiats, T. (2004). Impact of infertility on quality of life, marital adjustment and sexual function. *Urology, 63*, 126–130. https://doi.org/10.4103/0974-1208.86088

*Murkoff, H. & Mazel, S. (2016). *What to expect when you are expecting* (5th ed.). New York, NY: Workman Publishing Company.

Murphy, P., Hewitt, C., & BeLew, C. (2017). Contraception. In K. Schuiling and F. Likis (Eds.), *Women's gynecologic health* (3rd ed., pp. 209–260). Burlington, MA: Jones & Bartlett Learning.

National Institute of Mental Health (NIMH). (2015). *Major depression among adolescents*. https://www.nimh.nih.gov/health/statistics/prevalence/major-depression-among-adolescents.shtml

Newport, D. J., Fernandez, S. V., Juric S., & Stowe, Z. N. (2009). Psychopharmacology during pregnancy and lactation. In A. F. Schatzberg and C. Nemeroff (Eds.). *The American psychiatric publishing textbook of psychopharmacology (4th Ed.)*. http://www.psychiatryonline.org

Office of Women's Health, US Department of Health and Human Services (2017). *Homepage*. https://www.womenshealth.gov/

O'Hara, M. W., Stuart, S., Gorman, L., & Wenzel, A. (2000). Efficacy of interpersonal psychotherapy for postpartum depression. *Archives of General Psychiatry, 57*, 1039–1045. https://doi.org/10.1002/cpp.1778

Osborne, K. (2017). Health promotion. In K. Schuiling and F. Likis (Eds.), *Women's gynecologic health* (3rd ed., pp. 61–76). Burlington, MA: Jones & Bartlett Learning.

*Paulson, J. F., & Bazemore, S. D. (2010). Prenatal and postpartum depression in fathers and its association with maternal depression: a meta-analysis. *Journal of the American Medical Association, 303*, 1961–1969. https://doi.org/10.1001/jama.2010.605

Postpartum Support International. (2016). *You are not alone!* Retrieved from http://www.postpartum.net/

Rising, S. S. (1998). Centering pregnancy: An interdisciplinary model of empowerment. *Journal of Nurse Midwifery, 43*, 46–54. https://doi.org/10.1016/S0091-2182(97)00117-1

Shin, J. H., & Howard, F. M. (2011). Management of chronic pelvic pain. *Current Pain and Headache Reports, 15*, 377–385. https://doi.org/10.1007/s11916-011-0204-4

Soleimani, A. A., Najafi, M., Ahmadi, K., Javidi, N., Kamka, E. H., & Mahboubi, M. (2015). The effectiveness of emotionally focused couples therapy on sexual satisfaction and marital adjustment of infertile couples with marital conflicts. *International Journal of Fertility and Sterility, 9*, 393–402. https://www.ncbi.nlm.nih.gov/pmc/articles/PMC4671378/

Soltani, M., Shairi, M. R., Roshan, R., & Rahimi, C. (2014). The impact of emotionally focused therapy on emotional distress in infertile couples. *International Journal of Fertility and Sterility, 7*, 337–344. https://www.ncbi.nlm.nih.gov/pmc/articles/PMC3901179/pdf/Int-J-Fertil-steril-7-337.pdf

Stein, S. L. (2013). Chronic pelvic pain. *Gastroenterology clinics of North America, 42*, 785–800. https://doi.org/10.1016/j.gtc.2013.08.005

Stephenson, M., Awartani, K., & Robinson, W. (2002). Cytogenetic analysis of miscarriages from couples with recurrent miscarriage: A case-control study. *Human Reproduction, 17*, 446–451. https://doi.org/10.1093/humrep/17.2.446

Stuart, S. (2012). Interpersonal psychotherapy. In M. J. Dewan, B. N. Steenbarger, and R. P. Greenberg (Eds.), *The art and science of brief psychotherapies: An illustrated guide* (pp. 157–193). Arlington, VA: American Psychiatric Publishing.

Sullivan, M. J. L., Bishop, S. R., & Pivik, J. (1995). The pain catastrophizing scale: Development and validation. *Psychological Assessment, 7*, 524–532. https://doi.org/10.1037/1040-3590.7.4.524

Suri, R., Lin, A. S., Cohen, L. S., & Altshuler, L. L. (2014). Acute and long-term behavioral outcome of infants and children exposed in utero to either maternal depression or antidepressants: A review of the literature. *Journal of Clinical Psychiatry, 75*, 1142–1152. https://doi.org/10.4088/JCP.13r08926

*Tripp, D. A., & Nickel, J. C. (2013). Pain clinical updates: Psychosocial aspects of chronic pelvic pain. *International Association for the Study of Pain, 21*, 1–7. https://www.iasp-pain.org/files/Content/ContentFolders/Publications2/PainClinicalUpdates/Archives/PCU_21-1.pdf

Uguz, R., & Ayhan, M. G. (2011). Epidemiology and clinical features of obsessive-compulsive disorder during pregnancy and postpartum period: A review. *Journal of Mood Disorders*, (4), 178–186. https://doi.org/10.5455/jmood.20111219111846

Weissman, M. M., Markowitz, J. C., & Klerman, G. L. (2000). *Comprehensive guide to interpersonal psychotherapy*. New York, NY: Basic Books.

*Wenzel, A. (2014). *Coping with infertility, miscarriage, and neonatal loss: Finding perspective and creating meaning*. Washington, DC: American Psychological Association.

*Wenzel, A., & Kleiman, K. (2015). *Cognitive behavioral therapy for perinatal distress*. New York, NY: Routledge.

Wheaton, M. G., Galfalvy, H., Steinman, S. A., Wall, M. M., Foa, E. B., & Simpson, H. B. (2016). Patient adherence and treatment outcome with exposure and response prevention for OCD: Which components of adherence matter and who becomes well? *Behaviour Research and Therapy, 85*, 6–12. https://doi.org/10.1016/j.brat.2016.07.010

Wright, L. M., Watson, W. L., & Bell, J. M. (1996). *Beliefs: The heart of healing in families and illness*. New York, NY: Basic Books.

Chapter 7
Medical Family Therapy in Emergency Medicine

Rosanne Kassekert and Tai Mendenhall

Attention to the intersections of mental health and physical health in emergency medicine is long-standing. Patients' and families' emotional responses to the acute physical presentations that characterize this care context can be as diverse as the presentations themselves; common themes relate to struggling with ambiguities about what will happen to sick or injured patients, fears about one's own or a loved one's life and survival, and/or misplaced anger directed at each other, healthcare providers, or office staff. Behavioral health presentations per se – without clear physical components – are also commonplace here. Suicidality (and the severe depression that can fuel it), anxiety and panic, psychosis, and any variety of states defined by psychological decompensation can bring patients to the emergency department (ED). Moreover, the worries and fears maintained by the family members who bring them can echo those that we see in response to straightforward physical injuries or conditions.

Having long been dominated by the fields of psychology and social work, medical family therapists (MedFTs) represent a comparatively new discipline to join emergency medicine. They bring an orientation comfortable with the complexities of overlapping human and relationship systems and thereby add value to the nature in which care is conducted. To set the stage for our discussion of the practice of MedFT in this context, we begin by sharing the story of Justin. As a new MedFT employed in an urban-situated ED, the following account is representative of an "average" shift.

R. Kassekert
Regions Hospital, Saint Paul, MN, USA

T. Mendenhall (✉)
Department of Family Social Science, University of Minnesota, Saint Paul, MN, USA
e-mail: mend0009@umn.edu

Clinical Vignette
[Note: This vignette is a compilation of cases that represent treatment in emergency medicine. All patients' names and/or identifying information have been changed to maintain confidentiality.]

Justin arrived at the ED a few minutes before 6:00 PM; he was scheduled for a 12-hour shift and wanted to raid the coffee machine and check email before jumping-in.

"Justin! I'm glad you're here," said Dr. Drew Leger. "I'm attending tonight, and just inherited an old man from Drs. Smith and Roth. He's in room #4, and super-agitated. Go see what's up and I'll meet you there after I see the shoulder-patient in #7."

Going strong at 84 years old, Mr. Jones's family had explained to the MA (medical assistant) that he had not heretofore evidenced any significant psychiatric history. This afternoon he had grown increasingly irritable with his nursing home staff and was admitted to the ED when he became violent. Apparently, he hit one of the residents with a food tray three times.

"Hi there," Justin said. Mr. Jones and his adult daughter where arguing with each other when he came in. "My name is Dr. Ling; Justin Ling."

"I don't give a damn what your name is!" Mr. Jones growled. "I just want to get the hell out of here."

"Dad, we need to figure out what is going on with you! And you can't keep yelling at everyone like that." Mr. Jones' daughter's name was Jessica.

"I'm telling you that I am fine! He was talking bad about your mother; that's why I hit him. He deserved it!"

"Mom has been dead for six years," Jessica said. She was crying now.

"I can understand how angry you might feel with all of these folks keeping you here," Justin said. "How about I get some more information from you two about what's been going on so that we can figure out how to best help you, Mr. Jones?"

And maybe even get you out of here, Justin thought. This would ultimately be Dr. Leger's call; it was important for other ER staff to not prematurely communicate such hope.

"Hmph!" Mr. Jones grumbled. Then he was silent for a few moments. Finally, he nodded his head.

"Can I grab you something to drink?"

"How about a beer?"

"Wouldn't that be nice?" Justin smiled. "I'm sorry, though... How about water? Or maybe a Gatorade?"

"Water's good," Mr. Jones said.

"Jessica, do you want any?" Justin asked.

For the next 20 minutes, Justin talked with Mr. Jones and his daughter about the last several days leading up to the ED visit. It was not evident that Mr. Jones had any clear thoughts about wanting to harm himself or others.

What was evident, however, was that a combination of recent medication changes and (likely) onset of cognitive declines were working against him. Urinary tract infections (UTIs) in the elderly could cause symptoms like what Mr. Jones was presenting with, too. After explaining this to Dr. Leger, the two worked with Mr. Jones and Jessica to follow-up with indicated assessments on-site and (later) through family medicine and neurology.

From there Justin's shift continued. He was called in to assess two patients for possible delirium (one was off her schizophrenic medications; the other was intoxicated). Then he spoke at length with a young woman who had been violently attacked by her boyfriend; it was the fourth time Justin had seen her in the ED. This time was different, though. They worked with the hospital's social worker to secure emergency housing at a local shelter and then with local PD to formally file domestic violence charges. After that, Justin saw three patients in a row for suicidality; two had been brought in by worried family members, and one had called 911 after ingesting three bottles of NyQuil. All warranted compelling cases for 72 hour holds, which wasn't helping Dr. Leger's mood any. In-house psych beds were already full, and coordinating transfers with collaborating hospitals nearby was always a logistical nightmare.

"Let's try to send more of these folks home, instead." Dr. Leger fumed. "You know we need to save our rooms for people who are really sick."

And to help the flow of patients through the ED while it's under your watch, Justin thought.

"I know, Drew," Justin said. "But we've got to do it. I do not think that she is safe going home on her own accord. She still wants to die and her parents are, in my view, not able to monitor her effectively."

"We've got an MVA (motor vehicle accident) coming in three minutes," interrupted Chrissy. She was one of the most level-headed PAs (physician assistants) Justin had ever met. Her words communicated that the urgency of what was coming to the ED was more important than any paperwork burdens he (Justin) and Dr. Leger needed to work out.

And it was, indeed, bad. A drunk driver had run a light with his pickup truck, T-boning another car full of teenagers. And then a motorcyclist hit all of them. The biker was the worst. After an hour with the trauma team and three more in surgery, they lost him.

Oftentimes the ER uses chaplains to help in situations like this. But when they were busy, or sometimes just because he was closest, Justin was next in-line. It was close to the end of Justin's shift, too. He was remarkably tired.

Here we go, he thought. This is going to be rough.

After talking things through with the trauma surgeon, Justin made sure that one of the family rooms was available. Then he and one of the nurses went back into the waiting area.

"Maggie?" Justin asked. "We need to talk with you about Jim."

> "Oh my God, how is he doing?" she cried. "I have been asking and asking and asking and asking and nobody will tell me what is going on. I am going crazy here!" She was almost hyperventilating.
> "Can you come with me?"
> "Yes, yes, yes..." Maggie said. As she got up, she looked into Justin's eyes. They were teary.
> "No," she whispered. "No. No. No..."
> Supporting friends, family, partners, and other loved ones whose loved one has died was always one of the most difficult parts of this job for Justin. And as a newlywed, himself, he knew that this conversation was going to hit especially close to home.

What Is Emergency Medicine?

Emergency medicine is not defined by its focus on a particular body system (e.g., cardiology), disease type (e.g., oncology), or patient demographic (e.g., pediatrics). It is instead defined by the varied range of foci under its purview, all within an acute frame that requires urgent attention and response (American College of Emergency Physicians, 2014; Hughes & Cruickshank, 2011; Mahadevan & Garmel, 2012). In accord with Justin's experiences in the vignette, above, emergency medicine includes work with patients of all ages, health conditions, injury types, and diseases. The fact that these presentations represent an "unexpected event" in a patient's life is important to recognize, insofar as this experience alone differentiates the care experience from most other types (e.g., those for which patients and families arrive for prearranged appointments). Experiencing any care that is unexpected can foster and fuel a gamut of worries and fears beyond the health issues that are presented per se (Larkin et al., 2009; Larkin, Claassen, Emond, Pelletier, & Camargo, 2005; Marx, Hockberger, & Walls, 2014).

Emergency care is also defined by its nature as "single-issue" medicine. Attention is paid only to treating and stabilizing the presentation that prompted the admission (Adams, 2012; Wolfson, Hendey, & Harwood-Nuss, 2010). There is no expectation that patients will see a provider who is familiar with their medical history, like in family medicine, nor is it likely that follow-up or ongoing care will be provided by the provider(s) that patients and families encountered during the emergency visit. These same phenomena apply regarding behavioral health; providers' efforts are oriented to the immediacy of patients' and families' needs. Coordination of services immediately following stabilization can represent an essential component of doing this work well, but long-term behavioral health services are not generally provided by behavioral health personnel functioning within an ED.

Treatment Teams in Emergency Medicine

In accord with the diversity of things that emergency medicine providers will see and respond to during an average shift, the diversity of disciplines extant and available within ED teams is myriad. The following highlight key professionals who are involved in delivering care in this context (Capella et al., 2010; Kilner & Sheppard, 2010; Lemons et al., 2015; Sutton, 2015):

Emergency department physicians. Also called "attending physicians" or just simply "attendings," these doctors lead the broader healthcare team and its respective members in care provision. They assess and treat patients who present as the result of an acute illnesses, accidents, or traumatic injuries.

Physician assistants (PAs) and physician extenders. PAs and physician extenders (usually nurse practitioners) are trained to examine, diagnose, and treat a variety of healthcare conditions under the supervision of attending physicians. In emergency medicine, these activities can include preparing casts or splints, administering wound care (e.g., suturing), interpreting medical tests, and writing prescriptions.

Medical residents. These physicians are receiving additional and/or specialized training after completing medical school. Supervised by attending physicians, residents represent a gamut of baseline medical specialties (e.g., general surgery, family medicine, orthopedics, psychiatry, pediatrics, cardiology). They work to integrate said specialties with ED applications and/or presenting patient problems.

Nurses. Nurses employed in emergency medicine are certified beyond baseline training through at least 2 years of focused experience. They work with physicians to meet a variety of patient care needs. They administer medicine, use multiple types of medical equipment during testing and care sequences, perform minor medical procedures, monitor health conditions, and often provide psychoeducation to patients and their families about the illness or injury with which the patient is struggling.

Medical assistants (MAs). MAs perform a variety of functions to help the emergency department run smoothly. They assist with rooming patients, take vital signs, collect samples from blood or urine, gather data regarding health histories, prepare patients to see healthcare providers, and often carry out administrative duties related to charting, room setup, and room cleanup.

Pharmacists. Pharmacists work with care team members regarding patients' medications. They answer questions about dosages, possible interactions with other medications, side effects, and discharge planning. Trained to function in the fast-paced and complex contexts of emergency medicine, these pharmacists are key in medication errors, delays, and omissions that can otherwise occur in acute-care delivery.

Trauma teams. These small teams are ideally made up of a group of physicians, nurses, surgical assistants, radiologists (and radiology technicians), and other support personnel whose only commitment in the ED is to treat trauma patients. Secondary to their expense, these teams are generally only found within large hospital systems.

Trauma surgeons. These surgeons are trained to treat patients who have suffered a life-threatening trauma, oftentimes involving multiple organ systems simultaneously.

Emergency medical technicians (EMTs). EMTs are trained to stabilize patients in the field and transport them to a healthcare facility. Some EMTs are licensed to treat patients with medications and other emergency treatments during transport. Responsibility for care is transitioned to ED providers upon arrival.

Emergency room technicians (ERTs). ERTs work with on-site nurses, physicians, and physician extenders to provide care. They draw blood, place IV lines, transport patients to different locations in the hospital for sundry tests, perform EKG examinations, and/or carry out other tasks as directed.

Radiologists. Radiologists are physicians working in emergency medicine who are trained specifically in the diagnosis and treatment of the acutely ill and/or traumatized patients. They specialize in the use of imaging technologies to do this; said technologies include traditional x-ray, ultrasound, computerized tomography (CT), nuclear medicine, positron emission tomography (PET), mammography, and magnetic resonance imaging (MRI).

Radiology technicians. These technicians perform the imaging procedures ordered by radiologists and/or attending physicians. They prepare patients by explaining the procedures beforehand. They position patients so that the imaging equipment is most effective while at the same time protecting patients from unnecessary exposure to radiation.

Respiratory therapists (RTs). RTs evaluate and treat patients with acute respiratory issues such as asthma, pneumonia, and COPD. They also assist in the ED with patients who require life support ventilation (e.g., during times of heart attack, stroke, or respiratory arrest).

Police and other security personnel. The fast-pace of an ED, coupled with highly stressed nature of patients and family members who are there, can sometimes escalate into violent sequences between patrons and/or between patrons and ED personnel. It is also common for patients and family members to be violent by nature of alcohol or drug intoxication, and/or within more complex scenarios related to domestic violence or gang activity (e.g., an abusive spouse or rival gang member who shows up to do more harm). Police and other security personnel are thereby important to provide protection using graded management options like verbal or psychological interventions, displays of force, and physical restraints.

Sexual assault nurse examiners (SANEs). SANEs are registered nurses who specialize in providing medical forensic care to patients who have experienced sexual assault or abuse. They can conduct comprehensive medical forensic examinations, which include a detailed physical and emotional assessment, written/electronic and photographic documentation, collection and management of forensic samples, and the provision of emotional and social support and resources.

Chaplains. Chaplains represent spiritual practitioners (nondenominational) who work collaboratively with ED personnel, patients, and families to provide services for individuals and families in need. They can assist with the delivery of bad news, support family members during the immediate aftermath of a loved one's death, and provide encouragement in response to any variety of ambiguities or stressors. Their role in integrating patients/families' spirituality into the fast-paced and acute presentations commonplace in emergency medicine is an essential means of ensuring holistic care.

Social workers. Social workers are available to help with triaging patients to emergency and/or residential behavioral health hospitalizations, coordinate services between physical health and behavioral health providers (within and across locked and unlocked facility types), assess patients' safety vis-à-vis suicidality or homicidality, and/or connect patients and families with indicated hospital (e.g., chaplains, behavioral health providers) and/or community resources (e.g., public housing, emergency financial assistance). They can also determine which type(s) of outpatient care (e.g., partial hospitalization, intensive outpatient therapy, outpatient therapy) are appropriate.

Behavioral health providers. These practitioners aim to promote the behavioral health of individuals, couples, and families. While their roles can overlap with those aforementioned by social workers and chaplains (depending on the staffing and structure of the ED they are positioned within), these personnel maintain specialized training in baseline clinical therapies, psychological first aid, and other supportive interventions for common presentations like trauma, grief and loss, substance abuse, chronic illness, and domestic violence. They include psychologists, MedFTs, licensed independent clinical social workers (LICSWs), and counselors.

Child life specialists. These providers assist children and families with coping and stress management during an emergency visit. They also provide support (emotional, informational) during medical tests and procedures.

Case managers. Case managers work to improve patient flow and decrease inappropriate admissions in the ED. They coordinate services between multiple providers in care and connect patients with community resources upon discharge that align with indicated needs. They also connect uninsured and "frequent flyer" patients (i.e., those who present to the ED with an especially high regularity) to nonemergency resources to better support care needs and/or establish a healthcare home in primary care.

Financial teams. These personnel serve to connect uninsured patients to programs that will cover medical expenses. They work to liaison between patients and their families and the hospital facility and/or local, state, and federal government agencies.

Emergency medicine clerks. Clerks assist in a myriad of administrative duties. They greet patients and initiate registration through obtaining and verifying personal identification, insurance information, and any available healthcare records. They assist patients in navigating necessary paperwork and often serve in information liaison roles with other healthcare personnel.

Health unit coordinators (HUCs). HUCs register patients upon entry to the ED and collect insurance co-payments. They answer phones from within and outside of the hospital and work to share patients' and families' needs and requests with other members of the care team as necessary.

Scribes. Scribes are essential to increasing the efficiency of care provision. Often paired with a physician in a "shadowing" manner, they document elements of patient encounters in electronic medical records, track down ancillary health data, and facilitate communication between multiple care providers.

Patient sitters. Patient sitters work under the supervision of nursing staff; they help to monitor patients and provide ED providers with necessary status updates and reports. They are highly recommended for patients who represent flight risks and/or are a danger to themselves or others. Patient sitters can also be available to simply talk with, read to, and/or keep patients and families company while awaiting services.

Fundamentals of Care in Emergency Medicine

When working within the capacity of a MedFT provider in emergency medicine, specialized areas of content knowledge and skill sets are essential. The following represent those that are most important to this effort (McDonough et al., 2003; Schmitz et al., 2012; Sivakumar, Weiland, Gerdtz, Knott, & Jelinek, 2011).

Translator and Guide

MedFTs, alongside other providers in behavioral health, oftentimes assist patients and families in navigating the complex terrains of the ED and hospital system (Hodgson, Lamson, Mendenhall, & Crane, 2014; McDaniel, Doherty, & Hepworth, 2014). *Who does what? Why does this person need to talk with me? Why are they asking all of these questions that do not have anything to do with why I am here? How much longer do we have to wait to see the doctor? Who is that person standing behind the doctor but not talking to us?* Patients and families are oftentimes in psychological distress when they are at the ED, and it can be helpful to have a calm and compassionate presence to walk them through it. Similarly, physicians' and other healthcare providers' words and explanations can sometimes come across as hurried or esoteric; MedFTs often work to retell said words and explanations in ways that are more simple and understandable. For example, providing descriptions of how blood sugar crashes for a newly diagnosed diabetic patient caused the symptoms that prompted the ED visit, discussing the difference between an magnetic resonance imaging (MRI) and computerized axial tomography (CAT) scan, and why one or the other is preferred in light of the patient's injury, or taking patients and families through the admission process for an overnight stay are common fare for MedFTs in an ED. MedFTs might also work to ensure that language and cultural beliefs bestowed by patients and families are appropriately communicated and understood in the quick-paced environment of the ED, e.g., those regarding interpersonal "touch," gender of provider, and/or the role(s) and meaning(s) of blood or transfusions.

Assessment Skills in Behavioral Health

It is estimated that more than 10% of all ED visits involve a serious mental health or substance use condition (American Psychiatric Association [APA], 2016). Baseline familiarity with behavioral health diagnoses as outlined by DSM-5 (APA, 2013) is essential for any practitioner whose work is supported by third-party payers. In an ED environment, these skills are important in the conduct of a mental status exam and/or rapid assessment of presenting psychological symptoms (e.g., low mood, racing thoughts, suicidal ideation, delusions, hallucinations, depersonalization, cognitive flooding), concomitant behaviors (e.g., obsessive/compulsive sequences, non-suicidal self-injury, interpersonal violence), and formal diagnoses (e.g., major depressive disorder, post-traumatic stress disorder, schizophrenia). The execution of these skills serves to inform indicated courses of immediate treatment and stabilization of patients via psychopharmaceutic and/or talk therapy routes and inform key decisions regarding whether to hospitalize patients with or against their personal will to ensure the safety of said patients and others.

Assessment skills for suicidality and homicidality. While encompassed within the general assessment skills in behavioral health outlined above, it is important to highlight competencies in assessment for possible suicidality and homicidality in their own right (Bassett, 2010; Bernert, Hom, & Roberts, 2014; Granello, 2010). One of the most common scenarios in which an ED's attending physician and/or other personnel will act in accord with the MedFT's counsel is when a patient maintains high risk of intent to harm himself/herself or others. These types of situations can coexist with other behavioral health struggles (e.g., long-standing depression), but they do not have to. A distraught teenager whose girlfriend just broke with him, a drunk employee who just lost her job, an enraged parent who just discovered that his child was raped by a neighbor – and/or any number of other scenarios – can lead to a person carrying serious risk. Being able to quickly assess for said risk (e.g., plans, intents, means, identifiable victims) is a primary responsibility for MedFTs and other behavioral health providers in an ED. In doing this, it is also important to speak to the person who brought the patient in (or the person who called the police, mobile crisis team, etc.) – alongside family, friends, or other providers that the patient is willing to identify and/or permit contact with – to gain a holistic understanding of the patient's current situation, past experiences with care, potential barriers, and prospective resources.

Assessment skills for alcohol/drug abuse and dependency. Encompassed within the general assessment skills in behavioral health outlined above, it is important to highlight how MedFTs function vis-à-vis patient presentations around alcohol and drug use. These providers should be familiar with medical considerations surrounding assessment and triage for substance use (e.g., screenings that may be required for admittance to a particular program or hospital, different types of facilities that are available vis-a-vis the extent of a patient's physiological dependence). Research has shown that up to 50% of all trauma patients (defined as those requiring hospitalization and/or having sustained significant and acute injuries) screen positively for alcohol or drug use (Donovan & Marlatt, 2013; Pradel, Delga, Rouby, Micallef, & Lapeyre-Mestre, 2010). Even within the fast-paced context of an ED, screening for said use can inform responses via brief interventions (from 5 to 60 minutes) by behavioral health personnel. MedFTs trained in SBIRT(screening, brief intervention, referral, and treatment) will have knowledge such as the principles of motivational interviewing and skills to extend interventions that have been shown to help patients reduce unhealthy alcohol use and/or agree to follow-up treatment toward abstinence (Jensen et al., 2011; Lundahl et al., 2013; Substance Abuse and Mental Health Services Administration [SAMHSA], 2016).

Emergency Medicine Terminology

Familiarity with commonplace medical terminology (e.g., b.i.d., p.r.n., HEENT) is arguably necessary for any behavioral provider working within any healthcare context. A variety of terms and acronyms are used in emergency medicine that are unique in its context(s), and MedFTs are responsible for being appropriately conversant (Chabner, 2016; Ehrlich, 2014). Examples of these (also highlighted in this chapter's glossary) include ABCs (airway with cervical spine control, breathing, circulation with control of bleeding), AMA (against medical advice), BLS (basic life support), coag panel (test to assess blood clotting capability), dyspnea (shortness of breath), GSW (gunshot wound), MVA (motor vehicle accident), and NS (normal saline).

De-escalation Skills

When patients and/or family members escalate in anger, rage, or fear, ED personnel often rely on behavioral health personnel to assist in de-escalating the person(s) and situation(s) at hand. They usually do this in teams of two (not by one's self) through a combination of calm self-presentations (e.g., using low tones of voice, not being defensive), empathy (e.g., "I understand that you have every right to be mad about…"), and choice-giving (e.g., "Can I grab you water or a Coke?") – all the while moving the conversation outside or to another (and usually more quiet) location (Price & Baker, 2012; Richmond et al., 2012). External controls (e.g., hospital rules about waiting-room conduct, ED requirements that high-risk patients' stability is ensured) can be used in boundary setting, as these are not usually taken as personal. Attention to safety is the key (e.g., maintaining clear paths to a door and/or an unattainable distance to objects that can be used as weapons). If it is the behavioral provider's judgment that an agitated person will not calm down or is otherwise dangerous, police and/or other security personnel should be called.

Knowing When and How to Call Police or Security

Especially during de-escalation sequences, behavioral health providers must be careful to trust their instincts about whether to call police or other security personnel for assistance. If an agitated person is not responsive to the provider's attempts to calm him or her down, refuses to leave when asked, is disobedient to rule and/or boundary setting, makes hostile threats or posturing, or has any kind of weapon, then police or security should be called. Often these personnel are immediately on-site or close by and can be summoned by internal pager and/or alarm systems, telephone, or calling 911 from a landline (Oliva, Morgan, & Compton, 2010).

Delivering Bad News

Arguably one of the more difficult tasks for behavioral health providers in the ED, delivering bad news in an empathic and supportive manner is an essential skill to do well (Kaplan, 2010; Park, Gupta, Mandani, Haubner, & Peckler, 2010). These conversations proceed after a variety of events (e.g., meeting with a patient's family after she/he had died from his/her injuries or illness, informing a patient of his/her terminal disease diagnosis, confirming prenatal demise). Oftentimes done in the context of another provider with specific health knowledge about what has happened or specific administrative knowledge about what to do next, MedFTs and other behavioral providers colead these conversations. They take special care to prepare beforehand (e.g., becoming familiar with what has happened, arranging a space to have the conversation), building a therapeutic rapport (e.g., encouraging patients/families to gather supportive persons, foreshadowing that bad news is coming, determining how much patients/families want to know), communicating well (e.g., talking frankly but compassionately, avoiding euphemisms and medical jargon, allowing for silence and tears, going slowly), dealing with patients'/families' normative reactions (e.g., shock, disbelief, anger, blame, denial, intellectualization), and encouraging and validating emotions. It is also important to maintain familiarity with cultural norms regarding grief reactions and individual and family (and extended family and larger community) responses and to support and accommodate these to the extent(s) possible. Finally, it is important for the behavioral provider to work with patients and families to set the appropriate course for follow-up and collaborative services with other providers and indicated resources.

Coordinating Referrals for Long-Term Behavioral Healthcare

Many patients who present to the ED could benefit from long-term behavioral healthcare services. Simply encouraging this sans specific recommendations, names, and contact information is generally not effective, however. Behavioral providers in ED contexts should be familiar with local clinic sites that are staffed by competent clinicians, and they should be prepared to offer information about these resources in a manner that is personalized to the patients and families they encounter. For example, if a patient who is depressed, but not suicidal is amenable to follow-up and long-term care, the MedFT could offer specific names of providers who serve in that patient's geographic locale, who are of a preferred gender (if the patient has a preference), and who specialize in a particular challenge that the patient is struggling with (e.g., abuse survival, body image). If a patient can benefit from couple or family therapy (and many could), the ED provider should be prepared to offer systems-informed provider referrals in a similar manner. It is also important that the ED provider be able to offer three or more names and resources, as waiting times, insurance coverage, wait times, and personal "fit" with outside clinicians can vary (Druss et al., 2010; Hoffman, Haffmans, Spinhoven, & Hoencamp, 2015). Other barriers to care – like transportation, cognitive ability to adhere to a schedule or directions, etc. – are also important to take into account so that appropriately matched services are offered when possible.

Self-Care

Taking care of one's own psychosocial needs is a fundamental skill for MedFTs practicing in any environment (Lamson, Meadors, & Mendenhall, 2014). We highlight it here, however, on the grounds that emergency medicine's fast-paced, chaotic, unpredictable, and often emotionally charged nature represents a care context that can be especially dangerous to providers' behavioral health (Houry, Shockley, & Markovchick, 2000; Wrenn, Lorenzen, Jones, Zhou, & Aronsky, 2010). Effectively engaging in self-care requires that the MedFT recognizes himself/herself as a bio-psychosocial-spiritual (BPSS) being in the same ways that she/he sees her or his own patients (Engel, 1977, 1980; Wright, Watson, & Bell, 1996). Attending to biological/physical health can include regular and proper nutrition, hydration, sleep hygiene, and exercise. Psychological well-being can be maintained through peer and collegial support and debriefings following specific events (e.g., when a patient dies) or an exhausting shift (i.e., the cumulative effects of multiple cases can be overwhelming). Social well-being can overlap with this as colleagues engage with each other outside of work, but can – and often does – transpire with family and friends with whom the MedFT does not work professionally. Participating in church and faith-based communities, interest and hobby groups (e.g., hiking, motorcycling, boating), volunteering, etc. can go a long way. Spiritual health can come from these communities and activities, too, and/or represent very personal journeys through prayer, meditation, and/or other sequences. Fundamentally, if we take care of ourselves, we will be better equipped to provide care to others (Boyle, 2011; Cross, 2016; Hooper, Craig, Janvrin, Wetsel, & Reimels, 2010; Mendenhall, 2012).

Emergency Medicine Across the MedFT Healthcare Continuum

Medical family therapy serves as a useful framework for behavioral health and physical health providers in the care for individuals and families who are presenting for ED treatment and care. Specific training, practice, research, and policy competencies represent important facets of this work as professionals engage with these often-diverse populations. Tables 7.1 and 7.2 highlight specific skills that characterize MedFTs' involvement in ED contexts across Hodgson, Lamson, Mendenhall, and Tyndall (2014) MedFT Healthcare Continuum. As MedFTs grow along the continuum, so does their proficiency to incorporate BPSS and systemic care into each interaction through clinical practice, research, training, and policy.

At the beginning of the continuum, MedFTs at *Levels 1* and *2* should possess general understanding(s) of psychological and behavioral processes of patients and families who are highly distressed and/or traumatized (e.g., normative stress reactions to an acute situation versus post-traumatic stress disorder, typical psychological reactions to commonplace ambiguities extant within ED contexts and processes). MedFTs at these levels do not likely engage with ED personnel very often (e.g., maintaining a private practice while occasionally referring patients who are imminently suicidal or homicidal). They are able to effectively assess for risk and perform stabilizing interventions (e.g., psychological first aid) before ED admissions and are familiar with said admission processes. For example, a MedFT working with a suicidal teenager could explain his/her concern and responsibility to ensure the teen's safety. She/he could engage a supportive friend or family member

Table 7.1 MedFTs in Emergency Medicine: Basic Knowledge and Skills

MedFT Healthcare Continuum Level	Level 1	Level 2	Level 3
Knowledge	Basic knowledge about BPSS approaches to emergency behavioral health; sensitive to how stress responses and mood are mutually influential. Familiar with psychological first aid (PFA) as a baseline trauma intervention. Limited understanding ED admission processes.	Can differentiate between types of trauma reactions (e.g., normative stress responses, PTSD). Familiar with benefits of couple and family engagement in ED admission processes, post-emergency adjustments, and/or follow-up lifestyle changes and maintenance.	Working knowledge of specific team members (e.g., physician, chaplain) and terms in trauma response (e.g., DNR, GSW, MVA). Basic knowledge of common ED presentations (e.g., cardiac events, suicidality) and expected psychological reactions (e.g., hypervigilance, fear, irritability).
Skills	Can discuss (and psycho-educate) basic relationships between biological processes, psychological risk, and need to coordinate services with ED. Minimal collaborative skills with other providers; generally works in an individual practitioner model but collaborates with ED as necessary.	Able to apply systemic interventions in practice; assess patients for background issues such as family history and related risk factors to ED response. Adequate collaborative skills; works with ED personnel with some regularity; can coordinate referrals and follow-up with indicated specialists in patients' care.	Working within medical care clinics, able to integrate respective team members' expertise, and counsel into treatment decisions and planning. Can implement a systemic assessment of a patient and family with competencies in assessing for BPSS aspects of trauma and resources within the family; engage other professionals as indicated; skilled with standardized measures to assess patients' risk (e.g., for suicidality) as measured by symptoms of depression and anxiety – including, but not limited to, the PHQ-2, PHQ-4, PHQ-9, and diabetes distress scale (American Psychological Association, 2016; fisher, Hessler, Polonsky, & Mullan, 2012; Lowe et al., 2010).

Table 7.2 MedFTs in Emergency Medicine: Advanced Knowledge and Skills

MedFT Healthcare Continuum Level	Level 4	Level 5
Knowledge	Competent understanding of several trauma types and related clinical presentations. Adept in a range of trauma-focused treatments, medications, and terminologies. Conversant in nearly all terms, measures, and facets of ED care.	Understand treatment and care sequences for unique and/or challenging topics in ED (e.g., suicidality, intimate partner violence, alcohol and/or drug abuse); can consult effectively with professionals about medical topics from other fields. Conversant with evidence-based treatments regarding most trauma-related work and their role(s) in family therapy; has background to provide education to patients about a variety of symptoms, medications, and stress management. High content knowledge in clinical topics, research practice, policy, and administrative areas of ED response; proficient in developing a curriculum on PFA, behavioral health roles, and other supportive sequences to provide other professionals.
Skills	Able to deliver seminars and workshops about the BPSS complexities of ED work to a variety of professional types (e.g., behavioral health, biomedical). Can apply several BPSS interventions in ED response and follow-up care; can administer mood- and disease-specific assessment tools skillfully. Consistently collaborates with key team members (e.g., attending physician, chaplain); initiates team visits with multiple providers when working with patients and families.	Proficient in nearly all aspects of ED response efforts; able to synthesize and conduct research, engages in collaborative efforts to organize and advance team preparedness. Routinely engages in team-based approaches to care, with consistent communication through electronic health records, patient introductions, "curb-side consultations," and team meetings and visits. Engaged in advocacy efforts regarding third-party payer coverage and equity in hiring practices for LMFT providers positioned in ED contexts.

in this discussion and encourage them to take part in the admission process (e.g., making a phone call to the ED with the patient and his/her support person together, explaining the steps from transitioning from the private practice office to the hospital). Familiarity and competence through these processes, coupled with the patient's experience of traversing it with a loved one, will ease some of the common anxiety and fears that presenting to the ED can encompass.

A clinician equipped with knowledge and skills outlined in *Level 3* is arguably able to collaborate with and/or function within the ED team. In clinical practice, she/he would demonstrate most competence (in this level and the others beyond it) after the acute phases of an ED presentation, but the majority of his/her efforts are situated within said acute phases. This is important to note, insofar as the work provided by a MedFT within ED contexts is not the same as what is provided in ongoing therapy. This MedFT can readily implement systemic assessments of individuals and families impacted by trauma (broadly defined) and either respond with clinical competency in admitting patients to the ED, matching needs that they identify immediately, or coordinate follow-up services with others as indicated.

A MedFT functioning at *Level 4* maintains high competence and knowledge in caring for patients and families presenting with emergency issues and acute trauma, alongside intimate understandings about how the integrated behavioral healthcare teams that function within the ED work. Being adept with core content and terms essential to emergency medicine (see Glossary) enables him/her to effectively translate and track respective team members' efforts over the course of an admission (e.g., attending physician, radiologist, EMT). Maintaining clear understandings about said team members' training and scope of practice enables the MedFT to guide individuals and families through their care experience (e.g., Justin can explain to Mr. Jones and his daughter how sundry assessments will inform medication decisions, discharge planning, and follow-up evaluations and care).

A MedFT functioning at this level is thereby able to keep up with and contribute to more complex care plans with other providers engaged with patients (e.g., a survivor of a suicide attempt in therapy several weeks later) and families toward a shared vision of treatment goals and outcomes. This encompasses a working familiarity and competence with multiple treatment modalities (e.g., cognitive behavioral therapy [CBT], eye movement desensitization and reprocessing [EMDR]) performed in family-based contexts, alongside purposeful efforts to build relationships with other members of the care team (e.g., physician, chaplain). For example, in work with an adolescent during the weeks following the teen's suicide attempt, a MedFT could normalize and empathize with how challenging the acute and long-term stressors that led up the attempt were and how complex and overwhelming the medical system can be to navigate if/when/as concomitant symptoms like depression, anxiety, social isolation, insomnia, gastrointestinal distress, headaches, poor appetite, etc. are simultaneously present. Engaging this youth's parents and/or peers in supportive roles would be essential in this work, as well, especially in light of how social connections help to allay the profound sense of isolation that suicidal patients can oftentimes feel (Grav, Hellzèn, Romild, & Stordal, 2012; Lin, Dean, & Ensel, 2013).

MedFTs who function at *Level 5* generally have practiced at all levels of care and work in various roles within the ED context (e.g., clinical, administration, supervision, directing). As a clinician, proficiency in acute interventions and BPSS approaches includes competence and knowledge regarding other providers' contributions to care (e.g., medications, de-escalation and/or relaxation sequences, lifestyle management, follow-up coordination). This is evidenced in active and effective participation in, and leading of team-based collaboration, which often expands beyond the acute incident's timeframe and the ED's "walls" to include other specialties and indicated resources relevant to patients' and families' needs (e.g., grief work for Jessica or neurological testing for Mr. Jones in our vignette). As an educator and mentor, she/he is proficient in the didactic and supervisory instruction of these skill sets and knowledge – evidenced across live classroom and clinical sequences and/or in the construction of instructional materials (e.g., refereed journal articles, texts, conference workshops). Further, professionals at this level tend to be involved in research (e.g., testing and/or comparing interdisciplinary team-based methodologies, evaluating care efficiency across different team-based models), policymaking (e.g., advocacy for third-party recognition and payments for services provided by licensed marriage and family therapists [LMFTs] alongside licensed psychologists [LPs] and licensed independent clinical social workers [LICSWs]), and other administrative duties (e.g., overseeing behavioral health internships that include training for and experience in ED work). They do this with sensitivity to the three-world view of healthcare (Peek, 2008), concurrently addressing (a) common clinical challenges and problem-solving sequences, (b) operational processes that facilitate ED teams' effective and efficient functioning, and (c) financial considerations that are unique to the needs of specific communities (broadly) and within the clinic and health systems engaged to assist individual patients and families (narrowly).

Level 5 clinical efforts following the vignette provided in this chapter could engage MedFT trainees and/or medical residents in the care for patients who are struggling with the ambiguities of potential health declines (e.g., possible dementia) and/or acute loss (e.g., death of a loved one) to take active roles in co-owning and comanaging their psychological and/or relational health. As a researcher, a MedFT could seek in-depth understandings about patients' and families' experiences in the acute phases of care (e.g., a qualitative case study targeting what they did and did not like and/or what suggestions they have; a quantitative study regarding straightforward patient satisfaction). As an educator, the MedFT could use survivors' stories (either with their permission or in a manner appropriately disguised and potentially even with their coauthorship) as case examples in training manuals and/or professional presentations. As an advocate, she/he could present patients' and families' stories as examples – in tandem with research based analyses and/or health informatics – to persuade and/or guide indicated policy and administrative sequences facilitative of relationally trained providers working in emergency medicine.

Research-Informed Practices

Within the contexts of our increasingly integrated and interdisciplinary contemporary healthcare systems, MedFT has considerable face validity. It is a systemically oriented way of conducting clinical practice that connects the dots across multiple providers (professionally) and family members and loved ones (personally) involved in patients' lives. Most people directly connected to MedFT are able to see some, if not a great deal of, potential value. When experiencing the unexpected event(s) of an ED visit, it is natural for patients to want their families and loved ones there (and vice versa). MedFTs, as providers with expertise in human relationships (alongside baseline behavioral health per se), are readily able to navigate and work with families during times of crisis. Families are not "underfoot" or "in the way" of good care provision; they are essential to it.

Within an ED, MedFTs are equipped to elicit families' support for a variety of presentations and/or run interference between escalating members as indicated. They are able to work with multiple family members in the delivery of bad news, in conversations to challenge problematic health behaviors, and in discharge planning. Moreover, MedFTs' systemic orientation facilitates the effective communication and coordination of efforts between members of an ED's care team – all with different personalities, communication styles, interpersonal boundaries, and work habitats. Many have even cited MedFTs' support of their professional colleagues as a parallel "job duty" to their standard clinical role (e.g., Marlowe & Hodgson, 2014; Tyndall, Hodgson, Lamson, White, & Knight, 2014).

Objectively answering questions, however, like "Does MedFT work in ED contexts?" or "If it does work, in what ways?" is difficult. This is true for two primary reasons: First, collecting outcome data regarding MedFT conducted in emergency medicine is challenging because consistent health-related dependent variables that are comprehensively informative do not exist. For example, an ED – on any given day – sees patients who are presenting with diabetic events, migraine headaches, food poisoning, broken bones, drug overdoses, childbirth, heart attacks, suicide attempts, gunshot wounds, head trauma, and a myriad of other things. What, then, could a researcher measure to ascertain whether the inclusion of a MedFT on the ED team is effective? For one family, the MedFT is assisting with delivering bad news about a matriarch who was killed in a MVA. For another, she/he might be helping to brainstorm ways that a patient can connect to a diabetes group for education and support upon discharge. For another, she/he might be called in to de-escalate a couple who is fighting about whose fault it is that their child got into rat poison in their garage. What could a researcher measure across all of these cases to assess whether MedFT is effective?

The second reason that research regarding MedFT in emergency medicine is limited relates to a long-standing political impasse between behavioral disciplines in healthcare. Hiring practices (and third-party payer policies that support said practices) has long favored psychology (LP) and social work (LICSW) providers in ED contexts. The presence of MedFTs in emergency medicine is thereby limited, despite ongoing efforts across all 50 of the United States' states for equity in opportunity, access, and coverage (42 US Code §1395 l(a)(1)(F); American Association for Marriage and Family Therapy [AAMFT], 2005). And because these practices are regulated at the state level, considerable diversity in MedFT presence is extant, with some states categorically denying MedFTs entry. Collectively, these sequelae translate into a paucity of healthcare systems within which to engage MedFT research.

What we do know is as follows: family-based interventions for patients who are "high utilizers" or "frequent flyers" in healthcare – i.e., those who often present in the ED – are more effective than individually oriented approaches in reducing care-seeking for unnecessary services via urgent care. Boudreauz et al. (2002) found that patients presenting in emergency departments for invasive procedures and resuscitations fare better with family involvement and inclusion and that the family members themselves – while not identified "patients" per se – described their experiences as more favorable. Diamond et al. (2010) recognized considerably better change in self-reported suicidal ideation following emergency hospitalization by engaging family members as participants in team-based care. Walsh (2007) called attention to the utility of including families in trauma care, whether in clinic contexts or and community and field work. And to be sure, future efforts to extend and further substantiate this knowledge are indicated. For instance, researchers could evaluate ED processes (e.g., systems that include a MedFT from intake to discharge versus those whose team does not include a MedFT) and the ways that these predict overall experiences of patient satisfaction, baseline behavioral health functioning (e.g., PHQ-9 data for depression, GAD data for anxiety), and long-term ED utilization for nonemergency presentations.

In post-ED psychiatric care, which is essential in follow-up and discharge planning, Falloon (2003) described several studies that showed better outcomes for schizophrenic patients through family inclusion in care. Heru and Berman (2008) maintained that MedFTs' inclusion in psychiatry was helpful in engaging (versus excluding) family members; doing this also served to not demonize or blame families for patients' suffering. In alcohol and drug treatment, Szapocznik and Williams (2000) found that engaging families in care for adolescent youth showed promise in achieving and maintaining positive behavior change. Copello, Velleman, and Templeton (2005) and Gifford (2015) echoed these findings and went further to describe the importance of including family members' own needs as part of intervention sequences.

Specific interventions that we know to work in emergency contexts – whether advanced with individual patients or with patients and their families and loved ones together – include the following: *cognitive behavior therapy* (CBT), which is often employed to treat acute stress reactions to traumatic events and can be helpful in preventing the development of PTSD (Iverson et al., 2011; Kar, 2011). Several researchers have followed patients undergoing CBT for weeks or months after a traumatic event and have yielded consistently positive results. A thorough review of the literature concluded that early CBT "should be employed routinely as an early intervention for survivors of relatively discrete accidents who endorse significant, enduring posttraumatic difficulties" (Litz & Bryant, 2009, p. 128). While the use of CBT to prevent chronic PTSD following non-interpersonal accidents has strong support (Ehlers et al., 2003; Litz and Bryant, 2009), the support for CBT for PTSD resulting from interpersonal traumatic events – like intimate partner violence – is less conclusive. Some have shown positive results (e.g., Bryant, Moulds, & Nixon, 2006) and others have shown neutral results (e.g., Foa, Zoellner, & Feeny, 2006).

Psychological first aid (PFA) is an approach originally designed for fieldwork that advances supportive and practical help for surviving victims of a traumatic event (Ruzek, Brymer, Jacobs, & Layne, 2007; Ruzek, Young, Cordova, & Flynn, 2004). Its use has been extended to a variety of efforts situated within the contexts of acute care, including emergency medicine. PFA is guided by core actions wherein the provider works to engage distressed patients in a calm and empathic manner to promote safety, comfort, and stability while gathering information about current needs and concerns. The provider offers practical assistance, connects patients with indicated social and community supports, provides information about coping, and helps to link and coordinate follow-up services with indicated (non-acute) services. For more in-depth discussion about how PFA overlaps with MedFT practice, see *Chapter 15*.

Conclusion

Emergency medicine is a care context that is defined by its broad range of clinical foci, unpredictable and oftentimes chaotic nature, and "single-issue" care encounters that stand in marked contrast to the long-term clinical relationships and continuity of care ideals that most behavioral health providers are prepared for during graduate training. MedFTs – equipped with behavioral and relational skills in working with patients, families, and other providers within complex care systems – represent a relatively new addition to ED teams. Emerging evidence supports that their contributions and their participation in such acute-care environments will likely increase as more healthcare systems adopt integrated behavioral healthcare models.

Reflection Questions
1. As a MedFT working in emergency medicine, how can you appropriately and effectively take steps to mitigate personal risk(s) of compassion fatigue?
2. What ethnic and/or cultural considerations are important for you to think about when working with families who are facing an involuntary admission for one of their loved ones who is suicidal?
3. After reading this chapter, what areas of intervention(s) do you need to learn more about and/or increase skill within in order to provide better care?

Glossary of Important Terms for Care in Emergency Medicine

ABCs Essential steps and foci used by both medical professionals and lay persons when attending to a patient during an emergency; stands for airway with cervical spine control, breathing, circulation with control of bleeding.
Acute A sudden, unexpected, and often intense health condition.
Agonal A major negative change in a patient's health condition, usually preceding death (e.g., complete cessation of breathing, dire change in EKG).

ALS Advanced life support; includes life-saving protocols and skills that include both basic life support and efforts to facilitate circulation and provide an open airway and adequate ventilation for breathing.
AMA Against medical advice; refers to when a patient leaves a hospital and/or discontinues treatment against the advice of his or her care provider.
BLS Basic life support; refers to care provided to victims of a life-threatening illnesses or injuries until they can be admitted to a hospital for full medical attention.
BSA Burn surface area; refers to the total percentage area of a patient's body that is burned.
Chest film An x-ray of patient's chest.
Coag panel A test to assess blood clotting capability.
CPR Cardiopulmonary resuscitation; this is an emergency procedure that combines chest compressions and (often) artificial ventilation so as to manually preserve brain function until further measures can be taken to restore spontaneous breathing and blood circulation in a person who is experiencing cardiac arrest.
Crasher A person who passes out in the ED (often a family member who is upset about what is happening with their loved one).
DB Dead body; patient is deceased.
DNR Do not resuscitate; a directive that this formally requested or ordered for terminally ill or injured patients.
DOA Dead on arrival; patient arrived to care facility deceased.
Dyspnea Shortness of breath; refers to difficult and/or labored breathing. This condition is associated with a myriad of acute and chronic physical conditions.
GSW Gunshot wound.
LOC Loss of consciousness.
MVA Motor vehicle accident; can refer to incidents involving cars/trucks or motorcycles.
NS Normal saline; refers to a mixture of sodium chloride and water. NS is used for a variety of purposes, including (but not limited to) cleaning wounds, treating dehydration (when injected intravenously), wetting dry eyes, and diluting medications.
Rape kit A box or package containing envelopes hair, sperm, and blood samples from a rape victim; also contains formal reporting paperwork.

Additional Resources

Literature

Adams, J. (2012). *Emergency medicine: Clinical essentials.* Philadelphia, PA: Elsevier & Saunders.
Hughes, T., & Cruickshank, J. (2011). *Adult emergency medicine at a glance.* Hoboken, NJ: Wiley-Blackwell.

Mahadevan, S., & Garmel, G. (2012). *Introduction to clinical emergency medicine* (2nd ed.). New York, NY: Cambridge University Press.
Wyatt, J., Illingworth, R., Grahm, C., & Hogg, K. (2017). *Oxford handbook of emergency medicine* (4th ed.). New York, NY: Oxford University Press.

Measures/Instruments

Alcohol Use Disorders Identification Test (AUDIT). http://www.integration.samhsa.gov/AUDIT_screener_for_alcohol.pdf
CAGE Alcohol Questionnaire. http://www.integration.samhsa.gov/images/res/CAGEAID.pdf
Columbia-Suicide Severity Rating Scale. http://www.integration.samhsa.gov/clinical-practice/Columbia_Suicide_Severity_Rating_Scale.pdf
Patient Health Questionnaire (PHQ-9). http://www.integration.samhsa.gov/images/res/PHQ%20-%20Questions.pdf

Organizations/Associations

Substance Abuse and Mental Health Services Administration (SAMHSA)/Guide to Screening Tools. http://www.integration.samhsa.gov/clinical-practice/screening-tools
Substance Abuse and Mental Health Services Administration (SAMHSA)/Guide to Suicide Prevention. http://www.integration.samhsa.gov/clinical-practice/suicide-prevention
Suicide Prevention Resource Center. http://www.sprc.org/ed-guide

References[1]

*Adams, J. (2012). *Emergency medicine: Clinical essentials*. Philadelphia, PA: Elsevier & Saunders.
American Association for Marriage and Family Therapy [AAMFT] (2005). *Medicare coverage of marriage and family therapists*. Retrieved from https://www.aamft.org/iMIS15/AAMFT/Content/Advocacy/Medicare.aspx
American College of Emergency Physicians (2014). *Definition of emergency medicine*. Retrieved from https://www.acep.org/Clinical---Practice-Management/Definition-of-Emergency-Medicine/
American Psychiatric Association (2016). *Emergency room visits for mental health conditions: Expect long waits*. Retrieved from https://www.psychiatry.org/news-room/apa-blogs/apa-blog/2016/11/emergency-room-visits-for-mental-health-conditions-expect-long-waits

---

[1] Note: References that are prefaced with an asterisk are recommended readings.

American Psychiatric Association. (2013). *Diagnostic and statistical manual of mental disorders: DSM-5*. Washington, D.C: Author.
Bassett, D. L. (2010). Risk assessment and management in bipolar disorders. *Medical Journal of Australia, 193*(Suppl 4), S21–S23. Retrieved from https://www.mja.com.au/system/files/issues/193_04_160810/bas10132_fm.pdf
*Bernert, R. A., Hom, M. A., & Roberts, L. W. (2014). A review of multidisciplinary clinical practice guidelines in suicide prevention: Toward an emerging standard in suicide risk assessment and management, training and practice. *Academic Psychiatry, 38*, 585–592. https://doi.org/10.1007/s40596-014-0180-1.
Boudreauz, E., Francis, J., & Loyacano, T. (2002). Family presence during invasive procedures and resuscitations in the emergency department: A critical review and suggestions for future research. *Annals of Emergency Medicine, 40*, 193–205. https://doi.org/10.1067/mem.2002.124899
*Boyle, D. (2011). Countering compassion fatigue: A requisite nursing agenda. *Online Journal of Issues in Nursing, 16*(1), 2. https://doi.org/10.3912/OJIN.Vol16No01Man02.
Bryant, R., Moulds, M., & Nixon, R. (2006). Hypnotherapy and cognitive behavior therapy of acute stress disorder: A three year follow-up. *Behaviour Research and Therapy, 44*, 1331–1335. https://doi.org/10.1016/j.brat.2005.04.007
*Capella, J., Smith, S., Philp, A., Putnam, T., Gilbert, C., Fry, W., ... & Ranson, S. (2010). Teamwork training improves the clinical care of trauma patients. *Journal of Surgical Education, 67*, 439–443. https://doi.org/10.1016/j.jsurg.2010.06.006.
Chabner, D. (2016). *The language of medicine* (11th ed.). Atlanta, GA: Elsevier Health Sciences.
Copello, A., Velleman, R., & Templeton, L. (2005). Family interventions in the treatment of alcohol and drug problems. *Drug and Alcohol Review, 24*, 369–385. https://doi.org/10.1080/09595230500302356
Cross, A. (2016). Compassion fatigue: A personal perspective. *Emergency Medicine Australia, 28*, 104–105. https://doi.org/10.1111/1742-6723.12534
Diamond, G., Wintersteen, M., Brown, G., Diamond, G., Gallop, R., Shelef, K., & Levy, S. (2010). Attachment-based family therapy for adolescents with suicidal ideation: A randomized controlled trial. *Journal of the American Academy of Child & Adolescent Psychiatry, 49*, 122–131. https://doi.org/10.1016/j.jaac.2009.11.002
Donovan, D. M., & Marlatt, G. A. (Eds.). (2013). *Assessment of addictive behaviors*. New York, NY: Guilford Publications.
Druss, B. G., Silke, A., Compton, M. T., Rask, K. J., Zhao, L., & Parker, R. M. (2010). A randomized trial of medical care management for community mental health settings: The primary care access, referral, and evaluation (PCARE) study. *American Journal of Psychiatry, 167*, 151–159. https://doi.org/10.1176/appi.ajp.2009.09050691
Ehlers, A., Clark, D., Hackmann, A., McManus, F., Fennell, M., Herbert, C., & Mayou, R. (2003). A randomized controlled trial of cognitive therapy, a self-help booklet, and repeated assessments as early interventions for posttraumatic stress disorder. *Archives of General Psychiatry, 60*, 1024–1032. https://doi.org/10.1001/archpsyc.60.10.1024
Ehrlich, A. (2014). *Medical terminology for health professions*. Florence, KY: Delmar Publications.
Engel, G. (1977). The need for a new medical model: A challenge for biomedicine. *Science, 196*, 129–136. https://doi.org/10.1016/b978-0-409-95009-0.50006-1
Engel, G. (1980). The clinical application of the biopsychosocial model. *American Journal of Family Medicine, 137*, 535–544. https://doi.org/10.1176/ajp.137.5.535
Falloon, I. (2003). Family interventions for mental disorders: Efficacy and effectiveness. *World Psychiatry, 2*, 20–28. Retrieved from http://www.ncbi.nlm.nih.gov.ezp3.lib.umn.edu/pmc/articles/PMC1525058/?report=reader
Foa, E., Zoellner, L., & Feeny, N. (2006). An evaluation of three brief programs for facilitating recovery after assault. *Journal of Traumatic Stress, 19*, 29–43. https://doi.org/10.1002/jts.20096
Gifford, S. (2015). Family involvement is important in substance abuse treatment. *Psych Central*. https://psychcentral.com/lib/family-involvement-is-important-in-substance-abuse-treatment/

*Granello, D. H. (2010). The process of suicide risk assessment: Twelve core principles. *Journal of Counseling and Development, 88,* 363–371. https://doi.org/10.1002/j.1556-6678.2010.tb00034.x.

Grav, S., Hellzèn, O., Romild, U., & Stordal, E. (2012). Association between social support and depression in the general population: The HUNT study, a cross-sectional survey. *Journal of Clinical Nursing, 21,* 111–120. https://doi.org/10.1111/j.1365-2702.2011.03868.x

Heru, A., & Berman, E. (2008). Family meetings and integrated patient care. Medical family therapy in an inpatient setting. *Families, Systems, & Health, 26,* 181–184. https://doi.org/10.1037/1091-7527.26.2.181

Hodgson, J., Lamson, A., Mendenhall, T., & Crane, D. (Eds.). (2014). *Medical family therapy: Advanced applications.* New York, NY: Springer.

Hodgson, J., Lamson, A., Mendenhall, T., & Tyndall, L. (2014). Introduction to medical family therapy: Advanced applications. In J. Hodgson, A. Lamson, T. Mendenhall, and D. Crane (Eds.). *Medical family therapy: Advanced applications* (pp. 1–9). New York, NY: Springer.

Hoffman, T., Haffmans, J., Spinhoven, P., & Hoencamp, E. (2015). Collaborative mental health care versus care as usual in a primary care setting: A randomized controlled trial. *Psychiatric Services, 60,* 74–79. https://doi.org/10.1176/ps.2009.60.1.74

Hooper, C., Craig, J., Janvrin, D. R., Wetsel, M. A., & Reimels, E. (2010). Compassion satisfaction, burnout, and compassion fatigue among emergency nurses compared with nurses in other selected inpatient specialties. *Journal of Emergency Nursing, 36,* 420–427. https://doi.org/10.1016/j.jen.2009.11.027

Houry, D., Shockley, L. W., & Markovchick, V. (2000). Wellness issues and the emergency medicine resident. *Annals of Emergency Medicine, 35,* 394–397. https://doi.org/10.1016/S0196-0644(00)70060-6

*Hughes, T., & Cruickshank, J. (2011). *Adult emergency medicine at a glance.* Hoboken, NJ: Wiley-Blackwell.

Iverson, K. M., Gradus, J. L., Resick, P. A., Suvak, M. K., Smith, K. F., & Monson, C. M. (2011). Cognitive–behavioral therapy for PTSD and depression symptoms reduces risk for future intimate partner violence among interpersonal trauma survivors. *Journal of Consulting and Clinical Psychology, 79,* 193–202. https://doi.org/10.1037/a0022512

Jensen, C. D., Cushing, C. C., Aylward, B. S., Craig, J. T., Sorell, D. M., & Steele, R. G. (2011). Effectiveness of motivational interviewing interventions for adolescent substance use behavior change: A meta-analytic review. *Journal of Consulting and Clinical Psychology, 79,* 433–440. https://doi.org/10.1037/a0023992

Kaplan, M. (2010) SPIKES: A framework for breaking bad news to patients with cancer. *Clinical Journal of Oncology Nursing, 14,* 514–516. https://doi.org/10.1188/10.CJON.514-516

Kar, N. (2011). Cognitive behavioral therapy for the treatment of post-traumatic stress disorder: A review. *Neuropsychiatric Disease and Treatment, 7,* 167–181. https://doi.org/10.2147/NDT.S10389

*Kilner, E., & Sheppard, L. A. (2010). The role of teamwork and communication in the emergency department: A systematic review. *International Emergency Nursing, 18,* 127–137. https://doi.org/10.1016/j.ienj.2009.05.006.

Lamson, A., Meadors, P., & Mendenhall, T. (2014). Working with providers and healthcare systems experiencing compassion fatigue and burnout. In J. Hodgson, A. Lamson, T. Mendenhall, and D. Crane (Eds.), *Medical family therapy: Advanced applications* (pp. 107–123). New York, NY: Springer.

Larkin, G. L., Beautrais, A. L., Spirito, A., Kirrane, B. M., Lippmann, M. J., & Milzman, D. P. (2009). Mental health and emergency medicine: A research agenda. *Academic Emergency Medicine, 16,* 1110–1119. https://doi.org/10.1111/j.1553-2712.2009.00545.x

Larkin, G. L., Claassen, C. A., Emond, J. A., Pelletier, A. J., & Camargo, C. A. (2005). Trends in US emergency department visits for mental health conditions, 1992 to 2001. *Psychiatric Services, 56,* 671–677. https://doi.org/10.1176/appi.ps.56.6.671

Lemons, M., Berner, A., Baily, M., Huckins, D., Tils, B., & Leiter, E. (2015). *Emergency department leadership, physicians & staff.* Newton-Wellesley Hospital. Retrieved from http://www.nwh.org/departments-and-services/emergency/our-team/

Lin, N., Dean, A., & Ensel, W. (2013). *Social support, life events, and depression.* Cambridge, MA: Academic Press.
Litz, B., & Bryant, R. (2009). Early cognitive-behavior interventions for adults. In E. Foa, T. Keane, M. Friedman, and J. Cohen (Eds.), *Effective treatments for PTSD* (pp. 117–135). New York, NY: Guilford Press.
Lundahl, B., Moleni, T., Burke, B. L., Butters, R., Tollefson, D., Butler, C., & Rollnick, S. (2013). Motivational interviewing in medical care settings: A systematic review and meta-analysis of randomized controlled trials. *Patient Education and Counseling, 93,* 157–168. https://doi.org/10.1016/j.pec.2013.07.012
*Mahadevan, S., & Garmel, G. (2012). *Introduction to clinical emergency medicine* (2nd ed.). New York, NY: Cambridge University Press.
Marlowe, D., & Hodgson, J. (2014). Building relationships in integrated care. In J. Hodgson, A. Lamson, T. Mendenhall, and D. Crane (Eds.), *Medical family therapy: Advanced applications* (pp. 95–106). New York, NY: Springer.
Marx, J., Hockberger, R., & Walls, R. (2014). *Rosen's emergency medicine: Concepts and clinical practice.* Philadelphia, PA: Elsevier & Saunders.
McDaniel, S., Doherty, W., & Hepworth, J. (2014). *Medical family therapy and integrated care* (2nd ed.). Washington, DC: American Psychological Association.
McDonough, S., Wynaden, D., Finn, M., McGowan, S., Chapman, R., & Gray, S. (2003). Emergency department mental health triage and consultancy service: An advanced practice role for mental health nurses. *Contemporary Nurse, 14,* 138–144. https://doi.org/10.5172/conu.14.2.138
*Mendenhall, T. (2012). Practicing what we preach: Answering the call for responder self-care and resiliency. *The Dialogue* (SAMHSA/DTAC), *8,* 2–4. Retrieved from https://content.govdelivery.com/accounts/USSAMHSA/bulletins/3cd722
Oliva, J. R., Morgan, R., & Compton, M. T. (2010). A practical overview of de-escalation skills in law enforcement: Helping individuals in crisis while reducing police liability and injury. *Journal of Police Crisis Negotiations, 10,* 15–29. https://doi.org/10.1080/15332581003785421
Park, I., Gupta, A., Mandani, K., Haubner, L., & Peckler, B. (2010). Breaking bad news education for emergency medicine residents: A novel training module using simulation with the SPIKES protocol. *Journal of Emergencies, Trauma, and Shock, 3,* 385–388. Retrieved from http://www.onlinejets.org/text.asp?2010/3/4/385/70760
Peek, C. (2008). Planning care in the clinical, operational, and financial worlds. In R. Kessler and D. Stafford (Eds.), *Collaborative medicine case studies: Evidence in practice* (pp. 25–38). New York, NY: Springer.
Pradel, V., Delga, C., Rouby, F., Micallef, J., & Lapeyre-Mestre, M. (2010). Assessment of abuse potential of benzodiazepines from a prescription database using 'doctor shopping' as an indicator. *CNS Drugs, 24,* 611–620. https://doi.org/10.2165/11531570-000000000-00000
Price, O., & Baker, J. (2012). Key components of de-escalation techniques: A thematic synthesis. *International Journal of Mental Health Nursing, 21,* 310–319. https://doi.org/10.1111/j.1447-0349.2011.00793.x
*Richmond, J. S., Berlin, J. S., Fishkind, A. B., Holloman, G. H., Zeller, S. L., Wilson, M. P., … & Ng, A. T. (2012). Verbal de-escalation of the agitated patient: consensus statement of the American Association for Emergency Psychiatry Project BETA De-escalation Workgroup. *Western Journal of Emergency Medicine, 13,* 17–26. https://doi.org/10.5811/westjem.2011.9.6864.
Ruzek, J. I., Brymer, M. J., Jacobs, A. K., & Layne, C. M. (2007). Psychological first aid. *Journal of Mental Health Counseling, 29,* 17–49. 10.17744/mehc.29.1.5racqxjueafabgwp
Ruzek, J. I., Young, B. H., Cordova, M. J., & Flynn, B. W. (2004). Integration of disaster mental health services with emergency medicine. *Prehospital and Disaster Medicine, 19,* 46–53. https://doi.org/10.1017/S1049023X00001473
Schmitz, W. M., Allen, M. H., Feldman, B. N., Gutin, N. J., Jahn, D. R., Kleespies, P. M., … Simpson, S. (2012). Preventing suicide through improved training in suicide risk assessment and care: An American Association of Suicidology Task Force report addressing serious gaps

in US mental health training. *Suicide and Life-threatening Behavior, 42*, 292–304. https://doi.org/10.1111/j.1943-278X.2012.00090.x

Sivakumar, S., Weiland, T. J., Gerdtz, M. F., Knott, J., & Jelinek, G. A. (2011). Mental health-related learning needs of clinicians working in Australian emergency departments: A national survey of self-reported confidence and knowledge. *Emergency Medicine Australia, 23*, 697–711. https://doi.org/10.1111/j.1742-6723.2011.01472.x

Substance Abuse and Mental Health Services Administration [SAMHSA] (2016). *Screening tools.* Retrieved from http://www.integration.samhsa.gov/clinical-practice/screening-tools

Sutton, A. (2015). In case of emergency: Who's who in the ER. *Center for Advancing Health.* Retrieved from http://www.cfah.org/prepared-patient/prepared-patient-articles/in-case-of-emergency-whos-who-in-the-er

Szapocznik, J., & Williams, R. A. (2000). Brief strategic family therapy: Twenty-five years of interplay among theory, research and practice in adolescent behavior problems and drug abuse. *Clinical Child and Family Psychology Review, 3*, 117–134.

Tyndall, L., Hodgson, J., Lamson, A., White, M., & Knight, S. (2014). Medical family therapy: Charting a course in competencies. In J. Hodgson, A. Lamson, T. Mendenhall, and D. Crane (Eds.), *Medical family therapy: Advanced applications* (pp. 33–54). New York, NY: Springer.

Walsh, F. (2007). Traumatic loss and major disasters: Strengthening family and community resilience. *Family Process, 46*, 207–227. https://doi.org/10.1111/j.1545-5300.2007.00205.x

Wolfson, A., Hendey, G., & Harwood-Nuss, A. (2010). *Clinical practice of emergency medicine.* Philadelphia, PA: Lippincott, Williams, & Williams.

Wrenn, K., Lorenzen, B., Jones, I., Zhou, C., & Aronsky, D. (2010). Factors affecting stress in emergency medicine residents while working in the ED. *American Journal of Emergency Medicine, 28*, 897–902. https://doi.org/10.1016/j.ajem.2009.05.001

Wright, L. M., Watson, W. L., & Bell, J. M. (1996). *Beliefs: The heart of healing in families and illness.* New York, NY: Basic Books.

*Wyatt, J., Illingworth, R., Grahm, C., & Hogg, K. (2017). *Oxford handbook of emergency medicine* (4th ed.). New York, NY: Oxford University Press.

Chapter 8
Medical Family Therapy in Oncology

Talia Zaider and Peter Steinglass

Cancer diagnoses encompass a broad and varied group of diseases that share the feature of abnormal and uncontrolled cell growth. In the United States alone, an estimated 1.6 million new cases of cancer were diagnosed last year (American Cancer Society, 2016). Once considered a death sentence, many cancers are now treated as chronic illnesses that require long-term management (McCorkle et al., 2011). This shift from acute to chronic care for patients with cancer represents a culmination of continually evolving medical advances that have succeeded in prolonging survival and expanding the range of available treatment options.

Whereas the prevention, detection, and treatment of these diseases have been a focus of biomedical research for more than a century, interest in the psychosocial "human side" of cancer emerged only in the last half of the twentieth century (Holland, 2000). Historically, it was common for oncologists to withhold disclosure of a cancer diagnosis; they believed that patients would be harmed by such information. This view contributed to the exclusion of behavioral health professionals from cancer wards. As treatment advances promised a greater chance of survival, the stigma and fear surrounding cancer diminished. It became permissible to talk openly about the diagnosis, itself, alongside the psychological and social implications of living with cancer.

The National Cancer Institute and the American Cancer Society were established to promote cancer research and education in the early twentieth century. However, it was only in the mid-1970s that a new field called psycho-oncology was established to study and address the psychosocial challenges faced by patients and their families (Holland, 2000). Over the ensuing 40 years, a large body of research has

---

T. Zaider (✉)
Department of Psychiatry and Behavioral Science,
Memorial Sloan Kettering Cancer Center, New York, NY, USA
e-mail: zaidert@mskcc.org

P. Steinglass
Ackerman Institute for the Family, New York, NY, USA

accumulated that documents the extent of psychosocial burdens and distress experienced by cancer patients and their families. Consequently, it is now a routine to integrate support services into the cancer care delivery system (Pirl et al., 2014). There is greater recognition, too, that the impact(s) of a cancer diagnosis reverberates throughout the family system—with evidence about adverse effects across physical, emotional, and social functioning of caregiving family members many years past the onset of caregiving (Kim, Shaffer, Carver, & Cannady, 2015).

Psycho-oncology has been predominantly led and practiced by the more traditional disciplines of psychiatry, psychology, and social work. However, the systemic mind-set of medical family therapy (MedFT) is crucial to this field as patients and families navigate an increasingly complex and fragmented care experience. In this chapter, we orient MedFTs to the oncology setting and its key players and present an overview of the trajectory of cancer care from diagnosis to active treatment, surveillance, and advanced disease. We also describe evidence-based intervention models that have been developed to mitigate distress and optimize patient and family adjustment and coping.

We begin with the following clinical vignette; it illustrates common themes in patients' and families' experiences with the diagnosis and treatment of cancer and the multiple levels at which a MedFT can effectively intervene to help navigate this process.

Clinical Vignette

[Note: This vignette is a compilation of cases that represent treatment in oncology. All patients' names and/or identifying information have been changed to maintain confidentiality.]

Helen and Ray were married for 21 years, with a 16-year-old son and 19-year-old daughter. Ray was diagnosed with stage IV pancreatic cancer after an extensive workup for worsening back pain. When he was initially diagnosed, he and Helen were shocked to learn that the disease had already spread to his liver and lungs. Ray underwent a course of first-line chemotherapy, which initially appeared to contain tumor growth. Several months later, a follow-up scan showed that Ray's disease had spread. Ray then accepted enrollment in a trial of a new immunotherapy drug, although he and his wife were told that its success rate was not likely to be higher than 20%.

A number of weeks after starting the clinical trial, Ray's nausea, weight loss, and bone pain worsened. The couple began to decline social invitations and pressed their college-aged daughter to come home more often. Hearing about his symptom complaints, the oncologist referred the family to a palliative care team. The couple interpreted this suggestion as a signal that the oncologist had lost all hope of recovery, and when the palliative care physician suggested that they consider the pros and cons of continuing treatment, they "fired" her.

As Helen grew increasingly anxious, she asked for more frequent appointments with the oncologist and expressed frustration with what she perceived as Ray's treatment team's lack of responsiveness. Noticing Helen's mounting anxiety and being aware of the strain that it was placing on his nursing staff (who described Helen as "demanding," "in denial," and blocking her husband from expressing his wishes about possibly discontinuing treatment), the oncologist requested a MedFT consultation to add support for the family and to help facilitate better communication with the team.

In a meeting that the MedFT arranged with both the couple and the primary nurse assigned to them, he (the MedFT) was able to solicit from Ray and Helen their disappointment with the oncologist's decision to "delegate" Ray's symptom management to palliative care, feeling that he was abandoning them prematurely. They added that although the oncologist had not openly discussed Ray's prognosis, there was a palpable change in his demeanor recently. They noticed diminished enthusiasm when he talked with them.

Using a series of strategies designed to put the couple "back in charge" of the cancer experience, the MedFT facilitated a discussion with Ray and Helen about their preferences for communication about difficult illness and treatment topics—both with the oncologist and with each other—highlighting their changing needs as Ray's cancer care became more complex. Critical here was the ability of the MedFT to normalize the couple's reactions, highlighting their attachment to the oncologist and team and their fear that the palliative care referral represented abandonment by the team. The primary nurse was then able to assuage Ray and Helen's concerns by clarifying the role of the palliative care team within a larger, overall treatment approach.

Following this meeting, the MedFT completed the loop by speaking with the couple's oncologist about what he had learned, highlighting the couple's strong attachment to him. A plan was suggested for the primary nurse to arrange weekly check-in phone calls with the family to provide a more routine and structured means of addressing ongoing symptom management concerns. This plan was cemented by the oncologist, who reiterated his firm commitment to remain Ray's primary provider regardless of his involvement of other team members.

The MedFT continued to meet with the family to facilitate conversations about the future and to examine their choices in responding to the terrible uncertainty they faced. The couple's son and daughter were eventually drawn into these sessions. Their children's pointed questions about Ray's treatment options further pressed the couple to talk openly about the "what ifs."

Grief was shared as the MedFT normalized the sadness and worry that preoccupied each of them. Ray's daughter shared that she often cried alone and worried about burdening her mother with her fears. Ray was surprised to learn that his children wished to join him at his oncology visits and to accompany him to treatment. Over time, he was able to express to the family his understanding that his time left in the world was limited and that he wished for a "quiet" and "peaceful" death at home. The family was ultimately able to grant Ray these wishes when he died 2 months later.

What Is Cancer Care?

Choosing a specialist and treatment site is one of the first decisions made by families following a cancer diagnosis. The process by which families make this decision can itself offer clues as to how they will navigate future decision-making during care (e.g., the degree to which the family draws on their social networks, seeks multiple opinions, or divides roles). Approximately two-thirds of newly diagnosed cancer patients in the United States choose to be treated at an "accredited" cancer center. This designation is made by one of two overseeing agencies, including (a) the American College of Surgeons Commission on Cancer (COC), which has accredited 1500 hospitals in the United States on the basis of predetermined clinical care standards, and (b) the National Cancer Institute (NCI), which has accredited nearly 70 cancer centers on the basis of clinical care and academic standing. At an accredited cancer center, patients and families are typically navigating a large and very complex medical system. They are asked to interact with what feels like a dizzying array of specialists and treatment teams. They also may be asked to participate in ongoing cancer research trials or to submit to experimental protocols if patients do not respond to established treatment regimens.

Given the complexity inherent in modern cancer treatment, MedFTs working in a specialized cancer center must interface with a myriad of specialists and disciplines. Because the majority of cancer care takes place in an accredited cancer center, the concerns, issues, and clinical practices discussed in this chapter will reflect this particular context.

Treatment Teams in Cancer Care

The following highlight key professionals involved in cancer care teams:

Oncologists. The oncologist is the lead physician in a patient's care team; he or she is thereby responsible for diagnosing cancer and planning medical treatment. Because of the oncologist's central role in helping patients and families make sense of the disease and its management, the quality of communication between patients, families, and oncologists can have a significant impact(s) on various aspects of the care experience and has itself been a focus of much attention (Epstein et al., 2017; Kissane et al., 2012). There are three types of oncologists that may be involved in a patient's care: (a) medical oncologists who specialize in administering chemotherapy and other medications (e.g., targeted therapies, immunotherapies), (b) surgical oncologists who perform surgical procedures such as taking biopsies or resecting tumors, and (c) radiation oncologists who are trained to administer radiation therapies.

Oncology nurses. Oncology nurses perform a wide array of tasks, including the direct delivery of treatment (e.g., chemotherapy infusions) in the clinic setting, educating patients and families about how to manage treatment-related side effects, and coordinating access to services and resources across the treatment facility. As frontline providers, nurses routinely assess the practical and emotional support needs of patients and families, including general distress and caregiving needs. Nurses therefore serve as a kind of "relational bridge" (McLeod, Tapp, Moules, & Campbell, 2010, p. 6), linking the family with other helping systems. Furthermore, because of their close partnership with families over time, nurses are often privy to the intimate details and dynamics of family life and can thereby be a valuable resource to those providing psychosocial support.

Palliative care physicians and nurses. The palliative care team is a consultation service called upon by the primary oncologist to assist with symptom management for patients at any point along the treatment trajectory. Palliative care specialists focus their work on the relief of suffering, defined broadly to include physical concerns (e.g., lymphedema, nausea, shortness of breath, neuropathy) and psychological, social, and spiritual difficulties that threaten to diminish the patient's quality of life. Because of their holistic approach, palliative care providers are inclined to be patient- and family-centered and therefore collaborate frequently with behavioral health providers. Palliative care specialists are most often enlisted in caring for advanced cancer patients, whose symptom burden is greatest. However, there is a large body of research showing that early integration of palliative care into cancer treatment improves clinical outcomes for both patients and families (Bakitas et al., 2009; Smith et al., 2012).

There are persistent misperceptions about the role of palliative care among patients, families, and oncologists (e.g., the tendency to equate these services with hospice care), which unfortunately can impede referral and uptake of these services (Bauman & Temel, 2014; Schenker, Park, Maciasz, & Arnold, 2014). MedFTs may encounter these barriers when collaborating with a palliative care team (as in our vignette, above) and can play an important role in facilitating communication and understanding across teams and within the family about how to best use this service.

Behavioral health providers. Behavioral health providers in cancer treatment may include social workers, psychologists, psychiatrists, MedFTs, and others. All provide mental health services and collaborate with medical providers to provide comprehensive and integrated behavioral healthcare.

Oncology social workers. The oncology social worker helps patients and families manage distress and cope with cancer-related challenges. He or she may lead group support programs and/or provide psychoeducation about topics related to cancer management (e.g., communicating with children about a parent's illness). Social workers may also provide brief targeted counseling to patients or link patients and families to financial support and other resources. They are often colocated in the clinic setting and are thereby able to collaborate closely with oncologists, palliative care specialists, and nurses. However, they primarily see patients and families by referral. Because it would not be unusual for families to interact with all of these professionals, it often falls to MedFTs (see below) to ensure that contacts between the family and these different professionals are coordinated and consistent. Just as the medical oncologist is usually the person who acts as a "quarterback" for the patient's treatment plan, it may well be the MedFT who serves a comparable role in integrating the family into the overall treatment plan.

Psychiatrists. The psychiatrist is a medical doctor who treats clinically elevated levels of depression, anxiety, and other psychiatric conditions that either emerge or are exacerbated during cancer care. Psychiatrists are able to prescribe medications to alleviate symptoms of these presentations, alongside common patient struggles with insomnia and fatigue.

Psychologists. Clinical psychologists are involved in screening, identifying, and treating psychological distress among patients and families facing a cancer diagnosis and treatment. Psychologists are trained to deliver evidence-based psychotherapy interventions to address these concerns. Both psychologists and psychiatrists may provide supportive or cognitive-behavioral therapy to help patients or caregivers cope with cancer-related stresses. However, because they are not often well trained in couple/family therapy, it is more likely that a MedFT would be called upon to intervene with families when needed.

Medical family therapists. Oncology teams recognize that a supportive and well-functioning family is a key component of effective cancer care, but many acknowledge that collaborating with families can be challenging (Kissane, 2013; Zaider et al., 2016). When 912 hospital oncology nurses in the United States were asked to rank a list of obstacles to providing high-quality end-of-life care, the highest-ranked obstacle on average was working with anxious family members. Of the top ten primary obstacles perceived by nurses, seven pertained to families (e.g., families not accepting a patient's poor prognosis, nurses having to deal with angry family members) (Traeger et al., 2013).

In recent years, there have been numerous calls to integrate family-centered support services into cancer care and to more routinely assess the family's capacity to manage the chronic and often unpredictable demands of aggressive treatment and other illness-related stressors (Kent et al., 2016; Northouse, 2012). The unique value of MedFTs therefore lies in their ability to apply a broader biopsychosocial-spiritual (BPSS) lens to engaging and intervening with distressed families (Engel, 1977, 1980; Wright, Watson, & Bell, 1996) and to model the benefits of family-centered care for others in the oncology team. Often, this involves adding family-level assessment and intervention practices to routine care, such as gathering basic information about membership of the caregiving family, normalizing the family-level challenges that accompany cancer treatment, making contact with multiple family members when possible, and drawing on their perspectives and prior experiences in solving problems that arise during treatment.

This kind of family engagement has been well incorporated into many pediatric oncology and critical care settings (Kazak, Boeving, Alderfer, Hwang, & Reilly, 2005; Schaefer & Block, 2009), wherein providers rely heavily on family members as surrogate decision-makers. On the other hand, most adult oncology settings have not yet established the resources and protocols needed to routinely address family needs. Instead, most focus on the patient, alone. It is not surprising, then, that despite reporting a high number of unmet support needs, family members of adult cancer patients typically underutilize existing psychosocial care services (Sklenarova et al., 2015).

As in cancer care generally, the field of psycho-oncology has been oriented toward developing individually based interventions that target the patient's well-being and adjustment. Conjoint couple and family therapies in cancer remain sparse, although families who are offered the opportunity to convene for support together consistently report high satisfaction with this modality (Hodgson, McCammon, & Anderson, 2011; Ostroff, Ross, Steinglass, Ronis-Tobin, & Singh, 2004). MedFTs have the skills to provide more intensive family system-oriented interventions to address communication difficulties, conflict management, and other relational challenges that are not typically targeted in most psychotherapies for cancer patients.

Chaplains. Chaplains offer spiritual support; they provide patients and families with opportunities for prayer or engagement in religious rituals to address existential distress. They may serve patients and families who are admitted to the hospital and can be called upon to meet with patients at any time during care in the outpatient setting.

Radiologists. A radiologist is a medical doctor who uses medical imaging—such as X-ray, CT, MRI, or ultrasound—to examine internal bones or organs to facilitate making an accurate cancer diagnosis or determine the status of an existing cancer. Because such diagnostic procedures are administered by technicians, patients and families do not tend to directly interact with the radiologists who are interpreting the results. This is in contrast to the radiation oncologist (i.e., when radiation therapy is a component of the treatment plan).

Genetic counselors. Genetic counselors help patients and their families interpret results of genetic screening tests; they use this information, in combination with information from personal and family histories, to help family members understand their genetic risk factors for certain types of cancer. Because of the many challenges that arise in coping with genetic risks, genetic counselors often work collaboratively with psychosocial providers.

Fundamentals of Care in Oncology

MedFTs working in oncology and psycho-oncology must be familiar with a myriad of content, including common trajectories of care within this treatment context, indicated methods for family assessment, and helpful ways to support families after care has concluded.

Cancer Care Trajectory

To understand a family's experience with cancer, it is important to consider where they are in the physical and psychosocial timeline of the disease. As with many serious illnesses, cancer follows a developmental course with distinct psychosocial tasks and challenges accompanying each phase (Rolland, 2005). The course of cancer treatment can also be characterized by alternating periods of crisis (e.g., initial diagnosis, unplanned hospital admissions), chronicity (e.g., routine schedule of ongoing treatment or surveillance), and anticipatory grief (e.g., terminal phase of illness). It is thereby important for MedFTs to have a road map of the medical transitions and milestones associated with a particular disease group (e.g., the first 100 days after hematopoietic stem cell transplantation) so that they can anticipate and normalize periods of heightened anxiety and need(s) for mobilization.

In their published guidelines for distress management in oncology, the National Comprehensive Cancer Network (NCCN) identified a set of critical transition points in cancer treatment during which patients and families are especially vulnerable to distress and may benefit from psychosocial consultation (NCCN, 2017; Pirl et al., 2014). These include:

1. Initial period of diagnostic workup and decision-making
2. Preparation for treatment or surgery
3. Planned or unplanned changes in treatment modality
4. Planned or unplanned withdrawal of treatment
5. Discharge from the hospital
6. Transition from active treatment to long-term surveillance
7. Disease recurrence or progression
8. Transition to hospice and end-of-life care

In the clinical vignette above, Ray and Helen's transition from an initial treatment course to news about disease progression was distressing because of the resulting physical changes for Ray (e.g., fatigue, pain). It was disorienting, too, because of the changes made in his treatment regimen and in the number and type of providers involved in Ray's care. As families differ in their adaptability and manners in which they integrate changes in their environment, it can be useful to track whether and to what extent patterns of family life change in response to the demands of a particular illness phase. Such patterns can include how families allocate resources (e.g., time, effort, money), communicate with one another, negotiate and resolve differences, make plans for the future, and/or balance time together versus apart.

For example, at the time of an initial diagnosis (i.e., a crisis period), a family may dedicate more resources to researching treatment choices, seeking multiple opinions, and discussing cancer-related issues than would be necessary during a later phase of illness. In the vignette above, Ray's daughter, who typically spent her weekends away at college, came home more often to be with her parents. Ray, who may have been accustomed to expressing a difference of opinion with his wife, became more withdrawn and passive. At the same time, Helen became more protective and less inclined to argue with Ray. Often families are not aware of the degrees to which cancer has reorganized aspects of their lives and relationships. MedFTs can normalize these disruptions as an expected part of being in "cancer territory" and can empower families to evaluate and make choices about the accommodations they make.

Clinical course changes also precipitate changes in the nature of the relationship between the family and medical team: couples and family members may assume more passive "backseat" roles during a crisis period (e.g., when a patient is first admitted to an intensive care unit) but then shift into "copilot" roles during a chronic or long-term follow-up phase of care when oncologists rely on them to maintain vigilance and track symptoms (Reiss, Steinglass, & Howe, 1993). In the vignette above, Ray and Helen longed for their oncologist to maintain his position as the "captain of the ship," despite the need for consultation from other specialists.

Assessing Families in an Oncology Setting

Family members are ubiquitous in oncology clinics, interfacing with almost every provider and/or taking part in (or at least being present for) all consultations. However, and as previously noted, most cancer care settings do not yet have a systematic process for assessing the concerns of caregiving family members or for determining what support needs are warranted beyond those of the patient. Referrals to a behavioral health provider are often made at the request of the family or by another clinician (e.g., nurse, oncologist, chaplain) who perceives elevated distress, poor caregiving capacity, or other psychosocial risk factors among family members. Family assessments can occur during a single encounter in the inpatient or outpatient setting or across several sessions as part of a planned course of family therapy (Hudson, Thomas, Quinn, & Aranda, 2009; Kissane & Hempton, 2017; Rolland, 1994; Zaider & Kissane, 2009). Ideally, families are offered a psychosocial assessment or "checkup" with a MedFT during critical transition points throughout their cancer experience (Rolland, 2005), although this is seldom done in practice.

A single family consultation (also known as a "family meeting" or "family conference") is used routinely by medical staff in palliative care, critical care, or pediatric oncology settings to enlist the collaboration of family members in decision-making, clarify concerns or questions related to cancer and its management, and achieve consensus about treatment planning moving forward (Hudson, Thomas, Quinn, & Aranda, 2009). Although these meetings are typically led by the oncologist and other medical specialists, the presence of a MedFT ensures that psychosocial issues are addressed in addition to strict medical concerns. In helping to coordinate such a meeting, MedFTs should consult in advance with the medical team, patients, and family members about who should be invited. Families may need explicit permission to invite members who are not directly involved in caregiving tasks but nevertheless are key influences (e.g., close friends).

Particularly during a crisis period, family members may also ask to meet with a MedFT without the patient present. This is done usually with the intent to protect the patient from emotionally painful content or unresolved conflict. While such requests are common, they can raise worries about appropriately managing confidentiality or competing alliances. It is possible to honor this kind of request by allotting time for discussion with individuals and families together, underscoring that the goal of such sessions is to help the family find adaptive solutions to communication difficulties—rather than have the MedFT become a primary conduit of communication among them.

Guidelines for conducting a family meeting in an oncology setting have been put forth in research and clinical literature (e.g., Gueguen, Bylund, Brown, Levin, & Kissane, 2009; Hudson et al., 2009), usually with an emphasis on identifying and addressing caregiving needs. All assessment models emphasize general therapy techniques such as joining with each family member in the room and structuring the meeting from the outset by setting and eliciting a realistic agenda. Other components of a family assessment include (a) eliciting the family's "illness story," especially what they understand to be the current status of the disease and goals of treatment; (b) learning about prior experiences with illness, major transitions (e.g., immigration), or other adversity in the family's history; (c) identifying successful adaptation strategies that the family has used in the past; (d) pinpointing perceived strengths and vulnerabilities in their coping responses; and (e) discussing current and future support needs, both practical and emotional (Kissane & Hempton, 2017; Zaider & Kissane, 2009).

It is also important to listen for any implicit beliefs that a family might hold about what caused the disease (e.g., trauma, poor health habits, family history, religious sources) or beliefs about nonmedical factors that are assumed to be important to the patient's survival or protection from recurrence (e.g., positive thinking, low stress and conflict). An initial consultation might then conclude with a summary of the family's strengths and vulnerabilities, incorporating relevant psychoeducation about common challenges that families are expected to face when their lives are affected by illness. In the vignette above, for example, the MedFT may comment on the strong advocacy that Helen provides while, at the same time, highlighting the enormous responsibility that she feels toward keeping her husband well.

Normalizing and helping the family anticipate the emotional and relational tasks that lie ahead can be sufficient to empower them to forge ahead with good teamwork and communal coping. No matter how well functioning, many families navigate this experience without recognition of the choices they can make or of the internal and relational resources available to them. Thus, in addition to data collection, the conjoint family assessment will also affirm the unique values and skills that the family brings to this experience. Finally, as is with Ray and Helen, even 1 to 2 sessions focused on immediate concerns can facilitate conversations that are comparatively difficult for the couple or family to have on its own.

Supporting Families During the Posttreatment Phase of Cancer

Cancer is often thought of in popular culture as a single entity, but different cancers vary greatly in their clinical course(s). Consequently, a MedFT may be called upon to help with a wide array of issues depending on the type of cancer at hand. Although the most prevalent of these issues will be attendant to the diagnostic and treatment phases of cancer, increasing attention is being paid to two other issues: (a) late effects of otherwise successful cancer treatments and (b) posttreatment psychological sequelae. Prominent examples of treatment effects include infertility issues, impotence, permanent side effects from radiation scarring, and the like (Institute of Medicine Committee on the Future Health Care Workforce for Older Adults, 2008). Common psychological sequelae include chronic depression and PTSD-like symptoms (Brown, Madan Swain, & Lambert, 2003; Kazak, Boeving, Alderfer, Hwang, & Reilly, 2005).

Many presume that these issues are experienced primarily by patients, but research has shown that patients' family members also suffer significant posttreatment effects from the cancer experience (e.g., Kim, Kashy, Wellisch, Spillers, Kaw, & Smith, 2008). Further, sequelae like infertility or impotence impact relationships within the family. Particularly stressful are the issues raised when cancer occurs in

---

Clinical Vignette
[Note: This vignette is a compilation of cases that represent treatment in oncology. All patients' names and/or identifying information have been changed to maintain confidentiality.]

Walter is a 16-year-old adolescent who is 1-year posttreatment for leukemia that included a course of chemotherapy and a bone marrow transfusion. He is the oldest of three siblings in a family that had no prior experience with a serious medical illness in any of the children or their parents. Despite the oncologist's assurances that Walter is now "cancer-free," his parents continue to view him as at risk for a recurrence of the disease. Walter, for his part, wants to return to a "normal" life, including rejoining his soccer team and taking on a full academic schedule.

In a follow-up visit, the oncologist notes that Walter's parents seem unable to be reassured that all is well. They instead ask multiple questions about what to look for as early warning signs of cancer coming back. When she tries to take Walter's side in emphasizing that he is now fully capable of leading the life of a normal teenager, tension quickly arises between the oncologist and Walter's parents (and between Walter and his parents). Sensing that an escalating and counterproductive rift is developing right in front of her, the oncologist suggests that the family have to consult with the team's MedFT.

> When she met with the family, the MedFT was quickly able to assess the problem (i.e., hypervigilant parents who are experiencing unresolved PTSD symptoms typical of the posttreatment phase of leukemia in an adolescent family member and who are consequently in conflict with the said teenager who sees them as overly controlling). Maintaining the goal of helping to normalize what the family is going through, the MedFT refers Walter and his parents to a multiple-family discussion group (MFDG) program she has been running at the Cancer Center. This type of program typically brings together 4 to 6 families during the posttreatment phase of cancer to talk together about their experiences. Based on a combination of psychoeducational and family system principles, MFDG models are usually conceptualized as deriving their power from an ability to establish a non-pathologizing, collaborative environment within which a community of families who can share both challenges and coping strategies for dealing with cancer (Steinglass, 1998).
>
> During the first MFDG session, Walter's father expresses his feeling that the cancer diagnosis and the treatment experience were akin to "being taken hostage by a terrorist" and that he continues to have nightmares in which he is in Walter's hospital room crying uncontrollably. Parents from other families in the group immediately chime in with comparable feelings. A mother from another family talks about her confusion every time her daughter develops a mild cold. "Should I rush her back to the Cancer Center, or just call her pediatrician?" Heads nod around the room as other parents endorse this sense of fear and confusion.
>
> At the same time, adolescent patients in the group speak up forcefully for how they no longer want to be labeled as "cancer patients." They have thrown away the hats they used to wear to hide their post-chemotherapy hair loss, and they have gained back all of the weight that they lost. It is time to return to their lives.
>
> The MedFT leading the group is then able to use these "data" to normalize both reactions that are being expressed and to point out how the differing emotions expressed by patients versus parents is also part and parcel of typical reactions advanced within families as they progress through the posttreatment phases of cancer treatment.

children or young adults. In these situations, parents and spouses are often confused and distressed about the long-term implications of their family member having had cancer at a young age and about whether to think of the cancer as having been "cured" or to, instead, think (and worry) about it as "in remission" (Ostroff, Ross, & Steinglass, 2000).

Many cancer centers, aware of these issues, have established educational programs and support groups for family members. However, these programs typically do not bring patients and family members together. MedFTs, equipped with the biopsychosocial-spiritual (BPSS) orientations that define their efforts, can play an important role in shaping these programs to better reflect the needs of families as families.

Cancer Care Across the MedFT Healthcare Continuum

Although the oncology setting offers diverse opportunities to engage and support families, the level of intervention provided by MedFTs, and the degrees to which their roles are integrated with the patient's medical care, varies considerably. We use Hodgson, Lamson, Mendenhall, and Tyndall's (2014) MedFT Healthcare Continuum here to describe different levels at which the MedFT can be integrated into a cancer care system.

At *Levels 1 and 2*, the MedFT is familiar with a BPSS framework and applies it occasionally to his or her interactions with patients and their families but is nevertheless focused primarily on how the cancer patient is coping with immediate, disease-related concerns. He or she recognizes the important role(s) of caregiving families but will attend to the family only when needed to ensure the safety and well-being of the individual patient. Principal skills at these levels include providing acute, one-to-one support to a patient or distressed caregiver and serving as a liaison to the medical team on behalf of the patient and family when necessary.

MedFTs at this level intervene independently of any medical care provided, oftentimes in a separate location. They are not routinely introduced to patients and their families and have minimal contact with the primary oncologist except to exchange essential background information about a referred case. A MedFT working at this level will accept psychosocial care referrals for complex or "high-risk" cases from a member of the primary disease management team and will apply interventions that are oriented to short-term crisis management, psychoeducation, and practical problem-solving.

In our first clinical vignette, a MedFT working at this level may meet with Helen alone at the oncologists' request, hear and address any pressing questions about Ray's disease course and treatment, clarify the reasons for the oncologist's referral to palliative care, and provide information about a range of support services offered at the hospital. This MedFT would focus his or her interaction on de-escalating Helen's anxiety by providing empathic support, normalizing her worries, and problem-solving ways to meet caregiving needs.

At *Level 3*, MedFTs are embedded in a specific disease management team (e.g., a hematology or urology service). Working on-site, they interact directly with clinic staff and are routinely sought out by them for formal and informal consultation. Within inpatient units, MedFTs at this level will regularly join the oncologist and

Table 8.1 MedFTs in Oncology: Basic Knowledge and Skills

MedFT Healthcare Continuum Level	Level 1	Level 2	Level 3
Knowledge	Familiar with the biopsychosocial-spiritual (BPSS) framework as a general guide in care. Understands that cancer is associated with multiple biopsychosocial-spiritual challenges. Familiar with common complications resulting from cancer treatment (e.g., hair loss, fatigue). Aware of the importance of family members in caregiving and advocacy roles on behalf of the patient.	Understands how the BPSS framework pertains to the patient's and family's response to cancer. Can distinguish between BPSS challenges accompanying different phases of cancer treatment. Understands common treatment regimens and side effects associated with specific types of cancer (e.g., breast cancer, lung cancer, GI cancer). Familiar with family system concepts and can appreciate the aspects of family life that may impact and be impacted by cancer.	Understands psychosocial adjustments and critical transition points associated with specific cancers/diseases. Familiar with (and can anticipate) how certain patient- and family-level characteristics (e.g., history of loss, trauma) will contribute to the family's adjustment to a cancer diagnosis and treatment. Knows (and can identify) common marital or family relationship dynamics that arise in the context of coping with cancer and understands how these may impact the family's partnership with the oncology team.
Skills	Offers acute support or crisis management to patients and family members during times of high distress (e.g., after receiving bad news, changing treatment plans, anticipating surgery, or coping with an unplanned hospitalization), usually on a one-to-one basis. Accepts referrals for high-risk or complex patients and/or caregivers from the oncology team; can understand the basic nature of a patient's disease with access to his or her medical records and will follow cases in a separate site with only occasional contact with the oncology team.	Can anticipate and educate patients and families about common individual-, family-, and social-level challenges associated with cancer. Can engage and join with multiple family members in a conjoint consultation that is focused on the patient's caregiving needs. Can facilitate general support groups for individual patients and/or caregivers.	Proactively accesses families by attending case conferences and liaising with oncology team to identify those who may be at risk for elevated distress—or adjustment difficulties. Conducts family meetings or family therapy sessions with a dual focus on the patient's individual cancer care concerns and overall family functioning (e.g., communication, distribution of roles and responsibilities, intimacy or sexual functioning problems, parenting).

nurses on rounds so that they can present themselves to patients and families as part of the care team. In outpatient settings, MedFTs will participate in case conferences and team meetings to acquaint themselves with all active cases, regardless of psychosocial risk status.

MedFTs at *Level 3* may still see families primarily by referral from the medical team, but they are comfortable providing both short-term and long-term couple/family therapy. Because this MedFT is better known to care team's oncologists and nurses, he or she can more effectively advocate for the support needs of the family and will have more influence on the nature and quality of care delivered by other clinic staff. The MedFT may also participate more actively in research collaborations, using his or her systemic and biopsychosocial perspective to guide research questions.

Returning to our clinical vignette with Ray and Helen, a MedFT working at this level may introduce himself/herself to the couple early in their disease course and offer more frequent meetings to discuss the challenges that arise as Ray transitions to new care sequences. Because the MedFT is working with Ray's primary oncologist, he or she will more actively "translate" the perspectives of the family to the oncology team and vice versa. This MedFT will also be comfortable encouraging the couple to bring their young adult children to sessions and addressing the dynamics in the family system more broadly (Table 8.1).

At *Level 4*, MedFTs are consistently integrated into an oncology practice, providing consultation to patients and families routinely, and as an accepted part of standard cancer care. For example, instead of having the oncologist refer families to the MedFT when they are determined to be of high risk or at the point of crisis, the oncologist might introduce the MedFT at an initial visit or at a critical juncture in the patient's treatment course, with the intention of normalizing his or her supportive role on the team.

The MedFT working with Ray and Helen is using interventions most closely matching this higher level of involvement and integration. For example, he is likely to speak with Ray and Helen *alongside* their oncologist or primary nurse and convene multidisciplinary meetings with multiple team members at key transition points in their disease course. The MedFT may even anticipate the family's support needs by learning from the oncologist about new developments (e.g., scan results) in advance of their visit and planning time with the family to process bad news.

At *Level 5*, the MedFT will also provide training and supervision to medical and behavioral health trainees and providers in order to promote the use of family-centered care practices and to address the support needs of the healthcare team. He or she may conduct couple/family therapy sessions conjointly with the nurse, social worker, or oncologist involved in a given case to ensure that the perspectives of all family and team members are well represented and coordinated. This MedFT is also proficient in the conduct of research to better understand systemic factors impacting treatment in cancer care and/or to test interventions that advance integrated health services (Table 8.2).

Table 8.2 MedFTs in Oncology: Advanced Knowledge and Skills

MedFT Healthcare Continuum Level	Level 4	Level 5
Knowledge	Provider is affiliated with (and located within) a particular oncology clinic and thereby maintains adept understandings about disease management and treatment-related side effects and is familiar with the range of tests used to follow disease statuses. She or he is also familiar with how the oncology clinic operates, including the roles and relationships of all team members and various specialists. Adept knowledge regarding methods for assessing and intervening with couples and families who are dealing with more complex disease-related relational dynamics or psychosocial circumstances (e.g., comorbid psychiatric or medical conditions, language barriers).	Conversant with oncologists, nurses, and other team members and specialists regarding a myriad of disease-related complications and other aspects of care. Well versed in the sundry legal, medical, and ethical considerations involved in treatment decision-making, particularly during the advanced stages of illness. Familiar with widely disseminated empirically supported interventions for couples and families coping with cancer.
Skills	Able to offer training, supervision, and consultation to other oncology providers about the complexities of supporting patients and their families at all stages of cancer care. Plans and facilitates interdisciplinary family meetings to jointly address the patient's and family's BPSS concerns, as well as their potential impact(s) on one another. Skilled to conduct multiple family groups and to provide more intensive longer-term psychotherapy with couples and families when indicated.	Alongside direct clinical care is proficient in leading or coleading initiatives that advance integrated behavioral healthcare models within the oncology team and promote the routine engagement of families as part of patients' cancer treatment planning. Participates in hospital ethics committee, informs quality of care standards in the oncology clinics, and contributes to research regarding the implementation of family-centered care practices.

Research-Informed Practices

There is growing evidence that demonstrates that couple- and family-based interventions are associated with significant benefits. Brief (6–10 sessions) therapies have been developed and tested in research trials for couples and families across early and advanced stages of disease. Many of these interventions emphasize psychoeducation and skill enhancement (e.g., the therapist coaches couples and families in constructive communication and coping skills), whereas others are more exploratory and insight oriented. Common to all these interventions is the conjoint participation of both patient and family members and a focus on family-level management of the illness. We will highlight some of the most empirically supported interventions below for illustration.

Intimacy-Enhancing Couples Therapy (IECT) targets early phases of the cancer disease course, wherein the patient-partner dyad (not the whole family) is the more likely unit of care (Kissane et al., 2016; Manne, Kissane, Nelson, Mulhall, Winkel, & Zaider, 2011; Zaider & Kissane, 2011). IECT is one of a large number of therapies that have been designed and tested for couples coping with breast, prostate, lung, head, and neck cancers, as well as for couples facing advanced end-stage illness (Badr & Krebs, 2013; Dockham et al., 2016; McLean, Walton, Rodin, Esplen, & Jones, 2013; Scott, Halford, & Ward, 2004; Zaider & Kissane, 2011).

IECT was designed specifically for men with localized prostate cancer and their partners who are adjusting to postsurgical changes in sexual functioning. The treatment protocol consists of 4 to 6 sessions during which the IECT therapist guides couples through behavioral exercises intended to strengthen communication and problem-solving skills that will help them manage cancer-related concerns (e.g., erectile dysfunction, incontinence). Couples reflect on sources of physical and emotional intimacy pre- versus post-cancer, become aware of any identity-related losses that men may experience as a result of physical changes, and identify strategies for preserving intimacy despite the disruptions caused by treatment-related side effects. A pilot trial testing the efficacy of this intervention against a "usual care" control group found significant improvements among couples receiving the therapy in measures of communication, responsiveness, marital satisfaction, and intimacy (Manne et al., 2011).

Emotionally Focused Therapy (EFT) is based on principles of attachment theory; it targets couples' relationship functioning by working to repair and/or build secure interpersonal bonds between partners (Johnson, 2004; Wiebe & Johnson, 2016). EFT guides its participants through three distinct stages, including (a) de-escalation, wherein couples develop insights/understandings regarding negative interaction cycles that drive their distress; (b) restructuring interactions, wherein couples create new emotional experiences and exchanges that lead to more secure connections with each other; and (c) consolidation, wherein couples work together to solve problems as a team now equipped with secure attachment and improved relational functioning. Researchers have shown that EFT is effective in reducing a variety of individual (e.g., depression; Dessaulles, Johnson, & Denton, 2003; Denton, Wittenborn, & Golden, 2012) and relationship (e.g., forgiveness; Makinen & Johnson, 2006) concerns. Within the field of oncology, EFT has demonstrated effectiveness for couples coping with breast cancer (e.g., Naaman, 2008), terminal metastatic cancer (e.g., Mclean, Walton, Rodin, Esplen, & Jones, 2013), and cancer/chronic illnesses of their children (e.g., Cloutier, Manion, Walker, & Johnson, 2002; Walker, Johnson, Manion, & Cloutier, 1996; Walker, Manion, Cloutier, & Johnson, 1992).

Family-Focused Grief Therapy (FFGT) targets families coping with advanced, poor-prognosis cancers whose members were at elevated risk for psychological distress (e.g., depression, anxiety) during both the palliative care phase of treatment and later during bereavement. A family is determined to be "at risk" if at least one of its members reports significant impairment in family relationships on the Family Relationships Index, a well-validated screening tool that asks about the quality of family relationships (Schuler et al., 2014). Scores on this screening questionnaire have shown to be highly predictive of family members' long-term psychological adjustment, both during advanced illness and in ensuing bereavement (Kissane, Bloch, Onghena, & McKenzie, 1996; Schuler et al., 2017).

By identifying high-risk families and strengthening their capacity for mutual support in the months prior to a patient's death, FFGT aims to help families navigate the loss of their loved ones more adaptively and potentially prevent the emergence of prolonged grief disorder in the future. The therapy begins with the patient present and continues with surviving family members during bereavement. The continuity of care prescribed by this model is based on the observation that high-risk families are more likely to follow up with bereavement support when the therapist knew, and helped care for, the deceased member. Sessions are 90 minutes long and spaced 2–3 weeks apart so as to allow time to process clinical content and accommodate scheduling demands. During the early assessment stage of therapy, behavioral health providers use circular questions to understand how the family communicates about cancer, how roles and responsibilities are distributed, and how the family negotiates differences. A separate session is dedicated to constructing and exploring families' genograms. In addition to collecting "data" about family constellations, and about cross-generational experiences with illness and loss, this session is used to encourage reflection on which values and coping styles in a family's history will be preserved and which will be left behind.

Based on what emerges during these early assessment sessions, the behavioral health provider then works collaboratively to establish relational goals for the family. A central part of this "intervention stage" of therapy involves facilitating difficult conversations about death and dying. Having learned about their prior experiences with loss, a MedFT can help the family talk about what, in their view, constitutes a "good death." He or she helps family members acknowledge and express their grief, identify existential and spiritual concerns, and anticipate strengths and vulnerabilities that may arise in the aftermath of loss. Feelings of guilt, anger, disgust, and burden in the context of caregiving are named and normalized. Rather than act as a primary source of support and reassurance to family members, the behavioral health provider asks questions that redirect the family to providing empathic support for one another. Examples might include "Is it helpful for your daughter to cry when she thinks about your illness?" or "How will you know when dad is feeling lonely?" Because the therapy is time limited, a MedFT should remain focused on realistic goals and not necessarily attempt to resolve long-standing conflicts.

A multisite, randomized clinical trial demonstrated the efficacy of this therapy in reducing the prevalence of prolonged grief disorder in a group of 170 high-risk families. The prevalence of prolonged grief disorder by 13 months after loss was 15.5% in the group of families that received no intervention and only 3.3% among families who received 10 sessions of FFGT (Kissane & Hempton, 2017).

Conclusion

Oncology is a broad and varied field of healthcare wherein patients and their families interface with a myriad of specialists across the disease course. MedFTs can play a crucial role in helping families navigate this terrain, as they maintain skills needed to engage and intervene with distressed families, facilitate their partnership and participation with the treating team, and model benefits of family-centered care for other healthcare providers. Although there is widespread recognition that caregiving families are a crucial resource to cancer care, most oncology clinics do not routinely assess for the BPSS challenges experienced by adult patients and their families. The challenges that families face are best understood in connection with particular transition points in the disease trajectory, when distress and burden are felt more acutely (e.g., beginning of active treatment versus transition to survivorship versus end-of-life care). In addition to serving as a bridge between the family and oncology team, MedFTs may provide couple- and family-based interventions to strengthen mutual support among family members, encourage open sharing of grief, facilitate awareness about coping styles, and generate creative solutions to the commonplace adjustment difficulties that accompany cancer treatment. Research in this area has demonstrated that couple-/family-centered intervention models can significantly reduce distress for patients and their caregiving family members. Integrating these approaches into oncology practice settings—so that care for families is a standard part of cancer treatment planning—remains an important goal that MedFTs are particularly suited to address.

Reflection Questions
1. As a MedFT working with families who are experiencing profound loss, trauma, and existential distress due to cancer, what will you need to pay attention to in yourself? What might block versus facilitate your ability to be emotionally present while bearing witness to others' suffering?
2. How might relationship dynamics *within* a family (e.g., poor communication, rigidity in roles, low tolerance for uncertainty) impact, or be impacted by, the relationship dynamics *between* a family and oncology medical team with whom you are working?
3. While assessing a highly anxious family during cancer treatment, what questions could you ask to help differentiate cancer-related versus non-cancer-related sources of distress?

Glossary of Important Terms for Care in Oncology

Biopsy A surgical procedure to remove a segment of a tumor for the purpose of determining a precise diagnosis.
Carcinoma A cancer that begins in the skin or tissues that line the inside or cover the outside of internal organs.

Curative treatment Treatment intended (and expected) to destroy the cancer.

Disease-free survival (DFS) A measure of time following treatment during which no signs of cancer are discovered.

Localized A cancer that is confined to the area where it began; it has not spread to other parts of a patient's body.

Malignant A tumor is malignant when there is evidence of disease, as differentiated from a tumor said to be "benign" or noncancerous.

Metastasis The spread of cancer to organs beyond where it began (which is referred to as the "primary" or "original" site).

Palliative treatment Treatment intended to relieve symptoms and pain associated with the cancer.

Remission The disappearance of cancer signs and symptoms (but not necessarily the disease, itself); this can be temporary or permanent in duration.

Tumor markers Substances that can be measured in the blood, urine, or body tissues to indicate the presence of cancer.

Additional Resources

Literature

Breitbart, W. S., Breitbart, W., & Poppito, S. R. (2014). *Individual meaning-centered psychotherapy for patients with advanced cancer: A treatment manual*. Oxford, England: Oxford University Press.

Holland, J. C., Breitbart, W. S., Jacobsen, P. B., Butow, P. N., Loscalzo, M. J., & McCorkle, R. (Eds.). (2015). *Psycho-oncology* (3rd ed.). Oxford, England: Oxford University Press.

Kissane, D. W., & Bloch, S. (2002). *Family focused grief therapy*. Philadelphia, PA: Open University Press.

Kissane, D. W., & Parnes, F. (2014). *Bereavement care for families*. New York, NY: Routledge.

Rauch, P., & Muriel, A. (2005). *Raising an emotionally healthy child when a parent is sick*. New York, NY: McGraw Hill.

Watson, M., & Kissane, D. W. (Eds.). (2011). *Handbook of psychotherapy in cancer care*. Hoboken, NJ: Wiley-Blackwell.

Measures/Instruments

Family Relationships Index (FRI). https://www.ncbi.nlm.nih.gov/pubmed/15546124

National Comprehensive Cancer Network Distress Thermometer. https://www.nccn.org/patients/resources/life_with_cancer/pdf/nccn_distress_thermometer.pdf

Psychosocial Assessment Tool. https://www.psychosocialassessmenttool.org

Organizations/Associations

American Psycho-Oncology Society. https://apos-society.org
International Psycho-Oncology Society. http://ipos-society.org
Society for Behavioral Medicine. http://www.sbm.org

References[1]

American Cancer Society. (2016). *Cancer facts and cures 2016*. Retrieved from https://www.cancer.org/research/cancer-facts-statistics/all-cancer-facts-ures/cancer-facts-ures-2016.html
Badr, H., & Krebs, P. (2013). A systematic review and meta analysis of psychosocial interventions for couples coping with cancer. *Psycho-Oncology, 22*, 1688–1704. https://doi.org/10.1002/pon.3200
Bakitas, M., Lyons, K. D., Hegel, M. T., Balan, S., Brokaw, F. C., Seville, J., ... Byock, I. R. (2009). Effects of a palliative care intervention on clinical outcomes in patients with advanced cancer: The project ENABLE II randomized controlled trial. *Journal of the American Medical Association, 302*, 741–749. https://doi.org/10.1001/jama.2009.1198
Bauman, J. R., & Temel, J. S. (2014). The integration of early palliative care with oncology care: The time has come for a new tradition. *Journal of the National Comprehensive Cancer Network, 12*, 1763–1771. https://doi.org/10.6004/jnccn.2014.0177
*Breitbart, W. S., Breitbart, W., & Poppito, S. R. (2014). *Individual meaning-centered psychotherapy for patients with advanced cancer: A treatment manual*. Oxford, England: Oxford University Press.
Brown, R. T., Madan Swain, A., & Lambert, R. (2003). Posttraumatic stress symptoms in adolescent survivors of childhood cancer and their mothers. *Journal of Traumatic Stress, 16*, 309–318. https://doi.org/10.1023/A:1024465415620
Cloutier, P. F., Manion, I. G., Walker, J. G., & Johnson, S. M. (2002). Emotionally focused interventions for couples with chronically ill children: A 2 year follow up. *Journal of Marital and Family Therapy, 28*, 391–398. https://doi.org/10.1111/j.1752-0606.2002.tb00364.x
Denton, W. H., Wittenborn, A. K., & Golden, R. N. (2012). Augmenting antidepressant medication treatment of depressed women with emotionally focused therapy for couples: A randomized pilot study. *Journal of Marital and Family Therapy, 38*, 23–38. https://doi.org/10.1111/j.1752-0606.2012.00291.x
Dockham, B., Schafenacker, A., Yoon, H., Ronis, D. L., Kershaw, T., Titler, M., & Northouse, L. (2016). Implementation of a psychoeducational program for cancer survivors and family caregivers at a cancer support community affiliate: A pilot effectiveness study. *Cancer Nursing, 39*, 169–180. https://doi.org/10.1097/NCC.0000000000000311
Dessaulles, A., Johnson, S. M., & Denton, W. H. (2003). Emotion-focused therapy for couples in the treatment of depression: A pilot study. *American Journal of Family Therapy, 31*, 345–353. https://doi.org/10.1080/01926180390232266
Engel, G. L. (1977). The need for a new medical model: A challenge for biomedicine. *Science, 196*, 129–136. https://doi.org/10.1126/science.847460
Engel, G. L. (1980). The clinical application of the biopsychosocial model. *American Journal of Psychiatry, 137*, 535–544. https://doi.org/10.1176/ajp.137.5.535
Epstein, R. M., Duberstein, P. R., Fenton, J. J., Fiscella, K., Hoerger, M., Tancredi, D. J., ... Franks, P. (2017). Effect of a patient-centered communication intervention on oncologist-patient communication, quality of life, and health care utilization in advanced cancer: The VOICE randomized clinical trial. *JAMA Oncology, 3*, 92–100. https://doi.org/10.1001/jamaoncol.2016.4373

---

[1] Note: References that are prefaced with an asterisk are recommended readings.

Gueguen, J. A., Bylund, C. L., Brown, R. F., Levin, T. T., & Kissane, D. W. (2009). Conducting family meetings in palliative care: Themes, techniques, and preliminary evaluation of a communication skills module. *Palliative & Supportive Care, 7*, 171–179. https://doi.org/10.1017/S1478951509000224

Hodgson, J. L., McCammon, S. L., & Anderson, R. J. (2011). A conceptual and empirical basis for including medical family therapy services in cancer care settings. *American Journal of Family Therapy, 39*, 348–359. https://doi.org/10.1080/01926187.2010.537944

Hodgson, J., Lamson, A., Mendenhall, T., & Tyndall, L. (2014). Introduction to Medical Family Therapy: Advanced Applications. In J. Hodgson, A. Lamson, T. Mendenhall., and D. Crane (Eds.). *Medical family therapy: Advanced applications* (pp. 1–9). New York, NY: Springer.

*Holland, J. C. (2000). Improving the human side of cancer care: Psycho-oncology's contribution. *Cancer Journal, 7*, 458–471. Retrieved from http://europepmc.org/abstract/med/11769856

*Holland, J. C., Breitbart, W. S., Jacobsen, P. B., Butow, P. N., Loscalzo, M. J., & McCorkle, R. (Eds.). (2015). *Psycho-oncology* (3rd ed.). Oxford, England: Oxford University Press.

Hudson, P., Thomas, T., Quinn, K., & Aranda, S. (2009). Family meetings in palliative care: Are they effective? *Palliative Medicine, 23*, 150–157. https://doi.org/10.1177/0269216308099960

Institute of Medicine Committee on the Future Health Care Workforce for Older Adults. (2008). *Retooling for an aging America: Building the health care workforce*. Washington, DC: National Academies Press.

Johnson, S. (2004). *The practice of emotionally focused couple therapy: Creating connection*. New York, NY: Brunner-Routledge.

Kazak, A. E., Boeving, C. A., Alderfer, M. A., Hwang, W.-T., & Reilly, A. (2005). Posttraumatic stress symptoms during treatment in parents of children with cancer. *Journal of Clinical Oncology, 23*, 7405–7410. https://doi.org/10.1200/JCO.2005.09.110

*Kent, E. E., Rowland, J. H., Northouse, L., Litzelman, K., Chou, W. Y. S., Shelburne, N., ... Huss, K. (2016). Caring for caregivers and patients: research and clinical priorities for informal cancer caregiving. *Cancer, 122*, 1987–1995. https://doi.org/10.1002/cncr.29939.

Kim, Y., Kashy, D. A., Wellisch, D. K., Spillers, R. L., Kaw, C. K., & Smith, T. G. (2008). Quality of life of couples dealing with cancer: Dyadic and individual adjustment among breast and prostate cancer survivors and their spousal caregivers. *Annals of Behavioral Medicine, 35*, 230–238. https://doi.org/10.1007/s12160-008-9026-y

Kim, Y., Shaffer, K. M., Carver, C. S., & Cannady, R. S. (2015). Quality of life of family caregivers 8 years after a relative's cancer diagnosis: Follow-up of the National Quality of Life Survey for Caregivers. *Psychooncology, 25*, 266–274. https://doi.org/10.1002/pon.3843

Kissane, D. W. (2013). Marriage is as protective as chemotherapy in cancer care. *American Society of Clinical Oncology, 31*, 3852–3853. https://doi.org/10.1200/JCO.2013.51.5080

*Kissane, D. W., & Bloch, S. (2002). *Family focused grief therapy*. Philadelphia, PA: Open University Press.

Kissane, D. W., Bloch, S., Onghena, P., & McKenzie, D. P. (1996). The Melbourne Family Grief Study II: Psychosocial morbidity and grief in bereaved families. *American Journal of Psychiatry, 153*, 659–666. https://doi.org/10.1176/ajp.153.5.659

Kissane, D. W., Bylund, C. L., Banerjee, S. C., Bialer, P. A., Levin, T. T., Maloney, E. K., & D'Agostino, T. A. (2012). Communication skills training for oncology professionals. *Journal of Clinical Oncology, 30*, 1242–1247. https://doi.org/10.1200/JCO.2011.39.6184

*Kissane, D. W., & Hempton, C. (2017). Conducting a family meeting. In D. Kissane, B. Bultz, P. Butow, C. Bylund, S. Noble, and S. Wilkinson (Eds.), *Oxford textbook of communication in oncology and palliative care* (2nd ed., pp. 110–119). Oxford, England: Oxford University Press.

*Kissane, D. W., & Parnes, F. (2014). *Bereavement care for families*. New York, NY: Routledge.

Kissane, D., Zaider, T., Li, Y., Hichenberg, S., Schuler, T., Lederberg, M., ... Del Gaudio, F. (2016). Randomized controlled trial of family therapy in advanced cancer continued into bereavement. *Journal of Clinical Oncology, 24*, 1921–1930. https://doi.org/10.1200/JCO.2015.63.0582

Makinen, J. A., & Johnson, S. M. (2006). Resolving attachment injuries in couples using emotionally focused therapy: Steps toward forgiveness and reconciliation. *Journal of Consulting and Clinical Psychology, 74,* 1055–1064. https://doi.org/10.1037/0022-006X.74.6.1055

Manne, S. L., Kissane, D. W., Nelson, C. J., Mulhall, J. P., Winkel, G., & Zaider, T. (2011). Intimacy enhancing psychological intervention for men diagnosed with prostate cancer and their partners: A pilot study. *Journal of Sexual Medicine, 8,* 1197–1209. https://doi.org/10.1111/j.1743-6109.2010.02163.x

McCorkle, R., Ercolano, E., Lazenby, M., Schulman Green, D., Schilling, L. S., Lorig, K., & Wagner, E. H. (2011). Self management: Enabling and empowering patients living with cancer as a chronic illness. *CA: A Cancer Journal for Clinicians, 61,* 50–62. https://doi.org/10.3322/caac.20093

McLean, L. M., Walton, T., Rodin, G., Esplen, M. J., & Jones, J. M. (2013). A couple based intervention for patients and caregivers facing end stage cancer: Outcomes of a randomized controlled trial. *Psycho-Oncology, 22,* 28–38. https://doi.org/10.1002/pon.2046

McLeod, D. L., Tapp, D. M., Moules, N. J., & Campbell, M. E. (2010). Knowing the family: Interpretations of family nursing in oncology and palliative care. *European Journal of Oncology Nursing, 14,* 93–100. https://doi.org/10.1016/j.ejon.2009.09.006

Naaman, S. C. (2008). *Evaluation of the clinical efficacy of emotionally focused couples therapy on psychological adjustment and natural killer cell cytotoxicity in early breast cancer.* Doctoral dissertation, University of Ottawa (Canada). Retrieved from https://ruor.uottawa.ca/handle/10393/29526

National Comprehensive Care Network. (2017). *NCCN guidelines.* Retrieved from https://www.nccn.org/professionals/physician_gls/f_guidelines.asp (2017)

*Northouse, L. L. (2012). Helping patients and their family caregivers cope with cancer. *Oncology Nursing Forum, 39,* 500–506. https://doi.org/10.1188/12.onf.500-506.

Ostroff, J., Ross, S., & Steinglass, P. (2000). Psychosocial adaptation following treatment: A family systems perspective on childhood cancer survivorship. In L. Baider, C. Cooper, and A. De-Nour (Eds.), *Cancer and the family* (2nd ed., pp. 155–174). West Sussex, England: John Wiley & Sons.

*Ostroff, J., Ross, S., Steinglass, P., Ronis-Tobin, V., & Singh, B. (2004). Interest in and barriers to participation in multiple family groups among head and neck cancer survivors and their primary family caregivers. *Family Process, 43,* 195–208. https://doi.org/10.1111/j.1545-5300.2004.04302005.x.

Pirl, W. F., Fann, J. R., Greer, J. A., Braun, I., Deshields, T., Fulcher, C., … Lazenby, M. (2014). Recommendations for the implementation of distress screening programs in cancer centers: Report from the American Psychosocial Oncology Society (APOS), Association of Oncology Social Work (AOSW), and Oncology Nursing Society (ONS) joint task force. *Cancer, 120,* 2946–2954. https://doi.org/10.1002/cncr.28750

*Rauch, P., & Muriel, A. (2005). *Raising an emotionally healthy child when a parent is sick.* New York, NY: McGraw Hill.

*Reiss, D., Steinglass, P., & Howe, G. (1993). The family's organization around the illness. How do families cope with chronic illness. In R. Cole and D. Reiss (Eds.), *How do families cope with illness?* (pp. 173–213). Hillside, NJ: Laurence Erlbaum Associates.

Rolland, J. S. (1994). *Families, illness, and disability: An integrative treatment model.* New York, NY: Basic Books.

*Rolland, J. S. (2005). Cancer and the family: An integrative model. *Cancer, 104,* 2584–2595. https://doi.org/10.1002/cncr.21489.

Schaefer, K. G., & Block, S. D. (2009). Physician communication with families in the ICU: Evidence-based strategies for improvement. *Current Opinion in Critical Care, 15,* 569–577. https://doi.org/10.1097/MCC.0b013e328332f524

Schenker, Y., Park, S. Y., Maciasz, R., & Arnold, R. M. (2014). Do patients with advanced cancer and unmet palliative care needs have an interest in receiving palliative care services? *Journal of Palliative Medicine, 17,* 667–672. https://doi.org/10.1089/jpm.2013.0537

Schuler, T. A., Zaider, T. I., Li, Y., Hichenberg, S., Masterson, M., & Kissane, D. W. (2014). Typology of perceived family functioning in an American sample of patients with advanced cancer. *Journal of Pain and Symptom Management, 48*, 281–288. https://doi.org/10.1016/j.jpainsymman.2013.09.013

Schuler, T. A., Zaider, T. I., Li, Y., Masterson, M., McDonnell, G. A., Hichenberg, S., … Kissane, D. W. (2017). Perceived family functioning predicts baseline psychosocial characteristics in US participants of a family focused grief therapy trial. *Journal of Pain and Symptom Management, 54*, 126–131. https://doi.org/10.1016/j.jpainsymman.2017.03.016

Scott, J. L., Halford, W. K., & Ward, B. G. (2004). United we stand? The effects of a couple-coping intervention on adjustment to early stage breast or gynecological cancer. *Journal of Consulting and Clinical Psychology, 72*, 1122–1135. https://doi.org/10.1037/0022-006X.72.6.1122

Sklenarova, H., Krumpelmann, A., Haun, M. W., Friederich, H. C., Huber, J., Thomas, M., … Hartmann, M. (2015). When do we need to care about the caregiver? Supportive care needs, anxiety, and depression among informal caregivers of patients with cancer and cancer survivors. *Cancer, 121*, 1513–1519. https://doi.org/10.1002/cncr.29223

Smith, T. J., Temin, S., Alesi, E. R., Abernethy, A. P., Balboni, T. A., Basch, E. M., … Paice, J. A. (2012). American Society of Clinical Oncology provisional clinical opinion: The integration of palliative care into standard oncology care. *Journal of Clinical Oncology, 30*, 880–887. https://doi.org/10.1200/JCO.2011.38.5161

*Steinglass, P. (1998). Multiple family discussion groups for patients with chronic medical illness. *Families, Systems, & Health, 16*, 55–70. https://doi.org/10.1037/h0089842.

Traeger, L., Park, E. R., Sporn, N., Repper-DeLisi, J., Convery, M. S., Jacobo, M., & Pirl, W. F. (2013). Development and evaluation of targeted psychological skills training for oncology nurses in managing stressful patient and family encounters. *Oncology Nursing Forum, 40*, E327–E336. https://doi.org/10.1188/13.onf.e327-e336

Walker, J. G., Johnson, S., Manion, I., & Cloutier, P. (1996). Emotionally focused marital intervention for couples with chronically ill children. *Journal of Consulting and Clinical Psychology, 64*, 1029–1036. https://doi.org/10.1037/0022-006X.64.5.1029

Walker, J. G., Manion, I. G., Cloutier, P. F., & Johnson, S. M. (1992). Measuring marital distress in couples with chronically ill children: The Dyadic Adjustment Scale. *Journal of Pediatric Psychology, 17*, 345–357. https://doi.org/10.1093/jpepsy/17.3.345

*Watson, M., & Kissane, D. W. (Eds.). (2011). *Handbook of psychotherapy in cancer care*. Hoboken, NJ: Wiley-Blackwell.

Wiebe, S. A., & Johnson, S. M. (2016). A review of the research in emotionally focused therapy for couples. *Family Process, 55*, 390–407. https://doi.org/10.1111/famp.12229

Wright, L. M., Watson, W. L., & Bell, J. M. (1996). *Beliefs: The heart of healing in families and illness*. New York, NY: Basic Books.

Zaider, T. I., Banerjee, S. C., Manna, R., Coyle, N., Pehrson, C., Hammonds, S., … Bylund, C. L. (2016). Responding to challenging interactions with families: A training module for inpatient oncology nurses. *Families, Systems, & Health, 34*, 204–212. https://doi.org/10.1037/fsh0000159

*Zaider, T., & Kissane, D. (2009). The assessment and management of family distress during palliative care. *Current Opinion in Supportive and Palliative Care, 3*, 67–71. https://doi.org/10.1097/SPC.0b013e328325a5ab.

Zaider, T. I., & Kissane, D. W. (2011). Couples therapy in advanced cancer: Using intimacy and meaning to reduce existential distress. In M. Watson and D. Kissane (Eds.), *Handbook of psychotherapy in cancer care* (pp. 159–173). Hoboken, NJ: Wiley-Blackwell.

Chapter 9
Medical Family Therapy in Psychiatry

Kenneth Phelps, Jennifer Hodgson, Alison Heru, and Jakob Jensen

The term "Psychiatry," named first in 1808 by physician Johann Christian Reil, is derived from two Greek words: psyche (soul) and *iatros* (healer) (Marneros, 2008). Over the years, psychiatry has remained a specialty of medicine focused on the complexities of the human mind. While understanding the etiologic and remediating factors of mental illness has been a mainstay of psychiatric practice, clinical methods have varied over time. Psychiatry has seen shifts from Freudian psychoanalysis to more structured, manualized therapeutic approaches. Emerging science has taken the profession further away from its therapeutic roots, in favor of psychopharmacologic and neurologic discovery. Nevertheless, psychiatry continues to be a practice defined by interdisciplinary collaboration as well as conceptualization sensitive to familial and cultural factors. This is demonstrated through the American Psychiatric Association's (American Psychiatric Association, 2016a) values of "prevention, access, care and sensitivity for patients and compassion for their families; respect for diverse views and pluralism within the field; and respect for other health professionals" (para 3).

Psychiatry's interaction with family therapy is not new, as the foundational voices of family therapy can be traced to analytically oriented psychiatrists (e.g., Nathan Ackerman, Murray Bowen, Gregory Bateson; Beels, 2002). Early on, interest in how communication may influence an array of psychiatric disorders,

---

K. Phelps (✉)
Department of Neuropsychiatry and Behavioral Science, University of South Carolina, Columbia, SC, USA
e-mail: kenneth.phelps@uscmed.sc.edu

J. Hodgson · J. Jensen
Department of Human Development and Family Science, East Carolina University, Greenville, NC, USA

A. Heru
Department of Psychiatry, University of Colorado Denver, Denver, CO, USA

© Springer International Publishing AG, part of Springer Nature 2018
T. Mendenhall et al. (eds.), *Clinical Methods in Medical Family Therapy*, Focused Issues in Family Therapy, https://doi.org/10.1007/978-3-319-68834-3_9

particularly schizophrenia, spawned debate and inquisition among these originators of knowledge. Though decades have passed, the need for ongoing dialogue between clinicians representing varied lenses persists. The Group for the Advancement of Psychiatry's *Committee on the Family* made recommendations to residency programs to provide educational experiences that emphasize systems theory, life cycle development, and how families can contribute to psychiatric presentations or serve to remediate symptomatology (Berman et al., 2006). Various systemically oriented themes are also represented in the academic milestones for residents and fellows. Reciprocally, many family therapy programs underscore the need for students to obtain diagnostic competency and some degree of pharmacologic familiarity. Ideally, as psychiatrists and medical family therapists (MedFTs) collaborate with each other in integrated settings, this fundamental knowledge acquired in educational programs can grow through an exchange of expertise that arises from clinical partnership. In these circumstances, the integrated care setting serves as a crucible for furtherance of erudition alongside cohesive patient and family care. All names in this vignette are changed to maintain confidentiality.

Clinical Vignette

[Note: This vignette is a compilation of cases that represent treatment in psychiatry. All patients' names and/or identifying information have been changed to maintain confidentiality.]

I (KP), an outpatient MedFT that consults in the inpatient psychiatric unit, received a call from the inpatient social worker about Mr. Brandon Anderson, a 24-year-old male with recent five-day admission following a suicide attempt via overdose. To hear more about Mr. Anderson's care and current difficulties, I attended the multidisciplinary team meeting the following morning. Upon arriving at the hospital, Dr. Diaz, Brandon's treating inpatient psychiatrist, pulled me aside to share that they called on me to continue treatment on an outpatient basis due to the longstanding nature of Mr. Anderson's obsessive-compulsive disorder (OCD) paired with recent relational difficulties. Dr. Diaz revealed that Mr. Anderson had an onset of OCD at 18 years old during his transition to college. His primary symptoms fell into the contamination/cleaning and forbidden/taboo thought clusters. He obtained some prior supportive counseling at the college mental health clinic but never engaged in cognitive behavioral treatment for his symptoms. Over the last few years, Mr. Anderson's distress with intrusive thoughts, compulsive cleaning/washing, and repetitive mental rituals resulted in a more isolative existence. His withdrawal from social relationships also impacted his marriage to Mrs. Ashley Anderson. The couple were married for two years and dated since late college. Ashley felt frustrated with Brandon's insistence with how things must be kept in their household and bothered at his reluctance to engage in treatment. Additionally, she felt fearful of recently revealed obsessional thoughts concerning physical and sexual aggression. Prior to hospitalization, Brandon revealed that he had thoughts of harming her that were deeply disturbing for both members of the couple. The inpatient team confirmed the ego-dystonic nature of these thoughts. When Brandon shared his thoughts with Ashley, she insisted he obtain help and went to her parents' home to stay for the night, stating she "was not sure I can continue on like this in the marriage." At that point Brandon became increasingly down and hopeless, feeling like a burden. He took several old prescriptions but then called 911 due to feeling regretful about his behavior.

During the treatment team meeting, it was noted that Brandon's planned discharge was at the end of the week. He participated in dialectical behavior-oriented skills groups while on the unit. He interacted with others and demonstrated improvement in his overall mood symptoms. He currently denied any suicidal or homicidal ideations. He continued to have intrusive obsessional thoughts, but he had been trying to engage in fewer mental rituals since psycho-education had been provided by Dr. Diaz regarding the problematic outcome of thought suppression. He was adherent and willing to continue fluvoxamine with an outpatient psychiatrist. During the treatment team meeting, current responses of staff members to Brandon's request for reassurance were processed. The team also discussed possible exposures that could be conducted during Brandon's remaining time on the unit. Particular attention was paid to one team member's experience with their own adolescent living with OCD. The team formulated the plan of inpatient social work, inpatient psychiatrist, and MedFT to meet with Brandon and his wife later that day.

During the relational consultation, rapport building occurred with the couple and further education provided on the diagnosis and treatment of OCD/depression. Dr. Diaz discussed the efficacy of medication in these conditions and importance of exposure and response prevention (E/RP). I normalized some relational difficulties for couples' coping with OCD, using externalizing language. Additionally, the treatment team formulated an outpatient plan of enhanced E/RP using a couple-based approach, recently published in the literature. At the conclusion of the meeting, the couple received a written biopsychosocial plan of care. They were agreeable to continue in the hospital's outpatient clinic for medication management and psychotherapy the following week.

At the follow-up visit, a more detailed clinical interview occurred using the Yale-Brown Obsessive Compulsive Scale (YBOCS). Assessment of a variety of relational health constructs (i.e., communication, affective responsiveness, and relational patterns around the illness) also occurred. After obtaining a signed release, collaboration occurred with Brandon's new outpatient psychiatrist, Dr. Smith, so medication could be appropriately titrated. Brandon and Ashley engaged in 16 sessions of E/RP, including disorder-specific couple interventions and partner-assisted exposures. Between each session, Dr. Smith

> *and I discussed psychological and relational functioning. At period points in treatment, providers shared current diagnoses, medication changes, and treatment plans* via *a brief one-page collaborative form to Brandon's primary care doctor. After the initial treatment program, the couple continued on a maintenance schedule of therapy due to the waxing and waning nature of OCD. They currently follow up every three months to review coping skills, identify efficacious self-talk, brainstorm exposures, and discuss life transitions, such as recently reuniting in the same household and the couple's eventual hopes of expanding their family.*

What Is Psychiatry?

Psychiatry is a specialty of medicine, frequently cohabitating with other mental health professions, dedicated to the prevention and treatment of mental disorders. Psychiatrists commonly use subjective reports, collateral data, psychological tests, mental status examinations, and neuroimaging to identify diagnoses. However, even with such extensive information, the assessment of mental illnesses takes time and multiple stakeholders to move from ambiguity to an effective treatment plan. To become an adult psychiatrist, a person completes 4 years of medical school followed by a four-year general psychiatry residency program, which includes varied foci (e.g., inpatient, outpatient, pharmacology, psychotherapy, substance abuse). Following general training, some individuals pursue subspecialty training (e.g., child and adolescent psychiatry, geriatric psychiatry, forensic psychiatry), typically requiring the completion of a fellowship (APA, 2016a, 2016b).

Child and adolescent psychiatrists focus on the treatment of children from birth to young adulthood. These physicians complete an additional 2-year fellowship (1 year often replacing the final year of general psychiatry training). They commonly see youth with neurodevelopmental (e.g., autism spectrum disorders, attention-deficit hyperactivity disorder, motor disorders), anxiety (e.g., phobias, separation anxiety, social anxiety disorder), disruptive behavior (e.g., oppositional defiant disorder, conduct disorder), and emerging substance-related conditions. At the other end of the developmental spectrum, geriatric psychiatrists, who receive one additional year of fellowship training, often see individuals and families coping with neurocognitive disorders related to Alzheimer's disease or another medical condition.

The prevalence of a diagnosis within a particular context will depend greatly upon the demographic and phenomenological features of those who make up that context. For instance, a psychiatrist practicing in a Veterans Affairs (VA) hospital system may see more trauma- and stressor-related disorders, a consult-liaison, or psychosomatically trained psychiatrist will see more somatic symptoms disorders or delirium, and an emergency room psychiatrist may see more acute presentations of psychosis, suicidality, or substance abuse and/or withdrawal. Additionally, a forensic expert may practice in a prison setting where antisocial personality disorder is a common diagnosis maintained by inmates. They frequently see defendants opting for a "not guilty by reason of insanity plea" or the chronically mentally ill who inappropriately landed in a judicial system instead of community mental health. Regardless of the setting, identification of the correct diagnosis, alongside case conceptualization, serves to guide selection of therapeutic intervention and/or pharmacologic agent. The indicated treatment protocol ultimately determines which members of the interdisciplinary team may be involved for a given patient. General psychiatry and its subspecialties are a perfect example of science meeting art in clinical decision-making. These physicians and the MedFT are also reliant on other professionals to mobilize the patient and family into change.

Treatment Teams in Psychiatry

Given the complexities of treating psychiatric maladies, collaboration between individuals with a host of trainings and areas of expertise is likely to result in a more comprehensive, effective, and efficient treatment (Bustillo, Lauriello, Horan, & Keith, 2001). Because a family requires support in their care for the mentally ill patient throughout their journey, a team of providers is essential for preparing the family with the necessary resources to navigate physical, mental, emotional, and social challenges accompanying psychiatric illness (Heru, 2004). Despite the expectation that practitioners of psychiatry should integrate family factors into a biopsychosocial formulation and treatment plan (as previously mentioned), many psychiatry residencies do not spend significant time emphasizing practical family and relationship maintenance skills (Heru & Drury, 2006).

Therefore, as part of the psychiatric treatment team, MedFTs potentially fill vital gaps in treatment; they do this by facilitating effective communication between providers and health-care workers and in strengthening patients' family and social supports (Berman & Heru, 2005). Inpatient psychiatric patients have reported that MedFTs are critical members of their treatment team who helped them deal with complex family dynamics (e.g., maintaining an intimate connection with a partner throughout treatment, discussing the hospitalization in an age appropriate manner with children; Anderson, Huff, & Hodgson, 2008). Collaboration among various members of a psychiatric treatment team (e.g., psychiatrists, MedFTs, social workers, recreational therapists) may prove vital, given that when psychiatrists made use of family-based and social interventions (in addition to traditional psychiatric treatment), practitioners see reduced relapse rates and medical costs (Bustillo et al., 2001; Law & Crane, 2000). Consequently, stronger incentives are provided to third-party payment providers for the inclusion of family-based psychiatric treatment (Anderson et al., 2008). Therefore, providers who allow a biopsychosocial-spiritual (BPSS) framework to shape psychiatric treatment benefit from a more comprehensive vista of patient functioning, as well as offering more wide-ranging treatment

(Engel, 1977, 1980; Wright, Watson, & Bell, 1996). The following is a nonexhaustive list of important members of a typical psychiatric treatment team with whom MedFTs may encounter when working in psychiatric settings:

Psychiatrists. These providers are licensed medical physicians who specialize in the diagnosis and treatment of mental illness. They may prescribe medication for the treatment of a wide variety of mental illnesses. A psychiatrist is typically the primary/lead member of the treatment team and directs team meetings in collaboration with psychologists, nurses, MedFTs, social workers, etc. Taking into consideration input from all members of the treatment team, a psychiatrist ultimately decides when a patient is sufficiently stable to be released. He or she may refer a complex case to a psychologist for additional psychological testing, which aids in diagnosis and treatment. Psychiatrists may involve MedFTs if complex family dynamics are worsening a patient's mental functioning or, conversely, if family support may be a remediating factor in recovery.

Psychologists. These providers are trained to administer and interpret a number of screenings and assessments that can help diagnose a condition or reveal more about the way a patient thinks, feels, and behaves. Such tests may evaluate intellectual skills, cognitive strengths and deficits, vocational aptitude, personality characteristics, and neuropsychological functioning.

Psychiatric-mental health nurse practitioners. A psychiatric-mental health nurse practitioner (PMHNP) is a registered nurse who often performs similar roles to that of the psychiatrist, including ordering and interpreting tests, diagnosing mental illness, and prescribing medication (prescribing and ordering a commitment privileges may vary according to a PMHNPs state of practice). He or she may also provide psychoeducation and psychotherapy to the patient and family about how to best react in certain challenging situations (e.g., hallucinations, delusions).

Psychiatric care coordinators. Care coordinators may come from a variety of disciplinary backgrounds (e.g., social worker, licensed professional counselor). They collaborate with the psychiatrist and social workers to provide appropriate psychotherapeutic care to patients, offering input to the psychiatrist regarding each patient's progress toward greater mental stability (e.g., decrease in suicidal ideation). Care coordinators often lead process groups with multiple patients and may provide family members with psychoeducation during family visiting hours. They also complete initial screening measures and discharge planning.

Social workers. These providers advocate for the overall welfare of patients and their families. Social workers assist with monitoring behavioral progress of psychiatric patients, set up appointments for therapy and psychiatric visits, and schedule traditional medical visits. They may additionally assist patients with finding housing prior to discharge from an inpatient facility (e.g., for patients in need of assisted living or rehabilitation centers). Some social workers assist with finding community supports for patients, including social and recreational outlets, and offer psychotherapy.

Nurses or medical assistants (MA). These providers educate patients regarding illnesses, provide medication, and assess for treatment progression. In addition to collaborating with other providers regarding psychotherapy, they monitor sleep, diet, and basic vital indicators (e.g., blood pressure). Nurses or MAs are generally the first responders to assist a patient in crisis (e.g., via non-violent crisis intervention to prevent the patients from hurting themselves or someone else).

Mental health technicians. Mental health technicians collaborate extensively with nurses and MAs, as these providers are especially important for ensuring patient safety. They often sit in patients' rooms in cases of suicidal or homicidal ideation. They regularly perform room checks on the psychiatric unit to verify that every patient is present and safe. While employers may hire and train high school graduates to be mental health technicians/psychiatric aides, most hold a certificate or associate's degree in mental health technology.

Occupational therapists. These providers assist with patient activities of daily living (e.g., basic hygiene, grooming, dressing, and cleaning one's living space). Occupational therapists also perform safety evaluations to verify that patients are safe to return home after inpatient care and/or in accord with subsequent recommendations made by the psychiatrist.

Recreational therapists. Recreational therapists collaborate with the care coordinator and social workers to offer support to psychiatric patients through stress management and recreational activities. Such interventions may include meditation training, group outings, exercise classes, animal assisted therapy, aquatic activities, and biofeedback measurements and techniques.

Pharmacists. Most psychiatric units have a pharmacist on-call who collaborates extensively with the psychiatrist by providing expertise regarding prescriptions and possible emotional/behavioral side effects. These professionals also offer consultation concerning potential interactions between medications.

Fundamentals of Care in Psychiatry

When considering the ease of including a MedFT in collaborative psychiatric contexts, there are both strengths and cautions. The overlapping fundamentals between members of the treatment team, such as diagnostic language, may ease the tensions sometimes felt on interdisciplinary teams. However, the professionals' shared skill set (e.g., making a diagnosis, delivery of screening measures, treatment planning regarding therapeutic indications) can raise "turf wars," duplicate services, and questions regarding scope of practice. In the best of scenarios, the members of the treatment team collaborate in a way to bring forth the powerful influence of their complimentary skill sets. In this sense, the shared knowledge can serve to advance care by professionals speaking the same language. Undoubtedly, the value of a MedFT is to monitor the emotional climate of the treatment team, ensuring that the systemic process at play is collaborative and focused on the patient or family's best interest rather than letting competitive incidents take over. To effectively function on this team, MedFTs should be aware of fundamentals concerning the diagnosis and treatment of mental illness, especially information that may be lacking in some advanced training programs.

Diagnosis

One of the major differences in the diagnosis of psychiatric illnesses compared to other illnesses is that diagnoses are made without the benefit of definitive testing. Instead, psychiatric illnesses are diagnosed based on a pattern of symptoms that occur over time. It is not unusual for a patient to have a change in diagnosis as new information comes to light. Substance use and medical illness can act as etiological factors for various psychiatric symptoms, making the exact diagnosis more difficult. This can be frustrating for patients and their families, so clear explanations about how diagnoses are made are an important part of delivering care. Patients and families frequently "google their symptoms," so it is worth providing good written information or websites as soon as possible, especially since much misinformation exists within the online community.

The concept of psychiatric illness can be confusing for patients and family members as many psychological symptoms are part of normal life experience. For example, sudden changes in mood, transient anxiety symptoms, and panic when faced with a life-threatening situation can all occur as part of the normal human experience. It is the persistence of these symptoms, their association with other symptoms, and their interference with normal functioning that allows them to reach the threshold for diagnosis of a psychiatric illness. The Diagnostic and Statistical Manual of Mental Disorders—Fifth Edition (DSM-5; APA, 2013)—is frequently referred to as the "Bible of Psychiatry," but psychiatrists often disagree about the validity of some diagnoses. For example, many clusters of symptoms once considered pathological, such as homosexuality, have been removed and new diagnoses (e.g., premenstrual dysphoric disorder and hoarding) have been added. Conditions warranting more clinical research and experience, (e.g., internet gaming disorder), are listed in DSM-5, Sect. 3. It should also be noted that there is inherent human bias in making a diagnosis. Some diagnoses are made more commonly in women than men (e.g., borderline personality disorder), while others are made more commonly in men than women (e.g., antisocial personality disorder). This may be the result of study selection bias and that women voluntarily seek treatment more frequently than men (Bjorkland, 2006). Conversely, more men may be mandated for treatment secondary to violent behaviors comparable to women, resulting in an antisocial diagnosis in some cases. Epidemiological data and diagnostic descriptors must thereby be considered.

Treatment Setting

MedFTs will encounter patients with psychiatric illnesses in many settings, such as primary care, community mental health centers, specialty clinics, and inpatient medical or psychiatric hospitals. In primary care, patients usually have mild to moderate anxiety and depression, but some patients with more severe symptomatology may be reluctant to transition care to a psychiatric clinic. Within these outpatient mental health clinics, psychiatrists typically see patients with moderate to severe mood disorders and anxiety disorders and/or those with high complexity. Patients with complex mental disorders tend to have either treatment-resistant illnesses (e.g., mood or psychotic illnesses that persists through initial treatments), comorbid substance use disorders, or personality disorders. Additionally, many of these patients have had failed pharmacotherapy or psychotherapy trials, necessitating the involvement of a specialist. In the inpatient psychiatric setting, patients are admitted mostly for concern of safety toward self or others or grave disability. Suicidality is most likely in the context of depressive illnesses (e.g., major depression, bipolar disorder depressive phase, or adjustment disorder with depressed mood). Grave disability is usually associated with chronic serious mental illness (e.g., schizophrenia, bipolar disorder, or neurocognitive disorders).

Pharmacology and Associated Treatments

As previously noted, psychiatrists focus on difficult to treat or treatment-resistant illnesses. Treatment-resistant schizophrenia is the persistence of symptoms despite adequate pharmacological treatment and occurs in up to 60% of patients with schizophrenia (Miller, McEvoy, Jeste, et al., 2006). Adequate treatment is defined as two or more treatment trials of antipsychotics—such as olanzapine, risperidone, or haloperidol—at adequate dosages for 4–6 weeks (Silverman et al., 2016). Other strategies are then tried (e.g., clozapine and/or psychosocial treatments). Likewise, treatment-resistant depression (TRD) is defined as depression that is resistant to standard treatments. According to Papakostas and Fava (2010), 45% of patients with depression, when treated by a primary-care physician alone, do not respond. The next step is a reevaluation of the diagnosis and consideration of hitherto unexamined aspects of the case, such as family dysfunction, social location factors (e.g., struggles with gender sexual identity, racial/ethnic disparities, religious/spiritual crises), or other medical diagnosis not yet discovered or treated (e.g., diabetes, hypothyroidism, cancer, Parkinson's disease).

Thankfully, a significant portion of patients present with depressive disorders who are responsive to medication and/or psychotherapeutic intervention. For these patients, the initiation of a selective serotonin reuptake inhibitor (SSRI) or serotonin norepinephrine reuptake inhibitor (SNRI) leads to the resolution of most symptoms within 4–6 weeks (Silverman et al., 2016). Psychotherapeutic approaches to depression are outlined later in great detail within the research-informed practice subsection. Prescription of serotonergic medications for individuals with depression necessitates careful screening for manic symptoms, as to not cause iatrogenic effects in a bipolar individual. Bipolar disorder requires long-term management with mood stabilizers—such as lithium, valproic acid, and/or carbamazepine—and significant psycho-education of patients and families to ensure compliance and reduce the risk of hospitalization. Patients with anxiety, obsessionality, and compulsivity often benefit from serotonergic agents as well. Though effective treatment of anxiety disorders such as the SSRIs and cognitive-behavioral therapy (CBT) exist, about 40% of patients with anxiety disorders are partially or completely resistant to first-line treatment (Bystritsky, 2006). Advances in psychiatry and genetics have found that patients with a "short" arm of the serotonin transporter gene are significantly less likely to respond to maximally titrated SSRIs than patients with the "long" arm of this gene (Stein, Seedat, & Gelernter, 2006). Regarding Brandon, our patient with OCD, SSRIs, such as fluoxetine, fluvoxamine, or sertraline, are first-line medications. Clomipramine, a member of an older class of tricyclic antidepressants is also effective. Patients often require higher doses of these medications in the treatment of OCD compared to depression, and they may take longer to work: 8–12 weeks (Silverman et al., 2016). If symptoms do not improve with these types of medications, some patients may respond to an antipsychotic medication, such as risperidone. Psychotherapy, such as cognitive behavior therapy (CBT) and other related therapies such as exposure and response prevention (E/RP), is effective in reducing compulsive behaviors in OCD, even in people who do not respond well to medication. Innovative treatments include medication combinations as well as techniques, such as deep brain stimulation (DBS) (Silverman et al., 2016).

Most psychiatric illnesses are chronic and, rather than aiming for complete resolution of symptoms, require management (Keitner & Mansfield, 2012). Management requires adding a psychosocial approach, often with a strong family psychoeducation component and deemphasizing finding the "right drug." Nevertheless, most patients and families want information on medications; the National Institute of Mental Health website (http://www.nimh.nih.gov/health/topics/mental-health-medications/index.shtml) offers a good overview of all psychiatric medications, including those approved by the Food and Drug Administration (FDA) and those used as "off label."

In addition to medication options, neuromodulation programs that provide a range of services are emerging in psychiatry for treatment-resistant illnesses. In general, neuromodulation induces electrical current in peripheral or central nervous tissue, through various techniques such as electroconvulsive therapy (ECT), vagus nerve stimulation (VNS), transcranial magnetic stimulation (TMS), and deep brain stimulation (DBS). ECT has been used for many decades in psychiatry, and the evidence for its efficacy for specific indications (e.g., psychotic depression) is higher than the other modalities (e.g., VNS, TMS, DBS) (Silverman et al., 2016).

When engaging in treatment planning, it is important to remember that patients live in their own families and cultures, bringing specific and sometimes deeply personal beliefs about health and illness. It is not uncommon for patients and their families to consult with traditional and nontraditional healers in addition to Western

Stigma

Other factors likely influencing care-seeking behaviors, diagnosis, and treatment planning are the judgments often extended to people with mental illness. Stigma and discrimination have been described as sometimes having worse consequences than the conditions themselves (Thornicroft et al., 2016). Self-stigma occurs when patients accept negative stereotypes held against them (Corrigan & Watson, 2006). Stigma by association occurs with families who feel ostracized because their loved one has been diagnosed with a mental illness (Angermeyer, Schulze, & Dietrich, 2003). Patients with psychiatric illness are also subjected to unequal treatment in comparison to those with physical illnesses (Thornicroft et al., 2016), resulting in higher morbidity and mortality. Differences exist among ethnic groups regarding perceptions of stigma affecting access to support services (Smith et al., 2014). MedFTs, with their inherent strengths-based approach and attunement to subjugation, can assist families in building agency and communion in their health-care contexts rather than feeling victimized by the judgments of self or others. As these factors are addressed directly, they can enhance the experience of care and impact patients and their families' willingness to engage in treatment.

Psychiatry Across the MedFT Healthcare Continuum

Application of the MedFT Healthcare Continuum (Hodgson, Lamson, Mendenhall, & Tyndall, 2014) in a psychiatry context involves careful consideration of the role that the MedFT plays within the system. While some contexts afford the clinician a choice in how he or she integrates, others have a solid work flow and strict reimbursement system that challenges integration at more advanced levels. This section aims to highlight, using the case example at the beginning of this chapter, the various ways that MedFTs may be assimilated into psychiatric care settings. It builds off of Tables 9.1 and 9.2 wherein MedFT knowledge and skills across the continuum in this setting are provided.

Levels 1 and *2* of the continuum feature the skills one would expect to see from a clinician, researcher, and/or policy advocate or professional with some training in MedFT who executes components of a relational and BPSS framework (Engel, 1977, 1980; Wright et al., 1996) during assessment, diagnosis, and treatment phases. At these levels, the MedFT may or may not have the fluency, training, or "green light" within the outpatient or inpatient psychiatry system for moving to a more advanced level on the continuum. MedFTs in psychiatry settings are more commonly in roles where they provide both integrated behavioral health-care (IBHC) services and traditional psychotherapy services, alongside teaching and research. Their expertise is in working relationally and applying the BPSS framework, but at these levels this expertise is often sought after for "special cases" or "special situations" rather than as a routine service. For example, the MedFT in this

Table 9.1 MedFTs in Psychiatric Care: Basic Knowledge and Skills

MedFT Healthcare Continuum Level	Level 1	Level 2	Level 3
Knowledge	Basic knowledge about BPSS approaches to psychiatric services; sensitive to how mental health and biological conditions are mutually influential; advanced understanding of the diagnoses included in the most up to date version of the DSM. Familiar with psychiatry as a medical specialty; limited understanding of organic causes for psychiatric and comorbid health conditions that exacerbate psychiatric illnesses. Uncertain how and when to engage professional members, patients, and support system members, their unique and overlapping skills/roles, and the team's overall structure. Basic understanding regarding strategies for a healthy lifestyle when living with a psychiatric illness. If conducting research and/or policy/advocacy work is able to do it in collaboration with other disciplines related to psychiatry and include relational and/or BPSS aspects of health and well-being.	Can differentiate between DSM diagnoses and other comorbid health conditions; familiar with basic causes and symptoms of serious and persistent mental illnesses; can identify some disease-related complications. Familiar with benefits of couple and family engagement in health-related adjustments and/or lifestyle maintenance. Knowledgeable about how to use the electronic health record system or other forms of secured communication to collaboration with various team members. Is an occasional contributor to discussions about research design and policy/advocacy work that include relational and/or BPSS aspects of health and well-being.	Working knowledge of specific team members (e.g., psychiatrist, psychiatric nurses, recreational therapists, chaplains) and medical terminology with regard to side effects of medications (e.g., dyskinesia, akathisia, tics) and common comorbid medical conditions to psychiatric illnesses (e.g., diabetes, hypertension, TBI). Broad range of knowledge about research-informed family therapy and BPSS interventions; able to conduct couple and family therapy and incorporate BPSS health factors into treatment with minimal need to refer out due to limited expertise. When work permits, is knowledgeable and consistency committed to conducting research and constructing policy/advocacy work that identifies and intervenes on behalf of individuals, couples, families, and health-care teams toward the advancement of BPSS health and well-being.

(continued)

Table 9.1 (continued)

MedFT Healthcare Continuum Level	Level 1	Level 2	Level 3
Skills	Able to recognize the BPSS dimensions of health and apply a BPSS lens to practice, research, and/or policy/advocacy work. Can discuss (and psycho-educate) basic relationships between biological processes, personal well-being, and interpersonal functioning. Demonstrates minimal collaborative skills with psychiatry and other related health-care providers; prefers to work in an individual practitioner model but is able to contact/refer to other providers about services when needed.	Applies systemic interventions in practice usually; assesses patients and support system members present for background issues such as family history and related risk factors. Demonstrates adequate collaborative skills through (a) written and verbal communication mediums that are understandable to all team members and (b) coordination of referrals to specialty mental health providers and communication with the patient's primary care provider. Conducts separate treatment plan from other providers involved in the patient's care; goals and interventions can overlap with—or be informed by—a psychiatry team but not consistently.	Able to integrate respective team members' expertise and counsel into treatment planning. Implements successfully a systemic assessment of a patient and family with competencies in assessing for BPSS aspects of psychiatric illness and/or comorbid disease and resources within the family. Engages other professionals usually who are actively involved in the patient's care. Skilled with standardized measures to track patients' individual and relational strengths and challenges (e.g., PHQ9, GAD7, Relationship Dynamics Scale; Stanley & Markman, 1996). Attends and contributes usually to team meetings to help shape BPSS treatment plans for patients.

providers. This is especially noticeable when working with patients who are living with a psychiatric illness due to the high levels of stigma that many project unto such struggles. Some patients and families will be quite forthcoming with information about alternative medication or health behaviors, whereas others may be more guarded secondary to concerns about the perceptions that Western professionals may have about such practices. It is thereby vital to normalize this part of the clinical assessment and treatment plan.

Table 9.2 MedFTs in Psychiatric Care: Advanced Knowledge and Skills

MedFT Healthcare Continuum Level	Level 4	Level 5
Knowledge	Proficient understanding of DSM psychiatric illness and common comorbid conditions and their associated treatments, medications, and terminologies. Conversant in nearly all terms, measures, and facets of psychiatric care (e.g., medications, injections, normal lab values, electroconvulsive treatment, biofeedback). Understands how to implement and collaborate with other disciplines to implement evidence-based BPSS and family therapy protocols in traditional and integrated behavioral health-care contexts. Identifies self as a MedFT. Understands and can help design policies that govern BPSS-oriented inpatient and outpatient psychiatric care services. Aware of advocacy needs for patients and families in psychiatric settings.	Understands treatment and care sequences for unique and/or challenging topics in psychiatric practice (e.g., delirium, medication interaction effects, comorbidities); can consult effectively with professionals about medical topics from other fields. Conversant with evidence-based treatments regarding most mental health disorders and their role(s) in the family; has background to provide psychoeducation to patients and families about a variety of symptoms, medications, and behavioral health management. Knowledgeable in clinical topics, research design and execution, policy, and administrative areas of psychiatric care; proficient in developing a curriculum on integrated behavioral healthcare, BPSS applications, MedFT, etc., to mental health and other health professionals. Understands leadership strategies for building integrated behavioral health-care teams in outpatient and inpatient psychiatric settings. Supervises other MedFTs and health professionals who are integrating behavioral health services into psychiatric inpatient and outpatient settings.

(continued)

Table 9.2 (continued)

MedFT Healthcare Continuum Level	Level 4	Level 5
Skills	Able to deliver seminars and workshops about the BPSS complexities of a variety of DSM diagnoses to a variety of professional types (e.g., mental health, biomedical). Can apply several BPSS interventions in care (including most types of brief interventions); can administer mood- and disease-specific assessment tools proficiently. Consistently collaborates with key psychiatry team members (e.g., psychiatrist, psychiatric nurse, social worker, psychologist, rehabilitation counselor, substance abuse counselor, pharmacist, chaplain); initiates team visits with multiple providers when working with patients and families. Able to integrate effectively into inpatient and/or outpatient psychiatric contexts and adapt to the clinical, operational, and financial needs of the system. Can independently and collaboratively construct research and program evaluation studies that study the impact of BPSS interventions with a variety of diagnoses and patient/family units of care.	Able to synthesize and conduct research and clinical work; engages in community-oriented projects outside of tertiary clinic. Goes beyond interventions routine for this population; can integrate specific models of care into routine practice (e.g., family therapy, PCBH, Chronic Care Model). Routinely engages as an administrator/leader and supervisor in a team-based approach to inpatient and/or outpatient psychiatric care, with consistent communication through electronic health records, patient introductions, curb-side consultations, and team meetings/huddles/visits. Works proficiently as a MedFT and collaborates with other providers from a variety of disciples. Creates and executes curriculum related to DSM diagnoses and common comorbidities, MedFT, BPSS framework, and integrated behavioral healthcare to a variety of professional types (e.g., mental health, biomedical).

chapter was engaged by the inpatient social worker at a *Level 2*, via a referral, after she recognized that the patient was experiencing a relational crisis with his marriage. KP, the therapist, functioned at a *Level 2* when he incorporated the wife into the treatment during the "relational consultation." However, KP moved beyond *Level 2* when he incorporated the wife into the treatment plan versus maintaining her in a consulting role.

While MedFTs at *Levels 1* and *2* have a complementary skill set to other members of the team, they should also have a working knowledge of the pharmaceuticals more commonly being prescribed by the team and a familiarity with non-psychiatric diagnoses that may exacerbate or be a consequence of treatments for psychiatric conditions (e.g., medications for depression that cause weight gain or medications for hepatitis C that result in depression symptomatology). These skills should be executed more frequently and advance across the entire continuum as the MedFT becomes more fully integrated. As she/he becomes more integrated, she/he then moves beyond a siloed "mental health" or discipline-specific role into one where she/he is a member of the team wherein expertise among all members, including the patient and his support system member, is shared and respected collectively. Additionally, with regard to research and policy/advocacy, MedFTs operating at *Levels 1* or *2* may rarely to occasionally be asked or inspired to add to a study or policy addendum that taps into BPSS interactional dynamics. They may also advocate or be consulted with regarding relational and BPSS factors that influence the psychiatric setting's clinical, operational, financial, training/education policies and protocols. One example of this would be the modification of a policy on when and where support system members can visit with patients who are receiving treatment and who may participate in the patient's treatment per se.

At *Level 3* the MedFT is applying his use of MedFT knowledge and skills and is demonstrating how he can integrate effectively into the inpatient and outpatient psychiatric settings. He or she is known by the social worker as possessing skills in family therapy, which appears in our vignette to be the impetus for her referral to him for consultation. While not all MedFTs will have relational and BPSS research or policy/advocacy opportunities in psychiatric settings, this level of MedFT has the skills and experience necessary for participating in opportunities related to each and is able to contribute them effectively. In relation to the chapter's case example, something appears to be embedded in the procedures of the system wherein providers of different disciplines know about and refer to one another. At a *Level 3*, collaboration usually continues past the referral point and how frequently it occurs may depend upon the complexity of the case and how much the providers value it. The fact that KP collaborated with providers internal and external to his clinic and, not just in response to a crisis, demonstrated a *Level 3* application of MedFT clinical and collaborative knowledge and skills. He also worked to engage the spouse in treatment, acknowledging that she is important to the success of the patient's decrease in symptomatology, as well as caring about her own BPSS health.

MedFT at *Levels 4* and *5* highlights consistent and then proficient applications of MedFT knowledge and skills. At these levels the clinician, like KP, will identify as a MedFT professionally. He will be seen as part of the health-care team versus exclusively as a specialty care provider. Examples of this advanced level of skill would be when he offered guidance to team members about how to respond to Brandon, the patient, when he sought reassurance. Informing team members to label his reassurance seeking (e.g., "Do you think I might go to hell for having these thoughts or trying to take my life?" and "Do you know if these walls might have asbestos in them?") as his OCD talking was a means to begin some E/RP in the inpatient setting. It also ensured that all team members were responding similarly to his requests for comfort.

Additionally, KP was very attentive to one team member's personal narrative about what happened with her son, as well as beneficial ideas for "sitting with suffering" when Brandon was overwhelmed when reassurance did not occur. MedFTs, as systems thinkers, believe that caring for the team and acknowledging their personal and/or professional experiences with similar issues, is a part of good caring (Hodgson et al., 2014). *Level 5* skills were also evident with this case when KP led the team in developing a treatment plan that would be best for the couple, not just the patient. Both Brandon and Ashley were given a voice in this family consultation. Team members had access to each other's notes and everyone shared responsibility for encouraging the team's overall goals with the patient and his wife versus only the goals aligned with their individual treatment plans.

Research-Informed Practices

Frequently in psychiatric care, a multimodal treatment plan is utilized where medication management and individual and family therapy approaches coexist. While most therapeutic approaches to psychiatric care focus on psychosocial stressors, interpersonal functioning, emotional processing, cognitive patterns, and physiological soothing to some degree, where the provider places his or her primary focus, likely determine the type of therapy that is utilized. Clinicians often align with a certain school of therapy; however, it is recommended that MedFTs use a science-practitioner model. Using this mode, clinicians draw on techniques and strategies that have been shown to remediate suffering associated with the psychiatric illness and/or co-occurring relational distress (i.e., evidence-based modalities). Regardless of therapeutic approach employed, attunement to the patient-family provider dynamic is crucial for ongoing treatment engagement and progress.

Individual Approaches

Individual therapies in the twenty-first century are typically brief in nature, often lasting between 10 and 20 sessions (Steenbarger, Greenberg, & Dewan, 2012). This is dissimilar to some early psychotherapies, such as psychoanalysis, which were much more lengthy. As in family therapy, the developers of some individual psychotherapies started as psychoanalysts but decided to take a different, present-oriented approach to problems. Behavioral therapy was one of the first departures from psychoanalytic theory. Patients were asked to approach the feared stimuli using principles of systemic desensitization, taking graded steps toward ultimate exposure to avoided scenario. These behavioral principles have been applied to an array of psychopathology, including exposure and response prevention (E/RP) for obsessive-compulsive disorder or prolonged exposure therapy (PE) for post-traumatic stress disorder (Gillihan, Hembree, & Foa, 2012). Other more recent evidence-based approaches include exposure techniques for social or specific phobias and habit reversal approaches to body-focused repetitive disorders or tic disorders

(Comprehensive Behavioral Intervention for Tics; Woods et al., 2008). These behavioral treatments are commonly used in conjunction with selective serotonin reuptake inhibitors. Benzodiazepines are often not utilized as their use can perpetuate a patient's external locus of control and need to rid themselves of anxiety, which runs counter to the habituation necessary for treatment efficacy.

One of the most widely known therapeutic approaches commonly utilized alongside behavior therapy, called cognitive therapy, was developed by Aaron Beck in the mid-1960s. The cognitive model states that an individual's automatic thoughts influence and are influenced by his or her emotional, behavioral, and physiological experiences (Beck, 1964, 1995). Cognitive therapists develop a comprehensive conceptualization of the patient that guides intervention. Techniques include psychoeducation, cognitive restructuring (i.e., analyzing the validity and utility of thoughts), problem-solving, activity scheduling, and behavioral experimentation (Beck, Bieling, & Grant, 2012). When this therapy is combined with behavior therapy, it is called cognitive behavioral therapy, or CBT.

A recent comprehensive survey of 106 meta-analyses examining the efficacy of CBT demonstrated that this approach has the strongest support for anxiety disorders, somatic symptoms, bulimia, anger control, and overall stress management (Hofmann, Asnaani, Vonk, Sawyer, & Fang, 2012). In this review, CBT showed higher response rates than the comparison condition in the overwhelming majority of DSM diagnoses studied. Existing practice parameters by the American Academy of Child and Adolescent Psychiatry (AACAP, 2016) typically recommend the initiation of pharmacologic agents alongside cognitive behavioral therapy for severe mental disorders, whereas youth with mild to moderate distress should first obtain cognitive and/or behavioral intervention.

An outgrowth of CBT is dialectical-behavioral therapy (DBT), which was developed by Marsha Linehan. Due to the difficulty of applying existing therapeutic paradigms to borderline personality disorder, Linehan chose to merge traditional cognitive techniques with Eastern principles of mental wellness. This led to the structured and highly evidence-based approach. Patients involved in DBT programs attend individual outpatient psychotherapy, skills training, supportive process group therapy, and telephone consultations for approximately 1 year (Linehan, 1993, 2015). Content of this efficacious treatment involves four primary modules: mindfulness, distress tolerance, emotional regulation, and interpersonal effectiveness (Linehan, 1993, 2015). While brief cognitive therapy and the lengthier DBT are typically delivered in an outpatient context, the inpatient MedFT should still be familiar with their utility and efficacy as they are increasingly used during inpatient process groups and intensive outpatient programs (IOPs).

Another individual approach commonly used to ameliorate mental symptoms includes motivational interviewing (MI). This approach is utilized in many areas of medicine to change behavior (Miller & Rose, 2009). Beyond its efficacy with a number of mental disorders (particularly substance abuse), MI has been helpful in enhancing patient outcomes in other evidence-based treatments, such as cognitive therapy, when delivered early in care (Fischer & Moyers, 2012). Moreover, MI is useful to increase engagement in behavioral treatments that seem quite paradoxical (e.g., approach what makes you fearful).

Two other individual approaches are commonly used in outpatient psychiatric contexts: interpersonal psychotherapy and time-limited psychodynamic psychotherapy. Interpersonal psychotherapy (IPT) is a short-term psychotherapy wherein relationships and mood are the primary treatment foci. The therapist centers his or her assessment on three things—grief and loss, interpersonal disputes, and role transitions—using interpersonal inventories, communication analysis, and role plays to create change (Stuart, 2012). IPT is compatible with many other psychotherapies and shown to be effective for a number of depressive disorders (e.g., adolescent depression, geriatric depression, persistent depressive disorder, depressive phase of bipolar disorder, and perinatal depression; Cuijpers, van Straten, Andersson, & van Oppen, 2008; O'Hara, Stuart, Gorman, & Wenzel, 2000; Stuart, 2012). Time-limited dynamic psychotherapy shares IPT's focus on interpersonal relatedness and attachment theory but tends to focus more on early life experiences, repetitive maladaptive patterns, and transference/counter-transference (Levenson, 2012). Meta-analyses of short-term and long-term dynamic therapies have demonstrated large effect sizes for a number of mood, eating, and personality disorders (Leichsenring, Rabung, & Leibing, 2004; Leichsenring & Rabung, 2008). In an era of eclecticism in psychiatry, all of the abovementioned individual therapy techniques can be integrated with evidence-based family therapies.

Family Approaches

The role of the family has gone through a significant transformation in the field of psychiatry and among the broader therapeutic community. Early on, families were seen as an etiological and contributing factor in mental disorders, e.g., double binds (Weakland, 1960), communication deviance (Singer & Wynne, 1963), and the schizophrenogenic mother (Fromm-Reichman, 1948). However, over time families have been seen as an avenue of rehabilitation and support from the patient with mental illness (Falloon, 2003). Alongside this perspective shift, the concept of expressed emotion (EE), criticism, and overinvolvement emerged in the 1950s, 1960s, and 1970s (Brown, Carstairs, & Topping, 1958; Vaughn & Leff, 1976). Subsequent research on high EE families where one member has schizophrenia or bipolar disorder demonstrated a relapse rate ranging from 3 to 5 times higher than that of low EE families (Parker & Hadzi-Pavlovic, 1990; Yan, Hammen, Cohen, Daley, & Henry, 2004). This knowledge led to the advent of psycho-educational family groups, among other services offered through the National Alliance on Mental Illness (NAMI).

The effectiveness of family therapy and systemic intervention for psychiatric disorders has been carefully overviewed by Baucom, Shoham, Mueser, Daiuto, and Stickle (1998), Carr, (2009a, 2009b), Diamond and Josephson (2005), and Falloon (2003). A synopsis of these reviews is that behavioral family therapy (e.g., parent-child interaction therapy, Positive Parenting Program (Triple P), parent management training, Barkley model), functional family therapy, multidimensional therapy, and multisystemic therapy show utility in treating behavioral concerns of childhood and adolescence. While attention-deficit-hyperactivity disorder is most commonly treated with stimulant medication, behavioral approaches can be useful in addressing common co-occurring behavioral disturbances.

Recent investigators also encouraged integration partners and family members into cognitive and behavioral treatments to enhance efficacy (Baucom et al., 1998; Carr, 2009a, 2009b; Diamond & Josephson, 2005). Indeed, authors in a recent meta-analysis highlighted the interplay of family accommodation and OCD symptom severity (Strauss, Hale, & Stobie, 2015). Reflecting on Mr. Anderson from our case, literature is becoming rich with emerging couple-based approaches to anxiety difficulties, such as enhanced E/RP for OCD (Abramowitz et al., 2012). Pertaining to younger patients needing E/RP, CBT family treatment for childhood OCD, including a strong systemic component, was effective 7 years posttreatment (O'Leary, Barrett, & Fjermestad, O'Leary, Barrett, & Fjermestad, 2009). The benefits of relationally focused CBT extend beyond OCD, too. Empirical support for cognitive behavioral couple therapies (CBCT) was recently reviewed by Fischer, Baucom, and Cohen (Fischer, Baucom, & Cohen, 2016); findings showed evidentiary support in the treatment of mood disorders, substance use disorders, anxiety disorders, and post-traumatic stress disorder.

Another empirically supported couples treatment modality that incorporates behavioral, humanistic, and systemic principles is emotionally focused couples therapy (EFT; Johnson, 2004). Since the development of EFT in the 1980s, it has been found to meet or exceed the guidelines at the highest level (Sexton et al., 2011) as an evidence-based couple therapy approach with both efficacy and effectiveness studies to back it up. EFT is rooted in attachment theory and has been studied with several mental health issues such as general relational distress (as reviewed in Wiebe & Johnson, 2016), depressive disorders (Denton, Wittenborn, & Golden, 2012; Dessaulles, Johnson, & Denton, 2003), and post-traumatic stress disorder (Dalton, Greenman, Classen, & Johnson, 2013; MacIntosh & Johnson, 2008; Weissmann et al., 2017). It also has been found effective with high-risk couples caring for a chronically ill child (Cloutier, Manion, Walker, & Johnson, 2002; Walker, Manion, Cloutier, & Johnson, 1992), reducing pain and lowering neurological threats (Johnson et al., 2013), increasing partner's empathic caregiving (McLean, Walton, Rodin, Esplen, & Jones, 2013), and improving relationship satisfaction and quality of life for couples undergoing cancer treatment (Naaman, 2008).

Lastly, integrative behavioral couple therapy (IBCT), developed Jacobson and Christensen (1998), is a couple-based treatment modality for use in mental health settings. IBCT was developed out of behavioral acceptance-based therapies and has a research base rooted primarily in examining its impact on relationship distress and satisfaction (Roddy, Nowlan, Doss, & Christensen, 2016) with a few studies demonstrating positive impact on individual mental health symptoms (e.g., Christensen et al., 2004; Christensen, Atkins, Yi, Baucom, & George, 2006). While both IBCT and EFT therapists work with couples toward increasing emotional intimacy, IBCT approaches it more from a behavioral lens versus strengthening of the attachment bonds as in EFT. Also, while both IBCT and CBCT look at the intersection of cognitive and emotional changes to help reduce relational distress. IBCT focuses primarily on change through a new pattern of couple interaction, whereas CBCT works with couples to identify and correct cognitive errors in their thinking. Recently, Veteran Affairs Medical Centers endorsed integrative behavioral couple therapy (IBCT) for nationwide training and dissemination to all its centers (Roddy et al., 2016); however, more research is needed for its effectiveness and efficacy.

Another established approach that has received attention in the literature is a family-based approach (called the Maudsley method) for adolescents with anorexia nervosa; it has demonstrated superior effects when compared to individual treatment (Lock, Le Grange, Agras, & Dare, 2001). This approach pulls from structural family therapy, strategic family therapy, Milan systems therapy, and feminist theory. A final area of family intervention is attachment-based approaches, such as attachment-based family therapy (ABFT) and emotionally focused couple therapy (EFT). ABFT demonstrated considerable remission for adolescents with depression, alongside reductions in family conflict, anxiety, and hopelessness (Diamond, Reis, Diamond, Siqueland, & Isaacs, 2002; Diamond, Russon, & Levy, 2016). More recent inquiry shows reductions in depressive symptoms and suicidal ideation for high-risk youth (Diamond et al., 2010, 2016; Israel & Diamond, 2012).

Community Approaches

Since the de-institutionalization of psychiatric hospitals, patients who would have been in an inpatient setting have instead been in the least restrictive setting, residing in their communities. Given the volume of individuals with chronic and persistent mental illness paired with the hope to decrease repeated hospitalizations, many systems employ an Assertive Community Treatment (ACT) team. ACT is an individualized way of delivering care where patients with chronic and persistent mental illness, such as schizophrenia or schizoaffective disorder, receive psychopharmacologic treatment, individual supportive therapy, mobile crisis intervention, rehabilitation, and support services for family (NAMI, 2016).

Other resources for patients and families coping with mental health concerns include nonprofit organizations and foundations. These organizations are based at both the state and national levels, providing psychoeducational classes and support groups to families navigating an array of psychiatric difficulties. NAMI, the Depression-Bipolar Support Alliance, and the American Foundation for Suicide Prevention are examples of organizations offering guidance at a national level. Locally, organizations often have family-to-family support. In this model, families who have been coping with a mental illness for a considerable time are paired with families newer to the illness journey. The mentoring family offers an empathetic ear and education on prognosis or treatment options from a patient's perspective. Through this guiding role, the giving family receives altruistic benefits of sharing their knowledge and experience. Other groups, such as Alcoholics Anonymous and 12 step groups (e.g., Emotions Anonymous, Narcotics Anonymous, Overeaters Anonymous, Sex Addicts Anonymous), provide avenues for communion for those experiencing substance use disorders or impulse control difficulties in most geographic areas.

Conclusion

Psychiatry helped to give rise to the field of family therapy, recognizing that mental illness impacts and is impacted by the family system. While we have not been able to cure illnesses such as schizophrenia and bipolar disorder, we have figured out ways that family and support system members can facilitate gains in treatment. MedFTs are strong contributors to inpatient and outpatient settings helping the psychiatric team to design treatment plans that are patient and family centered. While colleagues bring a set of diagnostic and intervention skills that are more intra-individual, the MedFT encourages the team to think about how interventions will impact and be impacted by the patient's natural context(s).

Reflection Questions
1. As a MedFT working in a psychiatric setting, how will you define and make known your scope of practice when many other professionals (e.g., psychiatrist, psychiatric nurse, psychologist, social worker) may have similar skills sets?
2. How might a person or family's personal preferences, intergenerational patterns, or cultural beliefs impact their expression of mental health concerns, engagement in care, and willingness to participate in certain treatment approaches?
3. After reviewing the therapeutic approaches to mental illness outlined in this chapter, how do treatment providers go about determining the most efficacious treatment plan? For instance, should a person with major depressive disorder and alcoholism in a tumultuous marriage receive CBT, EFT, CBCT, AA, pharmacology, another treatment approach, or some combination of approaches? How might these decisions be made in light of the literature and practice restraints?

Glossary of Important Terms for Care in Psychiatry

Atypical antipsychotic Group of psychiatric drugs, also known as second-generation antipsychotics that block receptors in the brain's dopamine pathways; they are commonly used to treat psychosis, autism, and mood disorders.

Benzodiazepine Group of psychiatric drugs, also called "benzos" that lead to sedative and anxiolytic effects; they are commonly used to treat acute anxiety while other antidepressant drugs are taking effect.

Countertransference Emotional reactions of a therapist to a patient.

Ego-dystonic Thoughts (e.g., violent, sexual, religious, impulses) that are in conflict with the person's self-image, often seen in those with OCD.

Electroconvulsive therapy (ECT) Procedure where small electrical currents pass through the brain to trigger small seizure activity en route to relief from severe mental illnesses.
Emotional regulation Inhibiting and modulating one's emotional experience.
Enabling When family or friends, in an attempt to help resolve a specific problem (e.g., distress from cravings), perpetuate or exacerbate the problem (e.g., substance abuse) due to accommodation made for harmful behaviors (e.g., providing substances or money).
Expressed emotion Interactions in the family environment that are critical, hostile, or emotionally over-involved; these are known to exacerbate psychiatric illnesses.
Family accommodation Family members take part in compulsive rituals, avoidance patterns, or modifications of routines in an attempt to assist a patient with OCD.
Forensic interviewing Structured evaluation (not treatment) used to determine facts of a case related to child maltreatment, as well as the role of an individual's mental illness in criminal or civil litigation.
Intensive Outpatient Treatment (IOP) Part-time or full-time day treatment program used for those who do not meet criteria for hospitalization but need a higher level of care than traditional outpatient care.
Involuntary commitment Legal process where an individual who is determined to have symptoms of severe psychiatric illness (e.g., pose harm to self or others, lack self-care abilities) is court-ordered to treatment in an inpatient psychiatric hospital or outpatient community treatment program.
Mood stabilizer Group of psychiatric drugs used to treat mood disorders, such as bipolar disorders and schizoaffective disorder.
Psychological testing Evaluation of psychological symptoms by objective and standardized measures, commonly used in the diagnosis of neurocognitive and neurodevelopmental disorders.
Selective serotonin reuptake inhibitor (SSRI) Group of psychiatric drugs often used as a first-line pharmacologic treatment for depressive and anxiety disorders; they work by blocking the reuptake of serotonin in the brain.
Serotonin norepinephrine reuptake inhibitor (SNRI) Group of psychiatric drugs often used as a pharmacologic treatment for depressive disorders (occasionally anxiety and nerve pain as well) that block the reuptake of serotonin and norepinephrine.
Transference Unconscious redirection of feelings and desires from one person (often from one's family of origin) to another (often one's treatment provider).
Tricyclic antidepressant Group of early antidepressant medications that work by blocking the reabsorption of neurochemicals (e.g., norepinephrine, serotonin)] in the brain; this class of medications is rarely used nowadays due to high frequencies of associated side effects.
Typical antipsychotic Group of early antipsychotic medications often replaced by newer atypical antipsychotics due to side effects that are used in the treatment of psychosis and acute mania.
Urine toxicology screen (UTOX) Test that checks for drugs or other chemicals that could contribute to the presentation of psychiatric illness.

Additional Resources

Literature

Beck, J. (2011). *Cognitive therapy: Basics and beyond* (2nd ed.). New York, NY: Guilford Press.
Dewan, M. J., Steenbarger, B. N., Greenberg, R. P. (2012). *The art and science of brief psychotherapies: An illustrated guide* (2nd ed.). Arlington, VA: American Psychiatric Publishing, Inc.
Heru, A. M., & Drury, L. M. (2007). *Working with families of psychiatric inpatients: A guide for clinicians.* Baltimore, MD: Johns Hopkins University Press.
Keiter, G. I., Heru, A. M., & Glick, I. D. (2010). *Clinical manual of couples and family therapy.* Arlington, VA: American Psychiatric Publishing, Inc.
Linehan, M. M. (2015). *DBT skills training manual.* New York, NY: Guilford Press.

Measures/Instruments

Beck Scales. https://www.beckinstitute.org/get-informed/tools-and-resources/professionals/patient-assessment-tools/
Child/Adolescent Psychiatry Screen (CAPS). http://www2.massgeneral.org/school-psychiatry/childadolescentpscychiatryscreencaps.pdf
Generalized Anxiety Disorder 7-item scale (GAD-7). http://www.integration.samhsa.gov/clinical-practice/GAD708.19.08Cartwright.pdfMulti-Health Systems, Inc., http://www.mhs.com
Patient Health Questionnaire (PHQ-9). http://www.cqaimh.org/pdf/tool_phq9.pdf
Screen for Child Anxiety Related Disorders (SCARED). http://psychiatry.pitt.edu/sites/default/files/Documents/assessments/SCARED%20Child.pdf
Yale-Brown Obsessive Compulsive Scale Symptom Checklist. http://healthnet.umassmed.edu/mhealth/YBOCSymptomChecklist.pdf

Organizations/Associations

American Academy of Child and Adolescent Psychiatry. http://www.aacap.org
Association for Behavioral and Cognitive Therapies. http://www.abct.org/Home/
Association of Family Psychiatrists. http://familypsychiatrists.org
American Psychiatric Association. https://www.psychiatry.org
Beck Institute. https://www.beckinstitute.org
National Alliance on Mental Illness. https://www.nami.org

References[1]

Abramowitz, J. S., Baucom, D. H., Wheaton, M. G., Boeding, S., Fabricant, L. E., Paprocki, C., & Fischer, M. S. (2012). Enhancing exposure and response prevention for OCD: A couple-based approach. *Behavior Modification, 37,* 1–22. https://doi.org/10.1177/0145445512444596

*American Academy of Child and Adolescent Psychiatry. (2016). *Practice parameters.* Retrieved from http://www.aacap.org/aacap/resources_for_primary_care/practice_parameters_and_resource_centers/practice_parameters.aspx

American Psychiatric Association. (2013). *Diagnostic and statistical manual of mental disorders* (5th ed.). Arlington, VA: Author.

American Psychiatric Association. (2016a). *Vision, mission, values, and goals.* Retrieved from https://www.psychiatry.org/about-apa/vision-mission-values-goals

American Psychiatric Association. (2016b). *What is psychiatry?* Retrieved from https://www.psychiatry.org/patients-families/what-is-psychiatry

*Anderson, R., Huff, N., & Hodgson, J. (2008). Medical family therapy in an inpatient psychiatric setting. A qualitative study. *Families, Systems, and Health, 26,* 164–180. https://doi.org/10.1037/1091-7527.26.2.164.

Angermeyer, M. C., Schulze, B., & Dietrich, S. (2003). Courtesy stigma: A focus group study of relatives of schizophrenia patients. *Social Psychiatry Psychiatric Epidemiology, 38,* 593–602. https://doi.org/10.1007/s00127-003-0680-x

*Baucom, D. H., Shoham, V., Mueser, K. T., Daiuto, A. D., & Stickle, T. R. (1998). Empirically supported couple and family interventions for marital distress and adult mental health problems. *Journal of Counseling and Clinical Psychology, 66,* 53–88. https://doi.org/10.1037/0022-006X.66.1.53.

Beck, A. T. (1964). Thinking and depression: II. Theory and therapy. *Archives of General Psychiatry, 10,* 561–571. https://doi.org/10.1001/archpsyc.1964.01720240015003

Beck, J. (1995). *Cognitive therapy: Basics and beyond.* New York, NY: Guilford Press.

Beck, J., Bieling, P., & Grant, V. (2012). Cognitive therapy. In M. J. Dewan, B. N. Steenbarger, and R. P. Greenberg (Eds.), *The art and science of brief psychotherapies: An illustrated guide* (pp. 45–81). Arlington, VA: American Psychiatric Association.

*Beck, J. (2011). *Cognitive therapy: Basics and beyond* (2nd ed.). New York, NY: Guilford Press.

Beels, C. C. (2002). Notes for a cultural history of family therapy. *Family Process, 41,* 67–82. https://doi.org/10.1111/j.1545-5300.2002.40102000067.x

Berman, E., & Heru, A. (2005). Family systems training in psychiatric residencies. *Family Process, 44,* 321–335. https://doi.org/10.1111/j.1545-5300.2005.00062.x

Berman, E. M., Heru, A. M., Grunebaum, H., Rolland, J., Wood, B., & Bruty, H. (2006). Family skills for general psychiatry residents: Meeting ACGME core competency requirements. Group for the Advancement of Psychiatry Committee on the Family. *Academic Psychiatry, 30,* 69–78. https://doi.org/10.1176/appi.ap.30.1.69

Bjorkland, P. (2006). No man's land: Gender bias and social constructivism in the diagnosis of borderline personality disorder. *Issues Mental Health Nursing, 27,* 3–23. https://doi.org/10.1080/01612840500312753

Brown, G. W., Carstairs, G. M., & Topping, G. (1958). Post-hospital adjustment of chronic mental patients. *Lancet, 2,* 685–689. https://doi.org/10.1016/S0140-6736(58)92279-7

Bustillo, J., Lauriello, J., Horan, W., & Keith, S. (2001). The psychosocial treatment of schizophrenia: An update. *American Journal of Psychiatry, 158,* 163–175. https://doi.org/10.1176/appi.ajp.158.2.163

Bystritsky, A. (2006). Treatment-resistant anxiety disorders. *Molecular Psychiatry, 11,* 805–814. https://doi.org/10.1038/sj.mp.4001852

---

[1] Note: References that are prefaced with an asterisk are recommended readings.

*Carr, A. (2009a). The effectiveness of family therapy and systemic interventions for child-focused problems. *Journal of Family Therapy, 31*, 3–45. https://doi.org/10.1111/j.1467-6427.2008.00451.x.

*Carr, A. (2009b). The effectiveness of family therapy and systemic interventions for adult-focused problems. *Journal of Family Therapy, 31*, 46–74. https://doi.org/10.1111/j.1467-6427.2008.00452.x.

Christensen, A., Atkins, D. C., Berns, S., Wheeler, J., Baucom, D. H., & Simpson, L. E. (2004). Traditional versus integrative behavioral couple therapy for significantly and chronically distressed married couples. *Journal of Consulting and Clinical Psychology, 72*, 176–191. https://doi.org/10.1037/0022-006X.72.2.176

Christensen, A., Atkins, D. C., Yi, J., Baucom, D. H., & George, W. H. (2006). Couple and individual adjustment for 2 years following a randomized clinical trial comparing traditional versus integrative behavioral couple therapy. *Journal of Consulting and Clinical Psychology, 74*, 1180–1191. https://doi.org/10.1037/0022-006X.74.6.1180

Cloutier, P. F., Manion, I. G., Walker, J. G., & Johnson, S. M. (2002). Emotionally focused interventions for couples with chronically ill children: A 2-year follow-up. *Journal of Marital and Family Therapy, 28*, 391–398. https://doi.org/10.1111/j.1752-0606.2002.tb00364.x

Corrigan, P., & Watson, A. (2006). The paradox of self-stigma and mental illness. *Clinical Psychology Science and Practice, 9*, 35–53. https://doi.org/10.1093/clipsy.9.1.35

Cuijpers, P., van Straten, A., Andersson, G., & van Oppen, P. (2008). Psychotherapy for depression in adults: A meta-analysis of comparative outcome studies. *Journal of Consulting and Clinical Psychology, 76*, 909–922. https://doi.org/10.1037/a0013075

Dalton, E. J., Greenman, P. S., Classen, C. C., & Johnson, S. M. (2013). Nurturing connections in the aftermath of childhood trauma: A randomized controlled trial of emotionally focused couple therapy for female survivors of childhood abuse. *Couple and Family Psychology: Research and Practice, 2*, 209–221. https://doi.org/10.1037/a0032772

Denton, W. H., Wittenborn, A. K., & Golden, R. N. (2012). Augmenting antidepressant medication treatment of depressed women with emotionally focused therapy for couples: A randomized pilot study. *Journal of Marital and Family Therapy, 38*, 23–38. https://doi.org/10.1111/j.1752-0606.2012.00291.x

Dessaulles, A., Johnson, S. M., & Denton, W. H. (2003). Emotion-focused therapy for couples in the treatment of depression: A pilot study. *American Journal of Family Therapy, 31*, 345-353. https://doi.org/10.1080/01926180390232266

*Dewan, M. J., Steenbarger, B. N., & Greenberg, R. P. (2012). *The art and science of brief psychotherapies: An illustrated guide* (2nd ed.). Arlington, VA: American Psychiatric Publishing.

*Diamond, G., & Josephson, A. (2005). Family-based treatment research: A 10-year update. *Journal of the American Academy of Child and Adolescent Psychiatry, 44*, 872–887. https://doi.org/10.1097/01.chi.0000169010.96783.4e.

Diamond, G. S., Reis, B. F., Diamond, G. M., Siqueland, L., & Isaacs, L. (2002). Attachment-based family therapy for depressed adolescents: A treatment development study. *Journal of the American Academy of Child & Adolescent Psychiatry, 41*, 1190–1196. https://doi.org/10.1097/00004583-200210000-00008

Diamond, G. S., Russon, J., & Levy, S. (2016). Attachment-based family therapy: A review of the empirical support. *Family Process, 55*, 595–610. https://doi.org/10.1111/famp.12241

Diamond, G. S., Wintersteen, M. B., Brown, G. K., Diamond, G. M., Gallop, R., Shelef, K., & Levy, S. A. (2010). Attachment based family therapy for suicidal adolescents: A randomized controlled trial. *Journal of the American Academy of Child and Adolescent Psychiatry, 49*, 122–131. https://doi.org/10.1016/j.jaac.2009.11.002

Engel, G. L. (1977). The need for a new medical model: A challenge for biomedicine. *Science, 196*, 129–136. https://doi.org/10.1126/science.847460

Engel, G. L. (1980). The clinical application of the biopsychosocial model. *American Journal of Psychiatry, 137*, 535–544. https://doi.org/10.1176/ajp.137.5.535

Falloon, I. R. H. (2003). Family interventions for mental disorders: Efficacy and effectiveness. *World Psychiatry, 2*, 20–28. https://www.ncbi.nlm.nih.gov/pmc/articles/PMC1525058/pdf/wpa020020.pdf

*Fischer, M. S., Baucom, D. H., & Cohen, M. J. (2016). Cognitive-behavioral couple therapies: Review of the evidence for the treatment of relationship distress, psychopathology, and chronic health conditions. *Family Process, 55*(3): 423–442. https://doi.org/10.1111/famp.12227.

Fischer, D., & Moyers, T. B. (2012). Motivational interviewing as a brief psychotherapy. In M. J. Dewan, B. N. Steenbarger, and R. P. Greenberg (Eds.), *The art and science of brief psychotherapies: An illustrated guide* (pp. 27–41). Arlington, VA: American Psychiatric Association.

Fromm-Reichmann, F. (1948). Notes on the development of treatment of schizophrenics by psychoanalytic psychotherapy. *Psychiatry, 11*, 267–277. https://doi.org/10.1080/00332747.1948.11022688

Gillihan, S., Hembree, E., & Foa, E. (2012). Behavior therapy. In M. J. Dewan, B. N. Steenbarger, and R. P. Greenberg (Eds.), *The art and science of brief psychotherapies: An illustrated guide* (pp. 83–120). Arlington, VA: American Psychiatric Association.

Heru, A. (2004). Basic family skills for an inpatient psychiatrist: Meeting accreditation council for graduate medical education core competency requirements. *Families, Systems, & Health, 22*, 216–227. https://doi.org/10.1037/1091-7527.22.2.216

Heru, A., & Drury, L. (2006). Overcoming barriers in working with families. *Academic Psychiatry, 30*, 379–384. https://doi.org/10.1176/appi.ap.30.5.379

*Heru, A. M., & Drury, L. M. (2007). *Working with families of psychiatric inpatients: A guide for clinicians*. Baltimore, MD: Johns Hopkins University Press.

Hodgson, J., Lamson, A., Mendenhall, T., & Tyndall, L. (2014). Introduction to medical family therapy: Advanced applications. In J. Hodgson, A. Lamson, T. Mendenhall, and D. Crane (Eds.), *Medical family therapy: Advanced applications* (pp. 1–9). New York, NY: Springer.

Hofmann, S. G., Asnaani, A., Vonk, I. J. J., Sawyer, A. T., & Fang, A. (2012). The efficacy of cognitive behavioral therapy: A review of meta-analyses. *Cognitive Therapy Research, 36*, 427–440. https://doi.org/10.1007/s10608-012-9476-1

Israel, P., & Diamond, G. S. (2012). Feasibility of attachment based family therapy for depressed clinic referred Norwegian adolescents. *Clinical Child Psychology and Psychiatry, 18*, 334–350. https://doi.org/10.1177/1359104512455811

Jacobson, N. S., & Christensen, A. (1998). *Acceptance and change in couple therapy: A therapist's guide to transforming relationships*. New York, NY: Norton.

Johnson, S. M. (2004). *The practice of emotionally focused couple therapy: Creating connection* (2nd ed.). New York, NY: Brunner-Routledge.

Johnson, S. M., Burgess Moser, M., Beckes, L., Smith, A., Dalgleish, T., Halchuk, R., … Coan, J. A. (2013). Soothing the threatened brain: Leveraging contact comfort with emotionally focused therapy. *Public Library of Science One, 8*, 1–11. https://doi.org/10.1371/journal.pone.0079314

*Keiter, G. I., Heru, A. M., & Glick, I. D. (2010). *Clinical manual of couples and family therapy*. Arlington, VA: American Psychiatric Publishing.

Keitner, G. I., & Mansfield, A. K. (2012). Management of treatment-resistant depression. *Psychiatric Clinics North America, 35*, 249–265. https://doi.org/10.1016/j.psc.2011.11.004

Law, D., & Crane, D. R. (2000). The influence of marital and family interventions on professional health care services in a health maintenance organization. *Journal of Marital and Family Therapy, 26*, 281–291. https://doi.org/10.1111/j.1752-0606.2000.tb00298.x

Leichsenring, F., Rabung, S., & Leibing, E. (2004). The efficacy of short-term psychodynamic psychotherapy in specific psychiatric disorders: A meta-analysis. *Archives of General Psychiatry, 61*, 1208–1216. https://doi.org/10.1001/archpsyc.61.12.1208

Leichsenring, F., & Rabung, S. (2008). Effectiveness of long-term psychodynamic psychotherapy: A meta-analysis. *Journal of the American Medical Association, 300*, 1551–1565. https://doi.org/10.1001/jama.300.13.1551

Levenson, H. (2012). Time-limited dynamic psychotherapy: An integrative perspective. In M. J. Dewan, B. N. Steenbarger, and R. P. Greenberg (Eds.), *The art and science of brief psychotherapies: An illustrated guide* (pp. 195–237). Arlington, VA: American Psychiatric Association.

Linehan, M. M. (1993). *Cognitive-behavioral treatment of borderline personality disorder.* New York, NY: Guilford Press.

*Linehan, M. M. (2015). *DBT skills training manual* (2nd ed.). New York, NY: Guilford Press.

Lock, J., Le Grange, D., Agras, W. S., & Dare, C. (2001). *Treatment manual for anorexia nervosa: A family-based approach.* New York, NY: Guilford Press.

MacIntosh, H. B., & Johnson, S. (2008). Emotionally focused therapy for couples and childhood sexual abuse survivors. *Journal of Marital and Family Therapy, 34*, 298–315. https://doi.org/10.1111/j.1752-0606.2008.00074.x

Marneros, A. (2008). Psychiatry's 200th birthday. *British Journal of Psychiatry, 193*, 1–3. https://doi.org/10.1192/bjp.bp.108.051367

McLean, L. M., Walton, T., Rodin, G., Esplen, M. J., & Jones, J. M. (2013). A couple-based intervention for patients and caregivers facing end-stage cancer: Outcomes of a randomized controlled trial. *Psycho-Oncology, 22*, 28–38. https://doi.org/10.1002/pon.2046

Miller, A., McEvoy, J., Jeste, D., et al. (2006). Treatment of chronic schizophrenia. In J. Lieberman, T. S. Stroup, and D. Perkins (Eds.), *Textbook of schizophrenia* (pp. 365–381). Washington, DC: American Psychiatric Publishing.

Miller, W. R., & Rose, G. S. (2009). Toward a theory of motivational interviewing. *American Psychologist, 65*, 527–537. https://doi.org/10.1037/a0016830

Naaman, S. C. (2008). Evaluation of the clinical efficacy of emotionally focused couples. *Therapy on psychological adjustment and natural killer cell cytotoxicity in early breast cancer* (Doctoral Dissertation). University of Ottawa, Ottawa, ON.

National Alliance on Mental Illness (NAMI). (2016). *Mental health fact sheets.* Retrieved from https://www.nami.org/akaresources/factsheets

O'Hara, M. W., Stuart, S., Gorman, L., & Wenzel, A. (2000). Efficacy of interpersonal psychotherapy for postpartum depression. *Archives of General Psychiatry, 57*, 1039–1045. https://doi.org/10.1001/archpsyc.57.11.1039

O'Leary, E. M., Barrett, P., & Fjermestad, K. W. (2009). Cognitive-behavioral family treatment for childhood obsessive-compulsive disorder: A 7-year follow-up study. *Journal of Anxiety Disorders, 23*, 973–978. https://doi.org/10.1016/j.janxdis.2009.06.009

Papakostas, G. I., & Fava, M. (2010). *Pharmacotherapy for depression and treatment-resistant depression.* Hackensack, NJ: World Scientific.

Parker, G., & Hadzi-Pavlovic, D. (1990). Expressed emotion as a predictor of schizophrenic relapse: An analysis of aggregated data. *Psychological Medicine, 20*, 961–965. https://doi.org/10.1017/S0033291700036655

Roddy, M. K., Nowlan, K. M., Doss, B. D., & Christensen, A. (2016). Integrative behavioral couple therapy: Theoretical background, empirical research, and dissemination. *Family Process, 55*, 408–422. https://doi.org/10.1111/famp.12223

Sexton, T., Gordon, K. C., Gurman, A., Lebow, J., Holtzworth-Munroe, A., & Johnson, S. (2011). Guidelines for classifying Evidence-Based treatments in couple and family therapy. *Family Process, 50*, 377–392. https://doi.org/10.1111/j.1545-5300.2011.01363.x

Silverman, J. J., Fochtmann, L. J., Rhoads, R. S., Yager, J., Vergare, M. J., Anzia, D. J., et al. (2016). *The American Psychiatric Association practice guidelines for the psychiatric evaluation of adults* (3rd ed.). Arlington, VA: American Psychiatric Association.

Singer, M., & Wynne, L. (1963). Differentiating characteristics of parents of childhood schizophrenics, childhood neurotics, and young adult schizophrenics. *American Journal of Psychiatry, 120*, 234–243. https://doi.org/10.1176/ajp.120.3.234

Smith, M. E., Lindsey, M. A., Williams, C. D., Medoff, D. R., Lucksted, A., Fang, L. J., … Dixon, L. B. (2014). Race-related differences in the experiences of family members of persons with mental illness participating in the NAMI Family to Family Education Program. *American Journal of Community Psychology, 54*, 316–327. https://doi.org/10.1007/s10464-014-9674-y

Steenbarger, B. N., Greenberg, R. P., & Dewan, M. J. (2012). Introduction. In M. J. Dewan, B. N. Steenbarger, and R. P. Greenberg (Eds.), *The art and science of brief psychotherapies: An illustrated guide* (pp. 1–12). Arlington, VA: American Psychiatric Association.

Stein, M. B., Seedat, S., & Gelernter, J. (2006). Serotonin transporter gene promoter polymorphism predicts SSRI response in generalized social anxiety disorder. *Psychopharmacology, 187*, 68–72. https://doi.org/10.1007/s00213-006-0349-8

Strauss, C., Hale, L., & Stobie, B. (2015). A meta-analytic review of the relationship between family accommodation and OCD symptom severity. *Journal of Anxiety Disorders, 33*, 95–102. https://doi.org/10.1016/j.janxdis.2015.05.006

Stuart, S. (2012). Interpersonal psychotherapy. In M. J. Dewan, B. N. Steenbarger, and R. P. Greenberg (Eds.), *The art and science of brief psychotherapies: An illustrated guide* (pp. 157–193). Arlington, VA: American Psychiatric Association.

Thornicroft, G., Mehta, N., Clement, S., Evans-Lacko, S., Doherty, M., Rose, D., ... Henderson, C. (2016). Evidence for effective interventions to reduce mental-health-related stigma and discrimination. The health crisis of mental health stigma. *Lancet, 387*, 1123–1132. https://doi.org/10.1016/S0140-6736(15)00298-6

Vaughn, C. E., & Leff, J. P. (1976). The measurement of expressed emotion in the families of psychiatric patients. *British Journal of Social and Clinical Psychology, 129*, 125–137. https://doi.org/10.1111/j.2044-8260.1976.tb00021.x

Walker, J. G., Manion, I. G., Cloutier, P. F., & Johnson, S. M. (1992). Measuring marital distress in couples with chronically ill children: The dyadic adjustment scale. *Journal of Pediatric Psychology, 17*, 345–357. https://doi.org/10.1093/jpepsy/17.3.345

Weakland, J. (1960). The "double bind" hypothesis of schizophrenia and three-party interaction. In D. Jackson (Ed.), *The etiology of schizophrenia*. New York, NY: Basic Books.

Weissmann, N., Batten, S.V., Rheem, K.D., Wiebe, S.A., Pasillas, R.M., Potts, W., et al. (2017). The effectiveness of emotionally focused couples therapy with veterans with PTSD: A pilot study. *Journal of Couple and Relationship Therapy* (advance online publication). https://doi.org/10.1080/15332691.2017.1285261

Wiebe, S. A., & Johnson, S. M. (2016). A review of the research in emotionally focused therapy for couples. *Family Process, 55*, 1–18. https://doi.org/10.1111/famp.12229

Woods, D. W., Piacentini, J. C., Chang, S. W., Deckersbach, T., Ginsburg, G. S., Peterson, A. L., ... Wilhelm, S. (2008). *Managing Tourette Syndrome: Behavioral intervention for children and adults, therapist guide*. New York, NY: Oxford University Press.

Wright, L., Watson, W., & Bell, J. (1996). *Beliefs: The heart of healing in families and illness*. New York, NY: Basic Books.

Yan, L. J., Hammen, C., Cohen, A. M., Daley, S. E., & Henry, R. M. (2004). Expressed emotion versus relationship quality variables in the prediction of recurrence in bipolar patients. *Journal of Affective Disorders, 83*, 199–206. https://doi.org/10.1016/j.jad.2004.08.006

Part III
Medical Family Therapy in Tertiary Care

Chapter 10
Medical Family Therapy in Palliative and Hospice Care

Jackie Williams-Reade and Stephanie Trudeau

Contemporary advancements in health care and medical technology are allowing patients to live longer now than they ever have before. We are seeing these trends in longer life across all age groups—from increased survival during childhood from illnesses that were heretofore rapidly fatal to combating normative age-related declines (and thereby prolonging senescence) in the elderly. With these trends come marked increases in the likelihood of being diagnosed with a serious or terminal illness during one's lifetime (Centers for Disease Control and Prevention [CDC], 2011). Such illnesses and their unique health trajectories are generally treated under the medical specialties of Palliative and Hospice Care (CDC, 2010; Meier, 2011). Providers engaged in these treatment teams must attend to patients' physical functioning within a context where getting better is not presumed. Treatment teams must thereby attend to foci like quality of life, emotional suffering, loss, meaning making, and spirituality as part of everyday practice.

Medical Family Therapists (MedFTs) are well-equipped to engage in Palliative and Hospice Care teams by nature of the systemic orientations they bring in connecting biopsychosocial-spiritual (BPSS) facets of patients' and families' lives (Engel, 1977, 1980; Wright, Watson, & Bell, 1996). In this chapter, the authors describe key characteristics that distinguish and define work in Palliative and Hospice Care environments. We frame practical skills needed in these domains using Hodgson, Lamson, Mendenhall, and Tyndall's (2014) MedFT Healthcare Continuum and present research-informed recommendations for behavioral healthcare with patients, families, and other care providers situated in these interdisciplinary teams.

J. Williams-Reade (✉)
School of Behavioral Health, Loma Linda University, Loma Linda, CA, USA
e-mail: jwilliamsreade@llu.edu

S. Trudeau
Department of Family Social Science, University of Minnesota, Saint Paul, MN, USA

Clinical Vignette
[Note: This vignette is a compilation of cases that represent treatment in Palliative and Hospice Care. All patients' names and/or identifying information have been changed to maintain confidentiality.]

Megan is a 52-year-old woman who recently discovered a lump in her breast while on vacation with her husband, Joe. She was diagnosed with invasive stage 2C breast cancer, but it was still operable. A treatment plan was developed after advisement from her oncologist and medical team—which was comprised of surgeons, pathologists, radiation oncologists, plastic surgeons, oncology nurses, nurse breast care coordinators, medical social workers, a psychiatrist, and behavioral health clinician (MedFT). At this point, she also met with a Palliative Care consultant who talked to Megan to clarify the prognosis, goals of treatment, expectations, and preferred ways to maintain her quality of life. Megan underwent surgery for a double mastectomy and then began radiation. The second phase of her treatment included 12 rounds of chemotherapy and hormone therapy.

Both Megan and Joe were professionals in their careers. Megan ran a successful consulting firm, and Joe was an entrepreneur who had recently sold his business and was now investing in start-ups. Their daughter, Sophie, was a sophomore in college; she was living out of the state. Megan took a leave of absence from her firm with an unknown return date. Joe continued his investments and even began taking on more patients. Sophie continued at college with plans to come home during the summer break.

As time went on, the impact of treatment manifested in both physical and emotional exhaustion; the family began to meet regularly with the MedFT. Megan discussed feeling ashamed for not keeping up the appearance as the "fighter" that her husband, daughter, and family had come to expect. Sessions with the MedFT first involved only Megan but later included Joe. Individual and couple coping mechanisms were discussed, along with communication strategies for enhancing the couple's intimacy and ways to talk about Megan's illness with others included in Megan's social worlds.

Despite the aggressive treatments Megan underwent, her 6-month scan revealed metastasis to multiple organs. It was recommended that treatment be discontinued and that she begin seeing a Palliative Care team to address symptoms related to quality of life. Megan was furious and scared. She lacked the ability to communicate her emotions at the time and thereby placed blame on the healthcare system, its limits in scientific knowledge, and herself. Joe refused to take this as an option and began another passionate project—specifically, "shopping around" for different oncologists and treatment modalities (including homeopathic remedies).

Months later, the oncologist and Palliative Care consultant met with Megan and Joe to communicate that she likely had less than 6 months to live. The healthcare team met with the whole family to discuss Megan's prefer-

ences and allow for discussion around fears related to loss and the dying process. Family members assisting in care talked through strategies and created schedules to facilitate ease of transition from hospital-based Palliative Care to home-based Hospice Care. Visitation by family and friends, caregiver respite, and communication about Megan's progress and transitions via Caring Bridge were among the strategies discussed.

After the family meeting, Megan began her transition into Hospice Care. She is now in her home, receiving services from a community Hospice organization. Megan receives small doses of chemotherapy and increasing doses of pain medication to help alleviate the discomfort caused by spreading tumors.

The complex coordination needs of Megan's healthcare system engaged the MedFT to track the family throughout the process. Through meetings with Megan and her family at their home, the MedFT facilitated conversations to help them process existential beliefs and meaning making concerning illness and death. The family appreciates these additional psychosocial and spiritual services, framing them as helpful in preparing for Megan's impending death.

This case illustrates potential ways that a MedFT can function in Palliative and Hospice Care settings. Instead of working with a patient until his or her acute illness-related crisis has diminished, our work is more about accompanying patients during their suffering, helping them speak frankly with their healthcare team and loved ones, and helping to create and keep a web of supportive relationships that are meaningful. Managing life-threatening or life-limiting illnesses requires attention to issues of meaning making and the myriad of current and potential future losses that can be experienced with them. The MedFT's role can be to bring deeper insights and understandings to these complex psychosocial issues.

What Are Palliative and Hospice Care?

Palliative and Hospice Care have experienced significant growth and expansion in the United States over the past several years (Dumanovsky et al., 2015). Many opportunities thereby exist for the inclusion of MedFTs in contributing to and achieving the goals of these teams. Their involvement is particularly critical through attention and intervention on the larger psychosocial and spiritual issues experienced by patients, families, and healthcare teams (Babcock & Robinson, 2011). Because many illnesses in Palliative and Hospice Care are rare or complex, they are accompanied with a high level of uncertainty regarding their future trajectory(ies). This can cause additional stress and strain on relationships between patients, family members, and healthcare team members (Karlsson, Friberg, Wallengren, & Öhlén, 2014; Lobb et al., 2013; Oishi & Murtagh, 2014; Zambroski, 2006).

There is often misunderstanding among health professionals, patients, and family members about the definitions and goals of Palliative and Hospice Care and their relationship(s) to one another (Brickner, Scannell, Marquet, & Ackerson, 2004; Center to Advance Palliative Care [CAPC], 2011; Hanratty et al., 2006; Jones, 2006). While in other countries the terms Palliative and Hospice are typically synonymous, in the United States they are considered two distinct care services.

Palliative Care is a specialized type of medical care with the overall goal to reduce suffering and maintain or improve quality of life for both the patient and family. Oftentimes, it is offered alongside curative treatment and can be provided at any point along the illness trajectory of a serious illness, including those that are curable, chronic, or life-threatening (National Consensus Project for Quality Palliative Care, 2013). Palliative Care has been shown to increase quality of life (Armstrong, Jenigir, Hutson, Wachs, & Lambe, 2013; El-Jawahri, Greer, & Temel, 2012; Laguna et al., 2012; Sidebottom, Jorgenson, Richards, Kirven, & Sillah, 2015) and is increasingly being utilized earlier in the illness trajectory to help alleviate symptoms for patients diagnosed with chronic, progressive conditions such as pulmonary disorders, chronic heart failure, renal disease, and progressive neurological conditions (Curtis, 2008; Selecky et al., 2005; Selman, Beynon, Higginson, & Harding, 2007). *Hospice Care* refers to a philosophy of care that includes the alleviation of symptoms and enhancement of quality of life for patients whose life expectancy is less than 6 months and/or for those who have chosen to stop or are no longer benefitting from curative treatment (Center for Medicare & Medicaid Service, 2013). Eligibility for Hospice Care typically includes a cessation of curative treatment for a terminal illness with a continuation of treatments that enhance quality of life or treat symptoms.

To further understand the uniqueness of Palliative and Hospice Care, it is helpful to contrast them to our current model of *curative care*, which includes active treatment of disease in order to extend one's life-span (Kaur & Mohanti, 2011). Unlike Palliative or Hospice Care, curative care does not prioritize symptoms such as pain and suffering as much as it focuses on recovery from disease. Both Palliative and Hospice Care emphasize alleviating suffering and improving quality of life. Palliative Care focuses on the simultaneous acts of curing (active treatment) *and* maintaining the quality of life for those patients who have serious illness, while Hospice Care provides pain and symptom management in order to ensure patient comfort when a patient receives a terminal diagnosis, and cure is not possible. Additional similarities and differences between curative, Palliative, and Hospice Care can be found in Figure 10.1.

Treatment Teams in Palliative and Hospice Care

Both Palliative and Hospice Care include interdisciplinary, team-oriented approaches that attend to healthcare, pain and symptom management, patient and family goals, emotional and spiritual needs, and overall quality of life. The composition of

	Curative Care	Palliative Care	Hospice Care
Recipients of Care	Anyone with an acute, chronic, or serious illness	Anyone with a serious illness regardless of life expectancy	Anyone with an illness with a life expectancy of 6 months or less
Goals of Care	Cure the illness	Improve the quality of life while living with a serious illness	Improve the quality of life at the end-of-life
Treatments	Active treatment of the disease (e.g., surgery, treatments)	Pain and symptom management to reduce suffering alongside curative care	Pain and symptom management to reduce suffering
Locations	Hospitals, clinics	Hospitals, clinics, long-term care facilities, Hospice sites	Homes, long-term care facilities, hospitals
Treatment Teams	Typically includes physicians, nurses, behavioral health/mental health, and other health professionals based on the individual needs of each patient	Typically includes physician, nurses, behavioral health/mental health, chaplains, and other health professionals based on the individual needs of each patient	Typically includes physicians, nurses, behavioral health/mental health, chaplains, home health aides, volunteers, and other health professionals

Figure 10.1 Similarities and Differences between Curative, Palliative, and Hospice Care

Palliative and Hospice Care may extend from home-based outpatient to inpatient care in a large medical center that treats a wide variety of illnesses or conditions. In terms of delivery structure, Palliative Care is typically a team-based consultation service that may be comprised of a number of disciplines and offered across hospitals, outpatient medical clinics, and long-term care facilities (Campion, Kelley, & Morrison, 2015; Dumanovsky et al., 2015). Hospice is a more structured, organized care delivery system and is provided in hospitals, long-term care facilities, and patients' homes. Palliative Care team composition may vary in size and disciplines; Hospice teams are regulated to include physicians, nurses, behavioral health, chaplains, home health aides, and trained volunteers.

The current Palliative and Hospice Care workforce is inadequate due to lack of expertise and the growing population of those with serious illness (Hughes & Smith, 2014; Lupu, 2010). While many of the healthcare competencies required by Palliative or Hospice specialists are the same as those required by a general practitioner (e.g., assessing and managing physical and psychosocial symptoms, strong communication skills, and assistance with patient and family decision-making), some healthcare team members are able to receive additional training and credentialing in Palliative and Hospice specialties. Currently, additional credentialing is available for physicians, nurses, chaplains, and social workers.

Palliative and Hospice Care teams include a variety of professional disciplines (e.g., chaplains, child life specialists, pharmacists, physical and occupational therapists, and behavioral health/mental health specialists), alongside family caregivers and volunteers (who provide personalized support and caregiving). Complexities in billing and reimbursement for services, involving multiple professionals, disease-specific specialties, and multiple care provision sites, require that teams also include billing specialists, care coordinators, and a variety of other administrators (Claxton-Oldfield, 2015; Patterson, Peek, Heinrich, Bischoff, & Scherger, 2002; Peek & Heinrich, 2000). The following list describes typical roles of these care teams' most visible personnel:

Palliative/Hospice physician/medical directors. This director is someone with training in Palliative/Hospice Care and another area of specialty such as oncology or pediatrics. They provide medical directives into the management of patient symptoms and may have additional skills in communication and bioethics.

Personal physicians. It is common for the team to include the patient's physician who has cared for his or her underlying medical condition. This may include an oncologist, neurologist, primary care physician (PCP), or others.

Nurses. Nurses in Palliative and Hospice Care participate in administering medications, monitoring vital signs, and attending to activities of daily living (ADLs). They help guide families through the illness process, including hospitalizations, home care, and end-of-life care. Hospice and Palliative Care nurses are typically registered nurses.

Behavioral health providers (BHPs). The BHP is the behavioral health/mental health provider who helps to assess, diagnose, treat, and connect appropriate referrals specific to psychosocial, financial, discharge planning, and end-of-life psychosocial needs. Helping patients complete advance directives, educating about the psychosocial impact of illness and caregiving, and providing community resources are a few typical tasks.

Chaplains. The chaplain is a staff member who is trained in specific and general pastoral services and assists with spiritual and emotional needs of patients, families, and staff members. He or she helps support patients and families through connections in their religious or spiritual beliefs as they move through the course of the illness.

Child life specialists. Child life specialists provide support to the child, his or her siblings, and other family members while helping them understand a child's illness and the various treatments he or she need to undergo. They will also work with children who are directly involved with adults who are receiving Palliative or Hospice Care to help them understand on a developmentally appropriate level the treatments their family member may receive and the biopsychosocial changes they may be experiencing. Play, dialogue, art, music writing exercises, and other approaches are used to facilitate understanding.

Home health aides (Hospice). Hospice home health aides are trained to provide personal care to patients in their homes and can be hired privately or are offered through a home health or Hospice organization. They provide support in the following areas: nutrition, physical exercise and stretching, care for incontinence, bathing, grooming, oral hygiene, and communication with family and other medical staff. The home health aide offers education on patient care to family members/support persons so that they will feel comfortable providing day-to-day care to the patient.

Trained volunteers (Hospice). Hospice volunteers are commonly trained and provided by Hospice programs to extend support such as running errands, preparing meals, providing respite to the family members, and providing emotional support and companionship to patients and family members.

Complementary and alternative treatments. In various care settings, alternative treatment modalities such as acupuncture, chiropractic, imagery, hypnosis, and Reiki are being integrated alongside traditional biomedical treatments (Bardia, Barton, Prokop, Bauer, & Moynihan, 2006). In addition, animal-assisted therapy is sometimes used as a complementary intervention (Engelman, 2013).

Fundamentals of Palliative and Hospice Care

Fundamentals of Palliative and Hospice Care that a MedFT should know will differ depending on illness type, care team composition, service delivery format, and location of care. General considerations that supersede these specifics are detailed below:

Common Illnesses in Palliative and Hospice Care

Because Palliative and Hospice Care cover an array of conditions and illnesses, it is imperative that a MedFT understand the overarching typologies of various illnesses and their respective trajectories (Murray, Kendall, Boyd, & Sheikh, 2005; Rolland, 1994). Some of the most common diseases managed with Palliative Care are cancer, congestive heart failure, chronic obstructive pulmonary disease (COPD), Alzheimer's, Parkinson's, amyotrophic lateral sclerosis (ALS), and multiple sclerosis (MS). If an individual with any of these illnesses reaches a point in their progression at which they are determined to have 6 months or less to live, they will be transitioned to Hospice Care. About 60% of Hospice utilization is from individuals who are diagnosed with cancer, but increasingly more diseases are being included to include many that are seen in Palliative Care including stroke, coma, and kidney and liver diseases (Obermeyer et al., 2014).

Medications Used in Palliative and Hospice Care

While diagnoses in Palliative and Hospice Care can vary, being familiar with medications for common symptoms is helpful as many of the conversations among patients, family members, and medical team members are situated around the addition, discontinuation, or dosing of medications. Because of the focus on alleviation of suffering, treatment teams in both Palliative and Hospice Care work toward improving quality of life and easing painful symptoms of illness and treatment such as pain, fatigue, shortness of breath, nausea, loss of appetite, constipation, delirium, dehydration, difficulty sleeping, and malnutrition (Wilkie & Ezenwa, 2012). Becoming acquainted with the common medications used to treat these symptoms and illness-specific symptoms is best practice for MedFTs. A useful beginning resource is the World Health Organization's (WHO) *Essential Medicines in Palliative Care* (2013).

Psychosocial Care

Patients and family members in Palliative and Hospice Care face an increased emotional adjustment to the various symptoms, diagnoses, medications, treatments, uncertain prognoses, reactions of others, etc. To address these significant psychological impacts, the National Consensus Project for Quality Palliative Care (2013) recommends specific criteria for appropriate psychosocial care (see Figure 10.2), and meeting these quality care standards is an essential role of being a MedFT.

- Mental health professionals with specific skills and training in working with patients and families with serious illnesses
- Assessing for psychological needs
- Treating psychiatric diagnoses
- Promoting adjustment to the condition or illness
- Using validated and context-specific assessment tools to provide regular, ongoing assessments of psychosocial reactions to the illness
- Providing patient and family/support person education about the disease or condition and decision making and coping strategies
- Providing treatment of psychiatric diagnoses whether as a consequence of the illness or as a comorbid condition
- Family/support person education
- Regular assessment of treatment efficacy and patient-family preferences
- Appropriate referrals
- Grief and bereavement support

Figure 10.2 Criteria for Appropriate Psychosocial Care

Meaning making. Receiving a life-threatening diagnosis often causes an individual to reflect on the meaning of life and can bring up spiritual, religious, or existential questions (Chochinov et al., 2007; Grant et al., 2004; Harstäde, Andershed, Roxberg, & Brunt, 2013; Seibaek, Lise, & Niels, 2013). As patients and families face these challenges, they work to create personal meanings to help make sense of what is happening (Wright, 2009). These meanings are unique as they reflect each individual's own personal characteristics, experiences, social context, and cultural influences and inform how a patient and family will respond to the illness. To help alleviate patient suffering in this domain, issues of meaning and spirituality are an important consideration and need to be addressed by the entire healthcare team (Gordon & Mitchell, 2004; Richardson, 2014). MedFTs can participate in helping address these issues by conducting spiritual assessments and guiding conversations regarding these issues. Common assessments that can be used include the interview tool called FICA (*F*aith, *I*mportance/Influence of beliefs, *C*ommunity involvement, and *A*ddressing issues in providing care; Puchalski, 2006). Another is a standardized self-assessment called FACIT-Sp (*F*unctional *A*ssessment of *C*hronic *I*llness *T*herapy-Spiritual Well-Being; Peterman, Fitchett, Brady, Hernandez, & Cella, 2002) that focuses on meaning and faith. The SBI-15R (*S*ystems of *B*elief *I*nventory; Holland et al., 1998) attends to beliefs, practices, and support. Conducting an appropriate assessment, making connections and collaborating with chaplains and other community spiritual advisors, and providing continuing supportive efforts in this realm are recommended as part of a comprehensive care plan (National Quality Forum, 2006; Sulmasy, 2002).

Grief and bereavement. Grief and bereavement are primary themes in Palliative and Hospice Care; these must be attended to with both patients and surviving family members throughout an illness's course (Guldin, Vedsted, Zachariae, Olesen, & Jensen, 2011; Grassi, 2007; Milberg, Olsson, Jakobsson, Olsson, & Friedrichsen, 2008). Sadness from the myriad of losses is important to normalize as patients and family members may begin experiencing symptoms of anticipatory grieving at any point in the illness trajectory (D'Antonio 2014; Simon 2008). While in Palliative Care, death may not be imminent, anticipatory grief (Evans, 1994; Shore, Gelber, Koch, & Sower, 2016) is commonly experienced by both patients and family members as there are many losses that are deserving of grieving along the way. From the loss of a planned future to the day-to-day feelings of loss regarding changes in family structure or functioning, patients and family members may not be sure when it is appropriate to feel sadness. Providing psychoeducation regarding what emotional responses to expect, and normalizing these, can be helpful for both the patient and family members. As patients move closer to death, they may feel increased sadness, withdraw emotionally, and lose interest in connecting with loved ones or medical professionals. It is important to assess and differentiate between these types of behaviors in terms of typical responses and/or those suggesting clinical depression (Irwin et al., 2008; Rayner, Loge, Wasteson, & Higgson, 2009).

When death occurs, it can affect the psychological and physical well-being of loved ones for the duration of their lives (Hudson et al., 2012; Trudeau-Hern & Daneshpour, 2012). The *National Consensus Project for Quality Palliative Care, Third Edition* (2013) provides special considerations for grief and bereavement care. These include appropriate education and skill in this area; ongoing assessment regarding loss and grief in patients and families; initial and developmentally appropriate assessment to identify patients at risk for complicated grief, bereavement, and comorbid complications; intensive support and prompt referrals to appropriate professionals; follow-up bereavement support for a minimum of 12 months after the death of the patient; and culturally appropriate information and support that are sensitive to patient and family preferences. Focusing on end-of-life tensions, conflicts, and forgiveness of past neglects are important areas of family work throughout the illness process, death, and beyond (Kissane & Bloch, 2002).

The Dying Process

Beyond assisting patients and families in the psychosocial-spiritual aspects of the dying process, another fundamental of Palliative and Hospice Care concerns the biological process of dying (Persson, Ostlund, Wennman-Larsen, Wengstrom, & Gustavsson, 2008). And while not all Palliative Care patients are facing imminent death (like those in Hospice Care), their illnesses are serious enough that early death carries a potential likelihood. As a MedFT, it is helpful to have knowledge and experience in the process of dying as there are opportunities to assist patients, family members, and healthcare team members in the alleviation of emotional and psychosocial suffering related to it. Having witnessed the death of a seriously ill individual firsthand may provide perspective and understanding that can aid in helping the patient and family member's experience of death (Aoun, Currow, Hudson, Kristjanson, & Rosenberg, 2005; Hebert, Prigerson, Schulz, & Arnold, 2006; Kwak, Salmon, Acquaviva, Brandt, & Egan, 2007). Volunteering in Palliative or Hospice Care settings can also provide exposure to issues of death and dying, which can help in confronting personal biases, challenging previous experiences, and providing further insight into beliefs about death that are important to be aware of prior to entering these settings. By gaining exposure to these care environments, the MedFT can better learn to provide support in ways that can be both personally and professionally challenging (but also essential).

It is important for MedFTs to become more comfortable in talking about the topic of death and being able to support and explain these occurrences to loved ones. Exposure to death and dying brings with it a multitude of sights and sounds, for example, that most people are not familiar with. These sequences follow typical, but also unique, processes as a person's body begins to shut down organs and prepare for death (Berry & Griffie, 2010; Emanuel, von Gunten, & Ferris, 1999). Specific components of the dying process include changes in breathing (including long pauses between breaths and cycling between fast and slow breathing), decreases and/or cessation of appetite and thirst, increased restlessness and agitation, withdrawal from communicating, and increased periods of sleep. Patients may report seeing people who have already died in their dreams, through visions, and/or via hallucinations. They may begin talking actively about their deaths. Blood pressure can drop significantly, leading to the hands, arms, feet, and legs feeling cold to the touch and/or bluish in color. These biological processes (in part of in whole) provide signals that death is coming; they can be used to help prepare loved ones.

The process of death can be very draining for family members and friends, even when they are mentally prepared. Family members may need to receive comforting words about their concerns and to be encouraged to speak to the dying loved one even in situations wherein he or she is no longer in consciousness. Families should receive guidance, too, in discussing any rituals, prayers, traditions, and how a person's body is to be handled after the death. Advanced discussions about decision-making and goals of care can help families prepare for these experiences; they should be offered before death is imminent.

Decision-Making and Goals of Care

There are many issues to consider when engaged in decision-making and goals of care in Palliative and Hospice settings. For instance, patients, family members, and healthcare professionals may hold differing opinions regarding treatment goals (Bakitas, Kryworuchko, Matlock, & Volandes, 2011; Blank, Graves, Sepucha, & Llewellyn-Thomas, 2006; Erlen, 2005). Physicians may encourage a family to continue an aggressive course of treatment; patients and family members may be more concerned about the pain and suffering associated with such treatment. Alternatively, physicians may hold little hope for cure and encourage a transition to Hospice Care, whereas families may wish to exhaust every possible treatment option. These differing priorities can lead to misunderstandings and difficulties in making treatment decisions. MedFTs can be one of the multidisciplinary professionals who participate in family team meetings to help clarify, reframe, and normalize the myriad of ways in which those involved make decisions (Hudson, Quinn, O'Hanlon, & Aranda, 2008). Many of the terms used in these meetings are outlined in this chapter's glossary (e.g., advanced care planning, advance directive, living will, and death with dignity).

Cultural considerations in decision-making. While illness and death are universal human experiences, personal meanings and preferences around illness and dying are very much a cultural experience (Ho et al., 2013). Attending to issues of culture and diversity is a critical component of the decision-making considerations in Palliative and Hospice Care (López-Sierra & Rodríguez-Sánchez, 2015; Thompson, Bugbee, Meriac, & Harris, 2013). Culture can be understood to include ethnicity, gender, social class, family beliefs, religion, worldview, and other influences (Hardy & Laszloffy, 1995). All of these dimensions contribute to a person's cultural identity and can influence patients' and family members' behaviors, beliefs, and values in relation to illness and decision-making.

Culture can influence healthcare decision-making, preferences for communication, and specific processes of handling end of life (Galanti, 2015). While most patients want to be told when their illness becomes life-threatening (Lowey, Norton, Quinn, & Quill, 2013), some cultures prefer that patients not be included in these conversations as it can be believed to only add suffering or, perhaps, even hasten death. For example, individuals from the Hmong culture often believe that only God knows when someone will die, so attempts to warn of an impending death can be interpreted as meaning that medical team members are planning to kill the patient (Fadiman, 1997). Another consideration that often comes into play is religious beliefs, as some dictate which medical interventions are allowed and which are not. For instance, Jehovah's Witnesses do not approve of blood transfusions; they consider this an act that would be disobedient and disrespectful of God. Additionally, individuals from different regions and races have different preferences regarding end-of-life choices about drug treatments, utilizing (or not) assisted breathing devices, and/or where they die (Barnato, Anthony, Skinner, Gallagher, & Fisher, 2007). These differences in preferences for care can be very difficult for the healthcare team, as some decisions may feel unethical from their own cultural standpoint (especially when said standpoint is informed by Western values of patient autonomy in decision-making and Western medicine inclination to pursue all possible treatments). In these sensitive scenarios, it is helpful to have someone who can act as a "cultural broker" to help both sides understand the values and preferences more fully within a broader social and cultural context (Renzaho, Romios, Crock, & Sonderlund, 2013).

Working with Children

Another fundamental to understand relates to differences between adult and pediatric populations in Palliative and Hospice settings (Knapp, 2009; Meier & Beresford, 2007). Caring for children with serious illnesses requires unique skills and programs (Himelstein, Hilden, Boldt, & Weissman, 2004; NHPCO, 2015) and an understanding of children's physical, emotional, cognitive, and social development (Rushton, 2004). For example, children may lack the cognitive or emotional understanding of their condition and its consequences. Adolescents may be able understand these issues, but they are not legally able to make decisions regarding their own care. This presents parents with the additional role of healthcare advocate with the legal responsibility for healthcare decision-making (complicated by assessing the youth's ability—or not—to provide consent for said treatment). While pediatric Palliative Care is growing (Feudtner et al., 2013), unfortunately many local communities do not have the professional services needed to assess and treat these illnesses. This often results in families needing to travel long distances for treatment—separating them from essential social support and often disrupting parental employment and insurance coverage—which strains both finances and relationships (Williams-Reade et al., 2015).

Self of the Therapist and Compassion Fatigue Prevention

It is not uncommon for MedFTs working with serious illnesses to witness repeated long-term suffering and death. This necessitates vigilant attention to self-care practices, self-of-the-therapist reflection, and compassion fatigue prevention. Healthcare professionals must learn to help family members cope with grief and loss while at the same time face their own feelings about it (Edwards & Patterson, 2006; Kumar, D'souza, & Sisodia, 2013; Rolland, 1994). One of the professional side effects of working in this specialty area is the development of a deep awareness of mortality, grief, and loss in our own lives (Meier, Back, & Morrison, 2001). Put simply: because the potential for significant levels of stress is very high while working with this patient population, self-care should be tantamount (Mendenhall & Trudeau-Hern, 2013).

A potential consequence of avoiding self-care and/or not addressing self-of-the-therapist issues is compassion fatigue. Physical indicators of compassion fatigue include a chronic sense of exhaustion, insomnia, headaches, digestion issues, and other physical symptoms (Figley, 2002). Psychological indicators of compassion fatigue include feeling overwhelmed about the workload, case intensity, and case content and a slow progressive detachment from relational interactions. Over time, there is a risk of losing baseline compassion, along with declines in empathy and warmth toward patients and families (Mendenhall, 2006). There will be times that illness, loss, and death are a part of your personal life, and this can cause your professional work in Palliative and Hospice Care to feel additionally burdensome and isolating (Becvar, 2003). Recognizing and processing these feelings can be beneficial to both MedFTs and patients (Negash & Sahin, 2011; Sanchez-Reilly et al., 2013).

Palliative and Hospice Care Across the MedFT Healthcare Continuum

Patients and family members in Palliative and Hospice Care are in need of comprehensive services that can attend to their unique biopsychosocial-spiritual needs. The MedFT framework serves useful while guiding healthcare delivery from a biopsychosocial-spiritual, relational, and systemic lens. Providers delivering care from this lens possess unique skills which can significantly alleviate symptoms of suffering and improve overall coping mechanisms for patients and family members. Leading with a relational lens, MedFTs can help to foster improved communication with healthcare team members. As MedFT continues to develop as a sibling field to Marriage and Family Therapy (MFT), so will the depth of skills and involvement in directing tertiary care in core competencies that will further become guide research, policy, and practice. Tables 10.1 and 10.2 highlight the specific skills for healthcare professionals as they move across Hodgson, Lamson, Mendenhall, and Tyndall's (Hodgson et al., 2014) MedFT Healthcare Continuum.

Table 10.1 MedFTs in Palliative and Hospice Care: Basic Knowledge and Skills

MedFT Healthcare Continuum Level	Level 1	Level 2	Level 3
Knowledge	General understanding of chronic illness typology, disease trajectory, and the interplays between Palliative Care and Hospice Care. Recognition of the biopsychosocial-spiritual connection to a patient's overall health outcomes. Familiarity with typical psychosocial stressors associated with chronic illness, grief, and bereavement.	Knowledge of PCP, Palliative, and Hospice Care professionals within care settings. Aware of the differences and similarities between Palliative Care and Hospice treatment teams (and the types of illnesses most commonly present in each). Working relationship with mental health referral sources, support groups, and community resources. Ability to initiate and activate change within the healthcare system to create the inclusion of caregivers' health and well-being. Attends additional training and/or utilizes research-informed literature based on grief and loss in clinical practice.	Familiarity of illness genograms and BPSS interviews when working with individuals, couples, and families. Comfort in utilizing these in clinical practice (and in teaching these skills to healthcare team members).
Skills	Can deliver psychoeducation to healthcare team members, patients, and family members. Aware of and can utilize mental health screeners already in place at a care setting. Provides and maintains connections to referral sources. Utilizes strength-based models of practice and provides psychoeducation to patient, family, and healthcare professionals.	Encourages healthcare team members to screen for mental health issues. Conducts or coordinates support groups for caregivers and/or provides psychosocial resources for them. Actively participates in supervision that addresses self-care.	Actively incorporates family members into treatment plans and interventions. Regularly screens for common mental health conditions using instruments that include (but not limited to) the PHQ-2, PHQ-4, PHQ-9, and GAD-7.

Table 10.2 MedFTs in Palliative and Hospice Care: Advanced Knowledge and Skills

MedFT Healthcare Continuum Level	Level 4	Level 5
Knowledge	Utilizes advocacy practices for family members' preferences and values during decision-making times, and highlights systemic impacts of treatment throughout the family system. Understands and addresses illness meanings, tends to issues of blame and defenses, and facilitates processing losses associated with illness.	Works regularly with families from all diagnoses and phases along the continuum of illness trajectories as a fully integrated member of the healthcare team. Facilitates exploration, case consultation, and/or Balint groups to help attend to existential issues related to hope and the meaning of life and death with patients, families, medical team members, and oneself.
Skills	Adept in delivering short- and long-term therapy requiring a comprehensive team, keeps comprehensive progress notes, and provides updates at team meetings. Develops and advances self-care plans that recognize the risk of buildups of unprocessed feelings and responses to the depth of loss being dealt with. Administers screening assessments such as FICA, FACIT-Sp, and the SBI-15R.	Proficient in training and supervising interns, participates in administrative roles, and provides psychosocial education to hospital staff through formal and informal presentations. Actively participates in treatment team meetings, ethics committees, community volunteer organizations, support groups. Self-care plan moves beyond existential issues to balancing of time commitments and personal/professional boundaries.

MedFTs operating at *Levels 1 and 2* may not be part of an integrated behavioral healthcare team, but may see patients who have reached a non-critical status with their illness. They could see a family member of a patient who has reached non-critical status, too, or a loved one of somebody who has died from a serious illness. If a MedFT is in a practice in which they occasionally see patients or family members from Palliative or Hospice Care, it is important to collaborate with the primary physician and behavioral health providers who may be following this patient. This MedFT should possess a general understanding of chronic illness typology, disease trajectory, and the interplay between Palliative Care and Hospice Care. There should also be a recognition of the BPSS connection to a patient's overall health outcomes and typical psychosocial stressors. At these levels, care likely is not delivered past the individual patient level, but there should be a deeper understanding about the importance of the supportive role(s) that family and caregivers play. These MedFTs are also able to screen for symptoms of depression and anxiety, make appropriate referrals, and communicate these symptoms and/or plans to family members, caregivers, and the larger treatment team. For example, a MedFT working with Megan (in our clinical vignette) would be able to monitor and observe changes in her mood, recognizing that her levels of exhaustion are connected with the aggressive postoperative chemotherapy and radiation that she is undergoing. The MedFT would be able to recognize when changes could be potential indicators for depression and then relay that information to Megan's treatment team. Psychoeducation around typical individual, couple, and family emotional responses to chronic illness and prolonged treatment is important at these initial levels.

A clinician working in *Level 3* is likely to be co-located within a tertiary setting and has theoretical foundations of care rooted in family systems theory. He or she will go beyond holding the ideologies of the BPSS framework, put these into practice within their respective care teams. Clinicians at this level advocate for team-based care (e.g., consistent team meetings to discuss illness continuums with the medical team members, family members, and the patient). Skills extant at this level not only facilitate working with people in the same room; they help to create shared treatment goals by taking into account the dynamic interplays between medical, familial, and relational systems. For example, a MedFT would be able to facilitate a family meeting with both medical teams to discuss treatment plans and patient/family wishes to open the door for a deeper conversation regarding thoughts and feelings around treatment preferences and transitions of care. A MedFT would have the skills to empathize, normalize, and help process the anger, fear, confusion, and anxiety Megan and Joe are having regarding the news her treatment had been unsuccessful and Palliative Care was being suggested.

A MedFT functioning at *Level 4* would be advancing a higher degree of collaboration. MedFTs at this level consistently bring a family-centered approach to treatment team decisions, keeping family members' preferences and values in mind when decisions are made, and reminding treatment teams to think about the systemic impacts of treatment throughout the family system. Delivering short- and long-term therapy would be prudent and would require a comprehensive treatment plan. At this level, MedFTs are adept in care dynamics between Palliative and Hospice Care—recognizing that not all Palliative Care patients will transition to Hospice and that most all patients in Hospice will have had touches with a Palliative Care team. In the case of Megan, her treatment ended abruptly as the risks outweighed the benefits. A MedFT would be able to help the family process many of the existential and meaning-making questions that would arise—along with unspoken thoughts around death and dying. The MedFT will seek to provide emotional processing for healthcare team members as they deal with the vicarious trauma and grief associated with working with Megan's family (and other families like them). This can put MedFTs in a difficult position, as there may be no one to help process their own grief as they regarded to be a primary support person for other team members. MedFTs' self-care plans should be in place and include identifying colleagues or outside support persons who can regularly engage in discussions about the emotional aspect of this work.

MedFTs at *Level 5* regularly work with families from all diagnoses and phases along the continuum of illness trajectories, and they do this as fully integrated members of the Palliative and/or Hospice Care team. They may be sought out for their input at various treatment team meetings, ethics committees, community volunteer organizations, and support groups. MedFTs train and supervise interns and may participate in administrative and educational roles.

MedFTs at *Level 5* also provide psychosocial training to hospital staff and community partners through formal and informal presentations. They may still be actively involved in care, but may also be situated in clinical research and the operational aspects of care. For instance, a MedFT working within the tertiary care setting would be developing educational programming for providers and staff, attending and contributing to research and process improvement for clinical practices, as well as promoting health and well-being on a community level. In Megan's case, a MedFT at this level would likely be the behavioral health coordinator or director of a division of behavioral health services that oversees the coordination and supervision of providers meeting with the family. Self-care plans for these MedFTs now expand to include boundaries regarding how often they will manage time commitments to the myriad of professional commitments that they maintain and endeavors in which they take part.

Research-Informed Practices

Inclusion of mental health professionals on teams working with serious and terminal illness is not a new concept; chaplains and behavioral health providers have been by the bedsides of dying patients since the inception of Hospice Care (Doka, 1993). As MedFTs rapidly integrate into healthcare settings, the possibility of working with Palliative and Hospice patients is almost a certainty. Gaining evidence-based competencies in working with patients and families during these times is a suggested requirement of systemically trained therapists who are employed in healthcare settings (Gamino & Ritter, 2010). However, barriers to evidence-based practices in these specialties are in early stages of growth due to the sensitive nature and vulnerability of these patient populations. Large randomized control trials are not conducive, nor feasible, due to the unpredictability of illness and the dying processes of each disease. Adapting evidence-based or research-informed interventions within these fields is a first step in growing the body of Palliative and Hospice Care literature regarding this topic.

Individual Approaches

The primary focus of research done in Palliative and Hospice Care is targeted toward brief interventions that are psychoeducational and supportive in nature. Psychotherapeutic approaches to end-of-life and chronic illness care include person-centered techniques concentrating on meaning making and existentialism as an important resource for coping. From these come modalities such as meaning-centered psychotherapy (Breitbart, Gibson, Poppito, & Berg, 2004), existential psychotherapy (Chochinov, 2006), dignity therapy (Martínez et al., 2016), art therapy (Pratt & Wood, 2015), music and movement therapy (Gallagher, Lagman, Walsh, Davis, & LeGrand, 2006), and individual psychotherapy interventions such as CALM (Managing *C*ancer *a*nd *L*iving *M*eaningfully; Lo et al., 2014).

Along with these aforementioned approaches, therapeutic techniques with Palliative and Hospice Care populations attempt to address multifaceted concepts of grief and loss. Loss is a thread that runs through all illness experiences. Because it is not a task to complete, process-oriented models of care fit well into therapeutic care delivery structures advanced in Palliative and Hospice Care. MedFTs in these settings are encouraged to learn therapeutic models that teach skills related to meaning making (Wynne, Shields, & Sirkin, 1992), narrative framework (White & Epston, 1990; Williams-Reade, Freitas, & Lawson, 2014), illness beliefs (Wright, 2009), non-illness identity (Gonzalez, Steinglass, & Reiss, 1989), storytelling (Kleinman, 2009); legacy (Piercy & Chapman, 2001), agency and communion (McDaniel, Doherty, & Hepworth, 2014; McDaniel, Hepworth, & Doherty, 1992), and individual psychoeducation on distress and coping (Manne, Babb, Pinover, Horwitz, & Ebbert, 2004). McDaniel et al. (2014) provide a thorough and comprehensive overview of these specific modalities in their chapter entitled *Caregiving, End-of-life Care, and Loss.*

Family Approaches

When a patient is diagnosed with a serious illness, it is a stressful psychological event for themselves and, in some cases even more so, their family members (Edwards & Clarke, 2004; Mitschke, 2008; Rolland, 2005). Upon diagnosis, families are expected to assimilate an overwhelming amount of information; they are asked to rapidly make informed decisions about care options, negotiate ever-hanging healthcare service and insurance systems, and come to terms with the impact(s) of a seriously ill family member/loved one of themselves and others. For a family, illness brings with it new stressors—while at the same time it can exacerbate old and/or already existing stressors and difficulties (Kristjanson & Aoun, 2004; Schmitt, Santalahti, & Saarelainen, 2008). Normalization of family members' responses to these challenges (e.g., guilt, sadness, fear) is often the first step in MedFT care (McDaniel et al., 2014). Brief solution-focused therapy for couples aimed to elicit social support and feelings of equity (Kuijer, Bunk, Jong, Ybema, & Sanderman, 2004); couples psychoeducation to minimize negative emotional outcomes (Baucom et al., 2009); emotionally focused couples therapy to address attachment, empathy, and marital satisfaction (McLean, Walton, Rodin, Esplen, & Jones, 2013); and family focused grief models of care such as family focused grief therapy are used more readily in this population (Kissane et al., 2006; Kissane et al., 2003). Northouse, Katapodi, Song, Zhang, & Mood (2010) published a large meta-analysis aimed to examine randomized controlled trials (RCTs) that have been conducted regarding family caregivers of cancer patients; findings showed that interventions fell under three types: (a) psychoeducation, (b) skills training, and (c) therapeutic counseling. Interventions were aimed to reduce caregiver burden, improve patient and caregiver coping, increase self-efficacy, and improve quality of life. The need for further research regarding the impacts that cancer has on dyadic- and family- level functioning is ever present. This burgeoning scholarship—while still limited—is similarly supported as it relates to couples' work with dyads coping with cancer (Traa, De Vries, Bodenmann, & Den Oudsten, 2015).

Community Approaches

Community volunteers and family caregivers have been essential in the Palliative Care and Hospice Care movement. Recognition of psychosocial-spiritual aspects of care is taught to all lay persons who volunteer within these tertiary care settings. Support groups and peer support have been utilized as an important intervention for patients and families with the aim of alleviating distress. Many of these support groups are community-based and rely heavily on volunteerism (Hudson, Aranda, & McMurray, 2002; Ussher, Kirsten, Butow, & Sandoval, 2006; Weis, 2003). Whether professionally trained or skilled volunteers, typical concerns that should be addressed for patients and families include contexts such as culture, work, school, and housing—and how these contexts may impact each other and overall illness experiences (Evans & Ume, 2012; Johnson, 2013). In addition, it is important to remember that patients who have a serious illness often experience changes in social functioning. For children, participation at school or in extracurricular activities may be compromised. For adults, it may be their church community or work. Attending to these relationships can be an important aspect of care (Prince-Paul, 2008). All of these efforts, too, are advanced alongside working, raising children, caring for aging parents, and grieving the many day-to-day losses brought on by serious illness. Given the significant burden associated with caring for patients with serious illness, standards and policies for Palliative and Hospice Care provision—which focus on addressing psychosocial needs of family caregivers—have been established (Hudson & Payne, 2011). Embracing the energies and support from community members—as outlined here—is strongly supported and encouraged.

Conclusion

The number (and needs) of patients and families connected to Palliative and Hospice Care is growing. As health systems adopt paradigm shifts toward embracing patient- and family-centered philosophies of care, clinicians trained in MedFT will be at the forefront. With their systemic BPSS training, MedFTs have the knowledge and skills to participate as clinicians, researchers, educators, and policy makers. Along the way, the roles that they play will go beyond demonstrating competency in the abovementioned fundamentals of care. MedFTs are actively assisting in the development and testing of new systemic interventions that bring more relational understandings of Palliative and Hospice work. They are evaluating, refining, and advocating for evidence-based practices that ease patients' and family suffering, and they are training future generations of providers to carry forward this mission.

Reflection Questions
1. Look up the state-by-state report card on Palliative Care by the *Center to Advance Palliative Care* and the *National Palliative Care Research Center* (www.capc.org/reportcard/) to find out about your state's data. See how it compares to other states. In what ways could care in your state be improved?
2. Engage in the CDC's online course on advance care planning module called *Advance Care Planning: An Introduction for Public Health and Aging Services Professionals* (http://www.cdc.gov/aging/advancecareplanning/care-planning-course.htm). Reflect on the role you could play in your setting regarding advance care planning.
3. Create a medical genogram of your own family and then for a family you are already working with. A good clinical resource to read prior to doing this (to have available during the activity) is McGoldrick and Gerson's (1985) *Genograms in Family Assessment*. Consider such questions as: (a) How does observing death from illness in your family make you suited as a match for this family? (b) What understanding do you have about illness and loss that another clinician may not have? (c) As you were experiencing this in your own family, what do you wish would have been different? (d) What are patterns of coping have you witnessed that you would like to keep and build upon? (e) What are patterns of coping that you have witnessed that you would like to release? (f) How can you use your personal experiences to intervene with this family?
4. Beginning this work with an appreciation for its intensity means we need to be proactive about self-care and carving out times for self-reflection. Create a list of your best self-care activities, and look to see how often you are doing them and how realistically you can increase them. Then create another list of how you will know when you begin to feel compassion fatigue or burnout, and write down your indicators. Have a close friend or loved one fill out the same list for you. Create care plans for yourself based on your indicators, so you can get to self-care practices faster and more efficiently.

Glossary of Important Terms in Palliative and Hospice Care

Advanced care planning A process of communication between individuals and their healthcare agents to express wishes and preferences regarding care in the event they are unable to make their own decisions or speak for themselves

(Waldrop & Meeker, 2012). MedFTs can help patients and family members engage in advance care planning that can help prevent unnecessary suffering and improve quality of life toward the end of life and can aid caregivers in better understanding what the patient prefers (Houben, Spruit, Groenen, Wouters, & Janssen, 2014). Several documents and resources scan assist in this process and are listed at the end of this chapter. The decisions made in advanced care planning are reflected in an *advance directive*.

Advance directive A legal document that states your preferences regarding healthcare decisions in the event you are unable to speak for yourself. There are three main categories of advanced directives: "power of attorney," "healthcare proxy," and "living will."

Allow natural death (AND) A more recent terminology that can replace the DNR order. While a DNR/DNAR relates to CPR, an AND instructs that only comfort measures be taken to manage symptoms without interfering with the natural dying process.

Death with dignity A term commonly used to describe a physician-assisted death, physician-assisted dying, aid-in-dying, or medical aid-in-dying. It includes a process that allows for certain terminally ill patients (adults) to legally consult and request a lethal dose of medication from their primary care providers. Patients receive said medication from a pharmacist and then take it themselves (or have a family member administer it) in order to end life in a peaceful and dignified manner. This option is only available in certain areas (see Death with Dignity, 2016).

Do not resuscitate (DNR)/Do not allow resuscitation (DNAR) A medical order written by a primary care provider (Breault, 2011). It instructs healthcare providers not to do cardiopulmonary resuscitation (CPR) if a patient stops breathing or if his or her heart stops beating. The primary care provider writes the order only after talking about it with the patient (if possible), the proxy, or with the patient's family.

Healthcare proxy Designates an individual to make medical decisions on a patient's behalf if they are unable.

Living will Documents a patient's desired wishes about medical treatment at the end of life in the event they are unable to communicate. It can also be called a "directive," "healthcare declaration," or "medical directive."

Physician order for life-sustaining treatment (POLST) A more recent form developed to improve communication about goals of care, quality of life, diagnosis, prognosis, and treatment options between seriously ill or frail patients and healthcare professionals about wishes pertaining to life-sustaining treatments. (Polst Organization, 2016).

Power of attorney Authorizes an individual to make decisions on a patient's behalf in the event they become disabled or incapacitated. A medical power of attorney authorizes an individual to make medical decisions for a patient in the event he or she becomes unconscious or mentally incapable of decision-making.

Additional Resources

Electronic Resources

Advance Care Planning Conversation Guide. http://coalitionccc.org/tools-resources/advance-care-planning-resources/
Aging with Dignity (Five Wishes). http://www.agingwithdignity.org
American Academy of Pediatrics: Palliative Care for Children. pediatrics.aappublications.org/content/106/2/351.full
Caring Conversations. https://www.practicalbioethics.org/resources/caring-conversations
Consumer's Tool Kit for Health Care Advance Planning. http://www.americanbar.org/groups/law_aging/resources/health_care_decision_making/consumer_s_toolkit_for_health_care_advance_planning.html
GetPalliativecare.org. http://www.getPalliativecare.org
NHPCO Children's Project on Palliative/Hospice Services (ChiPPS). http://www.nhpco.org/resources/pediatric-Hospice-and-Palliative-care
Pediatric Supportive Care for Children with Cancer. http://www.cancer.gov/cancer-topics/pdq/supportivecare/pediatric/healthprofessional

Organizations/Associations

Association for Death Education and Counseling. http://www.adec.org/adec/default.aspx
Center to Advance Palliative Care's (CAPC) Pediatric Palliative Care. http://www.capc.org/Palliative-care-across-the-continuum/pediatric-Palliative-care
Children's Hospice and Palliative Care Coalition. www.chpcc.org
Hospice Action Network. http://Hospiceactionnetwork.org/
Hospice Association of America. www.Hospice-america.org/
Hospice Foundation of America. https://Hospicefoundation.org/End-of-Life-Support-and-Resources/Coping-with-Terminal-Illness/Hospice-Services
Initiative for Pediatric Palliative Care (IPPC). ippcweb.org
National Hospice and Palliative Care Organization. http://www.caringinfo.org/i4a/pages/index.cfm?pageid=1
National Hospice and Palliative Care Organization 2015. http://www.nhpco.org/sites/default/files/public/Statistics_Research/2015_Facts_Figures.pdf

References[1]

Aoun, S., Currow, D., Hudson, P., Kristjanson, L., & Rosenberg, J. (2005). The experience of supporting a dying relative: Reflections of caregivers. *Progress in Palliative Care, 13*, 319–325. https://doi.org/10.1179/096992605X75930

Armstrong, B., Jenigir, B., Hutson, S. P., Wachs, P. M., & Lambe, C. E. (2013). The impact of a Palliative Care program in a rural Appalachian community hospital: A quality improvement process. *American Journal of Hospice and Palliative Care, 30*, 380–387. https://doi.org/10.1177/1049909112458720

*Babcock, C. W., & Robinson, L. E. (2011). A novel approach to hospital palliative care: An expanded role for counselors. *Journal of Palliative Medicine, 14*, 491–500. https://doi.org/10.1089/jpm.2010.0432.

Bakitas, M., Kryworuchko, J., Matlock, D. D., & Volandes, A. E. (2011). Palliative medicine and decision science: The critical need for a shared agenda to foster informed patient choice in serious illness. *Journal of Palliative Medicine, 14*, 1109–1116. https://doi.org/10.1089/jpm.2011.0032

Bardia, A., Barton, D. L., Prokop, L. J., Bauer, B. A., & Moynihan, T. J. (2006). Efficacy of complementary and alternative medicine therapies in relieving cancer pain: A systematic review. *Journal of Clinical Oncology, 24*, 5457–5464. https://doi.org/10.1200/JCO.2006.08.3725

Barnato, A. E., Anthony, D., Skinner, J., Gallagher, P., & Fisher, E. (2007). Are regional variations in end-of-life care intensity explained by patient preferences? A study of the U.S. Medicare population. *Medical Care, 45*, 386–393. https://doi.org/10.1097/01.mlr.0000255248.79308.41

Baucom, D., Porter, L., Kirby, J., Gremore, T., Wiesenthal, N., Aldridge, W., . . . Keefe, F. (2009). A couple-based intervention for female breast cancer. *Psycho-Oncology, 18*, 276–283. https://doi.org/10.1002/pon.1395

*Becvar, D. S. (2003). The impact on the family therapist of a focus on death, dying, and bereavement. *Journal of Marital and Family Therapy, 29*, 469–477. https://doi.org/10.1111/j.1752-0606.2003.tb01689.x.

Berry, P., & Griffie, J. (2010). Planning for the actual death. In B. R. Ferrell and N. Coyle (Eds.), *Oxford textbook of palliative nursing* (pp. 629–644). New York, NY: Oxford University Press.

Blank, T., Graves, K., Sepucha, K., & Llewellyn-Thomas, H. (2006). Understanding treatment decision making: Contexts, commonalities, complexities, and challenges. *Annals of Behavioral Medicine, 32*, 211–217. https://doi.org/10.1207/s15324796abm3203_6

Breault, J. L. (2011). DNR, DNAR, or AND? Is language important? *The Ochsner Journal, 11*, 302–306. Retrieved from http://www.ochsnerjournal.org/doi/abs/10.1043/1524-5012-11.4.302?code=occl-site

Breitbart, W., Gibson, C., Poppito, S. R., & Berg, A. (2004). Psychotherapeutic interventions at the end-of-life: a focus on meaning and spirituality. *The Canadian Journal of Psychiatry, 49*, 366–372. https://doi.org/10.1177/070674370404900605

Brickner, L., Scannell, K., Marquet, S., & Ackerson, L. (2004). Barriers to hospice care and referrals: Survey of physicians' knowledge, attitudes, and perceptions in a health maintenance organization. *Journal of Palliative Medicine, 7*, 411–418. https://doi.org/10.1089/1096621041349518

Campion, E. W., Kelley, A. S., & Morrison, R. S. (2015). Palliative care for the seriously ill. *New England Journal of Medicine, 373*, 747–755. https://doi.org/10.1056/nejmra1404684

*Center to Advance Palliative Care. (2016). *About palliative care*. Retrieved from https://www.capc.org/about/Palliative-care/

Center to Advance Palliative Care. (2011). *Public opinion research on palliative care*. Retrieved from http://www.capc.org/tools-for-Palliative-care-programs/marketing/public-opinion-research/2011-public-opinion-research-on-Palliative-care.pdf

---

[1] Note: References that are prefaced with an asterisk are recommended readings.

Centers for Disease Control and Prevention. (2010). *End-of-life preparedness: An emerging public health priority*. Retrieved from www.cdc.gov/aging/endoflife/

Centers for Disease Control and Prevention. (2011). *Leading causes of death*. Retrieved from http://www.cdc.gov/nchs/fastats/leading-causes-of-death.htm

Centers for Medicare & Medicaid Services. (2013). *Medicare hospice benefits*. Retrieved from http://www.medicare.gov/pubs/pdf/02154.pdf

Chochinov, H. M. (2006). Dying, dignity, and new horizons in palliative end-of-life care. *CA: A Cancer Journal for Clinicians, 56*, 84–103. https://doi.org/10.3322/canjclin.56.2.84

Chochinov, H. M., Kristjanson, L. J., Hack, T. F., Hassard, T., Mcclement, S., & Harlos, M. (2007). Burden to others and the terminally ill. *Journal of Pain and Symptom Management, 34*, 463–471. https://doi.org/10.1016/j.jpainsymman.2006.12.012

Claxton-Oldfield, S. (2015). Hospice Palliative Care volunteers: The benefits for patients, family caregivers, and the volunteers. *Palliative & Supportive Care, 13*, 809–813. https://doi.org/10.1017/S1478951514000674

Engel, G. L. (1977). The need for a new medical model: A challenge for biomedicine. *Science, 196*, 129–136. https://doi.org/10.1126/science.847460

Engel, G. L. (1980). The clinical application of the biopsychosocial model. *American Journal of Psychiatry, 137*, 535–544. https://doi.org/10.1176/ajp.137.5.535

Curtis, J. R. (2008). Palliative and end-of-life care for patients with severe COPD. *European Respiratory Journal, 32*, 796–803. https://doi.org/10.1183/09031936.00126107

D'Antonio, J. (2014). Caregiver grief and anticipatory mourning. *Journal of Hospice & Palliative Nursing, 16*, 99–104. https://doi.org/10.1097/njh.0000000000000027

Death with Dignity National Center (2016). *FAQs about the Death with Dignity National Center*. Retrieved from: https://www.deathwithdignity.org/

*Doka, K. (1993). *Living with life-threatening illness: A guide for patients, their families and caregivers*. New York, NY: Lexington Books.

Dumanovsky, T., Augustin, R., Rogers, M., Lettang, K., Meier, D., & Morrison, R. S. (2015). The growth of palliative care in U.S. hospitals: A status report. *Journal of Palliative Medicine, 19*, 8–15. https://doi.org/10.1089/jpm.2015.0351

Edwards, B., & Clarke, V. (2004). The psychological impact of a cancer diagnosis on families: The influence of family functioning and patients' illness characteristics on depression and anxiety. *Psychoncology, 13*, 562–576. https://doi.org/10.1002/pon.773

Edwards, T., & Patterson, J. (2006). Supervising family therapy trainees in primary care settings: Context matters. *Journal of Marital and Family Therapy, 32*, 33–43. https://doi.org/10.1111/j.1752-0606.2006.tb01586.x

El-Jawahri, A., Greer, J. A., & Temel, J. (2012). Does palliative care improve outcomes for patients with incurable illness? A review of the evidence. *Journal of Supportive Oncology, 9*, 87–94. https://doi.org/10.1016/j.suponc.2011.03.003

Emanuel, L. L., von Gunten, C. F., & Ferris, F. F. (Eds.). (1999). *Module 12: Last hours of living in EPEC (Education on Palliative and End-of-Life Care) participant's handbook*. Princeton Township, NJ: Robert Wood Johnson Foundation.

Engelman, S. R. (2013). Palliative care and use of animal-assisted therapy. *Omega-Journal of Death and Dying, 67*, 63–67. https://doi.org/10.2190/OM.67.1-2.g

Erlen, J. A. (2005). When patients and families disagree. *Orthopaedic Nursing, 24*, 279–282. https://doi.org/10.1097/00006416-200507000-00009

Evans, A. J. (1994). Anticipatory grief: A theoretical challenge. *Journal of Palliative Medicine, 8*, 159–165. https://doi.org/10.1177/026921639400800211

Evans, B., & Ume, E. (2012). Psychosocial, cultural, and spiritual health disparities in end-of-life and palliative care: Where we are and where we need to go. *Nursing Outlook, 60*, 370–375. https://doi.org/10.1016/j.outlook.2012.08.008

Fadiman, A. (1997). *The spirit catches you and you fall down*. New York, NY: Farrar, Straus & Giroux.

Feudtner, C., Womer, J., Augustin, R., Remke, S., Wolfe, J., Friebert, S., & Weissman, D. (2013). Pediatric palliative care programs in children's hospitals: A cross-sectional national survey. *Pediatrics, 132*, 1063–1070. https://doi.org/10.1016/j.pcl.2014.04.007

Figley, C. R. (2002). Compassion fatigue: Psychotherapists' chronic lack of self care. *Journal of Clinical Psychology, 58*, 1433–1441. https://doi.org/10.1002/jclp.10090

*Galanti, G. A. (2015). *Caring for patients from different cultures* (5th ed.). Philadelphia, PA: University of Pennsylvania Press.

Gallagher, L. M., Lagman, R., Walsh, D., Davis, M. P., & LeGrand, S. B. (2006). The clinical effects of music therapy in palliative medicine. *Supportive Care in Cancer, 14*, 859–866. https://doi.org/10.1007/s00520-005-0013-6

Gamino, L. & Ritter, R. (2010). *Ethical practice in grief counseling*. New York, NY: Springer.

Gonzalez, S., Steinglass, P., & Reiss, D. (1989). Putting the illness in its place: Discussion groups for families with chronic medical illnesses. *Family Process, 28*, 69–87. https://doi.org/10.1111/j.1545-5300.1989.00069.x

Gordon, T., & Mitchell, D. (2004). A competency model for the assessment and delivery of spiritual care. *Journal of Palliative Medicine, 18*, 646–651. https://doi.org/10.1191/0269216304pm936oa

Grant, E., Murray, S. A., Kendall, M., Boyd, K., Tilley, S., & Ryan, D. (2004). Spiritual issues and needs: Perspectives from patients with advanced cancer and nonmalignant disease. A qualitative study. *Palliative & Supportive Care, 2*, 371–378. https://doi.org/10.1017/s1478951504040490

Grassi, L. (2007). Bereavement in families with relatives dying of cancer. *Current Opinion in Supportive and Palliative Care, 1*, 43–49. https://doi.org/10.1097/spc.0b013e32813a3276

Guldin, M., Vedsted, P., Zachariae, R., Olesen, F., & Jensen, A. B. (2011). Complicated grief and need for professional support in family caregivers of cancer patients in palliative care: A longitudinal cohort study. *Support Care Cancer Supportive Care in Cancer, 20*, 1679–1685. https://doi.org/10.1007/s00520-011-1260-3

Hanratty, B., Hibbert, D., Mair, F., May, C., Ward, C., Corcoran, G., ... Litva, A. (2006). Doctors' understanding of palliative care. *Palliative Medicine, 20*, 493–497. https://doi.org/10.1191/0269216306pm1162oa

Hardy, K., & Laszloffy, T. (1995). The cultural genogram: Key to training culturally competent family therapists. *Journal of Marital and Family Therapy, 21*, 227–237. https://doi.org/10.1111/j.1752-0606.1995.tb00158.x

Harstäde, C. W., Andershed, B., Roxberg, Å., & Brunt, D. (2013). Feelings of guilt: Experiences of next of kin in end-of-life care. *Journal of Hospice & Palliative Nursing, 15*, 33–40. https://doi.org/10.1097/njh.0b013e318262332c

Hebert, R. S., Prigerson, H. G., Schulz, R., & Arnold, R. M. (2006). Preparing caregivers for the death of a loved one: A theoretical framework and suggestions for future research. *Journal of Palliative Medicine, 9*, 1164–1171. https://doi.org/10.1089/jpm.2006.9.1164

*Himelstein, B., Hilden, J., Boldt, A., & Weissman D. (2004). Pediatric palliative care. *New England Journal of Medicine, 350*, 1752–1762. https://doi.org/10.1056/NEJMra030334.

Ho, A. H. Y., Cecilia, L. W. C., Pamela, P. Y. L., Chochinov, H., Neimeyer, R., Pang, S. M. C., & Tse, D. M. W. (2013). Living and dying with dignity in Chinese society: Perspectives of older palliative care patients in Hong Kong. *Age and Ageing, 42*, 455–461. https://doi.org/10.1093/ageing/aft003

*Hodgson, J., Lamson, A., Mendenhall, T., & Tyndall, L., (2014). Introduction to medical family therapy: Advanced applications. In J. Hodgson, A. Lamson, T. Mendenhall, and D. Crane (Eds.), *Medical family therapy: Advanced applications* (pp. 1-9). New York, NY: Springer.

*Hodgson, J., Lamson, A., & Reese, L. (2012). The biopsychosocial-spiritual interview method. In D. Linville and K. Hertlein (Eds.), *The therapist's notebook for family health care: Homework, handouts, and activities for individuals, couples, and families coping with illness, loss, and disability* (pp. 3–12). New York, NY: Haworth Press.

Holland, J. C., Kash, K. M., Passik, S., Gronert, M. K., Sison, A., Lederberg, M., ... Fox, B. (1998). A brief spiritual beliefs inventory for use in quality of life research in life-threatening illness. *Psycho-Oncology, 7,* 460–469. https://doi.org/10.1002/ (SICI)1099-1611(199811/12)7:6<460::AID-PON328>3.0.CO;2-R

Houben, C. H., Spruit, M. A., Groenen, M. T., Wouters, E. F., & Janssen, D. J. (2014). Efficacy of advance care planning: A systematic review and meta-analysis. *Journal of the American Medical Directors Association, 15,* 477–489. https://doi.org/10.1016/j.jamda.2014.01.008

Hudson, P., Aranda, S., & McMurray, N. (2002). Intervention development for enhanced lay palliative caregiver support: The use of focus groups. *European Journal of Cancer Care, 11,* 262–270. https://doi.org/10.1046/j.1365-2354.2002.00314.x

Hudson, P., & Payne, S. (2011). Family caregivers and palliative care: Current status and agenda for the future. *Journal of Palliative Medicine, 14,* 864–479. https://doi.org/10.1136/bmjspcare-2013-000500

Hudson, P., Quinn, K., O'Hanlon, B., & Aranda, S. (2008). Family meetings in palliative care: Multidisciplinary clinical practice guidelines. *Bio Med Central Palliative Care, 7,* 1–12. https://doi.org/10.1186/1472-684X-7-12

Hudson, P., Remedios, C., Zordan, R., Thomas, K., Clifton, D., Crewdson, M., ... Bauld, C. (2012). Guidelines for the psychosocial and bereavement support of family caregivers of palliative care patients. *Journal of Palliative Medicine, 15,* 696–702. https://doi.org/10.1089/jpm.2011.0466

Hughes, M. T., & Smith, T. J. (2014). The growth of palliative care in the United States. *Annual Review of Public Health, 35,* 459–475. https://doi.org/10.1146/annurev-publhealth-032013-182406

Irwin, S. A., Rao, S., Bower, K., Palica, J., Rao, S. S., Maglione, J. E., ... Ferris, F. D. (2008). Psychiatric issues in palliative care: Recognition of depression in patients enrolled in hospice care. *Journal of Palliative Medicine, 11,* 156–163. https://doi.org/10.1089/jpm.2007.0140

Johnson, K. S. (2013). Racial and ethnic disparities in palliative care. *Journal of Palliative Medicine, 16,* 1329–1334. https://doi.org/10.1089/jpm.2013.9468

Jones, B. L. (2006). Pediatric palliative and end-of-life care. *Journal of Social Work in End-of-Life & Palliative Care, 1,* 35–62. https://doi.org/10.1300/j457v01n04_04

Karlsson, M., Friberg, F., Wallengren, C., & Öhlén, J. (2014). Meanings of existential uncertainty and certainty for people diagnosed with cancer and receiving palliative treatment: A life-world phenomenological study. *BMC Palliative Care, 13,* 28–37. https://doi.org/10.1186/1472-684x-13-28

Kaur, J., & Mohanti, B. K. (2011). Transition from curative to palliative care in cancer. *Indian Journal of Palliative Care, 17,* 1–5. https://doi.org/10.4103/0973-1075.78442

Kissane, D. W., & Bloch, S. (2002). *Family focused grief therapy.* Philadelphia, PA: Oxford University Press.

Kissane, D., McKenzie, M., McKenzie, D., Forbes, A., O'Neill, L, & Bloch, S. (2003). Psychosocial morbidity associated with patterns of family functioning in palliative care: Baseline data from the family focused grief therapy controlled trial. *Palliative Medicine, 17,* 527–537. https://doi.org/10.1191/0269216303pm808oa

Kissane, D., McKenzie, M., Bloch, S., Moskowitz, C., McKenzie, D., & O'Neill, L. (2006). Family focused grief therapy: A randomized, controlled trial in palliative care and bereavement. *American Journal of Psychiatry, 163,* 1208-1218. doi: 10.1176/ajp.2006.163.7.1208

Kleinman, A. (2009). Caregiving: The odyssey of becoming more human. *The Lancet, 373,* 292-293. https://doi.org/10.1016/S0140-6736(09)60087-8

Knapp, C. (2009). Research in pediatric palliative care: Closing the gap between what is and is not known. *American Journal of Hospice and Palliative Care, 26,* 392–398. https://doi.org/10.1177/1049909109345147

Kristjanson, L. J., & Aoun, S. (2004). Palliative care for families: Remembering the hidden patients. *Canadian Journal of Psychiatry, 49,* 359–365. https://doi.org/10.3322/canjclin.56.2.84

Kuijer, R., Bunk, B., Jong, G., Ybema, J., & Sanderman, R. (2004). Effects of a brief intervention program for patients with cancer and their partners on feeling of inequity, relationship quality and psychological distress. *Psycho-Oncology, 13,* 321–334. https://doi.org/10.1002/pon.749

Kumar, S., D'souza, M., & Sisodia, V. (2013). Healthcare professionals' fear of death and dying: Implications for palliative care. *Indian Journal of Palliative Care, 19*, 196–198. https://doi.org/10.4103/0973-1075.121544

Kwak, J., Salmon, J. R., Acquaviva, K. D., Brandt, K., & Egan, K. A. (2007). Benefits of training family caregivers on experiences of closure during end-of-life care. *Journal of Pain and Symptom Management, 33*, 434–445. https://doi.org/10.1016/j.jpainsymman.2006.11.006

Laguna, J., Goldstein, R., Allen, J., Braun, W., Enguidanos, W., & Enguidanos, S. (2012). Inpatient palliative care and pain: Pre- and post-outcomes. *Journal of Pain and Symptom Management, 43*, 1051–1059. https://doi.org/10.1016/j.jpainsymman.2011.06.023

Lobb, E. A., Lacey, J., Kearsley, J., Liauw, W., White, L., & Hosie, A. (2013). Living with advanced cancer and an uncertain disease trajectory: An emerging patient population in palliative care? *BMJ Supportive & Palliative Care, 5*, 352–357. https://doi.org/10.1136/bmjspcare-2012-000381

Lo, C., Hales, S., Jung, J., Chiu, A., Panday, T., Rydall, A., . . . Rodin, G. (2014). Managing cancers and living meaningfully (CALM): Phase 2 trial of a brief individual psychotherapy for patients with advanced cancer. *Palliative Medicine, 28*, 234–242. https://doi.org/10.1177/0269216313507757

López-Sierra, H. E., & Rodríguez-Sánchez, J. (2015). The supportive roles of religion and spirituality in end-of-life and palliative care of patients with cancer in a culturally diverse context. *Current Opinion in Supportive and Palliative Care, 9*, 87–95. https://doi.org/10.1097/spc.0000000000000119

Lowey, S. E., Norton, S. A., Quinn, J. R., & Quill, T. E. (2013). Living with advanced heart failure or COPD: Experiences and goals of individuals nearing the end-of-life. *Research in Nursing & Health, 36*, 349–358. https://doi.org/10.1002/nur.21546

Lupu, D. (2010). American academy of hospice and palliative medicine workforce task force. Estimate of current hospice and palliative medicine physician workforce shortage. *Journal of Pain and Symptom Management, 40*, 899–911. https://doi.org/10.1016/j.jpainsymman.2010.07.004

Manne, S., Babb, J., Pinover, W., Horwitz, E., & Ebbert, J. (2004). Psychoeducational group intervention for wives of men with prostrate cancer. *Psycho-Oncology, 13*, 37–46. https://doi.org/10.1002/pon.724

Martínez, M., Arantzamendi, M., Belar, A., Carrasco, J. M., Carvajal, A., Rullán, M., & Centeno, C. (2016). Dignity Therapy: A promising intervention in palliative care. *Palliative Medicine, 31*, 492–509. https://doi.org/10.1177/0269216316665562

McDaniel, S. H., Hepworth, J., & Doherty, W. J. (1992). *Medical family therapy: A biopsychosocial approach to families with health problems*. New Yorkm NY: Basic Books.

*McDaniel, S., Doherty, W., & Hepworth, J. (2014). *Medical family therapy and integrated care* (2nd ed.). Washington, DC: American Psychological Association.

McGoldrick, M., & Gerson, R. (1985). *Genograms in family assessment*. New York, NY: Norton.

McLean, L. M., Walton, T., Rodin, G., Esplen, M. J., & Jones, J. M. (2013). A couple-based intervention for patients and caregivers facing end-stage cancer: outcomes of a randomized controlled trial. *Psycho-Oncology, 22*, 28–38. https://doi.org/10.1002/pon.2046

Meier, D., & Beresford, L. (2007). Pediatric palliative care offers opportunities for collaboration. *Journal of Palliative Medicine, 10*, 284–289. https://doi.org/10.1089/jpm.2006.9985

Meier, D. E., Back, A. L., & Morrison, R. S. (2001). The inner life of physicians and care of the seriously ill. *JAMA, 286*, 3007–3014. https://doi.org/10.1001/jama.286.23.3007

Meier, D. E. (2011). Increased access to palliative care and hospice services: Opportunities to improve value in health care. *Milbank Quarterly, 89*, 343–380. https://doi.org/10.1111/j.1468-0009.2011.00632

Mendenhall, T. (2006). Trauma-response teams: Inherent challenges and practical strategies in interdisciplinary fieldwork. *Families, Systems & Health, 24*, 357–362. https://doi.org/10.1037/1091-7527.24.3.357

Mendenhall, T. J., & Trudeau-Hern, S. (2013). Developing self-awareness in clinicians who work in medical settings: A guide for using medical genograms in supervision. In R. Bean, S. Davis, and M. Davey (Eds.), *Clinical activities for increasing competence and self-awareness* (pp. 141–148). Thousand Oaks, CA: Sage.

Milberg, A., Olsson, E. C., Jakobsson, M., Olsson, M., & Friedrichsen, M. (2008). Family members' perceived needs for bereavement follow-up. *Journal of Pain and Symptom Management, 35*, 58–69. https://doi.org/10.1016/j.jpainsymman.2007.02.039

Mitschke, D. B. (2008). Cancer in the family: Review of the psychosocial perspectives of patients and family members. *Journal of Family Social Work, 11*, 166–184. https://doi.org/10.1080/10522150802175159

Murray, S. A., Kendall, M., Boyd, K., & Sheikh, A. (2005). Illness trajectories and palliative care. *BMJ, 330*, 1007–1011. https://doi.org/10.1136/bmj.330.7498.1007

National Coalition for Hospice and Palliative Care. (2013). *Clinical practice guidelines for quality Palliative care* (3rd ed.). Retrieved from http://www.nationalcoalitionhpc.org/guidelines-2013/

National Consensus Project for Quality Palliative Care. (2013). *Clinical practice guidelines for quality palliative care* (3rd ed.). Pittsburgh, PA: Author.

National Quality Forum (NQF). (2006). *A national framework and preferred practices for palliative and hospice care quality.* Retrieved from http://www.qualityforum.org/Publications/2006/12/A_National_Framework_and_Preferred_Practices_for_Palliative_and_Hospice_Care_Quality.aspx

Negash, S., & Sahin, S. (2011). Compassion fatigue in marriage and family therapy: Implications for therapists and clients. *Journal of Marital and Family Therapy, 37*, 1–13. https://doi.org/10.1111/j.1752-0606.2009.00147.x

National Hospice and Palliative Care Organization. (2015). *NHPCO's facts and figures: Pediatric palliative and hospice care in America.* Retrieved from http://www.nhpco.org/about/Hospice-care

Northouse, L., Katapodi, M., Song, L., Zhang, L., & Mood, D. (2010). Interventions with family caregivers of cancer patients: Meta-analysis of randomized trials. *CA: A Cancer Journal for Clinicians, 60*, 317–339. https://doi.org/10.3322/caac.20081

Obermeyer, D., Makar, M., Abujaber, S., Dominici, F., Block, S., & Cutler, D. M. (2014). Associations between the Medicare hospice benefit and health care utilization and costs for patients with poor-prognosis cancer. *JAMA, 312*, 1888–1896. https://doi.org/10.1001/jama.2014.14950

Oishi, A., & Murtagh, F. E. (2014). The challenges of uncertainty and interprofessional collaboration in palliative care for non-cancer patients in the community: A systematic review of views from patients, carers and health-care professionals. *Palliative Medicine, 28*, 1081–1098. https://doi.org/10.1177/0269216314531999

Patterson, J., Peek, C. J., Heinrich, R. L., Bischoff, R. J., & Scherger, J. (2002). *Mental health professionals in medical settings: A primer.* New York, NY: Norton.

Peek, C. J., & Heinrich, R. L. (2000). Integrating behavioral health and primary care. In M. Maruish (Ed.), *Handbook of psychological assessment in primary care settings.* Mahwah, NJ: Lawrence Erlbaum.

Persson, C., Ostlund, U., Wennman-Larsen, A., Wengstrom, Y., & Gustavsson, P. (2008). Health-related quality of life in significant others of patients dying from lung cancer. *Palliative Medicine, 22*, 239–247. https://doi.org/10.1177/0269216307085339

Peterman, A. H., Fitchett, G., Brady, M. J., Hernandez, L., & Cella, D. (2002). Measuring spiritual well-being in people with cancer: the functional assessment of chronic illness therapy—Spiritual Well-being Scale (FACIT-Sp). *Annals of Behavioral Medicine, 24*, 49–58. https://doi.org/10.1207/S15324796ABM2401_06

Piercy, K., & Chapman, J. (2001). Adopting the caregiver role: A family legacy. *Family Relations, 50*, 386–393. https://doi.org/10.1111/j.1741-3729.2001.00386.x

Polst Organization. (2016). *About the national Polst program.* Retrieved from http://www.polst.org/

Pratt, M., & Wood, M. (Eds.). (2015). *Art therapy in palliative care: The creative response.* New York, NY: Routledge.

Prince-Paul, M. (2008). Understanding the meaning of social well being at the end-of-life. *Oncology Nursing Forum, 35,* 365–371. https://doi.org/10.1188/08.ONF.365-371

Puchalski, C. (2006). Spirituality and medicine: Curricula in medical education. *Journal of Cancer Education, 21,* 14–18. Retrieved from https://www.ncbi.nlm.nih.gov/pubmed/16918282

Rayner, L., Loge, J. H., Wasteson, E., & Higgson, I. J. (2009). The detection of depression in palliative care. *Current Opinion Supportive Palliative Care, 3,* 55–60. https://doi.org/10.1097/SPC.0b013e328326b59b

Renzaho, A., Romios, P., Crock, C., & Sonderlund, A. (2013). The effectiveness of cultural competence programs in ethnic minority patient-centered health care: A systematic review of the literature. *International Journal for Quality in Health Care, 25,* 261–269. doi: 10.1093/intqhc/mzt006

Richardson, P. (2014). Spirituality, religion and palliative care. *Annals of Palliative Medicine, 3,* 150–159. https://doi.org/10.3978/j.issn.2224-5820.2014.07.05

*Rolland, J. S. (2005). Cancer and the family: An integrative model. *Cancer, 104,* 2584–2595. https://doi.org/10.1002/cncr.21489.

*Rolland, J. S. (1994). *Families, illness, and disability: An integrative treatment model.* New York, NY: Basic Books.

Rushton, C. (2004). Integrating ethics and palliative care in pediatrics. *American Journal of Nursing, 104,* 54–63. https://doi.org/10.1016/2Fj.pcl.2007.10.011

Sanchez-Reilly, S., Morrison, L., Carey, E., Bernacki, R., O'neill, L., Kapo, J., ... deLima Thomas, J. (2013). Caring for oneself to care for others: Physicians and their self-care. *Journal of Supportive Oncology, 11,* 75–81. 10.12788/j.suponc.0003

Schmitt, F., Santalahti, P., & Saarelainen, S. (2008). Cancer families with children: Factors associated with family functioning: A comparative study in Finland. *Psycho-Oncology, 17,* 363–372. https://doi.org/10.1002/pon.1241

Seibaek, L., Lise, H., & Niels, C. H. (2013). Secular, spiritual, and religious existential concerns of women with ovarian cancer during final diagnostics and start of treatment. *Evidenced Based Complementary Alternative Medicine, 2013,* 1–11. https://doi.org/10.1155/2013/765419

Selecky, P. A., Eliasson, C. A., Hall, R. I., Schneider, R. F., Varkey, B., & McCaffree, D. R. (2005). Palliative and end-of-life care for patients with cardiopulmonary diseases: American College of Chest Physicians position statement. *Chest, 128,* 3599–3610. https://doi.org/10.1378/chest.128.5.3599

Selman, L., Beynon, T., Higginson, I. J., & Harding, R. (2007). Psychological, social and spiritual distress at the end-of-life in heart failure patients. *Current Opinion Supportive Palliative Care, 1,* 260–266. https://doi.org/10.1097/SPC.0b013e3282f283a3

Shore, J. C., Gelber, M. W., Koch, L. M., & Sower, E. (2016). Anticipatory grief. *Journal of Hospice & Palliative Nursing, 18,* 15–19. https://doi.org/10.1097/njh.0000000000000208

Sidebottom, A. C., Jorgenson, A., Richards, H., Kirven, J., & Sillah, A. (2015). Inpatient palliative care for patients with acute heart failure: Outcomes from a randomized trial. *Journal of Palliative Medicine, 18,* 134–142. https://doi.org/10.1089/jpm.2014.0192

Simon, J. L. (2008). Anticipatory grief: Recognition and coping. *Journal of Palliative Medicine, 11,* 1280–1281. https://doi.org/10.1089/jpm.2008.9824

Sulmasy, D. P. (2002). A biopsychosocial-spiritual model for the care of patients at the end-of-life. *The Gerontologist, 42*(Suppl. 3), 24–33. https://doi.org/10.1093/geront/42.suppl_3.24

Thompson, V. L. S., Bugbee, A., Meriac, J. P., & Harris, J. K. (2013). The utility of cancer-related cultural constructs to understand colorectal cancer screening among African Americans. *Journal of Public Health Research, 2,* e11–e18. https://doi.org/10.4081/jphr.2013.e11

Traa, M. J., De Vries, J., Bodenmann, G., & Den Oudsten, B. L. (2015). Dyadic coping and relationship functioning in couples coping with cancer: A systematic review. *British Journal of Health Psychology, 20,* 85–114. https://doi.org/10.1111/bjhp.12094

Trudeau-Hern, S., & Daneshpour, M. (2012). Cancer's impact on spousal caregiver health: A qualitative analysis in grounded theory. *Contemporary Family Therapy, 34,* 534–554. https://doi.org/10.1007/s10591-012-9211-9

Ussher, J., Kirsten, L., Butow, P., & Sandoval, M. (2006). What do cancer support groups provide which other supportive relationships do not? The experience of peer support groups for people with cancer. *Social Science & Medicine, 62,* 2565–2576. https://doi.org/10.1016/j.socscimed.2005.10.034

Waldrop, D. P., & Meeker, M. A. (2012). Communication and advanced care planning in palliative and end-of-life care. *Nursing Outlook, 60,* 365–369. https://doi.org/10.1016/j.outlook.2012.08.012

Weis, J. (2003). Support groups for cancer patients. *Supportive Care in Cancer, 11,* 763–768. https://doi.org/10.1007/s00520-003-0536-7

White, M., & Epston, D. (1990). *Narrative means to therapeutic ends.* New York, NY: W. W. Norton & Company.

World Health Organization. (2013). *Essential medicines in palliative care.* Retrieved from http://www.who.int/selection_medicines/committees/expert/19/applications/PalliativeCare_8_A_R.pdf

Wilkie, D. J., & Ezenwa, M. O. (2012). Pain and symptom management in palliative care and at end-of-life. *Nursing Outlook, 60,* 357–364. https://doi.org/10.1016/j.outlook.2012.08.002

Williams-Reade, J., Freitas, C., & Lawson, L. A. (2014). Narrative-informed medical family therapy: Using narrative therapy practices in brief medical encounters. *Families, Systems, and Health, 32,* 416–425. https://doi.org/10.1037/fsh0000082

Williams-Reade, J., Lamson, A., White, M. B., Knight, S., Ballard, S., & Desai, P. (2015). Paediatric palliative care: A review of needs, obstacles, and the future. *Journal of Nursing Management, 23,* 4–14. https://doi.org/10.1111/jonm.12095

*Wright, L., Watson, W., & Bell, J. (1996). *Beliefs: The heart of healing in families and illness.* New York, NY: Basic Books.

Wright, L. M. (2009). Spirituality, suffering and beliefs: The soul of healing with families. In F. Walsh (Ed.), *Spiritual resources in family therapy* (2nd ed., pp. 65–80). New York, NY: Guilford Press.

Wynne, L., Shields, C., & Sirkin, M. (1992). Illness, family theory, and family therapy: Conceptual issues. *Family Process, 31,* 3–18. https://doi.org/10.1111/j.1545-5300.1992.00003.x

Zambroski, C. H. (2006). Managing beyond an uncertain illness trajectory: Palliative care in advanced heart failure. *International Journal of Palliative Nursing, 12,* 566–573. 10.12968/ijpn.2006.12.12.22543

Chapter 11
Medical Family Therapy in Endocrinology

Max Zubatsky and Tai Mendenhall

Endocrinology is the study the body's endocrine system, which is responsible for the production of hormones that serve a variety of functions. The endocrine system normally controls the homeostasis of bodily systems and is responsible for growth, development, reproduction, and responses to various internal and external stimuli. Common types of disorders as a result of endocrine complications (e.g., diabetes mellitus, thyroid disease, Addison's disease, Cushing's disease, Grave's disease) are often related to improper functioning of the pancreas and/or pituitary, thyroid, and adrenal glands. These disorders can affect widespread complications such as increased heart rate, abnormal bone growth, skin changes, elevated blood glucose levels, and severe fatigue and weakness (Melmed, Polonsky, Larsen, & Kronenberg, 2015; Nelson, 2005). Life-threatening effects may include diabetic ketoacidosis, hypoglycemic coma, thyroid storm, acute pancreatitis, and pituitary apoplexy (National Adrenal Diseases Foundation, 2016; Savage, Mah, Weetman, & Newell-Price, 2004).

Effectively managing one's health in the face of an endocrine disorder can be extraordinarily stressful, carrying with it significant implications for patients' and their families' coping and adjustment that can be lifelong. As tertiary teams evolve to most successfully engage patients and families in this journey, integrated behavioral health teams that include a wide variety of professionals are becoming the rule (not the exception). To set the stage for our discussion of this as it relates to the practice of Medical Family Therapy (MedFT), we begin by sharing the story of a middle-aged patient, Joe, and his wife. They met Justin shortly after being referred to Endocrinology for diabetes care.

M. Zubatsky (✉)
Department of Family and Community Medicine, Saint Louis University,
St. Louis, MO, USA
e-mail: zubatskyjm@slu.edu

T. Mendenhall
Department of Family Social Science, University of Minnesota, Saint Paul, MN, USA

Clinical Vignette
[Note: This vignette is a compilation of cases that represent treatment in Endocrinology. All patients' names and/or identifying information have been changed to maintain confidentiality.]

Justin (MedFT) first met Joe after he was brought in by his wife following an acute state of diabetic ketoacidosis. He had been a patient of one of Justin's physician colleagues for about three months. He had not shown up regularly for many of his appointments.

Dr. O'Connell (Joe's endocrinologist) called Justin over and said, "His name is Joseph Albright. Goes by Joe. He's stable now; doing better. They've been here all night." He scrolled through his laptop. "At admission, Joe's blood glucose was 430; weight 300. His A1c came back at 14.5."

"Sounds like we need to learn if he's interested in improving his health." Justin said.

"Yeah; my hope is that we can talk with him together; figure out ways to help him be more compliant with his care regimen." Dr. Connell checked his laptop again. "He's only made it in twice so far; both times for acute presentations and upon his wife's insistence. I think this time really scared him."

"Third time's a charm," Justin said.

"I hope so. Before he got sent to Endocrinology, I know that Family Medicine went over diabetes-basics, but I just don't think that he wanted to hear it."

"What's his wife's name?", Justin asked.

Dr. O'Connell responded, "I don't know."

"Is she the one who does the grocery shopping?"

"I don't know."

"Oftentimes family members are not included in standard diabetes care, at least not at first." Justin said. "They should be, though, because day-to-day management of the disease is not done in our offices—it's done outside of the clinic within patients' family or social contexts. And family support—or lack of it—carries a great deal of influence on how well patients do."

Dr. O'Connell and Justin decided it would be best to meet with both members of the couple. They had communicated a strong want to do so, and Joe had already signed a consent form allowing his care team to communicate about his condition with his wife. At that encounter, I encouraged them to work as a couple in managing Tom's diabetes, and to do this as active members of the larger care team. It was clear that Joe's wife—Alice—wanted to be a part of Joe's recovery and ongoing health.

Justin asked Joe to complete a PHQ-4; his scores suggested considerable struggles with both depression and anxiety. He (Joe) explained how his disconnection from Alice—as his primary support person—was a driving factor behind his sense of feeling so overwhelmed. Justin and Dr. O'Connell noted (ironically) how earlier conversations that Joe had had with his doctors about

> diet had not included the person who buys and cooks most of his food. Justin normalized, too, how distressing diabetes can be even in the best of circumstances, and explained how its effective management—while including attention to diet—goes considerably further than this.
>
> "And to do this well, we need to create a treatment plan that includes more folks than just me and Dr. O'Connell," Justin explained. "I'd like us to talk about creating a new treatment plan that will involve a number of team-players—and I think that the two important members of this team are the two of you."
>
> Joe and Alice were up for the task. "Let's do it!," they exclaimed.
>
> "I'm not done in this world yet." Joe said.
>
> Alice laid her head on this shoulder and closed her eyes. Joe kissed her forehead.
>
> "No, you're not, Mr. Albright." She agreed. "We've got things to do."

This case is illustrative of how the practice of Medical Family Therapy within Endocrinology might begin. Instead of being shuffled off by a primary care provider to "mental health" when standard care is not working, care is explicitly and purposefully integrated. And just as we know that the words "stressed" and "desserts" are the same word spelled backwards, we know that managing diabetes well requires attention to a patient's physiological well-being within the context of his or her psychosocial well-being. Oftentimes, it is the MedFT who helps navigate patients and families on this journey—explaining how its respective parts fit together and even engaging those parts to do so. Justin's first discussion with Joe and Alice is illustrative of this.

In this chapter, we will further describe Endocrinology as a care setting-type. We characterize the common makeup(s) of our interdisciplinary teams and outline key knowledge and skill areas for MedFTs within these teams. We describe the practice of MedFT in Endocrinology teams in accord with Hodgson, Lamson, Mendenhall, and Tyndall's (2014) five-level MedFT Healthcare Continuum. We present common terminology, reflection questions, recommended readings, and resources in conclusion.

What Is Endocrinology?

As outlined above, Endocrinology is a medical specialty that focuses on the diagnosis and treatment of a variety of conditions that affect the endocrine system. This system includes many glands within our bodies whose primary function is to secrete hormones (e.g., thyroid, pancreas, testes, ovaries); when these glands do not work properly, we develop endocrine disorders. Endocrinologists—like Dr. O'Connell in the vignette described above—are primary care providers with specialized training to treat patients who are diagnosed with these types of conditions (Goodman, 2010; Lavin, 2012).

The most commonly diagnosed endocrine disorder, diabetes mellitus (DM), is a class of chronic illnesses that includes several endocrine disorders. These include—but are not limited to—Type 1 (immune-mediated diabetes mellitus), Type 2 (insulin-resistant diabetes mellitus), and gestational diabetes. Diabetes affects almost 30 million individuals in the United States, alongside an estimated 8.1 million people who have gone undiagnosed (Centers for Disease Control and Prevention [CDC], 2014). It is especially prevalent in minority groups, with trends showing that over 9% of Asian Americans, 12% of Hispanics/Latinos, 13% of non-Hispanic Blacks, and 20% of American Indians have been diagnosed with some type of diabetes (American Diabetes Association [ADA], 2016). These disparities are prevalent across both adult and pediatric populations (ADA, 2016; Raile et al., 2007; Seid, Sobo, Gelhard, & Varni, 2004). Earlier lifetime mortality rates are extant within persons living with diabetes compared to their non-diabetic counterparts and secondary to a host of comorbid physiological and health complications (Groop et al., 2009; Patterson et al., 2007). Emerging literature has suggested that a new form of diabetes, i.e., Type 3, represents a pathogenic mechanism of neurodegeneration in patients diagnosed with Alzheimer's disease (Suzanne & Wands, 2008; Rivera et al., 2005; Steen et al., 2005). The cognitive deficits and inability to use glucose effectively in these individuals is now said to be linked to several key features of diabetes localized specifically to the brain (de la Monte, 2012).

Attending to both individual (e.g., psychological, behavioral) and family (e.g., genetic predispositions, family functioning, and support) phenomena, the impact(s) of endocrine disorders cannot be overstated. The presence of depression and related mood symptoms, for example, is higher for those living with diabetes—and associated strongly with more serious and longer-lasting complications (ADA, 2016; Katon et al., 2004). These sequelae can greatly impact patients' utilization of services and compliance with recommendations for disease management (e.g., medications, insulin injections, diet, physical activity) (Anderson, Freedland, Clouse, & Lustman, 2001; Egede, Zheng, & Simpson, 2002), much like what we saw with Joe and Alice. Research teams in the United States and Europe found that the prevalence of diabetes in people with serious and persistent mental illnesses (e.g., schizophrenia, bipolar disorder) is 2 to 3 times that of the general population (Holt, Peveler, & Byrne, 2004; Oud & Meyboom-de Jong, 2009). Healthcare facilities are quickly discovering the need for more comprehensive services to adequately assess and treat the complexities of diabetes care.

In recent decades, the emergence of tertiary care in Endocrinology has offered additional resources and services often not provided in primary care. This work targets specific treatments, and—within these efforts—includes multiple providers representing multiple disciplines (Grone & Garcia-Barbero, 2001). For example, tertiary care for patients with diabetes ultimately aims to improve patients' lives through ongoing symptom- and disease- management. To this end, long-term attention to health complications, medications, injections, and lifestyle habits that accompany diabetes care are addressed by a team of healthcare professionals. These efforts are advanced through the coordination of personalized treatment plans that include both the patient and other members within his/her primary support system(s) (Sonino, 2008). Specialists attend to various aspects of the disease such as healthy eating, physical activity, medication adherence, problem-solving skills, risk-reduction behaviors, and spousal and family support and engagement (Gulabani, John & Issac, 2009; Rajasekharan et al., 2015). As more complications continue to arise in this population, MedFTs play a pivotal role as members on these teams.

Treatment Teams in Diabetes and Endocrinology Care

Collaboration in tertiary care settings—between providers and with each other, and between providers and patients and families—is essential (Foraida et al., 2003; Jefferies & Chan, 2004). Attending to the complexities of diabetes, for example, necessitates that providers (medical and behavioral) overlap their respective energies in care. As primary care providers probe questions regarding biomedical and pharmacological treatments, MedFTs and other professionals fill in critical gaps to address underlying challenges, conditions, connections, relationships, and resources playing a loud or silent role in diabetes management (or mismanagement). Providers who embrace these biopsychosocial-spiritual (BPSS) complexities maintain an advantage of holistically seeing how the patient functions (or not) within his/her family and social contexts (Engel, 1977, 1980; Wright, Watson, & Bell, 1996). Advancing care in accord to these complexities can ultimately improve both the patient's and family members' overall functioning and health.

Tertiary care teams tend to represent a broad range of disciplinary backgrounds and training—and in diabetes care, for example, produce better health outcomes (Levetan, Salas, Wilets, & Zumoff, 1995; Liau et al., 2010; Verlato et al., 1996). Diabetes and Endocrinology clinics are noticing, too, the importance of integrating specialty care professionals into their work with patients, families, and communities alike. High-quality teamwork among these providers includes effective patient introductions for initiating services, quality-of-care meetings for coordinating said services, curbside consultations (as indicated throughout treatment), and streamlining referrals through effective planning and discharge (Cook et al., 2009; Mitchell et al., 2012; Wrobel et al., 2003). The following highlight key professionals in and outside of tertiary care settings who are involved in delivering specific services and diabetes care education:

Primary care physicians (PCPs). These providers, usually within the context(s) of Family Medicine, see patients for regular checkups. They have a strong foundational knowledge regarding a variety of health and healthcare presentations and tends to function in key referral roles to connect patients to specialty providers, care teams, and/or community-based resources. The PCP may refer to or check in with the endocrinologist if the patient is not responding to evidence-based care and if his/her disease is progressing beyond the expertise available in the primary care setting.

Endocrinologists. These providers maintain specialized training in treating people with diabetes and other endocrine diseases. Most people with Type 1 diabetes will see an endocrinologist after their initial diagnosis and then continue to consult with him/her about disease management thereafter. Those living with Type 2 diabetes may see this professional when encountering ongoing difficulties with blood sugar management and/or other health issues. Patients diagnosed with Type 3 diabetes may see an endocrinologist in collaboration with a neurologist to track and attend to cognitive functioning and/or declines. Patients may seek a PCP for concomitant medical presentations.

Diabetes educators (often nurse practitioners). These providers possess comprehensive knowledge of prediabetes conditions (for diabetes prevention) and post-diagnosis disease management. They educate and support patients and families to understand and manage multiple facets of the condition and to develop personalized daily self-careplans.

Registered dieticians. These professionals are trained to help patients in their dietary and nutritional care around Type 1, Type 2, or gestational diabetes. They often are dual-certified as diabetes educators. Principal efforts center on assessing food needs, lifestyle history, weight management, and other benchmarks to coordinate appropriate care plans.

Pharmacists. Pharmacists help endocrine disorder patients with education about the use of insulin and/or other medication(s). They also work with women with gestational diabetes, addressing lifestyle habits and dietary management before and after birth of their child.

Behavioral health providers. Behavioral health providers in tertiary care are represented by a variety of disciplinary backgrounds, e.g., MedFTs, social workers, psychologists, counselors, and psychiatric nurses. They work collaboratively with each other and medical providers in the integration of psychosocial and psychotherapeutic services with biomedical care. Many are trained to deliver brief behavioral health assessments and interventions to patients and families while utilizing referrals and providers in their care teams to assist in the delivery of specific services. MedFTs, specifically, work purposefully to engage families as active members of the care team alongside behind-the-scenes (from patients' and families' perspectives) efforts in coordinating professionals' respective contributions and personal/interpersonal functioning and teamwork.

Although many patients with diabetes receive treatment in primary care clinics, there are numerous benefits to effective care coordination in tertiary care settings. Integrated behavioral healthcare services by both medical and behavioral health providers often work within one treatment plan for a particular patient or set of patients in a practice. When a protocol for care is established that includes multiple providers, behavioral health becomes a critical component of delivering the highest quality of care (Blount, 2003; Mullen & Funderburk, 2013; Talen & Valeras, 2013). Across different levels of integration (Doherty, McDaniel, & Baird, 1996), tertiary care normally operates in either a colocated or a partially integrated behavioral healthcare team.

Fundamentals of Care in Endocrinology

When working within the capacity of a MedFT provider in tertiary settings, specialized areas of content knowledge and concomitant skill sets are essential. The following represent those that are critical to Endocrinology (generally) and diabetes care (specifically).

Translating "Endocrinology"

Patients and families who are referred to a "specialist" are oftentimes fearful about what this means. They want to know why their primary care physician cannot "fix" them, whether they are "too sick" for a "usual doctor" to handle, etc. MedFTs are oftentimes in a role(s) whereby discussing the process(es) of referrals, and even the very definition of "Endocrinology" is important so as to assist patients and families in knowing what to expect. This is best done in a manner that is sensitive to patients' and families' distress and/or confusion, e.g., normalizing and empathizing how challenging diabetes can be to effectively manage how complex and overwhelming the medical system can be to navigate; how feelings of sadness, anger, hopelessness, worry, and/or a host of other emotions is normal for everyone (patients, families); and that interpersonal conflicts and discord (in general or specific to health-related foci) among spouses and/or family members is common.

Translating "Diabetes"

As complicated as diabetes can be on a physiological level, it is important to be able to explain (sometimes many times over the course of treatment) what it is in everyday language. Put simply, diabetes is a condition wherein the body is not able to break down or take in energy (carbohydrates) from the foods that we eat. This is because the hormone that is necessary to make our cells absorb sugar from our bloodstream—called insulin—is not produced by our pancreas, not produced enough, or produced but not "heard" by our cells. This then can lead to a buildup in blood sugar; our cells begin to starve, and a host of complications follow (ADA, 2016).

Type 1 diabetes is an autoimmune disorder wherein the insulin-producing cells are destroyed by one's body. Risk factors linked to it include family history and/or presence of autoantibodies, early exposure to viral illnesses, dietary factors (e.g., low Vitamin D consumption as an infant), and even geography. It usually onsets quickly during childhood and requires daily insulin replacement therapy for the patient to survive. Common symptoms include fatigue, weight loss, hunger, blurred vision, insatiable thirst, and frequent urination.

Type 2 diabetes is more common in adults, but it is increasingly prevalent in children. Risk factors linked to it include family history, being overweight, physical inactivity, race, and age. The onset is slow, usually with insulin resistance (i.e., our cells become less responsive to insulin), and carries with it many of the symptoms outlined above for Type 1 sans weight loss.

Other types of diabetes are extant but generally less prevalent. Gestational diabetes, for example, is a Type 2-like condition associated with pregnancy. Type 3 diabetes, as described above, is beginning to be understood as a correlate (and maybe causative agent) to dementia (Accardi et al., 2012; ADA, 2016).

Tests for Diabetes

There are four primary tests that MedFTs should be conversant with in diabetes care. The *random blood sugar test* assesses a patient's blood glucose at any time; sugar recorded and more than 200 milligrams per deciliter (mg/dL) suggests a diabetes diagnosis. The *fasting blood sugar test* assesses a patient's blood after several hours (usually overnight) of not eating. Sugar recorded at more than 126 mg/dL confirms a diabetes diagnosis. The *oral glucose tolerance test* encompasses ingesting a sugary liquid after fasting and then monitoring blood sugar changes over the following 2 hours. Readings more than 200 mg/dL at the conclusion of this time further confirm diabetes. Finally, the *glycated hemoglobin (A1c) test* measures a patient's average blood sugar over the preceding 2–3 months. Specifically, it measures the percentage of blood sugar attached to hemoglobin in red blood cells. An A1c of greater than 6.5% suggests a diabetes diagnosis. For patients with diabetes, the most common tests used for disease management are the random blood sugar test (up to several times per day) and the A1c test (usually 3–4 times per year) (ADA, 2016; Bradley, 2013). MedFTs functioning within Endocrinology should be able to read, interpret, translate, and discuss these tests with other members of the care team and with patients and families. This is important because they represent hallmark data regarding care effectiveness and patient improvements or declines.

Diabetes Management

Understanding the goals of diabetes management is essential for MedFTs, insofar as they permeate almost every clinical encounter, treatment plan, and problem-solving sequence related to the disease. Put simply, it is important for patients to maintain blood glucose (sugar) levels within an indicated range (not too high, not too low). Usually this means 90–190 mg/dL before meals, although this can vary by age and individual circumstances. This objective is achieved through a daily managing of insulin and/or medication (to lower blood sugar), physical activity (to lower blood sugar), and food intake (to increase blood sugar) (ADA, 2016; Garber et al., 2013).

MedFTs should be able to assist patients with setting up a log to track blood sugar testing, interpret trends in recorded values, and know when and how to collaborate with the endocrinologist or other team members (e.g., when values are trending in a negative manner).

It is important for MedFTs to be aware of—and to discuss, normalize, and mitigate—a number of common pitfalls to sticking with a diabetes management plan. For example, some patients and families initially experience a "honeymoon phase" post-diagnosis. They see diabetes as a "call" to be healthier, and they welcome its indicated changes in diet and physical activity routines. However, just like New Year's resolutions usually wane by February, so too do many of our diabetes "honeymooners" (Cogan, 2008).

Blood glucose monitoring. Regular monitoring of one's blood glucose is essential for diabetes management. MedFTs often help patients and families learn how to integrate this into their everyday routines, alongside developing ways to track patterns over time. Familiarity with different types of lancing devices (e.g., lancets, spring-loaded single-use devices, pen-types), meters (e.g., by ease of use, wait times), test strips (e.g., costs, availability), and procedures (e.g., assembly of supplies, methods blood application to test strips) is requisite in order to do this. MedFTs oftentimes—with access to on-site supplies—even demonstrate blood sugar checks on themselves and/or walk patients and families through it as a part of these sequences (ADA, 2016). MedFTs can teach patients how to record, retrieve, and read values stored in their (the patients') glucometers and recommend that they bring recording devices to meetings so as to keep indicated data current.

Hypoglycemia. Hypoglycemia is a condition wherein a patient's blood sugar is especially low. Causes include not having eaten enough food, having too much insulin, and/or exercising more than one should. Symptoms can onset suddenly, progress to unconsciousness if not treated, and can cause permanent brain damage or death. Mild symptoms can include fatigue, shakiness, blurry vision, sweating, hunger, weakness, and noticeable changes in anxiety and other behaviors. Moderate symptoms can include confusion, a "dazed" appearance, extreme fatigue, and/or marked irritability. Severe symptoms can include inability to swallow, seizures, and/ or coma. Responses to hypoglycemia should thereby be prompt; they can include consuming foods that are high in simple sugar (e.g., orange juice, honey, non-diet soda), ingesting tablets or gels with pre-measured amounts of pure glucose, or taking an injection of a hormone (e.g., Glucagon) that raises blood glucose (ADA, 2016). It is important for MedFTs to know where these supplies are kept on-site and that they be able to help access indicated interventions if/when necessary.

Hyperglycemia. Hyperglycemia is a condition wherein a patient's blood has too much sugar. Causes can include too little insulin, decreased physical activity, illness or injury, stress, and/or menstrual periods. While onset can be rapid when someone is on an insulin pump, it usually develops slowly. Mild symptoms include fatigue, thirst, frequent urination, stomach pains, poor concentration, skin flushing, and/or sweet "fruity" breath. Moderate symptoms include nausea and vomiting, stomach cramps, and dry mouth. Severe symptoms can include labored breathing, confusion, and unconsciousness. Responses should include verification of blood glucose via testing, exercising (unless ketones are present), insulin administration, and rapid hydration (ADA, 2016).

Glucagon administration. Glucagon is a naturally occurring hormone that, when injected, quickly raises patients' blood sugar. Its principal use is to reverse severe hypoglycemia. Any provider working with diabetic patients should be familiar with this treatment, insofar as discussing and preparing to use it if/when necessary should be a part of any diabetes management plan. The treatment process includes merging a powder and solution mixture and then injecting it into the patient with a syringe (ADA, 2016).

Insulin administration. MedFTs should maintain a baseline familiarity with the most commonly used insulin types (e.g., rapid-, short-, intermediate-, and long-acting) and methods of delivery (e.g., vial, syringe, pen, pump). They must be conversant regarding indicated ways to store insulin (e.g., refrigeration, room-temperature), timing of administration (e.g., before meals), dosage supplies (e.g., alcohol pads, gloves), and logarithms. This is important because it represents a common area of concern and negotiation among couples and families as they schedule patient- and/or family-centered care sessions in clinic and as they adapt to a diabetes-sensitive lifestyle outside of the clinic. It also represents an important developmental milestone for children and adolescents, i.e., managing insulin administration and/or insulin pumps on their own sans adult supervision (ADA, 2016).

Ketone monitoring. Ketones are acids that can build up in patients' bodies; they represent the principal culprit behind diabetic ketoacidosis (DKA), which is a leading cause of diabetes-related hospitalization, coma, and death. These acids are monitored through testing patients' urine with a specialized test strip. If/when ketones are moderate or high, it is important to not engage in physical activity, hydrate, and encourage frequent use of the restroom (ADA, 2016).

Complications. Thoroughly outlining all of the potential complications of diabetes is outside of this chapter's scope. However, it is important for MedFTs to be familiar with the most common ones associated with this disease when it is poorly managed; these include cardiovascular disease (e.g., signs of a possible stroke include facial droop, weakness in arms, and difficulties with speech; signs of a possible heart attack include feelings of pressure on the chest, chest pain, shortness of breath, and nausea), neuropathy (e.g., numbness, pain, and/or tingling in fingers and toes), nephropathy (e.g., signs of kidney damage include marked swelling—called edema—around the eyes, ankles, and feet, alongside foamy urine and/or weight gain secondary to fluid retention), retinopathy (e.g., signs of eye damage include seeing small black dots—called "floaters"—in one's forward vision and/or flashing lights—called "flashers" in one's periphery vision), and problems with the feet and skin (e.g., cuts and wounds that are very slow to heal, infections, itchy dry skin) (ADA, 2016). MedFTs should explain to patients how PCPs and endocrinologists may not ask about or see these symptoms in regular visits, and should communicate strongly that they (the patients) seek immediate medical attention if/when these types of symptoms manifest.

Nutrition. MedFTs must be conversant with the tenets of good nutrition, purposeful meal planning, food preparation, and portion sizes. A great storehouse of this information—for patients, families, and providers alike—is the American Diabetes Association's website(s): see www.diabetes.org. MedFTs should encourage patients to consume a variety of healthy foods, including produce (vegetables and fruits), grains, fish, and nuts—alongside talking about the importance of reducing intake of animal fats, trans fats, sodium, and alcohol. Working with patients and families with how to afford healthy foods (e.g., where and when to purchase these) and co-own new diets (e.g., we are in this together) is oftentimes something that MedFTs process and advance within team care (ADA, 2016).

Physical activity. MedFTs must work with patients and families toward making exercise a stalwart part of everyday life—and they are up against considerable resistance vis-à-vis modern day lifestyles of desk jobs, marathon television watching, videogames, and obesity (as almost normative) (ADA, 2016). Further, many patients are in no condition to simply begin lifting weights or go jogging. Familiarity with multiple strategies of light to moderate exercise (to begin with), chair aerobics (e.g., for those living with joint or back pain), and/or easy and indoor sequences (e.g., for those who cannot afford to go to a gym or do not feel safe being outside in their neighborhoods) is important so as to avoid commonplace impasses between primary care providers who say "You should exercise…" and patients who say "Yes, but…." Purposeful collaboration with patients' PCP, a physical therapist, and/or a sports medicine provider can further facilitate this care.

Sensitivity to diversity. MedFTs must maintain awareness of cultural and community phenomena that impact patients and families (Tyndall, Hodgson, Lamson, White, & Knight, 2012), especially in regard to well-known and documented health disparities among those suffering from diabetes. This is important, too, because patients' ethnicities and cultures play considerable roles in diabetes management and care (Counihan & Van Esterik, 2012; Nam, Chesla, Stotts, Kroon, & Janson, 2011). MedFTs must purposefully integrate these complexities into treatment teams' sights as interventions (medical, behavioral, or otherwise) are designed and implemented in collaboration with patients and their families. They must also be familiar with and honor different groups' conceptualizations of illness and disease (generally), diabetes (specifically), and traditions, habitudes, and meanings connected to food (e.g., ceremonial feasting with rice or fry bread—both very high-carbohydrate foods—as cultural staples) and physical activity (e.g., culturally-specific games) that directly impact disease management and course(s) (American Association of Diabetes Educators, 2015; Heisler, 2007). It is thereby important for a MedFT to research—and to learn through direct conversations with patients and families—about the culture(s) within which care is being advanced. For example, Tai Mendenhall's work in the American Indian (AI) community encompasses considerable attention to Indigenous peoples' historical trauma and (understandable) tendency to mistrust Western providers, common narratives about diabetes as an unstoppable plague, culturally framed conceptualizations of health within Medicine Wheel models and affiliated narratives about "walking in balance" (i.e., simultaneously attending to physical, emotional, interpersonal, and spiritual well-being), Native foods held in high-value, and drumming, dancing, and a host of culturally unique games and activities preferred as means of physical activity and exercise (Mendenhall et al., 2010; Mendenhall, Gagner, & Hunt, 2015; Mendenhall, Seal, GreenCrow, LittleWalker, & BrownOwl, 2012; Seal et al., 2016).

Stress management. MedFTs must be competent in working with patients and families to negotiate a variety of stressors in a manner whereby food or other substances are not used as coping mechanisms, exercise is not foregone for television watching, etc. Whether this is about general life functioning (e.g., prioritizing daily professional and personal responsibilities, effective time management) or specific problem solving (e.g., resolving marital conflict about money, creating a personalized self-care plan, substance use treatment), it is important to understand how diabetes health (e.g., metabolic control) and patients' mental health are highly associated (ADA, 2016). They must also be skilled with standardized measures to track patients' stress as measured by symptoms of depression and anxiety (like we saw with Justin's work with Joe and Alice); these include—but are not limited to—the Patient Health Questionnaire (PHQ-2, PHQ-4, and/or PHQ-9) and Diabetes Distress Scale (American Psychological Association, 2016; Fisher, Hessler, Polonsky, & Mullan, 2012; Löwe et al., 2010).

Attention to Ethics

MedFTs in any context must recognize challenges related to delivering mental health services within a broader healthcare system, negotiating and/or obtaining releases of information to discuss and consult regarding cases across multiple providers and/or provider teams, negotiating multiple providers' respective access (or not) to behavioral health notes, finding private space(s) for personal patient or family meetings, and decision-making regarding provider leadership and authority across different phases of care (e.g., acute physical crisis, discharge planning) and care episodes (e.g., during times of suicidal ideations and/or intent). Alongside these, MedFTs in Endocrinology and diabetes care must also be careful to not explicitly offer medical advice that is outside of their licensed scope of practice (e.g., giving specific suggestions regarding medication dosages, unilaterally advancing nutritional/dietary plans). Being equipped with the knowledge and information outlined above does not mean that a MedFT is qualified to overstep a primary care provider's counsel. MedFTs should thereby read about and be familiar with respective team members' disciplinary codes of ethics and be comfortable leading open and collaborative discussions regarding the above-referenced and related foci.

Diabetes Care Across the MedFT Healthcare Continuum

Medical Family Therapy serves as a useful framework for mental health and medical providers in the care for patients and families who live with diabetes. Specific training, practice, research, and policy competencies represent important facets of this work as professionals engage with this population. Tables 11.1 and 11.2 highlight specific knowledge and skills that characterize MedFTs' involvement across Hodgson, Lamson, Mendenhall, and Tyndall's (2014) MedFT Healthcare Continuum. As we move along the continuum, we carry greater expectations regarding roles, knowledge, and overall contributions to care (Willens, Cripps, Wilson, Wolff, & Rothman, 2011).

At the beginning of the continuum, MedFTs at *Levels 1* and *2* should possess general understanding(s) of Endocrinology and diabetes care and are able to advance biopsychosocial-spiritual sensitivity into their work. It is unlikely that they treat patients and families struggling with endocrine diseases in their everyday practices but are able to ask questions relevant to the maintenance of health vis-à-vis these struggles and/or coordinate referrals with outside providers who can assist with particular aspects of a holistic treatment plan. They maintain basic understandings about how diabetes and depression, for example, can be mutually exacerbating—and normalize and advocate said treatment plans upon this type(s) of insight. A clinician equipped with knowledge and skills outlined in *Level 3* is arguably able to function within a tertiary care team per se—keeping up with and contributing to more complex care plans with other providers engaged with patients (e.g., a newly diagnosed patient who is simultaneously overwhelmed with depression and an impending divorce, a long-term patient—like Joe—with consistently poor metabolic control despite several months of straightforward primary care interventions) and families toward a shared vision of treatment goals and outcomes. This encompasses a working familiarity with specific disease processes alongside purposeful efforts to build relationships with other members of the care team (e.g., physician, nurse practitioner, diabetes educator, endocrinologist, pharmacist, dietician).

A MedFT functioning at *Level 4* maintains high proficiency and knowledge in caring for patients and families living with endocrine disorders, alongside intimate understandings about how the integrated behavioral healthcare teams that function within this specialty area work. Being proficient with core content and terms essential to diabetes care (see Glossary) enables him/her to effectively translate and track biomarkers over the course of care (e.g., reading lab values and applauding patients' efforts over time as A1c, blood glucose, or diastolic/systolic blood pressure values improve; collaborating with prescribers regarding how to effectively orient patients to new routines with insulin and/or metformin regimens). Maintaining clear understandings about respective team members' training and scope of practice enables the MedFT to guide patients and families in their care journey—advancing explanations regarding who to go to for what (e.g., the dietician can help you to learn what to look for on food packaging labels, the pharmacist can explain how to calculate

Table 11.1 MedFTs in Endocrinology and Diabetes Care: Basic Knowledge and Skills

MedFT Healthcare Continuum Level	Level 1	Level 2	Level 3
Knowledge	Basic knowledge about BPSS approaches to diabetes care; sensitive to how disease management and mood are mutually influential. Familiar with Endocrinology as a medical specialty; limited understanding of endocrine disorders or team(s) structure. Basic understanding regarding most common Endocrinology presentations (e.g., diabetes) and concomitant strategies for healthy lifestyle.	Can differentiate between types of diabetes (as a common presentation in Endocrinology care); familiar with basic causes and symptoms. Familiar with benefits of couple and family engagement in health-related adjustments and/or lifestyle maintenance. Some differentiation of the primary endocrine disorders and their roles in the body; can identify some disease-related complications.	Working knowledge of specific team members (e.g., dietician, pharmacist) and terms in Endocrinology (e.g., blood glucose, hypoglycemia, insulin). Basic knowledge of biomarkers in endocrine disorders (e.g., hormone levels, thyroid levels, androgen, and testosterone).
Skills	Can discuss (and psycho-educate) basic relationships between biological processes, personal well-being, and interpersonal functioning. Minimal collaborative skills with Endocrinology providers; prefers to work in an individual practitioner model but is able to contact/refer to other providers about services when needed.	Able to apply systemic interventions in practice; assess patients for background issues such as family history and related risk factors; more diabetes cases seen in practice. Adequate collaborative skills; can coordinate referrals to a few specialists in patients' care; still conducts separate treatment plan; goals and interventions can overlap with—or be informed by—an Endocrinology team.	Working within a tertiary care clinic, able to integrate respective team members' expertise and counsel into treatment planning, contribute to some team meetings and consultations. Can implement a systemic assessment of a patient and family with competencies in assessing for BPSS aspects of disease and resources within the family; engage other professionals as indicated.

Table 11.2 MedFTs in Endocrinology and Diabetes Care: Advanced Knowledge and Skills

MedFT Healthcare Continuum Level	Level 4	Level 5
Knowledge	Proficient understanding of several endocrine disorders and their associated treatments, medications, and terminologies. Conversant in nearly all terms, measures, and facets of diabetes care (as one of Endocrinology's most common presentation), e.g., medications, injections, indicated biomarkers, dietary prescriptions, and tools/meters.	Understand treatment and care sequences for unique and/or challenging topics in endocrine practice (e.g., foot care, using insulin pumps); can consult effectively with professionals about medical topics from other fields. Conversant with evidence-based treatments regarding the most endocrine disorders and their role(s) in the family; has background to provide education to patients about a variety of symptoms, medications, and diet management. High content knowledge in clinical topics, research practice, policy, and administrative areas of endocrine disease care; proficient in developing a curriculum on diet, weight loss, family work, and/or mental health areas to provide other professionals.
Skills	Able to deliver seminars and workshops about the BPSS complexities of a variety of endocrine diseases (e.g., thyroid disorders, Grave's disease, Addison's disease) to a variety of professional types (e.g., mental health, biomedical). Can apply several BPSS interventions in care (including most types of brief interventions); can administer mood- and disease-specific assessment tools proficiently. Consistently collaborates with key Endocrinology team members (e.g., PCP, pharmacist, dietician); initiates team visits with multiple providers when working with patients and families.	Proficient in nearly all aspects of diabetes and endocrine disorders; able to synthesize and conduct research and clinical work; engages in community-oriented projects outside of tertiary clinic. Goes beyond interventions routine for this population; can integrate specific models of care into routine practice (e.g., PCBH, Chronic Care Model). Routinely engages in team-based approaches to care, with consistent communication through electronic health records, "patient introductions," "curbside consultations," and team meetings and visits.

insulin dosage vis-à-vis what you are about to eat, and a MedFT can work with you and your spouse regarding how to negotiate what feels supportive to you versus what feels like nagging); knowing how and when to advance diabetes-specific conversations (e.g., counseling about physical activity, weight management, connections between stress and dietary habits, connections between sleep apnea and blood glucose, connections between insomnia and weight gain); purposively scheduling joint meetings to manifest optimal synergy in overlapping and/or respective expertise areas (e.g., the PCP and MedFT can meet you together to discuss how to exercise safely vis-à-vis your physical limitations, and with your partner and/or other social support persons in the context of a neighborhood that may not feel safe or have easily accessible facilities or resources). Any and all of these sequences are likely to follow the care introduction(s) described above in Joe's and Alice's case.

MedFTs who function at *Level 5* generally have practiced at all levels of care and work in various roles across these respective contexts (e.g., administration, supervision, directing). As a clinician, proficiency in family therapy and BPSS approaches (including competence and knowledge regarding medications, nutrition, lifestyle management, and community approaches to care) extends now to include a comprehensive scope of all facets of diabetes care—including foot care, wound care, diabetic retinopathy, medication side effects, and interactions of sundry disease processes with diabetes per se (e.g., Crohn's disease, osteoporosis, thyroid disease, cancer, chronic pain). This is evidenced in active and effective participation in—and leading of—team-based collaboration, which often expands beyond the Endocrinology "walls" to include other specialties and indicated resources relevant to patients' and families' needs. As an educator and mentor, he/she is proficient in the didactic and supervisory instruction of these skill sets and knowledge—evidenced across live classroom and clinical sequences and/or in the construction of instructional materials (e.g., refereed journal articles, texts, conference proceedings). Further, professionals at this level tend to be involved in research (e.g., testing and/or comparing interdisciplinary team-based methodologies, tracking community-based interventions that purposively integrate patients' and families' lay wisdom and involvement in psychoeducation and support), policymaking (e.g., advocacy for team-based coverage by health maintenance organizations), and other administrative duties (e.g., overseeing behavioral health internships and residencies positioned with Endocrinology care, coordinating clinic sequences and personnel in accord to established or innovative care models). They do this with purposeful sensitivity to the three-world view of healthcare (Peek, 2008), simultaneously addressing (a) common clinical challenges and problem-solving sequences, (b) operational processes that facilitate care teams' effective and efficient functioning, and (c) financial considerations that are unique to the healthcare resources for patients (specifically) and within their clinic and health system (generally).

Research-Informed Practices

Pharmacological Approaches

Patients diagnosed with Type 1 diabetes require lifelong insulin therapy, with some requiring two or more insulin injections daily. Doses are adjusted according to blood glucose levels, set time intervals, and/or the patients' ability to self-monitor and administer dosages reliably (ADA, 2016). Common insulin therapies include Humalog (Insulin Lispro Injection), Novolog (Insulin Aspart), Levemir (Insulin Detemir), and Lantus (Insulin Glargine Injection).

Type 2 diabetes management through pharmacological therapies can be effective but oftentimes is challenging for both patients and family members. Controlling glycemic levels in Type 2 diabetes has become increasingly complex, with difficulties regarding adverse side effects and macrovascular complications (Inzucchi et al., 2012; Stone et al., 2010). Good management of Type 2 diabetes with both pharmacologic and non-pharmacological treatments requires specific education and self-management techniques for patients to learn over extended periods of time. Those with Type 2 diabetes often use oral therapies too (such as chlorpropamide, rosiglitazone, and Glucophage) to control blood glucose levels.

In gestational diabetes, women experience carbohydrate intolerance during the onset of pregnancy and, as a result, a failure to compensate with increased insulin secretion (Cheung, 2009). Pharmacology for this presentation brings with it a different set of guidelines and factors; medications must be deemed safe for the woman in controlling blood sugars while synchronously not harming the unborn fetus (Coustan, 2007). Commonly prescribed treatments, when indicated beyond baseline efforts to control blood sugar through diet and physical activity, include glyburide tablets and glyburide.

Individual Approaches

Several evidence-based approaches have addressed the psychosocial and lifestyle health habits of patients living with diabetes. Motivational interviewing (MI) is a common and effective way to help patients and family members find and access (and mobilize) motivational factors in their lives around chronic illness and disease management (Miller & Rollnick, 2012). Principles such as reflective listening, open-ended questions, motivational statements, guiding behaviors, and change talk can empower patients to explore solution-based options in practice (Rubak, Sandbaek, Lauritzen, & Christensen, 2005; West, DiLillo, Bursac, Gore, & Greene, 2007). MI has been used with patients with diabetes to help explore areas of change regarding a host of health habits and psychosocial challenges. Management of lifestyle habits (e.g., physical activity) and thought processes for exploring solutions have shown strong evidence for beneficent change (Rubak et al., 2005; West et al., 2007). For example, researchers have found strong support for MI with adolescents diagnosed with diabetes (Channon, Smith, & Gregory, 2003).

Cognitive behavioral therapy (CBT) represents another way to help patients learn effective ways of managing a variety of underlying issues that can make diabetes management difficult (e.g., depression, anxiety, weight gain). This, in conjunction with psychotropic medications, has been associated with improvements in metabolic control (Hamdy et al., 2008). Behavioral therapy, too, has demonstrated success in psychological adjustment around specific symptoms associated with diabetes. Patients also learn better coping skills and strategies to relate to family members and others around the disease (Wysocki et al., 2000). As MeFTs employ these methods with families (i.e., not just individual patients), they work to create shared mutual understandings regarding respective members' thoughts and narratives about disease management foci, alongside shared ownership for indicated behaviors in self-care.

Family Approaches

Family-based approaches to treatment have also been utilized by healthcare professionals around a number of issues in diabetes care. Researchers have shown strong support for parental involvement in treatment planning and disease management with children and adolescents (Wysocki et al., 2008). Systemic interventions that have incorporated a collaborative approach to patients' health have shown better disease- and family-related outcomes (Anderson, Brackett, Ho, & Laffel, Anderson, Brackett, Ho, & Laffel, 1999; Laffel et al., 2003; Peyrot et al., 2005). Integrating psychoeducation through family visits helps to promote co-ownership of new knowledge and joint problem solving (Delamater et al., 2001; Hood, Butler, Anderson, & Laffel, 2007). MedFTs should encourage family-based visits in tertiary care settings, where multiple perspectives of the disease can be processed and a systemic treatment approach to help the patient can be constructed. With Joe and Alice, for example, Justin engaged the couple from the moment of referral so as to mitigate Joe's sense of isolation, increase Alice's involvement, and facilitate the couple's sense of "being in this together."

Although less research has examined clinical interventions for couples living with diabetes (i.e., adult unions wherein one partner has the disease), we know that the quality of relationships per se and the health of the respective partners that inhibit these relationships are highly correlated (Trief et al., 2011). Partners of patients with diabetes often experience stress in trying to support their loved one's efforts to effectively manage the disease while at the same time finding ways to attend to and/or increase the quality of the relationship itself (Revenson, Abraído-Lanza, Majerovitz, & Jordan, 2005; August, Rook, Franks, & Parris Stephens, 2013). Psychoeducational interventions for couples that target diabetes care can offer couples new coping skills and strategies in co-owning disease management and achieving better health-related outcomes, and couples who demonstrate higher marital satisfaction and stronger tolerance for stress tend to evidence better health across both partners (Gilden, Hendryx, Clar, Casia, & Singh, 1992; Trief et al., 2003).

Community Approaches

The larger communities that patients and families reside within (e.g., neighborhood, faith, or cultural groups) represent a potentially powerful resource in diabetes management. Scholars and community members who have advanced projects informed by Community-based Participatory Research (CBPR) methods, for example, have evidenced considerable promise in improving the health of citizens and families alike (Hacker, 2013; Minkler & Wallerstein, 2011; Mendenhall, Doherty, Berge, Fauth, & Tremblay, 2013). In CBPR, all participants (e.g., primary care providers, MedFTs, patients, spouses) work together as collaborators across every stage of intervention design, implementation, and evaluation. This is different than conventional top-down, hierarchical methods of care wherein patients and families function in relatively passive roles (i.e., as recipients of services). Instead, everyone works together in the context of flattened hierarchies, with each contributing expertise to a larger mosaic of understanding. Research has demonstrated strong support for CBPR with American Indians (Mendenhall et al., 2010, 2012; Mendenhall et al., 2015) and other minority groups (Horwitz et al., 2009).

Community education and support groups also serve as a valuable opportunity for individuals seeking interpersonal connections and encouragement in managing diabetes. Patients at any stage of the disease can benefit from increased social support and knowledge from others with similar life circumstances. Research across a broad range of formats has evidenced support for these initiatives (e.g., Collinsworth, Vulimiri, Schmidt, & Snead, 2013; Philis-Tsimikas et al., 2004; Ramachandran et al., 2006; Venditti & Kramer, 2012). As Justin's work with Joe and Alice continues, for example, connecting them to others who share in similar struggles (and successes) could go a long way in terms of accessing support. Joe could gain from the wisdom of other patients like him who have figured out ways to stick with dietary or exercise regimens. Alice could learn from other spouses about the different ways to cope with stress while still working to support her husband. Both of them could share similar wisdom to others down the road.

Conclusion

The visibility of Endocrinology—and the integrated behavioral healthcare teams within this medical specialty—is growing. As more individuals continue to be diagnosed with all types of diabetes, for example, MedFTs' contributions to care models that attend holistically to patients' and families' well-being will grow in synchrony. MedFTs offer services (and perspectives) that address a number of underlying psychosocial features of endocrine disorders, alongside ways for patients and families to coordinate care with other professionals as they learn how to cope with (and effectively manage) these illnesses. As we do this, our team-based approaches in tertiary care will serve to connect the disciplinary dots between care provides who—when working together—offer a culmination of care that is more than the sum of its parts (Cavanaugh, White, & Rothman, 2007; Coleman, Austin, Brach, & Wagner, 2009).

Reflection Questions
1. As a MedFT working in an Endocrinology clinic, are you practicing what you preach? Can you, with integrity, engage patients and families toward a healthy lifestyle (e.g., good diet, regular physical activity) unless you are "walking the walk" as well?
2. What ethnic and/or cultural considerations are important for you to think about when working with patients and families who live with endocrine disorders? How might core tenets of some patients'/families' culture(s) influence decision-making in relation to seeking care and treatment options for endocrine-based health conditions?
3. After reading this chapter, what areas of care do you need to learn more about and/or increase skill within in order to provider better care?

Glossary of Important Terms in Endocrinology and Diabetes Care

A1c A laboratory test that shows the average amount of glucose in a patient's blood. This is usually measured every 3–6 months.
Blood glucose The principal sugar found in the blood; it serves as a key source of energy.
Diabetic ketoacidosis A serious condition in which very high blood glucose levels are detected, along with a severe deficiency of insulin in the body. This results in a breakdown of body fat for energy and accumulation of ketones in the blood (making it acidic). This condition can lead to diabetic coma or even death.
Glycemic index A rank order of foods based on the food's effect on one's blood glucose levels.
Impaired fasting glucose (IFG) A condition in which a patient's fasting blood glucose level is consistently elevated above what is considered normal. This is often called "prediabetes," insofar as blood sugar levels are high (100–125 mg/dL) but not yet high enough to indicate a diabetes diagnosis.
Insulin A peptide hormone produced in the pancreas; it regulates the metabolism of carbohydrates and fats by promoting glucose absorption from the blood to skeletal muscles and fat tissue and/or by enabling fat to be stored (rather than used for energy).

Lantus A common prescription medication approved to treat Type 1 or Type 2 diabetes; it acts as a long-acting form of insulin that is not human-made.
Metabolic syndrome Refers to several conditions that raise a patient's risk for heart disease, diabetes, and/or stroke. Said conditions include obesity, diabetes, prediabetes, hypertension, and/or high lipid levels.
Metformin An oral medicine that is used for Type 2 diabetes; it reduces the amount of glucose produced by the liver and helps the body respond better to insulin.

Additional Resources

Literature

Barnard, K., & Lloyd, C. (2012). *Psychology and diabetes care: A practical guide*. New York, NY: Springer.
Becker, G., & Goldfine, A. (2015). *The first year: Type 2 diabetes: An essential guide for the newly diagnosed*. Boston, MA: Da Capo Press.
Codario, R. (2011). *Type 2 diabetes, pre-diabetes and the metabolic syndrome*. New York, NY: Springer.
Hawthorne, G. (Ed.). (2011). *Diabetes care for the older patient: A practical handbook*. New York, NY: Springer Science & Business Media.
Hieronymous, L., & Geil, P. (2006). *101 tips for raising health kids with diabetes*. Alexandria, VA: American Diabetes Association.
Obrosova, I., Stevens, M., & Yorek, M. (2014). *Studies in diabetes*. New York, NY: Springer Science & Business Media.
Unger, J. (2013). *Diabetes management in primary care*. New York, NY: Lippincott Williams & Wilkins.

Measures/Instruments

Audit of Diabetes-Dependent Quality of Life. http://academicdepartments.musc.edu/family_medicine/rcmar/addqol.htm
CDC Pre-Diabetes Screening Test. http://www.cdc.gov/diabetes/prevention/pdf/prediabetestest.pdf
Diabetes Self-Management Questionnaire. http://www.ketteringhealth.org/diabetes/pdf/questionnaireKett.pdf
Diabetes Health Profile. http://www.diabetesprofile.com/63/133/dhp-18
Diabetes Quality of Life Measure. http://apntoolkit.mcmaster.ca/index.php?option=com_content&view=article&id=270:diabetes-quality-of-life-dqol-questionnaire&Itemid=62

Dyadic Coping Inventory. http://www.academia.edu/12572622/Dyadic_Coping_Inventory_DCI

Questionnaire on Stress in Diabetic Patients-Revised. http://academicdepartments.musc.edu/family_medicine/rcmar/qsdr.htm

Organizations/Associations

American Association of Diabetes Educators. www.diabeteseducator.org
American Diabetes Association. www.diabetes.org
Collaborative Family Healthcare Association. www.cfha.net
International Diabetes Federation. www.idf.org
Juvenile Diabetes Research Foundation. www.jdrf.org

References[1]

Accardi, G., Caruso, C., Colonna-Romano, G., Camarda, C., Monastero, R., & Candore, G. (2012). Can Alzheimer disease be a form of type 3 diabetes? *Rejuvenation Research, 15*, 217–221. https://doi.org/10.1089/rej.2011.1289

American Association of Diabetes Educators. (2015). Cultural considerations in diabetes education. *AADE Practice Synopsis*, July Issue. Retrieved from https://www.diabeteseducator.org/docs/default-source/default-document-library/cultural-considerations-in-diabetes-management.pdf?sfvrsn=0

*American Diabetes Association. (2016). *Diabetes basics*. Retrieved from http://www.diabetes.org/diabetes-basics/statistics/

American Psychological Association. (2016). *Patient Health Questionnaire* (PHQ-9 & PHQ-2). Retrieved from http://www.apa.org/pi/about/publications/caregivers/practice-settings/assessment/tools/patient-health.aspx

Anderson, B. J., Brackett, J., Ho, J., & Laffel, L. M. (1999). An office-based intervention to maintain parent-adolescent teamwork in diabetes management: Impact on parent involvement, family conflict, and subsequent glycemic control. *Diabetes Care, 22*, 713–721. https://doi.org/10.2337/diacare.22.5.713

Anderson, R. J., Freedland, K. E., Clouse, R. E., & Lustman, P. J. (2001). The prevalence of comorbid depression in adults with diabetes a meta-analysis. *Diabetes Care, 24*, 1069–1078. https://doi.org/10.2337/diacare.24.6.1069

*August, K. J., Rook, K. S., Franks, M. M., & Parris Stephens, M. A. (2013). Spouses' involvement in their partners' diabetes management: Associations with spouse stress and perceived marital quality. *Journal of Family Psychology, 27*, 712–721. https://doi.org/10.1037/a0034181.

*Barnard, K., & Lloyd, C. (2012). *Psychology and diabetes care: A practical guide*. New York, NY: Springer.

*Becker, G., & Goldfine, A. (2015). *The first year: Type 2 diabetes: An essential guide for the newly diagnosed*. Boston, MA: Da Capo Press.

Blount, A. (2003). Integrated primary care: Organizing the evidence. *Families, Systems, & Health, 21*, 121–133. https://doi.org/10.1037/1091-7527.21.2.121

---

[1] Note: References that are prefaced with an asterisk are recommended readings.

Bradley, C. (2013). *Handbook of psychology and diabetes: A guide to psychological measurement in diabetes research and practice*. New York, NY: Routledge.

Cavanaugh, K. L., White, R. O., & Rothman, R. L. (2007). Exploring disease management programs for diabetes mellitus. *Disease Management & Health Outcomes, 15*, 73–81. https://doi.org/10.2165/00115677-200715020-00002

Centers for Disease Control and Prevention. (2014). *National diabetes statistics report*. Retrieved from http://www.cdc.gov/diabetes/data/statistics/2014statisticsreport.html

Channon, S., Smith, V. J., & Gregory, J. W. (2003). A pilot study of motivational interviewing in adolescents with diabetes. *Archives of Disease in Childhood, 88*, 680–683. https://doi.org/10.1136/adc.88.8.680

Cheung, N. W. (2009). The management of gestational diabetes. *Vascular Health and Risk Management, 5*, 153–164. https://doi.org/10.2147/vhrm.s3405

Cogan, F. (2008). The honeymoon period in type 1 diabetes. *Health Central*, December Issue. Retrieved from http://www.healthcentral.com/diabetes/c/651280/50845/honeymoon-period/

Coleman, K., Austin, B., Brach, C., & Wagner, E. (2009). Evidence on the chronic care model in the new millennium. *Health Affairs, 28*, 75–85. https://doi.org/10.1377/hlthaff.28.1.75

*Collinsworth, A. W., Vulimiri, M., Schmidt, K. L., & Snead, C. A. (2013). Effectiveness of a community health worker-led diabetes self-management education program and implications for CHW involvement in care coordination strategies. *Diabetes Educator, 39*, 792–799. https://doi.org/10.1177/0145721713504470.

Cook, C., Seifert, K., Hull, B., Hovan, M., Charles, J., Miller-Cage, V., ... Littman, S. (2009). Inpatient to outpatient transfer of diabetes care: Planning for an effective hospital discharge. *Endocrine Practice, 15*, 263–269. https://doi.org/10.4158/ep.15.3.263

Counihan, C., & Van Esterik, P. (2012). *Food and culture* (3rd ed.). New York, NY: Routledge.

Coustan, D. R. (2007). Pharmacological management of gestational diabetes: An overview. *Diabetes Care, 30*(Suppl. 2), S206–S208. https://doi.org/10.2337/dc07-s217

de la Monte, S. M. (2012). Contributions of brain insulin resistance and deficiency in amyloid-elated neurodegeneration in Alzheimer's disease. *Drugs, 72*, 49–66. https://doi.org/10.2165/11597760-000000000-00000

Delamater, A., Jacobson, A., Anderson, B., Cox, D., Fisher, L., Lustman, P., Rubin, R., & Wysocki, T. (2001). Psychosocial therapies in diabetes: Report of the psychosocial therapies working group. *Diabetes Care, 24*, 1286–1292. https://doi.org/10.2337/diacare.24.7.1286

Doherty, W., McDaniel, S., & Baird, M. (1996). *Five levels of primary care/behavioral healthcare collaboration*. Behavioral HealthCare Tomorrow, Oct, 25–28. Retrieved from http://www1.genesishealth.com/pdf/mh_reynolds_resource_dohertybaird_051110.pdf

Egede, L. E., Zheng, D., & Simpson, K. (2002). Comorbid depression is associated with increased health care use and expenditures in individuals with diabetes. *Diabetes Care, 25*, 464–470. https://doi.org/10.2337/diacare.25.3.464

Engel, G. L. (1977). The need for a new medical model: A challenge for biomedicine. *Science, 196*, 129–136. https://doi.org/10.1126/science.847460

Engel, G. L. (1980). The clinical application of the biopsychosocial model. *American Journal of Psychiatry, 137*, 535–544. https://doi.org/10.1176/ajp.137.5.535

Fisher, L., Hessler, D. M., Polonsky, W. H., & Mullan, J. (2012). When is diabetes distress clinically meaningful? Establishing cut points for the Diabetes Distress Scale. *Diabetes Care, 35*, 259–264. https://doi.org/10.2337/dc11-1572

Foraida, M. I., DeVita, M. A., Braithwaite, R. S., Stuart, S. A., Brooks, M. M., & Simmons, R. L. (2003). Improving the utilization of medical crisis teams (Condition C) at an urban tertiary care hospital. *Journal of Critical Care, 18*, 87–94. https://doi.org/10.1053/jcrc.2003.50002

Garber, A., Abrahamson, M., Barzilay, J., Blonde, L., Bloomgarden, Z., Bush, M., ... Grunberger, G. (2013). AACE comprehensive diabetes management algorithm. *Endocrine Practice, 19*, 327–336. Retrieved from http://www.goodsamim.com/ resprog/internalmedicine/files/diabetes/AACE_2013_glycemic-control-algorithm[1].pdf

Gilden, J. L., Hendryx, M. S., Clar, S., Casia, C., & Singh, S. P. (1992). Diabetes support groups improve health care of older diabetic patients. *Journal of the American Geriatrics Society, 40,* 147–150. https://doi.org/10.1111/j.1532-5415.1992.tb01935.x

Goodman, H. M. (2010). *Basic medical endocrinology*. Boston, MA: Academic Press.

Grone, O., & Barcia-Barbero, M. (2001). Integrated care. *Journal of Integrated Care, 1,* 1–15. https://doi.org/10.5334/ijic.28

Groop, P. H., Thomas, M. C., Moran, J. L., Waden, J., Thorn, L. M., Makinen, V. P., ... Forsblom, C. (2009). The presence and severity of chronic kidney disease predicts all-cause mortality in type 1 diabetes. *Diabetes, 58,* 1651–1658. https://doi.org/10.2337/db08-1543

Gulabani, M., John, M., & Isaac, R. (2009). Knowledge of diabetes, its treatment and complications amongst diabetic patients in a tertiary care hospital. *Indian Journal of Community Medicine, 33,* 204–206. https://doi.org/10.4103/0970-0218.42068

Hacker, K. (2013). *Community-based participatory research*. Thousand Oaks, CA: Sage.

Hamdy, O., Goebel-Fabbri, A., Carver, C., Arathuzik, G., Shahar, J., Capelson, R., ... Mentzelopoulos, V. (2008). Why WAIT program: A novel model for diabetes weight management in routine clinical practice. *Obesity Management, 4,* 176–183. https://doi.org/10.1089/obe.2008.0206

*Hawthorne, G. (Ed.). (2011). *Diabetes care for the older patient: A practical handbook*. New York, NY: Springer.

Heisler, M. (2007). *Diabetes prevention and management: The challenge of cultural differences*. Medscape Diabetes & Endocrinology, July Issue. Retrieved from http://www.medscape.org/viewarticle/540922

*Hieronymous, L., & Geil, P. (2006). *101 tips for raising health kids with diabetes*. Alexandria, VA: American Diabetes Association.

Hodgson, J., Lamson, A., Mendenhall, T., & Tyndall, L. (2014). Introduction to medical family therapy: Advanced applications. In J. Hodgson, A. Lamson, T. Mendenhall, and D. Crane (Eds.), *Medical family therapy: Advanced applications* (pp. 1–9). New York, NY: Springer.

Holt, R. I. G., Peveler, R. C., & Byrne, C. D. (2004). Schizophrenia, the metabolic syndrome and diabetes. *Diabetic Medicine, 21,* 515–523. https://doi.org/10.1111/j.1464-5491.2004.01199.x

Hood, K. K., Butler, D. A., Anderson, B. J., & Laffel, L. M. (2007). Updated and revised Diabetes Family Conflict Scale. *Diabetes Care, 30,* 1764–1769. https://doi.org/10.2337/dc06-2358

Horwitz, C., Robinson, M., & Seifer, S. (2009). Community-based participatory research from the margins to the mainstream: Are researchers prepared? *Circulation, 119,* 2633–2642. https://doi.org/10.1161/CIRCULATIONAHA.107.729863

Inzucchi, S. E., Bergenstal, R. M., Buse, J. B., Diamant, M., Ferrannini, E., Nauck, M., ... Matthews, D. R. (2012). Management of hyperglycaemia in type 2 diabetes: A patient-centered approach. *Diabetologia, 55,* 1577–1596. https://doi.org/10.1007/s00125-012-2534-0

Jefferies, H., & Chan, K. K. (2004). Multidisciplinary team working: Is it both holistic and effective? *International Journal of Gynecological Cancer, 14,* 210–211. https://doi.org/10.1111/j.1048-891X.2004.014201.x

Katon, W. J., Simon, G., Russo, J., Von Korff, M., Lin, E. H., Ludman, E., ... Bush, T. (2004). Quality of depression care in a population-based sample of patients with diabetes and major depression. *Medical Care, 42,* 1222–1229. https://doi.org/10.1097/00005650-200412000-00009

Laffel, L. M., Connell, A., Vangsness, L., Goebel-Fabbri, A., Mansfield, A., & Anderson, B. J. (2003). General quality of life in youth with type 1 diabetes: Relationship to patient management and diabetes-specific family conflict. *Diabetes Care, 26,* 3067–3073. https://doi.org/10.2337/diacare.26.11.3067

Liau, K. H., Aung, K. T., Chua, N., Ho, C. K., Chan, C. Y., Kow, A., ... Chia, S. J. (2010). Outcome of a strategy to reduce surgical site infection in a tertiary-care hospital. *Surgical Infections, 11,* 151–159. Retrieved from http://online.liebertpub.com/doi/abs/10.1089/sur.2008.081

Lavin, N. (2012). *Manual of endocrinology and metabolism*. Baltimore, MD: Lippincott Williams & Wilkins.

Levetan, C. S., Salas, J. R., Wilets, I. F., & Zumoff, B. (1995). Impact of endocrine and diabetes team consultation on hospital length of stay for patients with diabetes. *American Journal of Medicine, 99*, 22–28. https://doi.org/10.1016/S0002-9343(99)80100-4

Löwe, B., Wahl, I., Rose, M., Spitzer, C., Glaesmer, H., Wingenfeld, K., ... Brähler, E. (2010). A 4-item measure of depression and anxiety: Validation and standardization of the Patient Health Questionnaire-4 (PHQ-4) in the general population. *Journal of Affective Disorders, 122*, 86–95. https://doi.org/10.1016/j.jad.2009.06.019

Melmed, S., Polonsky, K. S., Larsen, P. R., & Kronenberg, H. M. (2015). *Williams textbook of endocrinology*. Philadelphia, PA: Elsevier Health Sciences.

Mendenhall, T. J., Berge, J. M., Harper, P., GreenCrow, B., LittleWalker, N., WhiteEagle, S., & BrownOwl, S. (2010). The Family Education Diabetes Series (FEDS): Community-based participatory research with a Midwestern American Indian community. *Nursing Inquiry, 17*, 359–372. https://doi.org/10.1111/j.1440-1800.2010.00508.x

*Mendenhall, T., Doherty, W., Berge, J., Fauth, J., & Tremblay, G. (2013). Community-based participatory research: Advancing integrated health care through novel partnerships. In M. Talen and A. Valeras (Eds.), *Integrated behavioral health in primary care: Evaluating the evidence, identifying the essentials* (pp. 99–130). New York, NY: Springer.

Mendenhall, T., Gagner, N., & Hunt, Q. (2015). A call to engage youth in health research. *Families, Systems, & Health, 33*, 410–412. https://doi.org/10.1037/fsh0000163

Mendenhall, T. J., Seal, K. L., GreenCrow, B. A., LittleWalker, K. N., & BrownOwl, S. A. (2012). The Family Education Diabetes Series: Improving health in an urban-dwelling American Indian community. *Qualitative Health Research, 22*, 1524–1534. https://doi.org/10.1177/1049732312457469

Miller, W. R., & Rollnick, S. (2012). *Motivational interviewing: Helping people change*. New York, NY: Guilford Press.

Minkler, M., & Wallerstein, N. (Eds.). (2011). *Community-based participatory research for health: From process to outcomes*. New York, NY: John Wiley & Sons.

Mitchell, P., Wynia, M., Golden, R., McNellis, B., Okun, S., Webb, C. E., ... Von Kohorn, I. (2012). *Core principles & values of effective team-based health care*. Washington, DC: Institute of Medicine.

Mullen, D., & Funderburk, J. (2013). Implementing clinical interventions in integrated behavioral health settings: Best practices and essential elements. In M. Talen and A. Valeras (Eds.), *Integrated behavioral health in primary care* (pp. 273–298). London, England: Springer.

Nam, S., Chesla, C., Stotts, N. A., Kroon, L., & Janson, S. L. (2011). Barriers to diabetes management: Patient and provider factors. *Diabetes Research and Clinical Practice, 93*, 1–9. https://doi.org/10.1016/j.diabres.2011.02.002

National Adrenal Disease Foundation (2016). *Adrenal diseases*. Retrieved from http://www.nadf.us/adrenal-diseases

Nelson, R. J. (2005). *An introduction to behavioral endocrinology* (3rd ed.). Sunderland, MA: Sinauer Associates.

*Obrosova, I., Stevens, M., & Yorek, M. (2014). *Studies in diabetes*. New York, NY: Springer.

Oud, M. J., & Meyboom-de Jong, B. (2009). Somatic diseases in patients with schizophrenia in general practice: Their prevalence and health care. *BMC Family Practice, 10*, 1–9. https://doi.org/10.1186/1471-2296-10-32

Patterson, C. C., Dahlquist, G. F., Harjutsalo, V., Joner, G., Feltbower, R. G., Svensson, J., ... Rosenbauer, J. (2007). Early mortality in EURODIAB population-based cohorts of type 1 diabetes diagnosed in childhood since 1989. *Diabetologia, 50*, 2439–2442. https://doi.org/10.1007/s00125-007-0824-8

Peek, C. J. (2008). Planning care in the clinical, operational, and financial worlds. In R. Kessler and D. Stafford (Eds.), *Collaborative Medicine Case Studies* (pp. 25–38). New York, NY: Springer. https://doi.org/10.1007/978-0-387-76894-6_3

Peyrot, M., Rubin, R. R., Lauritzen, T., Snoek, F. J., Matthews, D. R., & Skovlund, S. E. (2005). Psychosocial problems and barriers to improved diabetes management: Results of the Cross

National Diabetes Attitudes, Wishes and Needs (DAWN) study. *Diabetic Medicine, 22,* 1379–1385. https://doi.org/10.1111/j.1464-5491.2005.01644.x

Philis-Tsimikas, A., Walker, C., Rivard, L., Talavera, G., Reimann, J. O., Salmon, M., & Araujo, R. (2004). Improvement in diabetes care of underinsured patients enrolled in Project Dulce: A community-based, culturally appropriate, nurse case management and peer education diabetes care model. *Diabetes Care, 27,* 110–115. https://doi.org/10.2337/diacare.27.1.110

Raile, K., Galler, A., Hofer, S., Herbst, A., Dunstheimer, D., Busch, P., & Holl, R. W. (2007). Diabetic nephropathy in 27,805 children, adolescents, and adults with type 1 diabetes: Effect of diabetes duration, A1C, hypertension, dyslipidemia, diabetes onset, and sex. *Diabetes Care, 30,* 2523–2528. https://doi.org/10.2337/dc07-0282

Ramachandran, A., Snehalatha, C., Mary, S., Mukesh, B., Bhaskar, A. D., & Vijay, V. (2006). The Indian Diabetes Prevention Programme shows that lifestyle modification and metformin prevent type 2 diabetes in Asian Indian subjects with impaired glucose tolerance (IDPP-1). *Diabetologia, 49,* 289–297. https://doi.org/10.1007/s00125-005-0097-z

*Rajasekharan, D., Kulkarni, V., Unnikrishnan, B., Kumar, N., Holla, R., & Thapar, R. (2015). Self-care activities among patients with diabetes attending a tertiary care hospital in Mangalore Karnataka, India. *Annals of Medical and Health Sciences Research, 5*(1), 59–64. https://doi.org/10.4103/2141-9248.149791.

Revenson, T. A., Abraído-Lanza, A. F., Majerovitz, S. D., & Jordan, C. (2005). Couples coping with chronic illness: What's gender got to do with it? In T. Revenson, K. Kayser, and G. Bodenmann (Eds.), *Couples coping with stress: Emerging perspectives on dyadic coping* (pp. 137–156). Washington, DC: American Psychological Association.

Rivera, E. J., Goldin, A., Fulmer, N., Tavares, R., Wands, J. R., & de la Monte, S. M. (2005). Insulin and insulin-like growth factor expression and function deteriorate with progression of Alzheimer's disease: Link to brain reductions in acetylcholine. *Journal of Alzheimer's Disease, 8,* 247–268. https://doi.org/10.3233/JAD-2005-8304

Rubak, S., Sandbaek, A., Lauritzen, T., & Christensen, B. (2005). Motivational interviewing: A systematic review and meta-analysis. *British Journal of General Practice, 55,* 305–312. Retrieved from https://www.ncbi.nlm.nih.gov/pmc/articles/PMC1463134/

Savage, M. W., Mah, P. M., Weetman, A. P., & Newell-Price, J. (2004). Endocrine emergencies. *Postgraduate Medical Journal, 80*(947), 506–515. https://doi.org/10.1136/pgmj.2003.013474

Seal, K., Blum, M., Didericksen, K., Mendenhall, T., Gagner, N., GreenCrow, B., . . . Benton, K. (2016). The East Metro American Indian Diabetes Initiative: Engaging indigenous men in the reclaiming of health and spirituality through community-based participatory research. *Health Education Research & Development, 4,* 1–8. https://doi.org/10.4172/2380-5439.1000152

Seid, M., Sobo, E. J., Gelhard, L. R., & Varni, J. W. (2004). Parents' reports of barriers to care for children with special health care needs: Development and validation of the barriers to care questionnaire. *Ambulatory Pediatrics, 4,* 323–331. https://doi.org/10.1367/a03-198r.1

Sonino, N. (2008). The need for rehabilitation teams in endocrinology. *Expert Review of Endocrinology & Metabolism, 3,* 291–293. https://doi.org/10.1586/17446651.3.3.291

Steen, E., Terry, B. M., J Rivera, E., Cannon, J. L., Neely, T. R., Tavares, R., ... de la Monte, S. M. (2005). Impaired insulin and insulin-like growth factor expression and signaling mechanisms in Alzheimer's disease–is this type 3 diabetes? *Journal of Alzheimer's Disease, 7,* 63–80. https://doi.org/10.3233/JAD-2005-7107

Stone, M. A., Wilkinson, J. C., Charpentier, G., Clochard, N., Grassi, G., Lindblad, U., et al. (2010). Evaluation and comparison of guidelines for the management of people with type 2 diabetes from eight European countries. *Diabetes Research and Clinical Practice, 87,* 252–260. https://doi.org/10.1016/j.diabres.2009.10.020

Suzanne, M., & Wands, J. R. (2008). Alzheimer's disease is type 3 diabetes: Evidence reviewed. *Journal of Diabetes Science and Technology, 2,* 1101–1113. https://doi.org/10.1177/193229680800200619

Talen, M., & Valeras, A. (2013). *Integrated behavioral health in primary care.* New York, NY: Springer.

Trief, P. M., Sandberg, J., Greenberg, R. P., Graff, K., Castronova, N., Yoon, M., & Weinstock, R. S. (2003). Describing support: A qualitative study of couples living with diabetes. *Families, Systems, & Health, 21*, 57–67. https://doi.org/10.1037/h0089502

Trief, P., Sandberg, J. G., Ploutz-Snyder, R., Brittain, R., Cibula, D., Scales, K., & Weinstock, R. S. (2011). Promoting couples collaboration in type 2 diabetes: The diabetes support project pilot data. *Families, Systems, & Health, 29*, 253–261. https://doi.org/10.1037/a0024564

Tyndall, L. E., Hodgson, J. L., Lamson, A. L., White, M., & Knight, S. M. (2012). Medical family therapy: Charting a course in competencies. *Contemporary Family Therapy, 34*, 171–186. https://doi.org/10.1007/s10591-012-9191-9

*Unger, J. (2013). *Diabetes management in primary care*. New York, NY: Lippincott Williams & Wilkins.

*Venditti, E. M., & Kramer, M. K. (2012). Necessary components for lifestyle modification interventions to reduce diabetes risk. *Current Diabetes Reports, 12*, 138–146. https://doi.org/10.1007/s11892-012-0256-9.

Verlato, G., Muggeo, M., Bonora, E., Corbellini, M., Bressan, F., & de Marco, R. (1996). Attending the diabetes center is associated with increased 5-year survival probability of diabetic patients: The Verona Diabetes Study. *Diabetes Care, 19*, 211-213. https://doi.org/10.2337/diacare.19.3.211

West, D., DiLillo, V., Gore, S., & Greene, P. (2007). Motivational interviewing improves weight loss in women with type 2 diabetes. *Diabetes Care, 30*, 108101087. https://doi.org/10.2337/dc06-1966

Willens, D., Cripps, R., Wilson, A., Wolff, K., & Rothman, R. (2011). Interdisciplinary team care for diabetic patients by primary care physicians, advanced practice nurses, and clinical pharmacists. *Clinical Diabetes, 29*, 60–68. https://doi.org/10.2337/diaclin.29.2.60

Wright, L. M., Watson, W. L., & Bell, J. M. (1996). *Beliefs: The heart of healing in families and illness*. New York, NY: Basic Books.

Wrobel, J. S., Charns, M. P., Diehr, P., Robbins, J. M., Reiber, G. E., Bonacker, K. M., ... Pogach, L. (2003). The relationship between provider coordination and diabetes-related foot outcomes. *Diabetes Care, 26*, 3042–3047. https://doi.org/10.2337/diacare.26.11.3042

Wysocki, T., Harris, M. A., Greco, P., Bubb, J., Danda, C. E., Harvey, L. M., ... White, N. H. (2000). Randomized, controlled trial of behavior therapy for families of adolescents with insulin-dependent diabetes mellitus. *Journal of Pediatric Psychology, 25*, 23–33. https://doi.org/10.1093/jpepsy/25.1.23

Wysocki, T., Nansel, T. R., Holmbeck, G. N., Chen, R., Laffel, L., Anderson, B. J., & Weissberg-Benchell, J. (2008). Collaborative involvement of primary and secondary caregivers: Associations with youths' diabetes outcomes. *Journal of Pediatric Psychology, 34*, 869–881. https://doi.org/10.1093/jpepsy/jsn13

Chapter 12
Medical Family Therapy in Alcohol and Drug Treatment

Kristy Soloski and Jaclyn Cravens Pickens

The prevalence rates of licit and illicit substances in the United States of America suggest that medical family therapists (MedFTs) and other behavioral health providers will undoubtedly encounter individuals or families struggling with substance use. In any given year, around half of Americans use alcohol, a quarter are binge alcohol users (i.e., five or more drinks on a single occasion), and about 6.5% are heavy alcohol users (i.e., those who binge 5 or more days in a 30-day period) (Substance Abuse and Mental Health Services Administration 2014). For illicit drugs, around 9.4% of Americans are current users, the majority of which are using marijuana (SAMHSA, 2014). A MedFT involved in an integrated behavioral healthcare (IBHC) team to treat alcohol, and drug issues will need to be aware of the complex physiological and social effects that substances can have, as well as the interplay of these factors on the disorder. In some cases, patients may see the use as benign and underreport it, and it may have unexpected effects on the patient or family system that are not immediately recognizable. Other patients may present for treatment for a different problem while at the same time having an undiagnosed or untreated substance use problem. MedFTs are crucial members of treatment teams who can attend to these intricacies.

Although alcohol and drug issues can present and be treated across a variety of different settings, treatment will require an IBHC team to achieve the best results. There is a complex interplay between substance use and physiological, social, and psychological outcomes. Alcohol and drugs act on the body's central nervous system (CNS) (Inaba & Cohen, 2014), and with repetitive use they can alter the body's homeostasis—which can potentially lead to physical or psychological dependency (American Psychiatric Association [APA], 2013). Excessive substance use can

---

K. Soloski (✉) · J. C. Pickens
Department of Community, Family, and Addiction Sciences, Texas Tech University, Lubbock, TX, USA
e-mail: Kristy.Soloski@ttu.edu

© Springer International Publishing AG, part of Springer Nature 2018
T. Mendenhall et al. (eds.), *Clinical Methods in Medical Family Therapy*,
Focused Issues in Family Therapy, https://doi.org/10.1007/978-3-319-68834-3_12

induce mental disorders, and disordered use can cause problems within the work, family, or other social systems (APA, 2013). The etiology of problematic substance use, sometimes referred to as addiction, has neurobiological, genetic, psychological, and social bases (Shaffer et al., 2004). Therefore, treatment for alcohol and drug problems is strengthened through the integration of multiple professionals (e.g., primary care providers [PCPs], social workers, probation officers, sponsors) while incorporating a biopsychosocial-spiritual (BPSS) (Engel, 1977, 1980; Griffiths, 2005; Wright, Watson, & Bell, 1996) and family systems approach (Gruber & Taylor, 2006). This integration is especially crucial, and even an ethical requirement, when the substance use has resulted in physical dependency or other physiological effects.

Throughout this chapter, we will discuss the collaboration of professionals in a variety of different settings. Some settings will have the IBHC team located on site; however, because of the nature of this particular disorder, in most cases at least some members of the team (e.g., probation officers) will not be located on site. It is our belief that the MedFT can, and should, successfully integrate a team approach for treatment of substance use problems in a variety of settings. To display how the practice of MedFT in alcohol and drug treatment is relevant to even patients not presenting for substance use issues, and outside of an integrated setting, we will share an example case study of Dustin and Elaina. They came to a university training clinic for couple services. In this training clinic, therapy rooms have one-way mirrors to allow for live supervision of cases. In this setting, it is standard practice for students to take mid-session breaks to receive feedback and direction from the supervisor to integrate during the remainder of the session. I (KS) was the supervisor on the case and Tom was the MedFT.

Clinical Vignette
[Note: This vignette is a compilation of cases that represent alcohol and drug treatment. All patients' names and/or identifying information have been changed to maintain confidentiality.]

Prior to the first session, my supervisee Tom came to me (KS) to consult about what areas he should be assessing in a new intake. He had been assigned a couple case, Elaina and Dustin, who called to request an appointment due to communication issues. In the intake, Elaina reported past addiction to drugs and present alcohol addiction that has affected the family, but that primarily the couple was interested in services for their relationship. I discussed areas of assessment with Tom, including identifying symptoms for a substance use disorder and assessing how much and how often the present alcohol use was and past drug use.

During the assessment, Dustin and Elaina reported that Dustin was drinking daily and having symptoms of withdrawal when he stopped use for several hours. He even required a drink when he got up in the morning. Dustin reported that he was vomiting up blood some mornings when he started to experience the withdrawal symptoms. Upon further assessment, Tom was able to identify that the couple became physically violent with one another during arguments at times and that it only happened at times when Dustin was drinking. The couple reported that Dustin would be going in for an appointment with his PCP during the next week. With concerns around the withdrawal symptoms Dustin was experiencing, the therapist and I were glad to hear an appointment had already been scheduled (otherwise we would have recommended it).

We requested a release to communicate with Dustin's PCP and then contacted her to collaborate and share assessment information. We described to the PCP the physiological symptoms that Dustin reported, alongside our concerns that the patient was physically dependent on alcohol and had a substance-related medical issue. The PCP gathered the clinic's information and after meeting with the patient ordered additional tests that led to the diagnosis of a stomach ulcer. With the results of these tests, the PCP advised that withdrawal from alcohol was not recommended without medical supervision and that Dustin should check in to an inpatient detoxification facility.

The couple did not make it back to therapy for 3 weeks following their intake because of work schedule conflicts. When they returned, Tom processed with Elaina and Dustin the findings from the appointment with the PCP. The couple identified that although inpatient detox was recommended, they did not see it as feasible at the time. Elaina reported that she just wanted Dustin to stop using alcohol, and they both discussed how he was able to quit using methamphetamine "cold turkey" 1 year ago.

Tom took a mid-session break and came back behind the mirror for his supervision consultation. I discussed with Tom the patterns reported by the patients, emphasizing that the withdrawal experiences Dustin was experiencing. I shared concerns about the potentially life-threatening dangers of withdrawing from alcohol without medical attention. I told Tom to reiterate to the couple the PCP's indication that it was not advised to go through alcohol withdrawal without being under medical supervision.

I instructed Tom to provide the couple with referrals for detoxification centers in the city. The couple resisted, indicating that if Dustin missed any work he would lose his job. With Dustin being the primary breadwinner in the family, they could not survive without his income. With the understanding of their challenges, we then identified the need to incorporate a case worker into our treatment team.

This case was multifaceted in both the number of challenges that the couple was facing and in terms of the professionals who should be involved. Given the severity of symptoms that Dustin was experiencing, it was not just a matter of whether we should collaborate with additional care providers—it was, instead, the only ethical means by which to continue treatment. The PCP was essential in establishing the patient's medical diagnosis. If left untreated, Dustin's level of alcohol use was potentially life-threatening. However, he also faced employment and financial challenges by seeking intensive care. Too invasive of a treatment recommendation without consideration of attending to his other challenges could have also been damaging, leading the patient to potentially drop out from treatment. A case worker was thereby necessary to coordinate treatment systems as the couple dealt with concomitant challenges related to Dustin's job and the couple's economic survival.

Amidst these issues, Dustin's partner began to pressure him to quit his alcohol use "cold turkey"—but alcohol is one of the few substances from which a patient can die during rapid withdrawal. The couple was not presenting for treatment for substance use issues and did not identify it as one of their primary concerns within their intake paperwork. Had the MedFT not directed assessment processes to inquire about substance use, Dustin's potentially life-threatening alcohol use might have gone unreported and unaddressed. Further, by attending to the relational and systemic factors affecting the case, the MedFT was able to identify and attend to challenges preventing the patient from pursuing treatment further. A MedFT in this type of tertiary care setting must be purposeful in integrating other systems of care into alcohol and drug treatment. Referral to additional professionals without such collaboration may not be adequate to properly manage substance use problems. In this chapter, we outline basic knowledge that MedFTs in these types of case settings need to have, as well as identify the interdisciplinary teams that could or should be involved in care across a range of treatment levels.

What Is Alcohol and Drug Treatment?

MedFTs can be involved in alcohol and drug treatment in a variety of settings, ranging from early intervention treatment to general outpatient treatment, intensive outpatient treatment, and residential or inpatient care. Treatment recommendations largely depend on the severity of the substance use that is occurring and its resulting consequences (see the "Fundamentals of Alcohol and Drug Treatment" section, below). Treatment approaches give focus to physiological, behavioral, and social causes or consequences of the substance use, as well as co-occurring mental health disorders. In residential and inpatient treatment centers, the MedFT will have an IBHC team that can include psychiatrists, medical directors, nurses, and other behavioral health providers on site. The MedFT working in outpatient treatment, on the other hand, will likely have an IBHC team of psychiatrists, PCPs, nutritionists, and—in some cases—probation officers or sponsors (some of whom may be located on site). The outpatient MedFT will likely have to be more purposeful with integrating different professionals into care processes.

The ability of a patient to access the most appropriate care can depend on financial resources, too, as not all medical insurance providers include coverage for alcohol and drug treatment. It is not uncommon for substance use problems to be discovered within a treatment setting that is not focused on alcohol and drug treatment per se. Behavioral health providers could be the first professionals in contact with the patient; comprehensive screening and assessment is thereby crucial to detect unrecognized problems with substances. Such screening and assessment can identify two types of psychopathology: internalizing types and externalizing types. Alcohol and drug use most commonly fit into externalizing sequences and often co-occur with other diagnoses like personality disorders, mood disorders, and anxiety disorders (Hasin & Kilcoyne, 2012).

The problematic use of alcohol or drugs can lead to a diagnosis of a substance use disorder (APA, 2013). However, not all alcohol and drug use coincides with a substance use disorder diagnosis. Alcohol and drug use moves into "disordered" use when psychological, social, and/or physiological problems arise that can be linked back to it. Substance use can induce other mental illnesses per se and can be related to disruptions in one's social system (APA, 2013). As noted above, repeated consumption of substances can affect the body's homeostasis. Compensatory adaptations occur to support continued functioning and survival (National Association for Addiction Professionals [NAADAC], 2009). These changes are what cause a physical dependency to substances. The body is affected by both these changes and the direct effects of the substance(s) itself. For example, alcohol can affect nutrition absorption, negatively impact liver functioning, and can cause bleeding in the digestive system. It can even cause nervous system impairment (Mirijello et al., 2015; Myrick & Anton, 1998).

When the effects of drug and alcohol use reach into biological, psychological, or social systems, the etiology of said use similarly has biopsychosocial (Zucker & Gomberg, 1986) and family systems roots (Gruber & Taylor, 2006). Those with other severe mental illnesses tend to be diagnosed with substance use disorders at a higher rate than the general population (RachBeisel, Scott, & Dixon, 1999). Family functioning is related to different substance use behaviors, including age of initiation of use, substance(s) of choice, and/or problematic use patterns (Gruber & Taylor, 2006). The family can buffer and protect against problematic use, with parent support and control factors being especially important (Barnes & Farrell, 1992; Gruber & Taylor, 2006). The family can also introduce risk for use, particularly when a parent is using alcohol (Kerr, Capaldi, Pears, & Owen, 2012). Genetic heritability of substance use has been documented, too. For alcohol, this may create differences in how people metabolize enzymes in alcohol and/or how they cope with stressful life experiences (Enoch, 2013). Addiction may also have underlying neurobiological basis; prefrontal cortex activity has been identified in imaging studies as playing a key role due to its regulation of rewards and involvement with higher-order thinking (e.g., self-control) (Goldstein & Volkow, 2011). The multifaceted impacts and origins of alcohol and drug use necessitate the involvement of multiple systems of care in recovery, with the MedFT playing an important role in these systems.

Whereas substance use disorders have biopsychosocial-spiritual and family systems etiology (Engel, 1977, 1980; Wright, Watson, & Bell, 1996), the underlying cause for the use is questioned. Models of addiction view the problems with substance use as a disease or as an adaptive process of coping (Alexander, 1987).

Members of the treatment team may differ in their perceptions of this disorder and may need to negotiate in finding common goals. For example, psychiatrists and psychologists may adhere to the disease model of addiction, specifically subscribing to a neurobiological basis to it (Noël, Brevers, & Bechara, 2013), whereas MedFTs may be more likely to additionally examine the relational influences on substance-seeking behaviors (Selbekk, Sagvaag, & Fauske, 2015). Moreover, different approaches to the treatment of alcohol and drug problems are debated in the field. Some recommend an abstinence-only approach as preferable; others recommend a harm-reduction approach (Marlatt & Witkiewitz, 2002).

Abstinence-only approaches (e.g., the 12-Step model) stress the importance of complete abstinence of the substances, indicating that any use could trigger cravings and a relapse into problematic use. The Center for Substance Abuse Treatment (1999) and Betty Ford Institute Consensus Panel (2007), for example, define this as essential for recovery. Harm-reduction approaches, on the other hand, focus primarily on reducing the negative impacts from substance use (i.e., not on eliminating the use altogether). This approach acknowledges differences among users and takes into account the stage of change a patient is presently in (Marlatt & Witkiewitz, 2002). By focusing on harm reduction, a broader range of patients may be engaged in treatment as it matches motivation level. This approach can also feel less stigmatizing to patients and thereby be more attractive treatment option for some. Ultimately, while a harm-reduction approach may be possible for those with a less severe alcohol or drug problem, abstinence may be a necessary goal to maintain recovery for those with more severe substance use disorders. There are some indications, too, that abstinence is a more stable recovery option than those seeking moderate drinking as a goal (Ilgen, Wilbourne, Moos, & Moos, 2008). In our view, the potential legal consequences related to continued drug use negate harm reduction as being a practical and ethical approach. The IBHC team should therefore work together to identify primary goal(s) for recovery.

Treatment Teams in Alcohol and Drug Treatment

MedFTs working with integrated treatment teams are necessary, as the safe and successful recovery of an alcohol or drug use patient may depend on the collaboration between multiple providers along with the patient and family (Marlowe, 2003; Myrick & Anton, 1998; Vanderplasschen, Rapp, Wolf, & Broekaert, 2004). The process of moving from active substance use to reduced use or abstinence is physically, emotionally, socially, and financially challenging. Reducing or eliminating substances from the body can have a variety of negative physical effects, especially when there has been physical dependency on the substance and the patient is experiencing withdrawal symptoms (Myrick & Anton, 1998). With reduced use or abstinence, a variety of other challenges present to the patient. Maintaining recovery often depends on integrating treatment for co-occurring behavioral health disorders (Drake, Mueser, Brunette, & McHugo, 2004) and can necessitate changes to other areas of one's life (e.g., access to employment or housing; Salyers & Tsemberis, 2007). If the patient is involved in the criminal justice system, recovery may also involve ongoing interactions with probation officers or other members of the court system (Marlowe, 2003). While each of these processes is being addressed and managed with the patient, members of the family system are also experiencing changes. Family members can be a supportive resource for the patient, and their involvement in treatment can provide useful information about triggers for relapse or indications of the patient's strength. Conversely, families may resist a change from the homeostasis or a change that involves something they do not quite understand (e.g., challenges associated with withdrawal from a substance). This resistance can undermine the work of the IBHC teams if it is not addressed purposively and systemically.

The tertiary care teams required for alcohol and drug treatment potentially involve different professionals not often encountered in other MedFT approaches. The nature of the presenting problem and the related issues necessitates a broader collaboration of disciplines. Professionals within the judicial system, if the patient is required to seek services because of legal charges, often require regular status updates. The integration of criminal justice supervision into treatment (Marlowe, 2003), along with case management (Cosden, Ellens, Schnell, Yamini-Diour, & Wolfe, 2003), shows support for improved recovery outcomes. Combinations of other services have also been examined; collaboration across multiple providers and resources (e.g., case management) consistently yields strong psychological, social, and treatment effects (Vanderplasschen et al., 2004). Not only are these types of collaborative or IBHC teams beneficial to the patient, but they also positively impact the team members involved enriching their professional and personal experience in the work (Akhavain, Amaral, Murphy, & Cardon Uehlinger, 1999). The following include professionals in tertiary care settings that could, and often should, be involved in integrated behavioral healthcare with MedFTs:

Psychiatrists. Substance use disorders can either induce another behavioral health disorder, including depressive disorders or neurocognitive disorders (APA, 2013), or co-occur with mental illness (RachBeisel, Scott, & Dixon, 1999). Psychiatrists can assess for co-occurring mental disorders and provide supportive care in treatment of those disorders, prescribing medications where necessary. Psychiatrists can report new prescriptions directly to probation officers, which can then be tracked for appropriate use. MedFTs can consult with the psychiatrist and report any potential substances actively being used that would be of relevance in prescribing or any substances that could prove to be a trigger for the patient's relapse into substance use. For example, a patient with a history of methamphetamine use may be triggered by being prescribed popular attention deficit hyperactivity disorder (ADHD) medications (e.g., Ritalin)—which are formally classified as amphetamines. Psychiatrists can be involved in the treatment planning process, too, identifying means of helping patients maintain abstinence from their substance(s) of choice. Pharmacotherapy can be used to assist in detoxification and maintenance therapy or to prevent overdoses (NAADAC, 2009). There are sensitizers that cause uncomfortable symptoms if taken with the substance of choice, antagonists that block the desired effects of the substance or that can prevent overdose, and other therapies that can decrease cravings for the substance of choice.

Primary care physicians (PCPs). Before patients make changes in their alcohol or drug use, it is important that they seek evaluation by their PCP to assess safety. The PCP can assess for a variety of health issues resulting from the substance use and anticipate any challenges that may be faced if the patient withdraws from the substance. For example, physical dependency on alcohol may be related to other conditions, including irregular heartbeat (i.e., arrhythmia), pancreatic disease (i.e., alcohol pancreatitis), or bleeding within the digestive system, to name a few (Myrick & Anton, 1998). The PCP can also assess for other health concerns that may have arisen because of the method for drug use. For example, the use of intravenous drugs is often associated with the reuse of dirty needles and a higher rate of human immunodeficiency virus (HIV) (Mathers et al., 2008). MedFTs' and PCPs' collaboration can help identify the necessary health tests to be conducted. Patients sometimes have difficulty in revealing their true level of use to the PCP and may not understand the importance of comprehensive reporting.

Nutritionists. The use of alcohol and drugs has physiological consequences, but also generally accompanies a lifestyle that neglects nutritional health (Islam, Hossain, Ahmed, & Ahsan, 2002). Those who use at clinically significant levels have used drugs over a longer period and are more likely to display nutritional deficiencies (Islam, Hossain, Ahmed, & Ahsan, 2002). Some substances serve as a replacement for food (e.g., alcohol), some undermine appetite (e.g., cocaine or methamphetamine), and others promote cravings for empty-energy foods leading to nutritional deficiencies (e.g., marijuana) (Islam et al., 2002; Lieber, 2003). Alcohol, for example, can interfere with the absorption of other nutrients (Lieber, 2003) and—during withdrawal—patients who have been using it may require nutrient supplementation to prevent life-threatening complications (Myrick & Anton, 1998). A nutritionist can assess for nutritional deficiencies in the patient and provide a dietary plan. They can work with the patient to understand the role of diet in healthy living and in their recovery. Nutritionists may also be employed as a supportive care along with outpatient alcohol withdrawal (Myrick & Anton, 1998).

Case managers. Patients who are struggling with substance use often present with a variety of other significant life problems (Vanderplasschen et al., 2004). This can include challenges with access to food, employment, housing, or transportation. Case managers assess and identify the services needed and coordinate the supportive care. This may include finding access to community resources, providing crisis intervention, or teaching specific skills. In alcohol and drug treatment, case managers can assist patients who do not have access to transportation to treatment (e.g., because an alcohol or drug charge resulted in revocation of driving privileges). Patients may have suffered a loss of employment following missed work because of treatment stays or incarceration. Patients may also be struggling financially, thereby benefitting from skills training for career advancement. Case managers can assist with each of these pieces and can collaborate with both probation officers and behavioral health providers in identifying necessary resources and tracking progress in accessing them.

Probation officers. Patients involved with the criminal justice system who are serving probation, or parole (if the patient has been incarcerated), will have supervised conditions for their release. If substances were involved in the charges, judges may require an alcohol and drug evaluation with stipulations that any clinical recommendations are followed. Probation officers generally (at a minimum) will require a monthly report from the treating psychotherapist that attests to patient participation in sessions and a brief summary about treatment progress or concerns. Probation officers can provide additional support to the therapeutic process, including drug testing in situations where patient relapse is a concern, require the patient come for a check-in, or conduct unannounced house visits. Probation officers may also monitor patient prescriptions, requiring new scripts be reported, and the medications brought in to be monitored (i.e., checked to ensure that medications are being taken as prescribed). They hold patients accountable for other actions, as well, including attending community support groups (e.g., Alcoholics Anonymous) or applying for jobs. In some situations, probation officers may even collaborate with the behavioral health provider regarding sentencing recommendations, and whether they should include specific treatment stipulations.

Fundamentals of Care in Alcohol and Drug Treatment

MedFTs who seek to have alcohol and drug use as a clinical area of interest can seek certifications or, potentially, state licensure in this specialty. The Association for Addiction Professionals (NAADAC) has a credential to acknowledge qualified addiction professionals. Some states have adopted a licensure to recognize these professionals, called licensed addiction counselor (LAC) or licensed chemical dependency counselor (LCDC). In some cases, being qualified for the Marriage and Family Therapy license (LMFT), or another master's level license (e.g., LICSW), also deems a behavioral health provider eligible to sit for the examination and licensure.

Terms in Alcohol and Drug Treatment Programs

Working as a MedFT with alcohol and drug use problems in tertiary care settings, specialized content knowledge is necessary to properly assess, treat, and collaborate with the interdisciplinary team.

Substance use disorder. The first area that the MedFT should be familiar with is the diagnostic criteria for a substance use disorder (SUD). This is fully described in the Diagnostic and Statistical Manual of Mental Disorders-5 (APA, 2013, pp. 481–589). A substance use disorder involves a pattern of behaviors surrounding the use of the substance that is pathological or results in clinically significant impairment. The diagnostic criteria for all substance use disorders include the following groupings: impaired control, social impairment, risky use, and pharmacological criteria.

With impaired control, the substance may be taken for a longer duration of time than was intended or more may be consumed than was originally intended (APA, 2013). There is an inability to successfully cut down on one's use, or an excessive amount of time may be spent to obtain the substance. Social impairment may occur as a result of the substance use. The user may fail to fulfill their obligations at work, school, or home or may have problems with those in their social network because of the substance. The user may also give up activities they once enjoyed because of the substance use. Risky use involves a pattern of substance use in circumstances in which it is dangerous or physically hazardous or despite knowledge that their physical or psychological health is affected by the substance use. Finally, pharmacological criteria involve both symptoms of tolerance (i.e., needing more of the substance in order to achieve the same effect or a reduction in the effect of the same dosage) and withdrawal symptoms (i.e., physiological effects of the marked reduction of the use of the substance). The presence of two or three symptoms is all that is required for a diagnosis of a substance use disorder specified with mild severity. The level of severity is diagnosed based on number of diagnostic criteria the patient meets, with levels of severity including mild (2–3 criteria), moderate (4–5 criteria), and severe (6 or more criteria).

Substance-induced mental disorders. One important factor that the MedFT should know about the repetitive use of a substance is that substance-induced mental disorders can present as a result (APA, 2013). Without taking into account present substance use, misdiagnosis can happen. This can include depressive disorders, anxiety disorders, and even schizophrenia spectrum and other psychotic disorders. Any co-occurring symptoms of another disorder that the patient presents with should be assessed for when they presented, whether before or after the onset of the substance use, and whether the symptoms sustained for more than a month of time following the withdrawal of a the substance. A co-occurring disorder diagnosis over a substance-induced mental disorder diagnosis should not be given unless the symptoms have been observed a month after cessation and withdrawal from the substance. Substance intoxication, dependence, and withdrawal can trigger other mental disorder symptomologies.

Polysubstance abuse. In assessing for what substances are being used by a patient, the MedFT should also assess for what substances are being used simultaneously. Polysubstance use occurs when more than one substance is consumed simultaneously or in succession of one another (NAADAC, 2009). Some substances, when taken together, heighten the intoxication experience (e.g., alcohol when combined with cocaine, benzodiazepines, marijuana, or heroin). Otherwise, some substances are used to manage symptoms of withdrawal from another substance (e.g., using marijuana to manage withdrawal from opioids).

Central nervous system depressants. Central nervous system (CNS) depressants are those psychoactive substances that work by depressing, or slowing, physiological functions including lung functioning, motor coordination, mental awareness, or heart rate (NAADAC, 2009). This includes alcohol, barbiturates, and benzodiazepines. When used or prescribed for medical purposes, CNS depressants are commonly taken to treat insomnia or anxiety. There is a potentiation effect for CNS depressants that are used together, meaning that the effect of each substance is magnified by the consumption of the other. Consider potentiation being depicted by the equation $2 + 2 = 8$. This effect can be life threatening, as it can result in a person's heart stopping. Alcohol when combined with an antianxiety medication like Xanax or Klonopin, for example, can produce these potentiation effects.

Other inventive nonconventional ways of consuming alcohol have emerged, and often attempted by underage minors, including soaking tampons in alcohol and inserting them, the use of alcohol through insertion of the rectum (i.e., "butt chugging"), soaking candy or fruit in alcohol, or even smoking alcohol in vaporized and inhaled forms. As outlined above, withdrawal from alcohol is different from most substances insofar as its detoxification process can be potentially life endangering (Myrick & Anton, 1998). Patients with symptoms of physical dependency to alcohol should be assessed medically before changing their pattern of use. These substances can be taken orally, intravenously, or intramuscularly (NAADAC, 2009).

Central nervous system stimulants. CNS stimulants—including nicotine, caffeine, amphetamine, and cocaine—work by exciting the CNS and arousing physiological functions even creating a sense of euphoria for the user (NAADAC, 2009). Medically, these can be used to treat narcolepsy, respiratory problems, or attention deficit hyperactivity disorder (ADHD). The withdrawal from CNS stimulants can cause fatigue, vivid or unpleasant dreams, insomnia or hypersomnia, increased appetite, dysphoric mood, or psychomotor retardation or agitation. The simultaneous use of the CNS stimulant cocaine with alcohol forms a metabolite called cocaethylene, which is a more lethal substance than cocaine alone (Hearn, Rose, Wagner, Ciarleglio, & Mash, 1991; McCance, Price, Kosten, & Jatlow, 1995). CNS stimulants can be taken orally, nasally, or intravenously.

Narcotics. The term "narcotics" is often misused to refer to any illegal substance. Formally, narcotics include any substance that was derived from the poppy (opium) plant (NAADAC, 2009). Opiates are extracted from the opium poppy or are a modified extract (e.g., morphine or codeine), whereas opioids are synthetic versions (e.g., hydrocodone, methadone, heroin). Narcotics are used medically to reduce or eliminate physical pain. They also can suppress anxiety, depression, and other physiological functions like coughing or diarrhea. The suppression of physiological functions that narcotics provide makes this psychoactive substance especially dangerous when combined with CNS depressants, such as alcohol. Respiratory functions could become so suppressed a person stops breathing when these substances are combined. Any patient taking pain medications should be made aware of the potential interactions of narcotics and CNS depressants. These substances can be taken orally, nasally, intravenously, or subcutaneously.

Hallucinogens. Hallucinogens act to produce an altered state of body and mind, where perceptions of thoughts and feelings are distorted (NAADAC, 2009). They include lysergic acid diethylamide (LSD), phencyclidine (PCP), and methylenedioxymethamphetamine (MDMA). Hallucinogens have no known withdrawal symptoms or risk for physical dependence, but can be psychologically addictive. Risk in using hallucinogens primarily comes from the user's behavior while intoxicated, as he or she can be erratic and/or behave in ways that are based on a delusion or hallucination (i.e., putting one's self in a dangerous situation). These substances are generally ingested orally, but they can be injected as well.

Cannabis. Psychoactive substances derived from the *Cannabis sativa* plant are part of the cannabis classification (NAADAC, 2009). Cannabis, commonly referred to as marijuana, is the most used illicit psychoactive substance in the United States (SAMHSA, 2009). By the end of 2016, marijuana was legal for recreational use in six places (Alaska, California, Colorado, Oregon, Washington DC, and Washington State) and was legal for medical use in some form in 44 states (Marijuana and the Law, 2016). When taken, marijuana creates feelings of euphoria, relaxation, and altered perceptions of space and time; it can also impair short-term memory, judgment, and reaction time (NAADAC, 2009). In some cases, hallucinations can result. Although not commonly accepted by the general public, marijuana use does have a potential for physical and psychological dependence (APA, 2013). Cannabis can affect testosterone levels in males (leading to increased secondary sex characteristics) and disrupt the reproductive cycle in females (NAADAC, 2009). Cannabis is primarily taken orally, either through smoking or as an edible when mixed with foods (NAADAC, 2009).

Solvents and inhalants. Solvents and inhalants are often used to produce psychoactive effects as an inexpensive and easily accessible alternative to other substances (NAADAC, 2009). Common household items can be used to create an instant feeling of being high, which results in euphoria, relaxation, excitement, hallucinations, and impaired thinking. Popular items used to create these effects include anesthetics (e.g., whipped cream propellant or chloroform), volatile solvents and sprays (e.g., nail polish remover, lighter fluid, hair sprays, or paint remover), and volatile nitrates (e.g., room deodorizers). These substances are generally breathed in orally, whether through "huffing," "sniffing," or "bagging," and can lead to permanent brain damage because of their ability to easily permeate the blood-brain barrier. No withdrawal effects have been discovered. Solvents and inhalants have not been found to cause physical dependence, but can result in psychological dependence.

Anabolic steroids. Anabolic steroids are synthetic and naturally occurring psychoactive substances generally used to build muscle by imitating the effects of androgens and testosterone (NAADAC, 2009). When taken, they result in significant gains in muscles and strength and can result increased secondary sex characteristics for females. Increased aggression, also known as "roid rage," can occur from use, alongside frightening dreams or hallucinations. When detoxing from anabolic steroids, behavioral health may be affected. Patients may experience severe depressive symptoms, even suicidal ideation. Anabolic steroids can be taken orally, topically in a cream or gel form, or injected.

Levels of Care

A substance use disorder is a chronic and progressive disease (American Society of Addiction Medicine [ASAM], 2011) and, depending on the severity, requires different intensities of treatment in different treatment settings. A MedFT can be involved in the integrated treatment of alcohol and drug use in each of these treatment settings. In relation to substance use or addiction recovery, levels of care refer to the appropriate treatment setting to best meet the needs of the patient. The most widely used guidelines in the treatment of alcohol and drug use is the American Society of Addiction Medicine Patient Placement Criteria (ASAM PPC; Mee-Lee, 2013). The ASAM PPC uses six dimensions to inquire about patient's strengths, systems of support, resources, risks, and deficits, to place the patient in a treatment setting ranging from early intervention (Level 0.5) to medically managed inpatient (Level 4)—with the options including inpatient or outpatient care. The six dimensions of the ASAM Criteria are (a) acute intoxication or risk of withdrawal; (b) biomedical conditions and complications; (c) emotional, behavioral, or cognitive conditions and complications; (d) readiness to change; (e) relapse, continued use, or continued problem potential; and (f) recovery/living environment.

It is critical that the MedFT or behavioral health providers working with alcohol and drug use understand when a patient is appropriate for outpatient services (i.e., withdrawal risk is minimal, medically stable, no safety concerns, supportive recovery environment) and when inpatient would be necessary (i.e., risk of withdrawal, immediate danger to self/others, medical concerns, lives in unsupportive recovery environment). The MedFT, or other behavioral health provider, can be the professional recommending a level of care for the patient. The level of care a patient is placed in will also influence the level of involvement of different professionals in the treatment process and may have to be coordinated by multiple professionals. The MedFT could be the provider of either individual therapy, group therapy, or couple and family therapy at any level of treatment.

Level 0.5 (early intervention) would be recommended or provided by the MedFT or other behavioral health providers when a patient displays a potential risk for developing a substance use disorder, but does not meet the diagnostic criteria for a SUD (ASAM, 2011; Mee-Lee, 2013). This treatment could be recommended as a standalone treatment or in addition to other behavioral health treatments focused on another behavioral health issue. This limited outpatient treatment, which can be as brief as a single 8-hour day class, focuses on psychoeducation of SUDs and related risk factors to allow the patient to make more informed choices about their substance use. Integration between the MedFT and other behavioral health providers would be warranted to ensure accurate risk was assessed. The MedFT could also integrate a PCP into treatment to assess physical health and a probation officer if applicable.

Level 1 outpatient treatment would be recommended when the patient meets the diagnostic criteria for a mild to moderate SUD (Mee-Lee, 2013). Substance use by the patient interferes with functioning in one or more areas of life (e.g., school, work, or family relationships). Typically patients are not experiencing withdrawal; do not have any biomedical conditions or complications as a result of the substance use; do not have any emotional, behavioral, or cognitive conditions or complications or are receiving mental health monitoring; display readiness to change or need motivation to strengthen readiness; are able to achieve abstinence or controlled use; and are able to cope with the recovery environment. Treatment is less than 9 hours per week for adults, and less than 6 hours per week for adolescents, and can be inclusive of individual therapy and group therapy. Treatment can be as few as a single hour of individual therapy per week, but the number of hours should be proportionate to symptomology. This treatment can also be provided as a step-down from a more intensive level of treatment. The IBHC team will include the MedFT, other behavioral health providers, the PCP, and possibly a psychiatrist and probation officer.

Level 2 intensive outpatient treatment (IOP) would be recommended when the patient meets the diagnostic criteria for a SUD as well as an emotional, behavioral, or cognitive condition that has the potential to interfere with treatment and should be monitored (Mee-Lee, 2013). Patients are at a minimal risk for severe withdrawal from the substance, either they have no biomedical conditions or complications or they are manageable at the outpatient level, display ambivalence or lack of engagement in treatment, have an increased risk of continued substance use or relapse without regular engagement and support in treatment, and are able to cope with the recovery environment. Treatment is at least 9 hours a week for adults and at least 6 hours a week for adolescents. Treatment will likely be inclusive of both group and individual therapy. This treatment can be provided as a step-down or step-up from a more or less intensive treatment. The integrated treatment team will likely be the same as above.

Level 3 medically monitored inpatient treatment would be recommended when a patient meets the diagnostic criteria for a moderate to severe SUD and when the elimination of the substance use requires a controlled environment and monitoring (Mee-Lee, 2013). The substance use results in significant interference with functioning in life. Patients are at minimal risk of withdrawal, or if it is present, it is not life threatening; may have biomedical conditions that require monitoring; may have emotional, behavioral, or cognitive deficits; may be in opposition to treatment; may need skill development to prevent relapse and continued use; and cannot cope with their recovery environment. Treatment will include at least 5 hours of clinical service, including therapy, a week. The length of treatment is determined on an individual basis and depending on the severity of the SUD. The IBHC team can include the MedFT or other behavioral health providers, psychiatrists, and nurses, with staff available and awake 24 hours a day, 7 days a week.

Level 4 medically managed inpatient treatment would be recommended when a patient meets the diagnostic criteria for a severe SUD, when the elimination of the substance use requires a controlled environment and monitoring, and when the patient has instability in symptoms in dimension 1, 2, or 3 of the ASAM criteria (Mee-Lee, 2013). Patients may be at risk of severe withdrawal; may have biomedical conditions that require monitoring; may have severe emotional, behavioral, or cognitive deficits that require monitoring (e.g., suicidal ideation); may be in opposition to treatment; may need skill development to prevent relapse and continued use; and cannot cope with their recovery environment. Therapy is available for patients in this setting. The IBHC team can include the MedFT or other behavioral health providers, psychiatrists, PCPs, and nurses, with staff available and awake 24 hours a day, 7 days a week.

Sensitivity to Diversity

MedFTs should be cognizant of and sensitive to issues of diversity that affect alcohol and drug treatment. Not only are there differences in the physiological influence of substances across different groups, but there are systemic factors affecting access to care across different communities. The use of alcohol and other substances is generally less among females as compared to males (SAMHSA, 2009; Nolen-Hoeksema & Hilt, 2006). Gender is an important factor to consider in treatment. Alcohol affects males and females differently. For example, females are more strongly affected by the same level of alcohol use as males, due to muscle mass, body fat, and activity of the enzyme gastric alcohol dehydrogenase (Nolen-Hoeksema & Hilt, 2006). Females generally experience more negative physiological and social consequences from drinking, which may deter heavier use as compared to males. Although females may use substances less, they are more likely to face barriers to seeking treatment for their alcohol or substance use, especially mothers (Finkelstein, 1994). Physiological effects of alcohol can also be more severe for those who have a specific genetic variant affecting metabolism of the substance, which disproportionately affects those of Asian descent (Li, Zhao, & Gelernter, 2011). Access to healthcare is less for racial and ethnic minorities; specifically African Americans and Hispanics have less access than White non-Hispanic with similar need for treatment (Wells, Klap, Koike, & Sherbourne, 2001). Cultural variables related to interpersonal relations (e.g., individualism-collectivism dynamics, respeto, or familism) and personal traits (e.g., acculturation, ethnic pride, or spirituality) are important to consider in treatment as they can potentially be protective or mediating factors against substance use (see Castro & Alarcón, 2002).

Alcohol and Drug Treatment Across the MedFT Healthcare Continuum

A MedFT's efforts in relation to—or within—an IBHC team working to treat patients with a substance use disorder will vary in accord his or her competency and care context. The MedFT Healthcare Continuum (Hodgson, Lamson, Mendenhall, & Tyndall, 2014) describes knowledge and skills across five different levels of practice application and complexity. Tables 12.1 and 12.2 highlight specific characterizations of MedFTs' work and involvement in alcohol/drug treatment across this continuum.

The first two levels of the MedFT Healthcare Continuum include a working knowledge of and ability to apply the BPSS model and an understanding of how the

Table 12.1 MedFTs in Alcohol and Drug Treatment: Basic Knowledge and Skills

MedFT Healthcare Continuum Level	Level 1	Level 2	Level 3
Knowledge	Basic understanding of clinical and lay person definitions of substance use disorder and its impact. Understands BPSS approaches to substance use care. Familiar with addiction recovery as a mental health field; limited understanding of evidence-based practice, treatment facilities, or team structure.	Understands the systemic impact of substance use disorders. Familiar with the role couple and family relationships play on sustained recovery. Basic knowledge about different substances of abuse; can identify some health complications associated to substances of abuse (e.g., cirrhosis, psychosis, cardiovascular disease). Can differentiate problematic substance use from clinically significant substance use; familiar with drug types.	Working knowledge of specific team members (e.g., case worker, psychiatrist, nutritionist) and terminology (e.g., detoxification, withdrawal, tolerance). Basic knowledge of the physiological impact of different substances of abuse. Understands theories of addiction, including the disease model of addiction.
Skills	Can explain the BPSS and how it applies to addiction recovery. Practices independent of treatment team. Adequate knowledge of referral sources when patient needs higher level of care.	Can conceptualize and treat substance use issues systemically; understands the circular role of families and substance use; routinely treats cases concerning substance use. Collaborates with professionals who specialize in addiction recovery and refers out appropriately; treatment of substance use issues is primarily separate from integrated behavioral healthcare.	Proficient in conceptualizing cases from multiple theories of addiction and the role different substances of abuse play in developing treatment plan. Practices primarily in a tertiary care setting, consistently integrating treatment team members in the treatment planning process; actively participates in treatment team meetings. Can implement a systemic assessment of a patient and family with competencies in assessing BPSS for addiction recovery and engage other professionals as indicated.

Table 12.2 MedFTs in Alcohol and Drug Treatment: Advanced Knowledge and Skills

MedFT Healthcare Continuum Level	Level 4	Level 5
Knowledge	Proficient understanding of drugs of abuse, their physical/mental/emotional effects, physiological responses (e.g., tolerance, withdrawal, tissue dependence), and drug-specific treatment.	Understands ASAM levels of care and the six dimensions of assessment (e.g., strengths, resources, risks) and can make appropriate treatment recommendations.
	Expert knowledge of addiction recovery field including terminology, assessment/diagnosis, measures, and treatment options.	Proficient knowledge of evidence-based treatments regarding addiction recovery and how to integrate family in treatment; experience in providing psychoeducation to patients and their systems of support about multiple areas of addiction recovery.
		Able to fulfill the role of clinician, researcher, policymaker, and administrator concerning addiction recovery.
		Skilled in providing community outreach concerning education on addiction recovery, including prevention, relapse, recovery skills, and family support.
Skills	Routinely collaborates with and conducts joint treatment sessions with other addiction recovery treatment team member providers (e.g., case worker, probation officer, nutritionist).	Ability to apply knowledge of substance use treatment related to complex issues such as drug interactions, pharmacotherapy, and role of detoxification.
	Able to deliver seminars and workshops about the BPSS complexities of a variety of substance use disorders (e.g., alcohol, methamphetamine, prescription opioids) to a myriad of professionals (e.g., mental health, judicial system).	Engages in cutting-edge research (e.g., neuroimaging techniques, biomarkers) using novel approaches to improve the understanding of addiction from a systemic lens.
		Provides community outreach, such as development of prevention programs, and work may extend to policymaking.
	Proficient in the application of evidence-based practice, and attends to systemic issues related to substance use disorders (e.g., intimate partner violence).	Established a standard of care that includes consistent interaction and communication with treatment team.

BPSS model relates to both relational and healthcare models. MedFTs working in alcohol and drug treatment at *Levels 1* and *2* should have basic knowledge concerning substance use disorder and drug and alcohol recovery, including both a clinical and lay person definition of SUD, how to assess for a substance use disorder, the difference between problematic and clinically significant substance use, and the role of family systems in addiction. MedFTs practicing at these first two levels of the continuum are unlikely to frequently treat patients for alcohol or drug use issues; however, they may rarely do so or will consult with other professionals on relational issues related to alcohol or drug use.

The *Level 1* and *2* MedFT may have experience conducting research concerning substance use, considering the role of systemic factors, but this research would not consider interdisciplinary healthcare teams. A MedFT working with our case example patients, Elaina and Dustin, would have the ability to assess for Dustin's history of drug use and assess for his current level of alcohol use. The MedFT's questions would be systemically focused, asking about how the use has impacted their relationship and how they are working together as a couple on the recovery process. Finally, the MedFT would evaluate whether outpatient therapy was the most appropriate level of care, working with Dustin's PCP to ensure medical risks are being properly addressed.

Moving to *Level 3*, this behavioral health provider will be able to utilize both family therapy and assess using a BPSS framework. We would expect MedFTs practicing at this level to be able to collaborate with appropriate medical and behavioral healthcare providers and be able to function in a tertiary care setting. The skills that would be demonstrated would be the ability to work with other treatment team members to create treatment plans and cocreate goals, as well as motivate both the patient and their family to be engaged in the treatment process. *Level 3* skills also encompass the ability to create strong working relationships with each of the treatment providers (e.g., PCP, nurse, case worker, probation officer, nutritionist, and psychiatrist). Considering our case example, Tom, the MedFT, was able to stress the importance of working with other providers for adequate care. Dustin expressed concerns around being able to take time off of work for treatment, prompting Tom to recommend Dustin work with a case worker around employment challenges. In collaboration with the PCP, the MedFT would suggest the use of a detoxification center and work with the patient to motivate him to engage treatment. A *Level 3* MedFT may speak directly to the PCP about the alcohol assessment and potential medical risks associated with Dustin's use. If the PCP was not able to work with Dustin on his withdrawal symptoms, the MedFT could then help explore the option of detoxification further, by working with Dustin and Elaina to discuss their fears, to validate their concerns, and to normalize that many patients worry about the financial burden associated with intensive care. This process is most commonly achieved by utilizing motivational interviewing techniques.

Dustin's readiness to change would be evaluated based on the stages of change model and the *Level 3* MedFT would be proficient at applying motivational interviewing (MI) techniques to help the patient prepare to make changes. The MedFT must work to be supportive but continue to stress the safety risk associated with quitting use without medical supervision. Finally, Tom would need to be prepared for questions relating to confidentiality with medical insurance and working with a PCP on alcohol and drug treatment issues, which is a common fear of patients who have insurance through their employers. Beyond clinical skills, the *Level 3* MedFT would be involved in research considering how integrated behavioral healthcare with the interdisciplinary healthcare team, as well as incorporating the patient's systems of support (e.g., family, friends), aids in reducing substance use and helping the patient move in to recovery. Policy work may also be addressed that urges for an understanding of addictive disorders as a medical condition, calling for insurance companies to provide better access to affordable care for the treatment of substance use disorders.

The MedFT who possesses the knowledge and skills outlined at *Level 4* will strongly identify as a MedFT and work primarily in a healthcare setting focused on alcohol and drug treatment. Common treatment settings that would have a diverse treatment team on site include both residential and inpatient treatment settings, as well as many outpatient treatment centers. This individual has an understanding of each of the treatment providers training, scope of practice, and role in accomplishing treatment goals. Further, the MedFT at *Level 4* will utilize treatment team members effectively, such as conducting joint treatment sessions with another provider and the patient, and would be active in attending. Their skills will also be enhanced by their knowledge of core content related to alcohol and drug treatment. Additionally, the *Level 4* MedFT will be engaged in conducting research related to the treatment of addiction in healthcare setting. This research would be informed by the biopsychosocial-spiritual model and would consider utilization of treatment teams for integrated behavioral healthcare. In our case example, Dustin shows signs of resisting Tom's recommendation to attend a detoxification center to monitor withdrawal symptoms. A MedFT functioning at *Level 4* would be able to help explain to Dustin the differences between what he experienced quitting methamphetamines last year and the serious medical risks associated with quitting alcohol when there are signs of physical dependence. Tom would be able to inform Dustin of what to expect at a detoxification center, the time investment required for this level of work, and how to better handle issues related to work absenteeism. Tom would coordinate with a case worker around employment options or community resources to make a stay from work more manageable. Additionally, Tom would also encourage Dustin to consider working with a psychiatrist if he was concerned about struggles with quitting alcohol, as the psychiatrist could prescribe medication that helps patients with alcohol use disorders. Finally, the MedFT at *Level 4* would also attend thoroughly to systemic issues related to substance abuse. Specifically, Tom would work with Elaina and Dustin to discuss how and when it will be appropriate for Elaina to ask about his abstinence from alcohol use and how they can support one another with the recovery process and most importantly address intimate partner violence and safety issues. The *Level 4* MedFT would recognize the benefit of incorporating behavioral couples therapy (BCT) for substance use, as it helps couples promote abstinence behaviors as well as improve positive relationship skills.

The fifth and final level of the continuum identifies a medical family therapist who has extensive practice in the treatment of alcohol and drug use and knows how to collaborate with treatment teams in different healthcare contexts (e.g., inpatient/residential, day treatment, outpatient). At *Level 5*, the MedFT would also have served in multiple roles, such as administration or supervision. Proficiency would be demonstrated in family therapy and BPSS approaches, and they would have comprehensive knowledge about substance use and recovery that extends beyond the basics of treatment—such as the effects of different classifications of substances of abuse, drug interactions, pharmacotherapy, and detoxification. These competencies would be seen in the MedFTs' ability to collaborate with all relevant professionals in the treatment of alcohol or drug use. This individual would also be widely engaged in the field of alcohol and drug use, engaging in mentoring activities related to supervision, connecting with their community to potentially facilitate prevention programs, and would be engaged in advancing the knowledge of this field through research. Their work may also extend to policymaking. The *Level 5* MedFT would be engaged in cutting-edge research, which would include using novel approaches (e.g., neuroimaging techniques, biomarkers) to improve understanding of the impact of addiction not only on the individual but their family system. The MedFT at this level would also be actively involved in policies that make funding available for research on addiction recovery.

Over the course of treatment, Tom could continue to work with Elaina and Dustin by providing additional recommendations for referral sources. For example, Tom may refer Dustin to a nutritionist to assess for nutritional deficiencies, which is common for patients who suffer from alcohol use disorder. The nutritionist would conduct an assessment, potentially prescribe nutrient supplements to correct issues related to issues of absorption, and then help create a meal plan that increases Dustin's likelihood of success with recovery. The supervisor on the case (KS) could use this case in the practicum setting to mentor students on how to effectively integrate the BPSS model in the treatment of alcohol and substance use and inform students of all the appropriate treatment team members that should be engaged in this process. This case could be utilized to inform future studies conducted by the supervisor or could be used to enhance educational opportunities at the supervisor's training program. The MedFT, Tom, as well as the supervisor (KS) could also be conducting research on the efficacy of substance use treatment. The MedFT and the supervisor could then use their findings to educate and work with local policymakers in establishing funding for both treatment and research in the area.

Research-Informed Practices

The establishment of MedFT and IBHC teams with alcohol and drug use treatment is a relatively new area of practice. Several different therapeutic approaches for behavioral health providers at both the individual (e.g., Barrowclough et al., 2009; Miller & Rollnick, 2002) and the systemic (e.g., Rowe, 2012) levels have been empirically validated, and IBHC team approaches incorporating various members have been identified as efficacious (e.g., Cosden, Ellens, Schnell, Yamini-Diouf, & Wolfe, 2003; de Shazer & Isebaert, 2003; Marlowe, 2003). Best practices for a MedFT working with an IBHC team, however, need further examination and validation.

Individual Approaches

Several evidence-based approaches exist to help individuals with recovery from drug or alcohol use. Motivational interviewing (MI) is a well-known approach associated with substance use treatment. MI is a goal-oriented, person-centered approach that focuses on the individual's perspectives and concerns (Miller & Rollnick, 2002). Behavioral health providers who practice MI describe this approach as a "way of being" with the patient that is directive but empathic with the patients' concerns for engaging in treatment and is most often used with another form of treatment (Hettema, Miller, & Steele, 2004). The use of motivational interviewing has been shown to increase participation in treatment, reduce consumption of drugs and alcohol, facilitate higher rates of abstinence, and aid in better social adjustment (Landry, 1996; Miller, Westerberg, & Waldron, 1995).

A MedFT may use MI in his or her early interactions with patients to explore patients' readiness to change and help them to identify the potential benefits of engaging in treatment. Further, the MedFT should work with the treatment team to ensure that all members of the treatment are working with the patient based on their readiness to change. Meeting the patients where they are in their readiness to change will validate their concerns and will prevent from pushing the patient beyond their view of their problem. The MedFT will then be able to better prepare the patients for the different types of treatment and treatment providers that they will engage and interact with. The MedFT may also find MI beneficial due to its ability to create change in brief sessions, as studies have found MI to be both statistically and clinically significant in 30 and 60 minute sessions (Callon et al., 2006; Kidorf, King, Gandotra, Kolodmer, & Brooner, 2012).

Another frequently used individual approach for the treatment of alcohol and drug use is cognitive-behavioral therapy (CBT; Beck, 1979; Magill & Ray, 2009). CBT has consistently been demonstrated as an effective model for reducing substance use (Barrowclough et al., 2009; Drummond et al., 2005; Glasner-Edwards et al., 2007; Maude-Griffin et al., 1998; Morgenstern, Blanchard, Morgan, Labouvie, & Hayaki, 2001). MedFT applications of CBT would include helping patients to identify negative thoughts that potentially trigger use, evaluating the positive and negative consequences related to their substance use, and developing new coping techniques to replace substance use behaviors (National Institute on Drug Abuse, 2012). For example, substance use can be a reinforcing behavior if it is effective at eliminating the patient's feelings of anxiety, and treatment can identify other means of achieving that outcome that are healthier for the patient. The exploration of triggering events may include assessing home environment stressors or other interpersonal relationships that trigger thoughts relating to the need to use the substance of abuse as well as emotional responses to these thoughts. The MedFT would work with the individual to identify faulty thinking or other core beliefs that influence substance use and then work to change substance use behavior by challenging automatic cognitions and changing the reinforcement schedule for the substance use (Center for Substance Abuse Treatment, 1999). With knowledge about faulty cognitions or behavioral triggers for the alcohol or drug use, the MedFT would work with the treatment team to be sure all providers are mindful of not contributing to any of the patient's cognitive distortions and are not triggering the substance use behavioral response.

Couple and Family Approaches

Couple- and family-based approaches have been extensively reviewed over the past 20 years (Liddle & Dakof, 1995; Rowe, 2012; Rowe & Liddle, 2003) with the general conclusion being that such models for the treatment of alcohol and drug use are among the most effective approaches for both adolescents and adults (Rowe, 2012). This should come as no surprise due to the extensive empirical support for the link between family function and substance use (Fals-Stewart, Lam, & Kelley, 2009). The overarching goal of couple- and family-based treatment models is to use the support and power of family members to reduce substance use and make lifestyle changes, as well as to improve family functioning and interactions to create an environment more conducive to long-term recovery promotion (Fals-Sterwart, Lam, & Kelley, 2009). Rowe (2012) identified three main categories of couple- and family-based treatment for alcohol and drug use: (a) behavioral (e.g., behavioral couples therapy (BCT); O'Farell & Fals-Stewart, 2006), (b) family systems (Brief Strategic Family Therapy; Szapoczink & Kurtines, 1989), and (c) multiple systems approaches (e.g., multidimensional family therapy (MDFT; Liddle, 2002). Fischer, Baucom, and Cohen (2016) more recently advanced specific attention to the utility of cognitive-behavioral couple therapies (CBCT) while still recognizing power of extending this to broader family inclusion.

All of these approaches have been designed to target alcohol and drug use at different stages of life, specifically adolescence and adulthood. Because drug and alcohol use typically becomes problematic in adolescence, a large amount of research exists on effective treatment approaches for teens. Multiple comprehensive reviews of adolescent substance abuse treatment have concluded that MDFT is identified as not only efficacious (Vaughn & Howard, 2004), but viewed as one of the highest-quality models for working with teens and substance use (Becker & Curry, 2008). MDFT is an integrative, outpatient treatment approach that is categorized as a multiple systems-ecological approach. Change in substance use is targeted by working with the teen, their subsystems (teen-sibling, teen-parent), family system, and extrafamilial systems (peers, school, juvenile justice system) to develop multiple alliances. MDFT has demonstrated an ability to have high retention rates in treatment

(Liddle, Dakof, Henderson, & Rowe, 2011) and to reduce teen drug use (Austin, MacGowan, & Wagner, 2005; Becker & Curry, 2008). For MedFT, MDFT presents a strong example of the power of collaborating with multiple providers and working as a treatment team, as evidenced by the integration of not only the teen and their parents, but by working with the school system, the community, and potentially the juvenile justice system. This could additionally include working with the teen's primary care physician or a psychiatrist for any co-occurring mental or medical health illness. The success of MDFT is based on its ability to address the teen's substance use at multiple levels in a collaborative model. A final model focused on addressing teen substance use that is noteworthy is functional family therapy (FFT; Alexander & Parsons, 1982). Integrating both behavioral therapy and systems-oriented approaches, FFT works to change maladaptive family interactions that are conceptualized as maintaining the teen's substance use. Behavioral interventions are used to create contingencies for promoting abstinence. Research has found that FFT can lead to improved family functioning and reduced recidivism among delinquent teens (Barton, Alexander, Waldron, Turner, & Warburton, 1985) and helps with reduction in substance use (Slesnick & Prestopnik, 2004).

Couple- and family-based models for the treatment of adult alcohol and drug users also have supporting evidence for their ability to reduce substance use (Stanton & Shadish, 1997). Researchers and behavioral health providers alike have recognized the power of these approaches for substance abuse due to the ability to create motivation to enter treatment, the recognition that all members of the family can be impacted due to substance use by one member, and that familial stress can create a barrier to recovery (Carlson, Smith, Matto, & Eversman, 2008; Dakof et al., 2010; Rowe, 2012). A well-researched model of adult treatment for addiction is behavioral couples therapy (BCT; O'Farell & Fals-Stewart, 2006; McCrady et al., 2016). BCT is an abstinence-based intervention for married or cohabitating substance abusers and their partners, which seeks to engage both partners in treatment, enhance relational dynamics, and support recovery efforts. BCT trials have found efficacy in comparison to individualized therapy models for outcomes related to relationship improvement, drug use, drug-related arrests, intimate partner violence, and hospitalizations (Fals-Stewart, Lam, & Kelley, 2009; McCrady et al., 2016).

Some insight gained from BCT research indicates that patients with comorbid disorders found greater improvement with BCT than individual treatment alone, those with a greater severity of drinking may reap the most benefits of treatment, and pretreatment relationship satisfaction may enhance the effects (McCrady et al., 2016). Particular active ingredients to the treatment have been examined, including partner skills training and relationship enhancement interventions, as have proposed mechanisms of behavior change (e.g., motivation, coping skills, couple interactions, and significant other supports; McCrady et al., 2016). It is worth noting that BCT has been examined more thoroughly in treating couples wherein the male partner is the identified patient (IP) and less so with female IPs (McCrady et al., 2016). Adaptations to account for different risk factors, societal influences, and consequences may be necessary in the treatment of women (McCrady et al., 2016). BCTs have been found to be efficacious with a wide variety of patient backgrounds and circumstances. Our case example therapist, Tom, could have considered the integration of BCT to help Dustin and Elaina negotiate daily check-ins for sobriety by creating a daily sobriety contract and safely addressed their reported intimate partner violence.

Solution-focused therapy (SFBT), another systemic approach to treatment, has been applied to the treatment of substance use (Berg & Miller, 1992; de Shazer & Isebaert, 2003). This particular approach can be used with individuals or families. Although this approach can be used with an individual, the intent of the approach is to have a relational and systemic clinical impact. The MedFT would work with a patient in a collaborative manner to identify goals they have for treatment. The MedFT employing SFBT would not force a patient to choose abstinence or harm reduction as goals for the substance use. The focus of treatment is on the times when the patient was more successful with meeting his or her goals (i.e., exceptions) and also identifying the patient's existing resources or skills that can be employed to achieve his or her goals (i.e., means) (de Shazer & Isebaert, 2003). For example, a patient may identify a goal of reducing alcohol use, and so the MedFT would focus on the times the patient was able to reduce or eliminate substance use and to identify what solutions the patient was applying. Treatment would focus primarily on the patient's success and the solutions, and if one solution did not work, the MedFT would help the patient find a new solution. The MedFT could also employ scaling questions and the miracle question, which are part of the SFBT approach (see de Shazer & Isebaert, 2003). This approach can also be applied to different intensities of substance abuse. SFBT has been employed as both an inpatient and outpatient treatment approach and has been used in conjunction with family therapy and an IBHC team composed of psychiatrists and nurses (de Shazer & Isebaert, 2003). The MedFT can work with the integrated treatment team to focus care at all levels on the successes of the patient and to focus on the solutions that have been established as effective. The MedFT can work with the IBHC team to work with the patient in a way that collaboratively identifies the treatment goals, potentially training the other professionals on how to use solution-focused language.

Community Approaches

Community-based/self-help programs have a strong history in the treatment of substance use disorders (Alcoholics Anonymous [AA], 2014). Differing from group therapy, self-help groups are peer-facilitated forums that do not include the presence of a licensed professional. These groups are community-based (i.e., not sponsored by a hospital, clinic, or other care sites). They are utilized to facilitate social support through group participation. The most recognized self-help group associated with substance use is *Alcoholics Anonymous* (AA, 2017). AA identifies as a spiritual, abstinence-based group that is based on members helping members. It is most readily known for the application of the 12 steps, but also has 12 traditions, including anonymity for all and self-sufficiency.

AA is recognized under SAMHSA's National Registry of Evidence-based Programs and Practices (2017). A randomized clinical trial supported AA's role in maintaining abstinence through recovery when combined with a structured treatment (Walitzer, Dermen, & Barrick, 2009). AA's 12-Step program aligns well with core tenets of the BPSS model, insofar as both stress the consideration of spirituality in treatment (in the case of AA, it is about seeking a higher power to find one's path to recovery). Other self-help groups have been modeled after AA, including Narcotics Anonymous (2017), Overeaters Anonymous (2017), Al-Anon Family Groups (2011–2017) for friends and families of problem drinkers, and Families Anonymous (2017).

Although AA and 12-Step groups are the most well-known self-help programs for substance abuse, other self-help options exist. For instance, Rational Recovery (RR, 2017) is a self-help group based on rational emotive therapy and does not require commitment to long-term abstinence to achieve recovery. The Secular Organization for Sobriety (SOS, 2016) was designed for individuals who have struggled with the spiritual integration found in AA practices, stressing personal responsibility to achieve sobriety and recovery. In recognition that women did not always benefit from the conflictual tactics used in substance abuse treatment, the Women for Sobriety (WFS, 2016) was developed as the first national self-help program for women alcoholics. Finally, SMART or self-management and recovery training (SMART Recovery, 1994–2017) was developed as a secular, science-based alternative to 12-Step groups, and it incorporates cognitive-behavioral and rational emotive behavioral therapy to build motivation, cope with cravings, problem solve, and create new balance in life.

Recommending self-help programs within patients' local communities will require the MedFT to be well versed in both the assumptions and traditions of each organization, alongside understanding the potential advantages and disadvantages of each organization. Programs should be recommended based on the consideration of the needs of each individual patient, as a one-size-fits-all model is ineffective. Our MedFT Tom could have recommended AA as a resource for Dustin, alongside Al-Anon or Families Anonymous for Elaina. Working the step process with a sponsor could be helpful to these patients, and any challenges experienced in AA or Al-Anon could be further incorporated into treatment with the MedFT.

Conclusion

The MedFT's role in alcohol and drug treatment can be varied depending on location of practice and intensity of the patient's use, among other factors. Alcohol and drug treatment is unique in the type of professionals who may be involved in a treatment team, including psychiatrists, nurses, case workers, probation officers, primary care physicians, nutritionists, sponsors, and other behavioral health professionals. In an IBHC treatment system, the MedFT will play a crucial role in assessment, treatment, and team coordination. Regardless of whether the MedFT is working in an already established IBHC team, this type of integrated behavioral healthcare can still be achieved, is encouraged, and is even an ethical matter. MedFTs may be the first point of contact for a patient with a need for alcohol and drug treatment. Substance use tends to go underreported by patients for various reasons, and it is sometimes seen as a separate issue from the presenting problem. Understanding the biopsychosocial-spiritual and family systems influences that affect and are affected by substance use will help the MedFT be a more effective treatment provider and treatment team member.

Reflection Questions
1. While working as a MedFT in alcohol and drug treatment contexts, under what conditions, if any, do you think that "moderate use" (rather than abstinence) is an appropriate patient goal?
2. When working with a patient who has both a physical dependency and financial challenges, what professionals would you integrate into a treatment team? How would you ethically balance the patient's financial concerns (e.g., limited health insurance) with his or her treatment needs for substance use/abuse?
3. What assumptions do you have about what it means to be a substance user, or an "addict"? How could these assumptions about the cause of use affect the direction you choose in your clinical work?

Glossary of Important Terms in Alcohol and Drug Treatment

Chemical dependency The physical and/or psychological dependence on one or more psychoactive drug.
Pharmacotherapy The practice of using drug action in the body to address/treat behavioral health issues; or, the field of medicine that addresses the use of medications to help treat or correct mental health illness and drug addiction.
Physical dependence The repeated use of licit or illicit substances can lead to a physiological reliance on the substance, which may include tolerance and withdrawal symptoms.
Polydrug abuse The use of several drugs either in succession or at the same time to achieve a certain effect.
Psychoactive substance Any substance that directly alters normal functioning of the central nervous system (CNS) when it is taken by means of injection, ingestion, inhalation, snorting, or absorbed by blood.
Psychological dependence A state of consciousness caused by substance use that will reinforce the dependence on substance use.
Psychotropic drugs Drugs used to treat behavioral health illnesses, including, but not limited to, antidepressants, antipsychotics, and anxiolytics.
Substance abuse The harmful or dangerous use of psychoactive substances, including alcohol and other licit or illicit chemical substances (e.g., prescription medication, marijuana, cocaine), that creates significant distress in the individual's life.

Tolerance The need for an increased amount of alcohol or drugs of abuse to experience an effect from use (this occurs after repeated use)—or the body's ability to consume greater amounts of a substance with the same physiological or psychological impact.

Withdrawal The abnormal physical or psychological response to the discontinuation of use of a licit or illicit substance that has the capability to produce physical dependence. Common withdrawal symptoms may include sweating, fever, vomiting, anxiety, insomnia, and muscle pain—or the body's attempt to reach homeostasis after a history of psychoactive drug use/abuse. Symptoms experienced by the individual will depend on several factors related to substance of abuse, frequency, and severity of use.

Additional Resources

Literature

American Psychiatric Association (2013). *Diagnostic and statistical manual of mental disorders* (5th ed.). Arlington, VA: American Psychiatric Association.

Inaba, D. S., & Cohen, W. E. (2014). *Uppers, downers, all arounders: Physical and mental effects of psychoactive drugs* (8th ed.). Medford, OR: CNS Publications.

Juhnke, G. A., & Hagedorn, W. B. (2013). *Counseling addicted families: An integrated assessment and treatment model.* New York, NY: Routledge.

Lieber, C. S. (2012). *Medical and nutritional complications of alcoholism: Mechanisms and management.* New York, NY: Springer Science & Business Media.

Mee-Lee, D. (Ed.) (2013). *The ASAM criteria: Treatment criteria for addictive, substance-related and co-occurring conditions* (3rd ed.). North Bethesda, MD: American Society of Addiction Medicine.

Measures/Instruments

Alcohol Screening and Brief Intervention for Youth: A Practitioner's Guide. http://www.integration.samhsa.gov/Alcohol_Screening_and_Brief_Intervention_for_Youth_Guide_and_Medscape_Promotion.pdf

Alcohol Use Disorders Identification Test (AUDIT). http://www.integration.samhsa.gov/AUDIT_screener_for_alcohol.pdf

AUDIT-C. http://www.integration.samhsa.gov/images/res/tool_auditc.pdf

CAGE-AID. http://www.integration.samhsa.gov/images/res/CAGEAID.pdf

Computer-based Tools for Diagnosis and Treatment of Alcohol Problems. http://pubs.niaaa.nih.gov/publications/arh291/36-40.htm

Drug Abuse Screening Test (DAST-10). http://www.emcdda.europa.eu/attachements.cfm/att_61480_EN_DAST%202008.pdf

Level 2, Substance Use, Adult (Adapted from the NIDA-Modified ASSIST). https://www.psychiatry.org/psychiatrists/practice/dsm/dsm-5/online-assessment-measures

Level 2, Substance Use, Child Age 11 to 17 (Adapted from the NIDA-Modified ASSIST). https://www.psychiatry.org/psychiatrists/practice/dsm/dsm-5/online-assessment-measures

Level 2, Substance Use, Parent/Guardian of Child Age 6–17 (Adapted from the NIDA-Modified ASSIST). https://www.psychiatry.org/psychiatrists/practice/dsm/dsm-5/online-assessment-measures

Measuring Codependency: Composite Codependency Scale. (Marks, Blore, Hine, & Dear, 2012)

Measuring Codependency: Spann-Fischer Codependency Scale. (Fischer, Spann, & Crawford, 1991)

NIDAMED: Medical & Health Professionals Evidence-Based Screening Tools and Resource Materials. https://www.drugabuse.gov/nidamed-medical-health-professionals/tool-resources-your-practice/screening-assessment-drug-testing-resources/chart-evidence-based-screening-tools-adults

Parent Motivation to Participate in Treatment: Parent Motivation Inventory. (Nock & Photos, 2006)

Readiness to Change Questionnaire. (Heather, Luce, Peck, Dunbar, & James, 1999)

Substance Use Screening & Assessment Instruments Database. http://lib.adai.washington.edu/instruments/

Organizations/Associations

Alcoholics Anonymous. http://www.aa.org/pages/en_US
Association for Addiction Professionals. http://www.naadac.org/
National Institute on Alcohol Abuse and Alcoholism. http://www.niaaa.nih.gov/
National Institute on Drug Abuse. https://www.drugabuse.gov/
Substance Abuse and Mental Health Services Administration. http://www.samhsa.gov/
U.S. Department of Health and Human Services. http://www.niaaa.nih.gov/

References[1]

Akhavain, P., Amaral, D., Murphy, M., & Cardon Uehlinger, K. (1999). Collaborative practice: A nursing perspective of the psychiatric interdisciplinary treatment team. *Holistic Nursing Practice, 13*, 1–11. https://www.ncbi.nlm.nih.gov/pubmed/10196897

Al-Anon Family Groups. (2011–2017). *Al-Anon family groups: Strength and hope for friends and families of problem drinkers*. Retrieved from http://www.al-anon.alateen.org/

---

[1] Note: References that are prefaced with an asterisk are recommended readings.

Alcoholics Anonymous. (2017). *What is A.A.?* New York, NY: Alcoholics Anonymous World Services. Retrieved from http://www.aa.org/pages/en_US/what-is-aa

Alcoholics Anonymous. (2014). *A brief history of the Big Book.* New York, NY: Alcoholics Anonymous World Services.

*Alexander, B. K. (1987). The disease and adaptive models of addiction: A framework evaluation. *Journal of Drug Issues, 17,* 47–66. https://doi.org/10.1177/002204268701700104.

Alexander, J., & Parsons, B. V. (1982). *Functional family therapy.* Monterey, CA: Brooks/Cole.

*American Psychiatric Association. (2013). *Diagnostic and statistical manual of mental disorders* (5th ed.). Arlington, VA: American Psychiatric Association.

American Society of Addiction Medicine. (2011). *The definition of addiction.* Retrieved from http://www.asam.org/docs/default-source/public-policy-statements/1definition_of_addiction_long_4-11.pdf?sfvrsn=4

Austin, A. M., MacGowan, M. J., & Wagner, E. F. (2005). Effective family-based interventions for adolescents with substance use problems: A systemic review. *Research on Social Work Practice, 15,* 67–83. https://doi.org/10.1177/1049731504271606

Barrowclough, C., Haddock, G., Beardmore, R., Conrod, P., Craig, T., Davies, L., ... Wykes, T. (2009). Evaluating integrated MI and CBT for people with psychosis and substance misuse: Recruitment, retention and sample characteristics of the MIDAS trial. *Addictive Behaviors, 34,* 859–866. https://doi.org/10.1016/j.addbeh.2009.03.007

Barton, C., Alexander, J., Waldron, H., Turner, C., & Warburton, J. (1985). Generalizing treatment effects of Functional Family Therapy: Three replications. *American Journal of Family Therapy, 13,* 16–26. https://doi.org/10.1080/01926188508251260

Barnes, G., & Farrell, M. (1992). Parental support and control as predictors of adolescent drinking, delinquency, and related problem behaviors. *Journal of Marriage and Family, 54,* 763–776. http://www.jstor.org/stable/353159

Beck, A. (1979). *Cognitive therapy and emotional disorders.* Madison, CT: Penguin Group.

Becker, S., & Curry, J. (2008). Outpatient interventions for adolescent substance abuse: A quality of evidence review. *Journal of Consulting and Clinical Psychology, 76,* 531–543. https://doi.org/10.1037/0022-006X.76.4.531

Berg, I. K., & Miller, S. D. (1992). *Working with the problem drinker: A solution-focused approach.* New York, NY: W. W. Norton.

Betty Ford Institute Consensus Panel. (2007). What is recovery? A working definition from the Betty Ford Institute. *Journal of Substance Abuse Treatment, 33,* 221–228. https://doi.org/10.1016/j.jsat.2007.06.001

Callon, C., Wood, E., Marsh, D., Li, K., Montaner, J., & Kerr, T. (2006). Barriers and facilitators to methadone maintenance therapy use among illicit opiate injection drug users in Vancouver. *Journal of Opioid Management, 2,* 35–41. Retrieved from https://www.researchgate.net/profile/David_Marsh3/publication/6487367_Barriers_and_facilitators_to_methadone_maintenance_therapy_use_among_illicit_opiate_injection_drug_users_in_Vancouver/links/56786f9008aebcdda0ebd8bf.pdf

Carlson, B. E., Smith, C., Matto, H., & Eversman, M. (2008). Reunification with children in the context of maternal recovery from drug abuse. *Families in Society, 89,* 253–263. https://doi.org/10.1606/1044-3894.3741

Castro, F., & Alarcón, E. (2002). Integrating cultural variables into drug abuse prevention and treatment with racial/ethnic minorities. *Journal of Drug Issues, 32,* 783–810. https://doi.org/10.1177/002204260203200304

Center for Substance Abuse Treatment. (1999). Brief cognitive-behavioral therapy. In *Brief interventions and brief therapies for substance abuse* (pp. 51–77). Rockville, MD: Substance Abuse and Mental Health Services Administration.

Cosden, M., Ellens, J. E., Schnell, J. L., Yamini-Diouf, Y., & Wolfe, M. M. (2003). Evaluation of a mental health treatment court with assertive community treatment. *Behavioral Sciences and the Law, 21,* 415–427. https://doi.org/10.1002/bsl.542

Dakof, G., Cohern, J., Henderson, C., Duarte, E., Boustani, M., Blackburn, A., Venzer, E., & Hawes, S. (2010). A randomized pilot study of the Engaging Moms Program for family drug court. *Journal of Substance Abuse Treatment, 38*, 263–274. https://doi.org/10.1016/j.jsat.2010.01.002

de Shazer, S., & Isebaert, L. (2003). The Bruges model: A solution-focused approach to problem drinking. *Journal of Family Psychotherapy, 14*, 43–52. https://doi.org/10.1300/J085v14n04_04

Drake, R., Mueserk K., Brunette, M., McHugo, G., (2004). A review of treatments for people with severe mental illnesses and co-occurring substance use disorders. *Psychiatric Rehabilitation Journal, 27*, 360–374. http://dx.doi.org/10.2975/27.2004.360.374

Drummond, C., Kouimtsidis, C., Reynolds, M., Russell, I., Godfrey, C., McCusker, M., … Porter, S. (2005). The effectiveness and cost effectiveness of cognitive behaviour therapy for opiate misusers in methadone maintenance treatment: A multicentre, randomised, controlled trial. *Drugs: Education, Prevention & Policy, 12*, 69–76. Retrieved from https://kar.kent.ac.uk/id/eprint/16974

Engel, G. L. (1977). The need for a new medical model: A challenge for biomedicine. *Science, 196*, 129–136. https://doi.org/10.1126/science.847460

Engel, G. L. (1980). The clinical application of the biopsychosocial model. *American Journal of Psychiatry, 137*, 535–544. https://doi.org/10.1176/ajp.137.5.535

Enoch, M. (2013). Genetic influences on the development of alcoholism. *Current Psychiatry Reports, 15*, 412–421. https://doi.org/10.1007/s11920-013-0412-1

Fals-Stewart, W., Lam, W., & Kelley, M. (2009). Learning sobriety together: Behavioral couples therapy for alcoholism and drug abuse. *Journal of Family Therapy, 31*, 115–125. https://doi.org/10.1111/j.1467.2009.00458.x

Families Anonymous. (2017). *Families Anonymous recovery fellowship*. Des Plaines, IL: Families Anonymous. Retrieved from http://www.familiesanonymous.org/

Finkelstein, N. (1994). Treatment issues for alcohol- and drug- dependent pregnant and parenting women. *Health & Social Work, 19*, 7–15. https://doi.org/10.1093/hsw/19.1.7

*Fischer, M. S., Baucom, D. H., & Cohen, M. J. (2016). Cognitive-behavioral couple therapies: Review of the evidence for the treatment of relationship distress, psychopathology, and chronic health conditions. *Family Process, 55*, 423–442. https://doi.org/10.1111/famp.12227.

Fischner, J. L., Spann, L., & Crawford, D. (1991). Measuring codependency. *Alcoholism Treatment Quarterly, 8*, 87–100. https://doi.org/10.1300/J020V08N01_06

Glasner-Edwards, S., Tate, S. R., McQuaid, J. R., Cummins, K., Granholm, E., & Brown, S. A. (2007). Mechanisms of action in integrated cognitive-behavioral treatment versus twelve-step facilitation for substance-dependent adults with comorbid major depression. *Journal of Studies on Alcohol and Drugs, 68*, 663–672. 10.15288/jsad.2007.68.663

Goldstein, R., & Volkow, N. (2011). Dysfunction of the prefrontal cortex in addiction: Neuroimaging findings and clinical implications. *Nature Reviews Neuroscience, 12*, 652–669. https://www.ncbi.nlm.nih.gov/pmc/articles/PMC3462342/

Griffiths, M. (2005). A 'components' model of addiction within a biopsychosocial framework. *Journal of Substance Use, 10*, 191–197. https://doi.org/10.1080/14659890500114359

Gruber, K. J., & Taylor, M. F. (2006). A family perspective for substance abuse: Implications from the literature. *Journal of Social Work Practice in the Addictions, 6*, 1–29. https://doi.org/10.1300/J160v06n01_01

Hasin, D., & Kilcoyne, B. (2012). Comorbidity of psychiatric and substance use disorders in the United States: Current issues and findings from the NESARC. *Current Opinion in Psychiatry, 25*, 165–171. https://doi.org/10.1097/YCO.0b013e3283523dcc

Hearn, W. L., Rose, S., Ciarleglio, A., & Mash, D. C. (1991). Cocaethylene is more potent than cocaine in mediating lethality. *Pharmacology Biochemistry and Behavior, 39*, 532–533. https://doi.org/10.1016/0091-3057(91)90222-N

Heather, N., Luce, A., Peck, D., Dunbar, B., & James, I. (1999). Development of a treatment version of the Readiness to Change Questionnaire. *Addiction Research, 7*, 63–83. https://doi.org/10.3109/16066359909004375

Hettema, J., Miller, W., & Steele, J. (2004). A meta-analysis of motivational interviewing techniques in the treatment of alcohol use disorders. *Alcoholism-Clinical and Experimental Research, 28*, 74A–74A (supplement).

Hodgson, J., Lamson, A., Mendenhall, T., & Tyndall, L. (2014). Introduction to medical family therapy: Advanced applications. In J. Hodgson, A. Lamson, T. Mendenhall, and D. Crane (Eds.), *Medical family therapy: Advanced applications* (pp. 1–9). New York, NY: Springer.

Ilgen, M., Wilbourne, P., Moos, B., & Moos, R. (2008). Problem-free drinking over 16 years among individuals with alcohol use disorders. *Drug and Alcohol Dependence, 92*, 116–122. https://doi.org/10.1016/j.drugalcdep.2007.07.006

*Inaba, D. S., & Cohen, W. E. (2014). *Uppers, downers, all arounders: Physical and mental effects of psychoactive drugs* (8th ed.). Medford, OR: CNS Publications.

Islam, S. K. N., Hossain, K. J., Ahmed, A., & Ahsan, M. (2002). Nutritional status of drug addicts undergoing detoxification: Prevalence of malnutrition and influence of illicit drugs and lifestyle. *British Journal of Nutrition, 88*, 507–513. https://doi.org/10.1079/BJN2002702

*Juhnke, G. A., & Hagedorn, W. B. (2013). *Counseling addicted families: An integrated assessment and treatment model.* New York, NY: Routledge.

Kerr, D., Capaldi, D., Pears, K., & Owen, L. (2012). Intergenerational influences on early alcohol use: Independence from the problem behavior pathway. *Development and Psychopathology, 24*, 889–906. https://doi.org/10.1017/S0954579412000430

Kidorf, M., King, V. L., Gandotra, N., Kolodner, K., & Brooner, R. K. (2012). Improving treatment enrollment and re-enrollment rates of syringe exchangers: 12-month outcomes. *Drug Alcohol Dependence, 124*, 162–166. https://doi.org/10.1016/j.drugalcdep.2011.12.008

Landry, M. J. (1996). *Overview of addiction treatment effectiveness. HHSPub. No. (SMA) 96–3081.* Rockville, MD: Diane Publishing.

Li, D., Zhao, H., & Gelernter, J. (2011). Strong association of the alcohol dehydrogenase 1B gene (ADH1B) with alcohol dependence and alcohol-induced medical diseases. *Biological Psychiatry, 70*, 504–512. https://doi.org/10.1016/j.biopsych.2011.02.024

Liddle, H. A. (2002). *Multidimensional family therapy for adolescent cannabis users, cannabis youth treatment (CYT) series (Vol. 5).* Rockville, MD: Center for Substance Abuse Treatment (CSAT). Retrieved from http://files.eric.ed.gov/fulltext/ED478685.pdfhttp://files.eric.ed.gov/fulltext/ED478685.pdf

Liddle, H., & Dakof, G. (1995). Efficacy of family therapy for drug abuse: Promising but not definitive. *Journal of Marital and Family Therapy, 21*, 511–544. https://doi.org/10.1111/j.1752-0606.1995.tb00177.x

Liddle, H., Dakof, G. A., Henderson, C. E., & Rowe, C. L. (2011). Implementation outcomes of mutli-dimensional family therapy-detention to community (DTC): A reintegration program for drug-using juvenile detainees. *International Journal of Offender Therapy and Comparative Criminology, 55*, 587–604. https://doi.org/10.1177/0306624X10366960

*Lieber, C. S. (2012). *Medical and nutritional complications of alcoholism: Mechanisms and management.* New York, NY: Springer.

Lieber, C. S. (2003). Relationships between nutrition, alcohol use, and liver disease. *Alcohol Research & Health, 27*(3), 220–231. Retrieved from https://pubs.niaaa.nih.gov/publications/arh27-3/220-231.htm?ref=vidupdatez.com/image

Magill, M., & Ray, L. A. (2009). Cognitive-behavioral treatment with adult alcohol and illicit drug users: A meta-analysis of randomized controlled trials. *Journal of Studies on Alcohol and Drugs, 70*, 516–527. 10.15288/jsad.2009.70.516

Marijuana and the Law. (2016). *Marijuana and the law.* Retrieved from http://www.marijuanaandthelaw.com/

Marlatt, G. A., & Witkiewitz, K. (2002). Harm reduction approaches to alcohol use: Health promotion, prevention, and treatment. *Addictive Behaviors, 27*, 867–886. https://doi.org/10.1016/S0306-4603(02)00294-0

Marlowe, D. (2003). Integrating substance abuse treatment and criminal justice supervision. *Addiction Science & Clinical Practice, 2*, 4–14. https://www.ncbi.nlm.nih.gov/pmc/articles/PMC2851043/?report=reader

Mathers, B. M., Degenhardt, L., Phillips, B., Wiessing, L., Hickman, M., Strathdee, S. A., ... Mattick, R. P. (2008). Global epidemiology of injecting drug use and HIV among people who inject drugs: A systematic review. *The Lancet, 372*, 1733–1745. https://doi.org/10.1016/S0140-6736(08)61311-2

Maude-Griffin, P. M., Hohenstein, J. M., Humfleet, G. L., Reilly, P. M., Tusel, D. J., & Hall, S. M. (1998). Superior efficacy of cognitive behavioral therapy for urban crack cocaine abusers: Main and matching effects. *Journal of Consulting and Clinical Psychology, 66*, 832–837. https://doi.org/10.1037/0022-006X.66.5.832

McCance, E. F., Price, L. H., Kosten, T. R., & Jatlow, P. I. (1995). Cocaethylene: Pharmacology, physiology and behavioral effects in humans. *Journal of Pharmacology and Experimental Therapeutics, 274*, 215–223. Retrieved from http://jpet.aspetjournals.org/content/jpet/274/1/215.full.pdf

McCrady, B. S., Wilson, A. D., Muñoz, R. E., Fink, B. C., Fokas, K., & Borders, A. (2016). Alcohol-focused behavioral couple therapy. *Family Process, 55*, 443–459. https://doi.org/10.1111/famp.12231

*Mee-Lee, D. (Ed.) (2013). *The ASAM criteria: Treatment criteria for addictive, substance-related and co-occurring conditions* (3rd ed.). North Bethesda, MD: American Society of Addiction Medicine.

Miller, W. R., & Rollnick, S. (2002). *Motivational interviewing: Preparing people for change, vol. 2*. New York, NY: Guilford.

*Miller, W. R. & Clunies, S. (Eds.) (2000). *Enhancing motivation for change in substance abuse treatment*. Rockville, MD: Diane Publishing.

Miller, W. R., Westerberg, V. S., & Waldron, H. B. (1995). Evaluating alcohol problems in adults and adolescents. In R. Hester and R. Miller (Eds.), *Handbook of alcoholism treatment approaches: Effective alternatives* (2nd ed., pp. 61–88). Boston, MA: Allyn & Bacon.

Mirijello, A., D'Angelo, C., Ferrulli, A., Vassallo, G., Antonelli, M., Caputo, F., ... Addolorato, G. (2015). Identification and management of alcohol withdrawal syndrome. *Drugs, 75*, 353–365. https://doi.org/10.1007/s40265-015-0358-1

Morgenstern, J., Blanchard, K. A., Morgan, T. J., Labouvie, E., & Hayaki, J. (2001). Testing the effectiveness of cognitive-behavioral treatment for substance abuse in a community setting: Within treatment and posttreatment findings. *Journal of Consulting and Clinical Psychology, 69*, 1007–1017. https://doi.org/10.1037/0022-006X.69.6.1007

Myrick, H., & Anton, R. F. (1998). Treatment of alcohol withdrawal. *Alcohol Research and Health, 22*, 38–43. Retrieved from http://login.ezproxy.lib.umn.edu/login?url=http://search.proquest.com/docview/222384220?accountid=14586

Narcotics Anonymous. (2017). *Narcotics Anonymous world services*. Van Nuys, CA: NA World Services. Retrieved from https://na.org/

*National Association for Addiction Professionals. (2009). *The basics of addiction counseling: Desk reference and study guide. Module 1: The pharmacology of psychoactive substance use, abuse and dependence* (10th ed.). Alexandria, VA: NAADAC.

*National Institute on Drug Abuse. (2012). *Principles of drug addiction treatment: A research based guide*. Retrieved from http://www.drugabuse.gov/publications/principles-drug-addiction-treatment

Nock, M. K., & Photos, V. (2006). Parent motivation to participate in treatment: Assessment and prediction of subsequent participation. *Journal of Child and Family Studies, 15*, 333–346. https://doi.org/10.1007/s10826-006-9022-4

Noël, X., Brevers, D., & Bechara, A. (2013). A neurocognitive approach to understanding the neurobiology of addiction. *Current Opinion in Neurobiology, 23*, 632–638. https://doi.org/10.1016/j.conb.2013.01.018

Nolen-Hoeksema, S., & Hilt, L. (2006). Possible contributors to the gender differences in alcohol use and problems. *Journal of General Psychology, 133*, 357–374. https://doi.org/10.3200/GENP.133.4.357-374

*O'Farell, T. J., & Fals-Stewart, W. (2006). *Behavioral couples therapy for alcoholism and drug abuse*. New York, NY: Gilford Press.

Overeaters Anonymous. (2017). *Overeaters anonymous: You are not alone anymore!* Rio Rancho, NM: Overeaters Anonymous. Retrieved from https://oa.org/

RachBeisel, J., Scott, J., & Dixon, L. (1999). Co-occurring severe mental illness and substance use disorders: A review of recent research. *Psychiatric Services, 50*, 1427–1434. https://doi.org/10.1176/ps.50.11.1427

Rational Recovery (2017). *Rational recovery: How to quit your addiction right now—for life.* Rational Recovery Systems, Inc. Retrieved from https://rational.org/index.php?id=94

*Rowe, C. L. (2012). Family therapy for drug abuse: Review and updates 2003–2010. *Journal of Marital and Family Therapy, 38*, 59–81. https://doi.org/10.1111/j.1752-0606.2011.00280.x.

Rowe, C. L., & Liddle, H. A. (2003). Substance abuse. *Journal of Marital and Family Therapy, 29*, 97–120. https://doi.org/10.1111/j.1752-0606.2002.tb00386.x

Salyers, M. P., & Tsemberis, S. (2007). ACT and recovery: Integrating evidence-based practice and recovery orientation on assertive community treatment teams. *Community Mental Health Journal, 43*, 619–641. https://doi.org/10.1007/s10597-007-9088-5

SAMHSA's National Registry of Evidence-based Programs and Practices. (2017). *Intervention summary: Twelve step facilitation therapy.* Retrieved from http://legacy.nreppadmin.net/ViewIntervention.aspx?id=358

Secular Organizations for Sobriety. (2016). *SOS: Together we can recover.* Los Angeles, CA. Retrieved from http://www.sossobriety.org/what-we-do

Selbekk, A. S., Sagvaag, H., & Fauske, H. (2015). Addiction, families and treatment: A critical realist search for theories that can improve practice. *Addiction Research & Theory, 23*, 196–204. https://doi.org/10.3109/16066359.2014.954555

Shaffer, H. J., LaPlante, D. A., LaBrie, R. A., Kidman, R. C., Donato, A. N., & Stanton, M. V. (2004). Toward a syndrome model of addiction: Multiple expressions, common etiology. *Harvard Review of Psychiatry, 12*, 367–374. https://doi.org/10.1080/1067322090905705

Slesnick, N., & Prestopnik, J. L. (2004). Office versus home-based family therapy for runaway, alcohol abusing adolescents: Examination of factors associated with treatment attendance. *Alcoholism Treatment Quarterly, 22*, 3–19. https://doi.org/10.1300/J020v22n02_02

SMART Recovery. (1994–2017). *SMART Recovery: Self-management and recovery training.* Retrieved from http://www.smartrecovery.org/intro/

Stanton, M. D., & Shadish, W. R. (1997). Outcome, attrition, and family-couples treatment for drug abuse: A meta-analysis and review of the controlled, comparative studies. *Psychological Bulletin, 122*, 170–191. https://doi.org/10.1037/0033-2909.122.2.170

Substance Abuse and Mental Health Services Administration. (2014). *Results from the 2013 National Survey on Drug Use and Health: Summary of national findings, NSDUH Series H-48, HHS Publication No. (SMA) 14-4863.* Rockville, MD: Substance Abuse and Mental Health Services Administration. Retrieved from https://www.samhsa.gov/data/sites/default/files/NSDUHresultsPDFWHTML2013/Web/NSDUHresults2013.pdf

Szapocznik, J., & Kurtines, W. M. (1989). *Breakthroughs in family therapy with drug-abusing and problem youth.* New York, NY: Springer.

Vanderplasschen, W., Rapp, R. C., Wolf, J. R., & Broekaert, E. (2004). The development and implementation of case management for substance use disorders in North America and Europe. *Psychiatric Services, 55*, 913–922. https://doi.org/10.1176/appi.ps.55.8.913

Vaughn, M. G., & Howard, M. O. (2004). Adolescent substance abuse treatment: A synthesis of controlled evaluations. *Research on Social Work Practice, 14*, 325–335. https://doi.org/10.1177/1049731504265834

Walitzer, K. S., Dermen, K. H., & Barrick, C. (2009). Facilitating involvement in Alcoholics Anonymous during out-patient treatment: A randomized clinical trial. *Addiction, 104*, 391–401. https://doi.org/10.1111/j.1360-0443.2008.02467.x

Wells, K., Klap, R., Koike, A., & Sherbourne, C. (2001). Ethnic disparities in unmet need for alcoholism, drug abuse, and mental health care. *American Journal of Psychiatry, 158*, 2027–2032. https://doi.org/10.1176/appi.ajp.158.12.2027

Women for Sobriety. (2016). *Women for sobriety*. Quakertown, PA: Women For Sobriety. Retrieved from http://womenforsobriety.org/beta2/

Wright, L., Watson, W., & Bell, J. (1996). *Beliefs: The heart of healing in families and illness*. New York, NY: Basic Books.

Zucker, R. A., & Gomberg, E. S. (1986). Etiology of alcoholism reconsidered: The case for a biopsychosocial process. *American Psychologist, 41*, 783–793. http://dx.doi.org/10.1037/0003-066X.41.7.783

Part IV
Medical Family Therapy in Unique Care Contexts and Populations

Chapter 13
Medical Family Therapy in Community Health Centers

Jennifer Hodgson, Angela Lamson, Rola Aamar, and Francisco Limon

Community health centers (CHCs) provide affordable, accessible care to patients in urban and rural areas across the nation. Health centers must be located in underserved locales, governed by a community-majority board, provide a core set of primary care services, and offer a sliding fee scale to patients under 200% of the federal poverty level (National Associations of Community Health Centers, 2017a). Based on most recent figures, health centers serve more than 25 million patients (1 out of every 15 Americans), 71% of whom are at the 100% federal poverty level and below and 83% are uninsured or publicly insured (NACHC, 2017a). Health centers employ over 8400 mental health and substance abuse staff and provide access to these services in the most underserved communities in the nation. In 2015, over 8.3 million clinic visits were provided for mental health or substance abuse issues; this represents a 56% growth in behavioral health visits since 2010 (NACHC, 2017b).

CHCs often operate as patient- and family-centered healthcare homes; they also function as community-centered healthcare homes due to their integration of behavioral health, oral care, and medical health services. CHCs often tend to (a) be culturally proficient; (b) offer team-based care; (c) provide enabling services, which offer enhanced access to care; and (d) be highly attuned to community accountability and governance. Many of the services provided through CHCs are not reimbursed at the same level as those in private primary care contexts, yet CHCs who engage in collaborative and integrated behavioral healthcare are able to highlight their cost-effectiveness, cost-offset, and positive effects on quality of care, patient satisfaction,

---

J. Hodgson (✉) · A. Lamson · R. Aamar
Department of Human Development and Family Science, East Carolina University, Greenville, NC, USA
e-mail: hodgsonj@ecu.edu

F. Limon
Green County Health Care, Snow Hill, NC, USA

and health outcomes (Mukamel et al., 2016), in part due to the four factors mentioned above.

Providers trained in Medical Family Therapy (MedFT) offer a unique lens in CHCs that bridges medical and behavioral health assessments, diagnoses, and treatment via a collaborative, transdisciplinary team and approach to care. In this context, MedFT is described as the practice of treating patients and their families (i.e., support persons) in relation to health, illness, loss, or trauma using a biopsychosocial-spiritual (BPSS; Engel, 1977, 1980; Wright, Watson & Bell, 1996) and systemic approach to care (Hodgson, Lamson, Mendenhall, & Crane, 2014). The BPSS framework is essential for MedFTs in CHCs because patients come from diverse social locations and are treated outside of a traditional medical model through an integration of biological, psychological, social, and spiritual components of their life. Patients in some healthcare contexts may not be asked how their health decisions are informed through their religious/spiritual beliefs. However, due to the cultural diversity reflected in CHC patient panels, MedFTs commonly consider the role of spirituality in tandem with physical and psychosocial health. Thus, in order for a MedFT to understand how a patient makes sense of health, the MedFT must also work to capture the way in which patients make sense of life (whether that is aligned with a higher power, nature, or freedom to have agency in decision-making).

In addition to MedFTs working from a BPSS approach to care, they are inclined to promote behavioral health to be just as important as physical health concerns and, furthermore, support the importance of relational health as a part of overall wellness. Unfortunately, across many healthcare systems, behavioral healthcare is underutilized, mental illnesses and behavioral health conditions are underdiagnosed, and patients are under-, over-, or mistreated for their complex diagnoses (Fagiolini & Goracci, 2009). Behavioral healthcare is often not well coordinated with medical care, especially for low-income populations. This is partly because providers and clinicians are not maximizing collaborative communication or treatment plans. As such, the window for BPSS care can become compromised, and the opportunity and accountability to work collaboratively with patients who are likely representative of underserved social locations (e.g., lower socioeconomic status, physical/mental ability challenges, ethnic minority) are minimized or closed. In addition, in disrupted or disjointed healthcare systems, there is little inclusion of the family as part of a patient's treatment process—despite the ravaging effects that an untreated or mistreated medical or behavioral health illness has on families (Rolland, Emanuel, & Torke, 2017). The literature is summarized well in several systematic reviews that show the reciprocal effects of family relations on health, both physical and behavioral (e.g., Hartmann, Bäzner, Wild, Eisler, & Herzog, 2010; Martire, Schulz, Helgeson, Small, & Saghafi, 2010), yet few healthcare systems aim to incorporate families as part of everyday healthcare practices.

MedFTs see these BPSS and relational complexities as an opportunity to work with patients and families while they are receiving care in CHCs. There are various ways that behavioral health has been received in medical contexts, including collaborative, colocated, and integrated care (Blount, 2003). Having behavioral and medical health providers colocated or, better yet, extending integrated behavioral healthcare (IBHC) increases the likelihood that patients will attend their behavioral health visit and reduces patient barriers to healthcare treatment (Krupski et al., 2016). However, IBHC alone does not ensure that providers will communicate on a regular basis, construct collaborative patient-centered care plans, or safeguard that integration will occur beyond the clinical world (i.e., extend into the operational world (e.g., systemic procedures)) or the financial world (e.g., billing systems) (Peek, 2008). Moving toward integrated behavioral healthcare models with maximum collaboration between healthcare providers, operating officers, and billing specialist professionals must be purposeful. Assessments and treatment plans must be coordinated, medical records streamlined, and reimbursement for services conducted in a way that ensures that all patient needs are cared for with equity (i.e., that physical health needs are not perceived as more important than behavioral health needs).

CHCs across the nation have different methods for addressing the BPSS needs of their patients. Therefore, "if you have seen one health center, you have seen one health center" (National Association of Community Health Centers, 2011, p. iv). This chapter was prepared by a team of MedFTs who are all involved with behavioral health services within a CHC system. Throughout, we describe the model we use and our approach to addressing patients' health. The following vignette presents an example of high-level integration between behavioral and primary care providers, family members, and integrated procedures that helped to maximize care delivery.

Clinical Vignette
[Note: This vignette is a compilation of cases that represent treatment in a Community Health Center. All patients' names and/or identifying information have been changed to maintain confidentiality.]

In 2006, JH and AL designed and delivered integrated behavioral healthcare (IBHC) for a community health center (CHC) in eastern North Carolina. Since then, the CHC system has grown its IBHC program from 1 to all 5 medical clinics in the CHC system. Each of these locations included MedFT services integrated in tandem with medical health services. In 2013, additional funding allowed the IBHC service to start including health coaches (HC) along with MedFT services. This approach maximized the full extent of our MedFTs' clinical skill sets (e.g., assessing, diagnosing, and intervening with severe mental health symptoms and concerns) while, at the same time, providing support and education to patients at risk for chronic health conditions via health coaching services.

Our protocol for HCs and MedFTs was to prepare for each encounter before meeting the patient, including (a) reviewing the patient's medical chart to identify whether there was a history of a mental health diagnosis or symptoms based on a previous mental health assessment and, if indicated, the patient was to be seen by the on-site MedFT; (b) determining what chronic health concerns existed for the patients, given that most had at least one chronic health condition (e.g., diabetes, hypertension, hyperlipidemia, obesity), and any corresponding biomarkers on management of the condition (e.g., hemoglobin A1c, blood pressure, cholesterol levels, body mass index); and (c) evaluating progress made on a patient-constructed goal from a previous integrated care visit.

In early 2013, a MedFT supervisor was scheduled to provide live supervision for a HC who was still in training. Together they reviewed the patient's chart and noted that he was a fairly new patient to the clinic. In the chart, they could see that Jamar self-reported and identified as a 19-year-old African American male. He was 5'11" and weighed 386 pounds. His body mass index (BMI) was 53.8, meeting the criteria for severe obesity. He had not been previously seen by one of the clinic's HCs or MedFTs. The HC and supervisor knocked on the exam room door and entered together. Given that the HC was shadowing her that day, the HC supervisor modeled the introduction:

The HC supervisor opened the encounter stating, "Good morning Jamar. We are health coaches and a part of your health care team. We work with patients on ways to improve health by getting better sleep, changing eating or activity habits, reducing stress, working on smoking cessation, and finding ways to improve family support. We also try to set health goals with each patient and share this information in the same chart as the one kept by your primary care provider (PCP). Would it be okay if we talked for a bit today about your health?"

Jamar agreed, whereupon the supervisor had another question for him. "Jamar, who do you have with you today?"

Jamar pointed to his mother in the room. The HC supervisor asked if it would be okay for her to talk with him while his mother was in the room or if he preferred that she step out. He consented to have his mother present.

Behavioral health team members begin every health coaching and MedFT visit in the same way: by completing the Patient Health Questionnaire-3 (and PHQ-9 if necessary; Kroenke, Spitzer, & Williams, 2001) and Generalized Anxiety Disorder-2 (and GAD-7 if necessary; Spitzer, Kroenke, Williams, & Lowe, 2006) to determine if there are any concerns related to mental health (e.g., symptoms of depression or anxiety). Jamar's score was a zero on both screeners.

The HC trainee then asked Jamar if he had any concerns that he would like to give attention to in relation to his health. His mother quickly jumped in with a concern about his weight. Jamar quietly mentioned—under his breath—that he was not concerned with his weight.

"I wish I slept better," he said with confidence.

Based on their approach of meeting patients where they are at, the HC supervisor and trainee began to assess Jamar's sleep through our screener and engaged his mother in the conversation as much as we could (e.g. "Do you remember Jamar having this concern when he was younger?"). Through

> that process, they learned that he drank four 2-liter bottles of a highly caffeinated and sugary soda each day. The HC supervisor asked him if anyone had ever told him that caffeine can disrupt his sleep. He said that he started drinking a lot of soda while in high school and that he had never really thought about it in relation to his sleep. More recently, Jamar shared that he was realizing that he was having a hard time getting to sleep and staying asleep.
>
> Jamar's mother became tearful during the conversation as she heard about his struggles with sleep and, again, reiterated her concerns about his health. Jamar also talked about getting up in the middle of the night several times to use the restroom.
>
> The HC supervisor asked Jamar what he thought he could do to improve his sleep that might also help him improve his overall health. Their discussion included conversations about behaviors that sometimes complicate sleep (e.g., screen time before bed, setting a regular sleep schedule, and caffeine intake). Jamar decided on a goal to cut back to one 2-liter bottle per day.
>
> While the HC supervisor and trainee were excited by his motivation, they also understood the research about withdrawal from caffeine and wanted to set a more realistic goal that Jamar could sustain. His mother became passionate about how to help him cut back on his soda intake, which was more related to her concomitant want for him to lose weight. Together, Jamar and his mother constructed a health goal that ultimately addressed his sleep hygiene concerns. Soon thereafter, the PCP entered the room and the HC supervisor and trainee shared Jamar's goal with her while also informing her of a concern that he shared about getting up to urinate several times throughout the night (which triggered the PCP's attention to check for diabetes).

Our primary concerns in CHC range from managing mental health presentations (e.g., depression and anxiety) and chronic health conditions (e.g., diabetes and hypertension education) to lifestyle issues (e.g., sleep and stress), all of which require consistent collaboration between medical and behavioral health providers (BHPs). Recently, services have ramped up even further as we have begun providing care in the dental wings of these clinics as well as through the local school system. In every instance, we use motivational interviewing (MI; Rollnick, Miller, & Butler, 2007) as a framework for health coaching interactions and solution-focused care (e.g., De Shazer et al., 2007) when delivering MedFT (see more detailed discussion below). All providers document care in the same electronic health record (EHR) to facilitate interdisciplinary collaboration and coordination of care. Inclusion of family members, as well as others from the patient's support system, is encouraged so as to maximize success with each patient's health goal(s). Respecting the support system and community that surround the patient, as well as delivering the highest quality services to those who are underserved and underinsured, represents core values of CHCs (Taylor, 2014). While some providers may choose to take an aggressive approach to treatment for significant health concerns, our team is inclined to take a BPSS and systemic approach that is strength based, and through realistic goals, we move patients toward sustainable wellness.

What Are Community Health Centers?

CHCs serve as a laboratory for innovation. This innovation includes the integration of MedFT on-site, whereby patients are seen in the context of their families and treatment is offered in ways that are sensitive to diverse family and cultural belief systems. Including MedFTs in community health centers (e.g., Federally Qualified Health Centers) has resulted in positive outcomes for families and, perhaps as important, positive outcomes among providers (Aamar, Lamson, & Smith, 2015; Phelps, Hodgson, Lamson, Swanson & White, 2012; Phelps et al., 2009). And while some CHCs choose to contract with off-site behavioral health services (e.g., specialty mental health services such as psychiatry, psychotherapy, case management), in this chapter, we focus primarily on contexts that advance on-site integrated behavioral healthcare. Behavioral health providers (BHPs) working as members of an IBHC team may include any mental health professional with specialized training in IBHC. Herein MedFTs are featured in this role.

Community healthcare centers have a significant outreach potential that includes sending medical providers, nurses, BHPs, and specially trained lay persons (e.g., promotoras) into the community to work with patients in their homes and/or at their work settings. Some BHPs are colocated in a CHC clinic, which means that they are available on-site, but are not typically providing patient care in the exam rooms. Instead, they are seeing their own scheduled patients for traditional 45–50 minute psychotherapy sessions. Other BHPs in a CHC may help PCP care for patients who are experiencing mental health crises but primarily see their own scheduled patients a majority of the time. Lastly, some CHCs are advanced in their integration of behavioral health and have their BHPs go into the exam room before, during, or after the PCP to screen for and treat behavioral health issues related to wellness, mental illness, chronic illnesses/conditions, and/or an acute general medical condition. These BHPs typically carry smaller "traditional therapy" caseloads; the majority of their work in IBHC is in tandem with other healthcare providers (e.g., PCPs, nurses, dentists, hygienists, case managers, nutritionists). This permits them to see more patients and improve access to behavioral healthcare that is otherwise a challenge for patients with minimal financial resources, fear of stigma associated with seeing a behavioral health provider off-site, limited time, and/or transportation difficulties for additional doctor appointments.

As with any healthcare setting, membership of a CHC treatment team is critical to its success, insofar as each member fulfills an important role. The following represent key contributors in CHCs.

Treatment Teams in Community Health Centers

Teams in CHCs are charged with the task of meeting a wide variety of simple to complex healthcare needs. They treat pediatric to geriatric patients from a wide variety of socioeconomic, educational, and cultural/ethnic backgrounds. In addition, these teams function under tremendous pressure due to limited time, resources, and high patient volume. Therefore, they must function as a well-oiled machine with clear and effective leadership. In a CHC, too, it is beneficial to have team members who are bilingual and bicultural to help ensure patients' healthcare needs are addressed with minimal opportunities for misunderstandings secondary to language or cultural differences.

Behavioral health providers (BHPs). These professionals may provide 45–50 minute scheduled traditional mental health visits and/or integrated behavioral healthcare visits (15–30 minutes) working alongside PCPs. They may include providers who screen for mental health conditions and provide brief interventions and/or work with patients to set health goals toward optimizing health or managing a chronic illness(es) effectively. BHPs most common to CHC settings include health coaches and/or providers from a variety of mental health disciplines (e.g., medical family therapy, health psychology, clinical social work, psychiatric nursing, psychiatry).

Care managers/coordinators. Care managers are members of the team who assess, plan, organize, and monitor patients' health. They assess for particular challenges that the person is experiencing (e.g., access to food, medication, shelter), listen to patients'/families' concerns, and help problem-solve issues associated with basic needs. Among underserved and underinsured populations, these members of the team are critical because they reduce healthcare barriers common to the population(s) they serve and are prepared with resources from the community that may meet a range of bilingual and bicultural needs.

Diabetes health educators. Often certified, diabetes educators are healthcare professionals who are trained to have comprehensive knowledge of and experience in educating on the topics of (a) prediabetes, (b) diabetes prevention, and (c) diabetes management. Their role is to educate and support individuals and families who are affected by diabetes. They help patients and families understand and self-manage the disease through individualized treatment plans for health outcome promotion (National Certification Board for Diabetes Educators, 2017). They are prepared with educational materials available in the language (and at the literacy level) of the CHC patients served.

Front desk staff. These staff check patients in and out of the clinic, answer the phones, collect payments, and help to schedule appointments. They oftentimes serve as cultural brokers to ensure that patients and their support persons feel a sense of quality and safety provided within the CHC center. These individuals are frequently bilingual and bicultural (reflecting the more dominant languages and cultures in the community) to help communicate with patients and to ensure understanding about care offered and processes for being seen.

Health coaches (HCs). HCs work with the PCP and BHPs to provide coaching around common health behaviors that may lead to or lessen the impact of chronic conditions (e.g., healthy eating, physical activity, stress management, sleep hygiene). They may help with basic screenings for mental health issues (e.g., depression, anxiety) and report to the PCP and BHPs on the team the results of any brief screens. HCs in a CHC are trained to assess and address health risk behaviors associated with toxic stress, too. They also are prepared to identify uncontrolled health behaviors common to uninsured and underinsured patients, as well as screen for stress and resources needed due to recent local traumas (e.g., floods, earthquakes, tornados).

Lab technicians. Lab techs work under the supervision of PCPs to conduct lab tests (e.g., strep, flu, exposure to common environmental toxins found in the fields where workers are exposed). They may also be trained as phlebotomists (i.e., to draw blood for analysis).

Medical office assistants (MOAs). MOAs are often the first and last point of contact after the patient checks in for an appointment. They perform a variety of administrative tasks, including (but not limited to) managing a patient's medical record, file insurance forms, schedule appointments, and arrange clinical procedures such as X-rays. MOAs sometimes gather patients' vital signs and record the data in medical records. At times, they will administer basic mental health screenings (e.g., depression, substance abuse) and pass that information onto the BHP or PCP treatment team member. They escort the patient to his or her exam room and notify the PCP that the patient is ready to be seen. At times, MOAs may be called upon by the PCP for other skills (e.g., translating).

Nurses. Nurses work alongside the PCP to assist with the collection of patient information and patient vitals (e.g., height, weight, blood pressure, blood glucose levels). Nurses perform diagnostic tests, interpret and/or report to the PCP in-house test results (e.g., strep, hearing, blood glucose, blood pressure), administer PCP-recommended medication/treatment, and interact with patients to help allay concerns during medical visits. They also answer the phones and relay information to and from the PCP to patients and other healthcare collaborators. They may administer vaccinations and other health screenings. In a CHC, nurses may be bilingual or bicultural to further ensure that patients' healthcare needs are addressed with minimal opportunities for misunderstandings.

Primary care providers (PCPs). This is a healthcare practitioner who sees people with common medical problems and is responsible for diagnosing and treating medical and mental health conditions. This person may be a medical doctor, nurse practitioner, or physician's assistant. He or she oversees the patient's medical care visit, prescribes any pharmaceutical treatment, orders necessary labs or tests, refers to specialists, and documents findings in the patient's medical record.

Referral specialists. These team members process referrals made by the PCP to other healthcare providers in the community. Some of the more common referrals include dental services, specialty medical and mental health services (not offered on-site), and lab and imaging services. Referral specialists' efforts may be particularly complicated due to a lack of bilingual and/or affordable services for underserved and uninsured patients commonly seen in a CHC.

X-ray technicians. These technicians use imaging methods to visualize the inside of the human body (e.g., bones, teeth). The pictures they create help PCPs diagnose and treat sundry illnesses or injuries.

Fundamentals of Care in Community Health Centers

Using a BPSS framework (Engel, 1977, 1980; Wright, Watson & Bell, 1996), MedFTs collaborate with medical and other healthcare professionals to improve patient outcomes and enhance patient satisfaction while addressing a variety of common behavioral and mental health topics. To address these concerns, MedFTs working in a CHC should be prepared to:

1. Join with patients, support persons, and the healthcare system in an ethical manner, especially given that the delivery of behavioral health via IBHC models is still relatively new.
2. Recognize and deliver a wide range of screenings and assessments across the lifespan, including for those associated with managing psychosocial crises (e.g., child or elder abuse, intimate partner violence, suicidal/homicidal ideation).
3. Formulate an accurate diagnosis for common DSM-5 psychiatric disorders (American Psychiatric Association, 2013) with knowledge about the International Classification of Disease coding system (World Health Organization, 1992).
4. Identify ways in which collaborative processes can be improved by the inclusion of MedFT in a CHC setting.
5. Extend research-informed and best practice interventions indicated for diverse populations and in the context of a variety of complex or chronic conditions.

While the information below may be applied to other primary care settings, we have found this content to be especially helpful when collaborating with patients and providers in CHCs. This is not a comprehensive map of services; it instead provides a general overview of the types of care and concerns that MedFTs may address at different phases of a CHC healthcare visit.

Pre-visit Work

Before entering the room, MedFTs should review the patient's EHR and consult with the PCP to become acquainted with the patient's health history. Reviewing the patient's vitals (e.g., blood pressure, blood glucose, weight, height, age), problem/diagnosis list, list of medications, and recent health visit treatment plans will assist with the MedFT's joining, assessing, and intervening accurately. It will also assist with promoting continuity of care. Please note, though, that there are some scenarios in which it is not appropriate or advisable for a MedFT to enter the exam room. Examples include:

- If the patient has the flu, high fever, a quarantined contagious condition, is actively vomiting, or is unclothed
- If notes in the chart indicate that the patient has consistently declined MedFT interventions for non-circumstantial reasons
- If the PCP has requested that the MedFT wait to see the patient until after the PCP or another member of the team completes a task
- If the patient does not speak the same language as the MedFT and no translator is available at that time

Joining

Joining is an ongoing experience that starts from the beginning through the end of an encounter. When deemed appropriate to enter the patient's room, the MedFT should begin with (a) offering an introduction, (b) explaining one's role at the clinic with consideration for the patient's social location (e.g., age, ethnicity), (c) outlining the purpose of one's visit, (d) obtaining verbal consent from the patient, and (e) explaining the limits of confidentiality. Several of these factors are discussed in more detail below. Joining behaviors may include nonverbal interactions like maintaining direct eye contact and leaning forward slightly while the patient and any support persons are talking. Joining is also done through a variety of verbal interactions, including reflectively listening and repeating back what is heard throughout the encounter, being transparent with one's purpose and collaborative partnership with the healthcare team, and concluding the interview with a summary that acknowledges the patient's reason for the health visit, health goal(s), and any interventions or resources discussed.

Explaining One's Role with Consideration for Patient's Social Location

Joining, particularly in a CHC, should include acknowledgment of any factors (e.g., cultural, financial, housing, occupational) that the MedFT, additional healthcare team member, or the patient/support person(s) thinks may present a possible barrier to successfully carrying out a treatment plan. For example, if working in a CHC setting with a high percentage of Spanish-speaking patients, ask the patient if he or she is comfortable communicating in English before beginning the encounter. Some patients may be comfortable speaking English minimally but would prefer a translator or bilingual MedFT for this part of the visit. Acknowledging what may help the patient to be more comfortable is an important part of the joining process and in the patient understanding the MedFT's role as a part of his or her healthcare. Support persons may also help by explaining whether the patient hears better in one ear over another or can see best if the MedFT sits closer to him or her.

Joining with children is a separate skill to master; MedFTs should make sure to acknowledge children in the room and tailor their work and description of their role so that it is age appropriate. For example, joining aides with children may include puppets, magic markers, crayons, coloring books, etc. It is also helpful to modify one's voice, vocabulary, and location in the room (i.e., make yourself eye-level if the child is the patient), when joining with children.

Obtaining Consent

If there are support persons in the room, it is important to get permission from the adolescent or adult patient to include them in the encounter before moving to the assessment phase. On occasion, the person in the exam room is not someone that the patient wants to have heard his or her health history. That person should be asked to step out of the room for the visit, upon the patient's request.

Note that getting a child's assent is important to joining successfully, even if the adult in the room says that it is okay to talk to the child. With smaller children, the MedFT should make attempts to adjust one's position in the room to appear less intimidating. For example, sitting on the small step connected to the exam table will put the MedFT more at eye-level with a young patient who is seated on a chair.

Explaining the Limits of Confidentiality

Building a successful relationship with a patient in any IBHC context can be expedited when the primary care provider or another member of the healthcare team introduces the MedFT to the patient during a healthcare visit. Typically, the PCP and MedFT describe the limits of confidentiality pertaining to the patient's presenting concern (e.g., that the patient's concern will be discussed by the PCP and MedFT and that both providers document in the same charting system). While it is not always possible for a healthcare team member to stop workflow to do this, the MedFT can also borrow the rapport already established with the healthcare team by mentioning that he or she is also a member of the patient's healthcare team and works to see all patients coming into the CHC. This may help to reduce a patient's uncertainty or stigma about having a mental health professional on board his or her healthcare team. Once the MedFT has begun to join with the patient, he or she should then consider how to prioritize screening or assessment as a part of the visit.

Assessing

As a MedFT, you may deliver both behavioral and mental health services as part of a traditional therapy appointment or as an IBHC visit (i.e., in conjunction with a medical encounter). Priority should be given to IBHC visits and to behavioral health issues, first and foremost. MedFTs use a variety of common adult and pediatric mental health screeners (see Table 13.1) to aid in assessment and diagnosis. MedFTs should be aware that screeners are not designed to be purely diagnostic but rather aid in assessment and determining symptom severity. For example, a clinically significant PHQ-9 (Kroenke, Spitzer, & Williams, 2001) score does not automatically mean that a patient has major depressive disorder. However, the information gathered from the PHQ-9 can assist in understanding which symptom(s) a patient is experiencing, the severity of specific symptoms, and severity of the overall depression. Depending on the patient's chief complaint, other brief mental health screenings may be indicated. All assessments/screeners should be documented in the patient's EHR and revisited to track changes in symptom severity. They serve as a secondary line of assessments to a more thorough mental health assessment in accordance with the DSM-5 (APA, 2013).

When an assessment suggests that mental health issues are not present, the MedFT should then assess for how patients are managing with any current and/or previously diagnosed chronic conditions (as seen in the patient's EHR or through prior consultation with the PCP). If everything is well managed, then the MedFT

Table 13.1 Examples of Behavioral Health Screening Tools

Adult		Pediatric	
Depression	PHQ-9 (Kroenke et al., 2001)	**Behavioral and emotional development**	ECSA—Early Childhood Screening Assessment (Gleason, Zeanah, & Dickstein, 2010)
Anxiety	GAD-7 (Spitzer et al., 2006)	**Behavioral and emotional health**	PSC—Pediatric Symptom Checklists (Jellinek et al., 1988)
Cognitive functioning	MoCA—Montreal Cognitive Assessment (Nasreddine et al., 2005)	**ADHD**	Vanderbilt-NICHQ Assessment for ADHD (Wolraich et al., 2003)
Bipolar disorder	MDQ—Mood Disorder Questionnaire (Hirschfeld et al., 2000)	**Pediatric development**	Ages and Stages Questionnaire (Squires, Bricker, & Potter, 1997)
PTSD	SPRINT—PTSD screener (Connor & Davidson, 2001)	**Trauma**	Adverse Childhood Experience (Felitti et al., 1998)
Alcohol use	AUDIT—Alcohol Use Disorder Identification Test (Babor, Higgins-Biddle, Saunders, & Monteiro, 2001)	**Alcohol and drug use**	CRAFFT Screening Interview (Knight et al., 1999)
Substance use	DAST-10—Substance Use Screening Tool (Skinner, 1982)		
Domestic violence	AAS—Abuse Assessment Screen (Weiss, Ernst, Cham, & Nick, 2003)		

Table 13.2 Examples of Health Behavior Screeners

	Adult	Pediatric
Healthy eating	PAN—Physical Activity and Nutrition Behaviors Monitoring Form (Eat Smart, Move More NC, 2005)	PAN—Physical Activity and Nutrition Behaviors Monitoring Form (Eat Smart, Move More NC, 2005)
Sleep	ESS—Epworth Sleepiness Scale (Johns, 1991)	BEARS Sleep Interview (Owens & Dalzell, 2005)
Physical activity	RAPA—Rapid Assessment of Physical Activity (Topolski et al., 2006)	PAN—Physical Activity and Nutrition Behaviors Monitoring Form (Eat Smart, Move More NC, 2005)

will assess for opportunities for health behavior change. In the model that we use, every patient is supported in designing a health goal to promote his or her own health. For example, patients may want to modify/improve their eating, stress management, or sleeping patterns to prevent or lessen the effects of chronic health conditions (e.g., obesity, diabetes, hypertension, hyperlipidemia). Some patients also take this opportunity to engage in steps toward smoking cessation. All MedFTs (in our model) are trained in motivational interviewing (Rollnick et al., 2007) and on how to construct SMART (i.e., specific, measurable, assignable, realistic, and time related) goals (Doran, 1981). This helps to ensure that the process is patient centered and that the health goal is directly relevant to the patient's concern. These goals are documented in the patient's EHR so that they can be tracked in the system and followed up on by any member of the healthcare team.

The following tools are available for assessing specific patient health behavior issues and needs. They are not to be used as a first step in assessment, but rather as a means to gain more depth, when necessary. These instruments, like the ones in Table 13.1, can be found in English and Spanish and in some cases other languages as well. While Table 13.2 is not exhaustive, it reflects the screeners for some of the more commonly presented issues to the authors who work in the CHC setting.

Diagnosing

Working in a CHC setting affords MedFTs the opportunity to engage with patients who are managing acute and chronic conditions, as well as simple to complex mental and/or medical diagnoses. Each patient encounter should be coded by the MedFT with a mental health diagnosis and/or behavioral health screening/assessment code. The diagnosis should be based on information given during the patient interview, reviewed in the patient's EHR, discussions with support persons present, results of screening assessments, and conversations with the PCP. Not all mental health encounters will result in a DSM-5 (American Psychiatric Association, 2013) psychiatric diagnosis. In such cases, you may choose to give a provisional diagnosis or use the ICD-10 code (World Health Organization, 1992) when screening for depression (Z13.89). Provisional diagnoses are used when a MedFT feels that he or she has insufficient data for determining a diagnosis. Codes are also available for instances when a behavioral health screening is done and no formal diagnosis is identified. It is advisable for MedFTs to secure training in coding and billing when working in a CHC, even if the MedFTs' services are not billed for directly (e.g., Medicare or Medicaid). Using the correct codes and tracking them are important to identifying trends in presenting concerns among the patient population and using that data to advocate for policy and training for the healthcare teams.

Intervening

When intervening in an IBHC model, MedFTs function as both mental and behavioral health specialists. In this capacity, they may offer traditional 45–50 minute therapy sessions to patients and families, but generally their interventions take place during brief 15–30 minute encounters. During these visits, MedFTs collaborate with patients, families, and healthcare providers in order to join, assess, diagnose, intervene, and/or initiate healthy lifestyle modifications through the use of health goals. MedFTs may make referrals to other specialty behavioral health interventionists and/or community resources when the patient's needs are outside of the CHC offerings (e.g., substance abuse treatment, severe mental health concerns). Outside referrals are made because not all behavioral health interventions are suitable, available, or manageable in a CHC or brief traditional therapy service. For example, treatment for schizophrenia and other psychotic disorders, feeding and eating disorders, substance use and addictive disorders, and/or other complex mental health issues may need longer-term evidence-based care off-site with continued collaboration involving members of the on-site CHC healthcare team.

The main objective of behavioral health interventions is to support and encourage patient health through lifestyle modification and research-informed treatment for acute and/or chronic conditions. Interventions may include (a) patient psychoeducation, (b) crisis interventions, and (c) interventions at the individual, family, and/or community system levels. Research-informed practices aimed at the individual, family, and/or community system levels are addressed later in this chapter. Here we focus on the psychoeducation and crisis intervention levels.

Patient Psychoeducation

Patient psychoeducation includes (a) ensuring that patients understand the implications of their chronic illness (if they have one) and/or (b) ensuring that patients understand how their own behaviors affect their health. Both of these factors are necessary requirements for developing and maintaining healthy lifestyle changes and lay the foundation for setting health goals with patients and their support person(s).

Patients must be aware of the implications of their health condition(s). MedFTs should initially spend time assessing the patient's/family's level of understanding of an illness. For example, a patient who has recently been diagnosed with diabetes may know very little about how stress, nutrition, sleep, physical activity, or medication management will affect insulin levels. In cases where patients have lower health literacy, less social support, and/or higher anxiety blocking their understanding and retention of information, it is paramount that MedFTs educate them on how health behaviors affect specific illnesses. Otherwise, there will be little success with health goals created at the visit. MedFTs should also become well informed of common major chronic diseases (e.g., diabetes, hypertension, obesity, asthma) seen and treatments delivered in their CHCs. This will help the MedFTs, in collaboration with the PCPs, prepare and/or disseminate educational materials that increase patients' and support persons' health literacy (and address areas where more psychoeducation is needed).

Crisis Interventions

MedFTs working in a CHC may encounter patients with severe mental health issues and/or who are living in dangerous settings (e.g., suicidal ideation, child abuse, domestic violence, substance abuse). For example, encountering suicidal ideation (SI) is not uncommon when working in a CHC setting. Researchers in one study found that approximately 64% of patients who had attempted suicide had visited their primary care provider within 1 month of their attempt (Ahmedani, 2015). MedFTs should be especially cognizant of populations who are at increased risk for SI; these may include American Indians (Middlebrook, LeMaster, Beals, Movins, & Manson, 2001), LGBTQ adolescents and young adults (Haas et al., 2010), men and women after a relationship breakup (Wyder, Ward, & De Leo, 2009), older men (over 80 years; Conwell, Duberstein & Caine, 2002), patients with history of a mood disorder (Tidemalm et al., 2011), and persons who are unemployed (Classen & Dunn, 2012). Understanding the context for any crisis, indicated screenings/assessments (e.g., Columbia Suicide Severity Rating Scale for suicidal ideation; Posner et al., 2011), and research-informed interventions pertaining to populations who experience said crisis is an incredibly important skill for MedFTs. Once screened, follow-up communication and visits are essential for those who have experienced a crisis. Further, adequate and accurate documentation is required to help reduce patients from falling through the cracks, especially those who are not seen often or routinely at the CHC.

Documentation

Once the MedFT has joined, assessed, diagnosed, and intervened, it is imperative that he or she clearly and thoroughly document the details of the encounter. Proper documentation of encounters is not only an essential part of patient care and ethical practice; it also enables CHCs to adequately assess patient needs, cost/outcome effectiveness, and quality of care through quality improvement endeavors. Proper documentation ensures that the MedFT receives credit in the monthly encounter totals (see Glossary for more details). MedFTs working in a CHC should have awareness and knowledge of (a) the EHR system (where one records what happened during a patient visit), (b) patient management systems (where one enters the information needed to support the billable encounter charge slips, current procedural terminology (CPT) codes, etc.), and (c) any required documents that still exist in hard copy (i.e., paper forms).

The EHR is an electronic version of a patient's medical history that is maintained and managed by designated members of the treatment team (e.g., PCP, BHP, nurses). This record will contain information about a patient such as demographics, medical and mental health diagnoses, lab and test results, progress notes, and medication lists. MedFTs have access to patients' medical charts, thus ensuring that providers are accountable to using the EHR effectively and efficiently as they provide care and protect patients' privacy (i.e., only accessing data in private areas and logging off after each use). Table 13.3 includes information about the EHR and the fundamentals of its use that MedFTs should master.

Table 13.3 Fundamentals of EHR usage for MedFTs

MedFTs should know how to	Specific Tasks
Customize your EHR	It is recommended that MedFTs customize their EHR. In most EHRs they can do this by setting user preferences. Through this process, the MedFT will create an electronic signature, common lists for encounters, and access and import important documents to personal folders.
View the daily schedule	MedFTs should be able to view the daily appointment schedule by provider and/or by facility. This will help prepare for and target patients who would benefit most from MedFT services.
Send/receive internal mail	All non-face-to-face correspondence about patients must occur via the internal mail system. Through this system, MedFTs may collaborate with PCPs, nurses, and other BHPs.
Set reminders	MedFTs will want to set reminders about following up on patient's goals and needs. They may do this through setting reminders and deciding how often the reminder will pop up.
Practice with fake patient charts	If the MedFT does not feel confident documenting in the EHR, practice using fake patient charts that are often already created in the system provides training.
Document a behavioral health encounter	MedFTs should document a behavioral health encounter by using the behavioral health template. Recommended templates include those for patients managing blood pressure, cholesterol, diabetes, depression, stress, smoking, healthy eating, physical activity, family support, medication, and health promotion. MedFTs will want to record the scores of all assessments used, diagnoses given, and information relevant to the treatment and plan.
When a patient declines services and calls, contact the patient to follow-up	MedFTs should consider documenting in the EHR even when a patient declines services. All calls and attempts to contact the patient for follow-up should also be logged to track patient engagement attempts.

When working collaboratively with medical providers in CHCs, it is important to consider the type of information documented in the EHR. Documentation should be used to provide integrated healthcare providers with meaningful information about the patient's treatment plan. With that in mind, behavioral health providers should seek to include language about the patient's visit that is familiar to other providers on the team, as well as being consistent with the language that other providers use in treatment planning. Rather than solely focusing on building therapy narratives about the patient's behavioral health encounter, it is equally important to include adequate information about the diagnosis, including the status and severity of the diagnosis and the progress of the patient's treatment. Including information about relevant biomarkers, screening tools, and interventions implemented during the visit can also be helpful in bridging the treatment plans between the biomedical and behavioral/mental healthcare teams. Finally, behavioral health providers in CHCs should consider writing easy-to-understand goals in the EHR. Aforementioned SMART goals are frequently used across healthcare disciplines; they are an efficient way to streamline treatment planning efforts across a care team. It is thereby helpful to the collaborative process if these goals were easily accessible by (and visible to) other healthcare providers in the CHC.

Common Challenges and Considerations

Delivering IBHC services in a CHC setting has some unique challenges. In this section, we address time and space limitations, potential ethical issues, meeting the needs of minority and non-English-speaking patients, and challenges associated with the basics of collaboration.

Time and Space Limitations

To be able to work effectively with time and/or space limitations, it is important to know the environment and other members of the treatment team well. The CHC team is designed to work as efficiently as possible to maximize care for a high volume of patients every day. It is the MedFT's responsibility to understand and work in context of the patient flow. Working with time limitations requires awareness of how quickly the PCP is moving between patients and how many patients have been checked in and are waiting to be seen. Communicating with the PCP, the nurse, or a medical assistant before you begin a patient encounter may help maximize the workflow and ensure patients are seen in a logical order. Generally, providers see patients for 10–15 minutes and visit rooms based on check-in order. MedFTs should plan accordingly to strategize which rooms to visit and when (i.e., have reviewed their chart for signs of concern from previous visit or patient goal that deserves continuity in care).

Regarding space, it is important to know what other spaces around the clinic could be used to visit with patients if an exam room is not available. This is particularly important if the provider asks the MedFT to meet with the patient after the visit but needs the room for his or her next patient. MedFTs should ask the medical provider how much time is available to meet with the patient or if they would prefer that the patient be moved to another unused clinic room/office. It is important that the MedFT not delay clinic workflow, as this will be a deterrent for providers to use IBHC with their patients. However, sometimes patients need longer sessions with the MedFT, so communication with the PCP or nurse is important to resolving workflow challenges and achieving optimal patient care. In some clinics, there are designated spaces for the MedFT to meet with patients when there are longer IBHC or traditional sessions; these spaces are typically larger in size, too, so as to allow for caregivers or family members to be present.

Ethical Considerations

Navigating different codes of ethics in an IBHC setting, especially when it applies to confidentiality and obtaining patients' consent, can be especially complicated. The following discussion provides guidance on how to respect limits of confidentiality and obtaining consent while following established codes of ethics and meeting HIPAA (Health Insurance Portability and Accountability Act of 1996) requirements:

Confidentiality. Confidentiality of all patients' medical information must be protected. Fundamentally, confidentiality is achieved when a patient's private, personal medical information is guarded from disclosure to unauthorized individuals. As a general rule, all medical information for a given patient must remain private, unless (a) permission to share said information has been granted by the patient and/or (b) a compelling and legal reason to break confidentiality is extant (e.g., life-or-death emergency, imminent potential for self-harm via suicide or harm to others via homicide). Procedures for guarding confidentiality may include:

1. Making sure that doors are closed in exam rooms and that conversation volumes are kept low to prevent others from hearing private information.
2. Explaining to the patient during the encounter that his or her information will not be shared with anyone except for their PCP, nurse(s), or other CHC staff directly involved with the patient.
3. Securing the EHR and not leaving patients' records unattended on a computer or otherwise available for viewing on an unlocked device.
4. Sharing information with the PCP that is pertinent/relevant to the patient's situation.
5. Remaining cognizant of new or additional individuals (e.g., friends, family) who have joined the patient room and not disclosing information from current or previous visits without first receiving consent from the patient to proceed with visitor(s) present.

Consent. Before beginning an IBHC or colocated traditional mental health encounter, consent must be obtained from each patient. Adult patients may give their own consent, whereas minors (or others who are incapable of giving consent) must receive consent from a legal guardian (know state law exceptions to providing emergency care to minors). At some healthcare settings, wherein IBHC has been offered previously and consent is embedded in the initial registration paperwork, patients are often unfamiliar with all the stipulations of receiving behavioral health services. As such, it is important to have a clear conversation with each patient to ensure understanding of what may result from an encounter (e.g., a mental health diagnosis from MedFTs) and to explain the limits of confidentiality. Once this has been explained, it is also part of the consent process to let the patient know that the information from the encounter will be documented in the EHR to be shared with the patient's PCP.

Serving Minority and Non-English-Speaking Patients

One major issue that CHCs were designed to address is combatting health disparities in medically underserved areas, many of which tend to serve ethnic minority and non-English-speaking populations (Geiger, 1984; Taylor, 2014). These populations also tend to be more vulnerable to the social, cultural, psychological, financial issues related to health, including lower socioeconomic status, fewer opportunities for consistent employment, limited proficiency with the English language, issues related to immigration status, and social marginalization (Derose, Escarce, & Lurie, 2007). Ultimately, these issues can result in seeking out healthcare services less often, lower compliance with and adherence to medical recommendations, less trust in the healthcare team, and poorer treatment outcomes. Attentiveness to these issues is crucial to providing quality care for all patients in CHCs, and healthcare providers can better attend to this by engaging minority and non-English-speaking patients through culturally sensitive healthcare practices (Brach & Fraserirector, 2000).

Culturally sensitive healthcare practices should include learning about (and educating other members of the treatment team about) how chronic illnesses and behavioral health needs might differ for ethnic minority populations (e.g., implications, indications, and contraindications of treatment may vary based on the cultural practices and identities of patients). One of the foremost culturally sensitive practices healthcare providers can use to attend to the needs of non-English-speaking populations is to make sure that handouts and resources about behavioral health and chronic illnesses are available in multiple languages (Israel et al., 2005). This can help to ensure that information about a patient's health or condition is available in a language that the patient is comfortable with. Also, learning key medical or treatment terminology in other languages may help healthcare providers to bridge language barriers and provide better overall care (Derose, Escarce, & Lurie, 2007). One of the most helpful resources that CHCs can implement to better serve minority and non-English-speaking patients is to include staff members who represent the target patient population (Cabral & Smith, 2011; Wu & Windle, 1980). For example, Spanish-speaking physicians, medical assistants, receptionists, behavioral health providers, etc. should be present in a clinic that serves a predominately Latino community. There is also some evidence to suggest that matching the staffing of clinics to the patient population (e.g., hiring bilingual and bicultural staff members) can promote better health outcomes (Cabral & Smith, 2011).

Finally, with populations served by CHCs (e.g., highly uninsured or underinsured), it is important to consider the impact of limited literacy skills when exploring culturally sensitive practices, particularly because low literacy skills have been found to be associated with significantly higher healthcare costs among underserved populations (Weiss & Palmer, 2004) and health disparities in geriatric populations (Sudore et al., 2006). Assessing for literacy level is an important culturally sensitive practice because individuals with limited literacy might use coping tools to show comprehension of the handouts, pamphlets, or information sheets provided, despite having limited reading abilities (Cowan, 2004). Literacy is not an indication of high intelligence; it is thereby important to not assume that a patient with lower literacy skills is less intelligent and/or less capable of compliance. Once assessment has been completed, healthcare providers can teach patients with low literacy skills by using techniques such as (a) providing verbal instructions, (b) teaching information using only a few sentences at a time and then repeating or reviewing instructions, and (c) using demonstrations. Also, for patients with low literacy skills, written materials should be avoided unless the materials are at the patient's reading level (Cowan, 2004).

Engaging in Collaboration

Engaging in effective collaboration means contributing to all parts and members of the system. The information below includes methods for engaging the support systems of both patients and members of the patients' healthcare team. Not all patients, support persons, or healthcare team members were socialized or trained to work alongside behavioral health professionals in a healthcare setting. This requires the MedFT to lean heavily on his or her relational skills to help build trust in the system while at the same time respecting the learning curves of those who are not as familiar with IBHC.

Family Collaboration

Family members, support persons, and other caretakers are important in the work that MedFTs do in a CHC setting. Because of their unique training, MedFTs excel at working with patients and their support persons. The challenge, though, is oftentimes getting said support persons to attend a healthcare visit. Asking patients if anyone accompanied them to a visit is a common way to begin. Many family members/support persons wait in the car or waiting room to give the patient privacy. Sometimes the patient does not know that it is okay or beneficial to invite support persons into the exam room. Oftentimes just asking if the patient would or could invite a partner or support person in, when appropriate, is a quick process with tremendous gains. Another way to engage with support persons is to have the patient call or text the individual to communicate his or her health status and components of the treatment plan (including ways in which the support person can help to meet needs or extend support). Lastly, inviting the patient to bring in his or her primary support person to the next visit is an important strategy for expanding the system and inviting support persons to be a continuous part of the patient's healthcare team.

It is important that any family member/support person attending the appointment with the patient be acknowledged and engaged at the start of the visit. Tips for ethically engaging family members into visits include the following:

1. Obtain consent from the patient to discuss the patient's issues in front of others in the room.
2. Ask the patient to introduce you to each person in the room, and ask why he or she accompanied the patient to the visit.
3. Seek information from the visitor about the chief complaint (e.g., family members can help clarify the patient's story, add valuable information, and will tell you things that the patient may omit).
4. View the visitor(s) as collaborators in your work vs. impediments (e.g., parents can help children with emotional self-regulation).
5. Ask the patient to identify how the visitor can support him or her in achieving his or her health goals.
6. Encourage the patient and the visitor to summarize the next steps that will be taken to continue progress on the treatment plan.

Provider Collaboration

Primary care providers generally serve as patient gatekeepers. If a provider is not comfortable with a MedFT or IBHC, it is unlikely that the MedFT will be able to access the patient. MedFTs should, therefore, cultivate relationships with providers if they are interested in increasing their interactions with patients. Building relationships with support staff can also help increase patient encounters. This is particularly useful when each provider works with a designated medical assistant (MA) or registered nurse (RN). Being able to communicate well with MAs/RNs will help MedFTs to determine the best time(s) to enter a room and to be aware of the provider's timeline and approach to care for each visit.

Typically when MedFTs begin in a new work context, one of their roles is to respectfully introduce other providers to IBHC and the BPSS framework. Providers may not be accustomed to planning patient care and treatment planning with other clinicians. It is therefore important that MedFTs be aware of the level of integrated care (e.g., Doherty, McDaniel, & Baird, 1996) established at the CHC site and also of the level of integration that respective providers are comfortable with (this often varies from provider to provider, even at the same location). Engaging providers in interactions around patient care begins with MedFTs modeling said interactions. This can begin with MedFTs initiating conversations with providers about shared patients.

After each encounter, MedFTs should follow up with the PCP to relay pertinent information about the visit and overall treatment planning. MedFTs should be aware that providers often have limited time for conversations between patients, so this may be a brief transfer of information. The following are some useful guidelines for follow-up: (a) keep it brief (15–30 seconds), (b) report salient information only (e.g., assessment scores, psychological, social, and spiritual issues—including financial and access to care issues—impacting treatment planning), (c) address red flag issues (e.g., suicidality, homicidality, child abuse, interpersonal violence), (d) design and deliver appropriate interventions (e.g., briefly explain mindfulness exercises, brief evidence-based psychotherapy or family therapy, interviewing strategies for motivating change), and (e) offer modified and/or additional treatment recommendations.

If a MedFT is having difficulty joining with a particular healthcare team member, he or she should consider finding a time to speak with the said team member to build more of a relationship (e.g., after patient appointments or during a lull in patient flow). In this conversation, the MedFT may consider (a) explaining to the provider the types of services that MedFTs offer, (b) asking the provider if there are particular services that he or she would like the MedFT to extend, (c) asking the provider if there are any particular patients with whom the MedFT could assist, (d) asking the provider how he or she would like the MedFT to follow up after patient care (including the type of information to be relayed), and (e) getting to know the provider better by asking about things that the team member enjoys and values as a way to develop a successful partnership. Afterward, MedFTs should be consistent in following up with providers about MedFT-patient interactions. It is important that MedFTs show an appreciation for the opportunity to collaborate and occasionally check in with providers about the collaborative process and how it may be improved—all the while maintaining an appropriate demonstration of confidence and competence. This will help MedFTs to increase rapport and build ongoing trust.

Community Health Centers Across the MedFT Healthcare Continuum

Skills and knowledge in medical family therapy can extend from primarily focusing on psychosocial issues presented by an individual or family with very limited integration of BPSS or systemic factors in the sessions to advanced relational and BPSS skills and knowledge who function as a part of collaborative teams in diverse CHC contexts. Tables 13.4 and 13.5 highlight specific knowledge and skills that

Table 13.4 MedFTs in Community Healthcare Centers: Basic Knowledge and Skills

MedFT Healthcare Continuum Level	Level 1	Level 2	Level 3
Knowledge	Familiar with CHC as a system of care beneficial to the community but rarely engages in opportunities to collaborate with healthcare team members about patients' BPSS health. Limited knowledge about BPSS impacts of a few common population health conditions seen at CHC clinics. Rarely engages professional members, patients, and support system members collaboratively in joining, assessing, diagnosing, planning, and/or intervening. Basic understanding regarding strategies for a healthy lifestyle when living with and/or with someone who has a health condition. If conducting research and/or policy/advocacy work, on rare occasions will collaborate with other disciplines related to CHC care and consider relational and/or BPSS aspects of health and well-being.	Can recognize the disease processes and differentiate between some of the more common ones and other comorbid BPSS health conditions and impacts on the CHC population served. Familiar with benefits of couple and family engagement in health-related adjustments and/or lifestyle maintenance but tends to refer more than provide this service. Knowledgeable about how to use the electronic health record system or other forms of secured communication to collaborate with various team members. Is an occasional contributor to discussions about research design and policy/advocacy work that include relational and/or BPSS aspects of health and well-being.	Working knowledge of specific team members (e.g., allopathic and osteopathic physicians, nurse practitioners, physicians, assistants, nurses, medical office assistants, phlebotomists, pharmacists, nutritionists, physical therapists, other behavioral health disciplines), medical terminology with regard to medications and EHR charting (e.g., prn, qd, BGL, TSH), and common comorbid medical conditions to commonly seen illnesses in a CHC (e.g., anxiety, asthma, depression, diabetes mellitus, hypertension, hyperlipidemia, substance use disorders). Broad range of knowledge about research-informed family therapy and BPSS interventions; able to and usually will conduct couple and family therapy and incorporate BPSS health factors into treatment with minimal need to refer out due to limited expertise. When work permits, is knowledgeable and consistency committed to conducting research and constructing policy/advocacy work that identifies and intervenes on behalf of individuals, couples, families, and healthcare teams toward the advancement of BPSS health and well-being.

(continued)

Table 13.4 (continued)

MedFT Healthcare Continuum Level	Level 1	Level 2	Level 3
Skills	Able to recognize at a basic level the BPSS dimensions of health and apply a BPSS lens to CHC practice, research, and/or policy/advocacy work. Can discuss (and psychoeducate) basic relationships between biological processes, personal well-being, and interpersonal functioning. Demonstrates minimal collaborative skills with CHC and other related healthcare providers; prefers to work independently, but when care is complex enough will contact/refer to other providers on- or off-site about additional services.	Knowledgeable about how to apply systemic interventions in practice but does it occasionally; capable of assessing patients and support system members present for background health issues such as family history and risk-related factors. Demonstrates adequate and occasional collaborative skills through (a) written and verbal communication mediums that are understandable to all team members and (b) coordination of referrals to specialty behavioral health providers and communication with the patient's CHC primary care provider. Conducts separate treatment plan from other providers involved in the patient's care; goals and interventions can overlap with—or be informed by—a CHC team member, but BPSS goals and collaboration with the team are not consistently done.	Able to and usually will integrate respective CHC team members' expertise and counsel into treatment planning. When done can successfully conduct a systemic assessment of a patient and family with competencies in assessing for BPSS aspects of illnesses and/or comorbid diseases and resources within the family. Usually engages other professionals within and outside of the CHC center who are actively involved in the patient's care. Skilled with standardized measures to track patients' individual and relational strengths and challenges, and makes them available in the patient's dominant language. Attends and contributes to team meetings to help shape BPSS treatment plans for patients.

characterize MedFTs' involvement in CHC contexts across Hodgson, Lamson, Mendenhall, and Tyndall's (2014) MedFT Healthcare Continuum.

MedFTs at *Level 1* rarely apply relational or biopsychosocial-spiritual (BPSS) practices and/or include partners, families, or healthcare systems into their work. This level often includes professionals from many different disciplines who recognize that working from a relational perspective is beneficial, although they might only take a relational perspective in certain settings (e.g., hospice, pediatrics) or situations (e.g., when needing to make a referral, when one family member is the healthcare proxy for another family member). In CHCs, the range of skills or desire for collaboration with providers from other disciplines can be quite diverse. In this instance, a MedFT at *Level 1* may focus on a health concern and rely on BPSS only when its systemic nature drives the need to consider all of the BPSS domains, as can be the case with health coaching. In other instances, a MedFT at this level may consider the BPSS strengths and consequences associated with a diagnosis, but not attend well to the systemic relationships that can benefit or be influenced by the diagnosis. A strength at this level could be that attention is given with precision to the presenting concern. The vignette in this chapter illustrates a MedFT who moved

Table 13.5 MedFTs in Community Healthcare Centers: Advanced Knowledge and Skills

MedFT Healthcare Continuum Level	Level 4	Level 5
Knowledge	Consistently applies understanding of the more commonly treated health conditions and BPSS impacts in CHC centers. Knowledgeable about BPSS benefits and risks of associated treatments of the more commonly seen biological and mental health conditions across the lifespan in CHC centers (e.g., anxiety, asthma, depression, diabetes mellitus, hypertension, hyperlipidemia, substance use disorders). Understands how to implement and collaborate with other disciplines to implement evidence-based BPSS and family therapy protocols in traditional and integrated behavioral healthcare contexts. Identifies self as a medical family therapist. Knowledgeable about designing and advocating for policies that govern BPSS-oriented CHC services.	Understands and educates others about treatment and care sequences for unique and/or challenging topics in CHC practice (e.g., trauma, citizenship issues, geographic separation from family, unfamiliar cultural beliefs/practices); can consult proficiently with professionals about BPSS topics from other fields. Proficient at explaining evidence-based treatments regarding most mental health disorders and their role(s) in the family; has background to provide psychoeducation to patients and families about a variety of symptoms, medications, and behavioral health management. Very knowledgeable about BPSS research designs and execution, policies, and advocacy needs as relevant to CHC care. Proficient in developing a curriculum on integrated behavioral healthcare, BPSS applications, MedFT, etc. to mental health and other health professionals. Understands leadership and supervision strategies for building integrated behavioral healthcare teams in CHC settings.

(continued)

Table 13.5 (continued)

MedFT Healthcare Continuum Level	Level 4	Level 5
Skills	Able to deliver seminars and workshops to a variety of professional types (e.g., mental health, biomedical) about the BPSS complexities of a variety of commonly reported health and wellness topics found in CHC settings. Can apply several BPSS interventions in care (including most types of brief interventions); can administer mood- and disease-specific assessment tools as the CHC context requires. Consistently collaborates with key CHC team members (e.g., primary care providers, nurses, medical assistants, behavioral health providers, pharmacists, dieticians); initiates and facilitates team visits with multiple providers when working with patients and families. Can independently and collaboratively construct research and program evaluation studies that study the impact of BPSS interventions with a variety of diagnoses and patient/family units of care.	Proficient in nearly all aspects of commonly seen presenting problems in a CHC setting; able to synthesize and conduct research and clinical work; engages in community-oriented projects outside of the CHC center. Goes beyond intervention routine for this population; can integrate specific models of integrated behavioral healthcare into routine practice (e.g., PCBH, chronic care model). Works proficiently as a MedFT and collaborates with other providers from a variety of disciples serving within the CHC center. Leads, supervises, and/or studies success of the implementation and dissemination of BPSS curriculum on integrated behavioral healthcare, BPSS applications, MedFT, etc. Explains at a high level of skill evidence-based treatments regarding most commonly seen CHC presenting problems and their impact on family systems; has background to provide psychoeducation to patients and families about a variety of symptoms, medications, and behavioral health management techniques that facilitate managing chronic illnesses well, returning to optimal health, or managing one's health successfully.

well past *Level 1* by demonstrating value in exploring the patient's BPSS health and constructing a treatment plan accordingly.

Level 2 does not deviate dramatically from the skills in *Level 1*, except in the frequency that BPSS or relational health is addressed as a part of each encounter. In our vignette, Jamar is a 19-year-old patient accompanied by his mother to a healthcare visit. The MedFT supervisor and trainee work from the start of the visit to explain the model of care adopted at the CHC and how it may benefit his goals for care at that visit. It is clear that the supervisor and trainee share the value of BPSS health and skills in explaining and engaging the patient and his mother in discussing it. They also have collaborative skills in communicating with the patient, family member, and PCP to help construct a BPSS treatment plan.

At *Level 3*, the MedFT is usually applying a relational and BPSS practice in each encounter, as well as through conversations with other providers or collaborators. At this level, the MedFT can showcase that he or she is specifically trained to apply a broad range of family therapy interventions and conduct family therapy in the healthcare context. MedFTs at this level are providing care with consideration of data-driven or research-based information on relational and/or BPSS care. Given the frequency of using BPSS and relational healthcare at this level, a growing competence in diverse uses of MedFT is apparent to the supervisor's eye (similar to what was encountered by the supervisor described in the vignette). The MedFT is able to easily weave comments pertaining to biological health into concerns related to social stressors or psychological challenges. Furthermore, the MedFT is able to justify choices in care due to evidence-based research knowledge. In the vignette, the MedFTs are highlighting how effective they are in joining, assessing, and treating from a family-centered intervention level. They work to set a health goal that is not only identified as important to the patient, in this instance sleep patterns, but is also supported through a goal that was constructed in collaboration with the patient's mother. Not all family members share the same concern about weight or sleeping habits, so encouraging change and intervening in this type of conversation are something that one needs specialized training in order to deliver successfully. At *Level 3,* MedFTs will have had some of this training, alongside more extensive family therapy intervention skills.

Level 4 represents the MedFT who is consistently applying relational and/or BPSS knowledge and skills into his or her practice, research, policy, and/or advocacy work. The MedFT is experienced in using his or her knowledge and skills in both traditional mental health (i.e., the typical 50 minute couple/family or larger system session) and integrated behavioral healthcare contexts (i.e., MedFTs who work in tandem with biomedical and spiritual health providers when extending care/research/training). *Level 4* MedFTs in CHCs are recognized as part of the healthcare team, attend conjoint meetings and trainings, and are clearly identified as a MedFT in their work context. The medical assistants, dental team, or other medical providers know that the MedFT is a strong collaborator and contributor in addressing social determinants that may disrupt continuous care. The MedFT is recognized for attending to behavioral health concerns, symptoms, and diagnoses, along with stressors associated with a new diagnosis and/or anxiety associated with a medical procedure (e.g., a tooth extraction or receiving an injection). In these instances, the MedFT is able to extend evidence-based knowledge by providing a relaxation technique or determining whether brief therapy is a good option for the patient and his or her partner/family.

Finally, *Level 5* represents proficiency as a MedFT. At this level, the MedFT is able to serve as an administrator, supervisor, educator, researcher, and trainer in either a behavioral health or healthcare context and is trained and experienced in family therapy and MedFT practice, research, policy, and/or administration (including the interface with diverse healthcare providers and staff, diagnoses, research, complications across BPSS domains, and ethical standards). At this level, MedFTs have the knowledge and skills to mentor new MedFT, healthcare, and IBHC providers on models of integrated behavioral healthcare. They are also able to ensure that the level of collaboration is held to the highest standard by integrating care at the clinical, operational, and financial levels (e.g., attending to quality care, shared documentation processes, and working to improve cost-effectiveness and cost-offset). The vignette showcases a MedFT supervisor functioning at this level on the continuum.

Research-Informed Practices

CHCs generally serve populations who have less access to healthcare options (Taylor, 2014). These populations often include racially and ethnically diverse patients or those with less access to educational and financial resources (Derose, Escarce, & Lurie, 2007). Therefore, behavioral health models used in CHCs should be appropriate for and empirically validated with populations from diverse social locations.

Individual Approaches

Given that CHCs offer a variety of healthcare services, with primary care services being a priority, BHPs working in CHC settings need to be prepared to help patients within the context of infrequent and brief interviews that typically last between 15 and 30 minutes (McDaniel, Doherty, & Hepworth, 2014). To effectively address the mental health needs and health behaviors of patients in CHCs, BHPs need to work from a theoretical approach that can effectively help individuals in the context of brief and infrequent face-to-face interactions with patients. Fortunately, there is a growing body of scientific evidence that supports the use of several clinical approaches within the context of primary care settings.

Motivational Interviewing

Motivational interviewing (MI) has been recognized as an effective approach to health behavior management for use in healthcare settings (Rollnick et al., 2007). It is also widely recognized as being a patient-centered approach to healthcare and has shown higher rates of success in promoting health behavior changes among patients in comparison to the traditional "recommendation-giving" practices of healthcare providers (Britt, Hudson & Blampied, 2004). The basic principles of MI suggest that individuals are more likely to change when they can associate the desired change to something of intrinsic value and that the motivation to engage in behavior change grows when people feel safe to explore their reasons for change in the context(s) of what they value (Hecht et al., 2005; Miller & Rollnick, 2002).

Motivational interviewing can be a particularly useful intervention for patients served by CHCs because its principles are centered on assessing patients' current level of motivation, access to resources, willingness to make actionable change, and feasibility of the change (Emmons & Rollnick, 2001). MI's techniques encourage healthcare providers to take into account patient factors that may promote or limit change and thereby offer MedFTs and other providers the opportunity to explore social locations and cultural influences that have a role in shaping the patient's engagement in treatment. Lundahl et al. (2010) also found that MI was effective in increasing patients' engagement in treatment and promoting healthy behaviors. Finally, an additional advantage of MI is that it has been studied for use with mental health illness (e.g., Miller & Rose, 2009; Schoener, Madeja, Henderson, Ondersma, & Janisse, 2006) and chronic illness (e.g., Spencer et al., 2011). Therefore, a variety of healthcare providers can apply MI practices to their areas of focus to build collaborative treatment plans with consistent treatment approaches.

Transtheoretical Model for Change

A complementary tool that MedFTs might consider using in conjunction with motivational interviewing are the stages of change captured in the transtheoretical model for change (DiClemente, & Prochaska, 1998; Prochaska, Diclemente, & Norcross, 1992); after all, the two models are well-known for "growing up together" in the 1980s (Miller & Rollnick, 2009). The transtheoretical model for change presents five stages of change that a patient might move through during treatment: *precontemplation*, *contemplation*, *planning*, *action*, and *maintenance*. By assessing a patient's readiness to change, healthcare providers in CHCs are better able to identify how concerning the presenting problem is to the patient and whether the patient is interested in making changes to address his or her presenting problem. It can also be used to ensure that healthcare providers are appropriately engaging patients in the treatment process. When used along with MI, the transtheoretical model for change can be beneficial to populations served by CHCs because it allows for patient agency in the treatment process while encouraging providers to work from patients' respective stages of change (DiClemente & Velasquez, 2002; Norcross, Krebs, & Prochaska, 2011). This model has been found to be effective at increasing physical activity in adults with diabetes (e.g., Avery, Flynn, Wersch, Sniehotta, & Trenell, 2012), reducing dietary fat intake in underserved patients (e.g., Parra-Medina et al., 2011), and reducing substance use and other addictive behaviors (e.g., alcohol, tobacco, marijuana, gambling) (e.g., Lundahl, Kunz, Brownell, Tollefson, & Burke, 2010). Along with being an effective tool for individual treatment, the transtheoretical model can be used to engage partners and families of the patient in the treatment process (Tambling & Johnson, 2008).

Cognitive Behavioral Therapy

In mental health fields, cognitive behavioral therapy (CBT) is hailed as the gold standard for behavioral health interventions. The body of empirical evidence in support of CBT as an effective treatment option for an array of mental illnesses is vast (e.g., Fischer, Baucom, & Cohen, 2016; Otte, 2011; Safren et al., 2010). While CBT is easily recognizable to multidisciplinary healthcare providers, it is still more commonly regarded as a psychological approach for mental health treatment, rather than a behavioral health treatment option. Emergent literature suggests that CBT is effective in the treatment of chronic illness (e.g., Katon et al., 2010) and lifestyle changes (e.g., Trockel, Manber, Chang, Thurston, & Taylor, 2011); however, this body of literature is young, and the treatment of chronic illness using CBT is frequently studied along with a comorbid mental illness.

Cognitive behavioral therapy was designed to be a brief approach for symptom resolution, which makes it appropriate for individual patients at CHCs who may have few, sporadic appointments. Furthermore, evidence of CBT's effectiveness in primary care settings is beginning to emerge, showing CBT to be effective with anxiety disorders, depression, medication adherence, chronic illness management, and parent management skills for parents of children with externalizing symptoms (e.g., Weisberg & Magidson, 2014), depression, anxiety, and physical health quality of life in primary care patients (e.g., Cully et al., 2010), chronic obstructive pulmonary disease, chronic heart failure, depression, and anxiety (e.g., Mignogna et al., 2014). However, there remains some concern that CBT-effectiveness researchers have not investigated the model's adequacy for use with diverse patients, such as those presenting to community healthcare centers (CHCs). For example, while Serfaty and colleagues (2009) found that CBT was effective in reducing depression scores in older adults treated in primary care, only 6% of their sample was non-White and no sample socioeconomic factors (SES) were reported. Therefore, MedFTs in CHCs should actively implore a culturally sensitive and patient-centered lens when engaging patients in CBT treatment techniques.

Family Approaches

Engaging families of underserved patients in treatment at CHCs can help to expand resources available to the patient, encourage shared responsibility for management of the presenting problem, and educate healthcare providers about the meaning of the presenting illness for the patient and family (Hu, Amirehsani, Wallace, McCoy, & Silva, 2016). While opportunities for traditional family therapy services may be available in some CHC settings, the primary focus of MedFTs in CHCs should be to engage available family members during IBHC visits while working collaboratively with other healthcare providers (Marlowe, Hodgson, Lamson, White, & Irons, 2012). Each of the approaches suggested for family-based intervention is used to offer support to patients by engaging their family or social support system in the treatment process.

Solution-Focused Therapy

Solution-focused therapy (SFT) is a strength-based approach to behavior change that focuses on solutions rather than deficits (Gingerich & Peterson, 2013). And while there is value to more frequent sessions (as is the case with any treatment), even a single session of SFT can assist in getting a patient and family engaged in care and thinking about change (Bloom, 2001; Lamprecht et al., 2007; Perkins, 2006). Additionally, a main assumption in SFT is that patients are the experts of and in their own lives. This assumption is instrumental to engaging marginalized individuals and families in treatment, thereby making SFT a valuable clinical model in CHCs.

Another major advantage of using SFT with families in CHCs is that its proponents assume competence and strength in the patient's and family's skill sets to address presenting illnesses (Berg, & De Jong, 1996; Grant, 2012). There are several reports of SFT being used to address lifestyle foci, chronic illness, and mental illness—including physical activity, diet, sleep hygiene (Valve et al., 2013), diabetes and obesity (Rudolf, Hunt, George, Hajibagheri, & Blair, 2010; Viner, Christie, Taylor, & Hey, 2003), and depression and anxiety disorders (Gingerich & Peterson, 2013; Grant, 2012). SFT has also been shown to be effective in engaging families and caregivers in the treatment of pediatric diabetes management (Christie, 2008), stroke survivors (Plosker & Chang, 2014), patients with psychosis (Priebe et al., 2015), and mothers with postpartum depression (Ramezani, Khosravi, Motaghi, Hamidzadeh, & Mousavi, 2017).

Patient-Centered Communication

Narrative approaches, specifically patient-centered communication, have been found to promote the development of shared meaning between providers, patients, and families about the presenting illness and the role of the said illness in the patient's and family's lives (Charon, 2001; Sakalys, 2003). There is evidence to suggest that patient-centered communication in family treatment promotes motivational enhancement and family engagement to reduce mental health symptoms of underserved parents and children in primary care settings (Cooper et al., 2011; Wissow et al., 2008).

Patient-centered communication may be particularly valuable in addressing the spiritual domain of the BPSS—i.e., the meaning-making domain of health (Sulmasy, 2002). By helping families make meaning about a presenting illness, providers can be more attuned to patients' and families' needs and limitations (Street, Makoul, Arora, & Epstein, 2009). Engaging in meaning-making communication can also help providers develop treatment plans that are aligned with unique values, needs, concerns, and resources.

With the diverse and often marginalized populations served in CHCs, the importance of allowing families and patients to explain the significance and impact of illness on their individual and shared lives cannot be understated. Underserved groups often have a different lived experience than as compared to their healthcare providers (Rao, Anderson, Inui, & Frankel, 2007), not to mention different access to information about and resources to treat their illness (Nam, Chesla, Stotts, Kroon, & Janson, 2011). Patient-centered communication can be used to develop a relationship between healthcare providers, patients, and families that strengthens alliance, creates meaning about the illness, and encourages more active participation from families in care.

Community Approaches

Community health centers grew out the Civil Rights Movement and the War on Poverty (Taylor, 2014). They were designed with the intent of bringing services to impoverished communities, especially inner cities and rural communities. A primary goal of CHCs was (is) to promote community-oriented care, wherein members of the community simultaneously access and shape the services that they engage with (Geiger, 1984; Gibson, 1968). CHCs were developed to be a community resource for populations with limited access to and options for healthcare; this highlights how CHCs lend themselves naturally to community-based approaches to care.

Community Involvement

Health and illness narratives are a collective endeavor. Patients do not exist in isolation; their health and illness thereby have significance across personal levels and with those whom they interact with across friendship, family, and professional spheres and within the communities they inhabit (Murphy, 2015). Institutions in and surrounding the communities that CHCs serve can be another source of intervention. These community resources might include schools, churches, banks, local businesses/companies, and universities that have a vested interest in the health of their community population. Banks and local businesses/companies can be engaged to provide financial support for community health initiatives, particularly if the community is struggling with or at risk for a health disparity (Horowitz & Lawlor, 2008). Schools may be the next frontier in connecting potential patients to CHCs, encouraging the consistent practice of health behaviors, and providing space for behavioral health services in nonclinical settings (Keeton, Soleimanpour, & Brindis, 2012; Rosenthal et al., 2010). Universities have a long history of being strong supporters of CHCs. From providing the research expertise to engage CHCs in community-based participatory research (Wallerstein & Duran, 2006) to extending clinical support to patients and CHCs through providers in training (Cashman & Seifer, 2008; Seifer, 1998), the relationship between CHCs and local universities is one of the longest-standing and mutually beneficial community resources.

Community-Based Participatory Research

Community health centers are particularly well-suited for community-based participatory research (CBPR)—a collaborative research approach in which local organizations and residents are directly involved in the design and implementation of investigative pursuits (Israel et al., 2005; Wallerstein & Duran, 2006). These studies are designed to address concerns that are important to—and support initiatives that will—directly benefit community members (AHRQ, 2003; Rhodes, Malow, & Jolly, 2010). A strength of CBPR is its focus on building sustainable community partnerships to increase capacity of community organizations to better serve their constituents (Dulmus & Cristalli, 2012; Minkler & Wallerstein, 2011). CBPR can be particularly valuable when the research is service oriented, providing not only an opportunity for knowledge about the population through research but also providing the patients with access to additional healthcare services and options for treatment.

For example, Mendenhall et al. (2010) used CBPR to provide better quality diabetes education and treatment to urban-dwelling American Indian (AI) populations. By engaging the AI community in and throughout the research and treatment process, the healthcare team was able to move away from conventional top-down models of providing care toward an approach where healthcare providers and researchers were learning from and responding to the needs of the target population as co-owners and coproducers of the work. This included facilitating and empowering the target population's involvement in the design of the research, advancing the intervention(s), and even writing and publishing the results. Ultimately, the use of CBPR improved the health outcomes for the AI community across several diabetes-relevant indicators (Berge, Mendenhall, & Doherty, 2009; Mendenhall et al., 2012; Seal et al., 2016). When implemented with the support and interest of the target population in mind, CBPR—and/or any of the aforementioned treatment approaches—can be used by healthcare teams to provide more patient-centered and culturally aware care to (and indeed, with) those who are often marginalized and overlooked in the healthcare system.

Conclusion

Community health centers are incubators for innovation in healthcare delivery, including the integration of primary medical treatment with oral care, care management, substance use/abuse, and behavioral health services. They have been shown to be cost-effective and are designed to serve the needs of underserved families and individuals. Furthermore, CHCs are ideal for integrating MedFTs, as they are trained to treat patients and their families in relation to health, illness, loss, or trauma using a biopsychosocial-spiritual (BPSS) and systemic approach to treatment. MedFTs are trained to assess, diagnose, and treat a wide array of concerns that patients bring to primary care, ranging from lifestyle issues, chronic mental health conditions, and other health concerns in concert with the primary care team.

Common evidence-based interventions embraced by MedFTs include motivational interviewing, transtheoretical model/stages of change, cognitive behavior therapy, family (support system) engagement, solution-focused therapy, narrative approaches, and interventions developed from community-based participatory research. MedFTs embrace intervention models that honor patients' cultural values, beliefs, and preferences as they engage with the healthcare team through their illness and recovery/management processes.

Reflection Questions
1. What are some ways that MedFTs are able to deliver culturally appropriate services to underserved families and individuals?
2. Identify some of the challenges that MedFTs might experience (and possible solutions) when delivering services in a community health center context.
3. What are some of the research-informed approaches that MedFTs may want to practice when working in community health centers?

Glossary of Important Terms for Care in Community Health Centers

Collaborative care The process of working with healthcare providers across disciplines to discuss patient's diagnoses, treatment options, and interventions and to develop a treatment plan.

Cost report Often used for Medicaid and Medicare reimbursements, a report that includes information about the provider system (e.g., an FQHC), including utilization of services, charges to patients, and cost of services.

Encounters A face-to-face visit between a patient and healthcare provider that must include a treatment intervention and proper documentation.

Encounter rate A facility-specific rate that is paid to an FQHC to cover the cost of services for each valid encounter.

Federally Qualified Health Center (FQHC) A comprehensive healthcare center designed to service underserved populations, typically in areas with limited health resources. FQHCs must offer a sliding fee option to patients without insurance and are eligible for enhanced reimbursement from Medicare and Medicaid.

Health behaviors Practices, habits, and knowledge that can improve a patient's health.

Health disparities The differences in health status that socially disadvantaged populations experience. Factors that contribute to health disparities include access to healthcare, socioeconomic status, geographic location, race/ethnicity, and gender.

Population health Factors contributing to the health of (and the health outcomes of) a group of individuals who share a common illness, environment, or social identity.

Promotora A Hispanic/Latino community member who provides basic health education to the population as a trained lay person (not as a professional healthcare worker).

Rural health clinics Public, profit, or nonprofit clinics located in rural, underserved areas to provide primary care services to rural populations.

Social determinants of health The social, cultural, economic, and environmental factors that contribute to an individual's health status, including marital status, education, socioeconomic status, and immigration (see PRAPARE in Resources for more details).

Additional Resources

Literature

Engel, J. (2006). *Poor people's medicine: Medicaid and American charity care since 1965*. Durham, NC: Duke University Press.

Hoffman, B. (2012). *Health care for some: Rights and rationing in the United States since 1930*. Chicago, IL: University of Chicago Press.

Lefkowitz, B. (2007). *Community health centers: A movement and the people who made it happen*. New Brunswick, NJ: Rutgers University Press.

Minkler, M., & Wallerstein, N. (Eds.). (2011). *Community-based participatory research for health: From process to outcomes*. San Francisco, CA: Wiley.

Ward Jr., T. J., & Geiger, H. J. (2016). *Out in the rural: A Mississippi health center and its war on poverty*. New York, NY: Oxford University Press.

Electronic Resources

Agency for Healthcare Research and Quality: The Role of Community-Based Participatory Research. https://archive.ahrq.gov/research/cbprrole.htm

Community-Campus Partnerships for Health: Community-Based Participatory Research. https://depts.washington.edu/ccph/commbas.html

Health Resources Services Administration: Federal Office of Rural Health Policy. https://www.hrsa.gov/ruralhealth

Measures/Instruments

Alcohol Use Disorders Identification Test (AUDIT). https://www.drugabuse.gov/sites/default/files/files/AUDIT.pdf

Anxiety: Generalized Anxiety Disorder 7-Item Scale (GAD-7). http://www.phqscreeners.com/sites/g/files/g10016261/f/201412/GAD-7_English.pdf
CAGE AID Questionnaire. http://www.integration.samhsa.gov/images/res/CAGEAID.pdf
Depression: Patient Health Questionnaire 9 (PHQ-9). http://www.phqscreeners.com/sites/g/files/g10016261/f/201412/PHQ-9_English.pdf
Drug Abuse Screen Test (DAST—10). https://www.drugabuse.gov/sites/default/files/dast-10.pdf
Duke Population Health Profile (Duke-PH). http://www.integration.samhsa.gov/clinical-practice/DukeForm.pdf
Social Determinants of Health/Protocol for Responding to and Assessing Patient Assets, Risks, and Experiences (PRAPARE). http://www.nachc.org/research-and-data/prapare/
Suicide Risk: Columbia-Suicide Severity Rating Scale (C-SSRS). http://cssrs.columbia.edu/the-columbia-scale-c-ssrs/about-the-scale/, http://www.integration.samhsa.gov/clinical-practice/Columbia_Suicide_Severity_Rating_Scale.pdf
Trauma: PTSD Checklist—Civilian version (PCL-C). https://www.mirecc.va.gov/docs/visn6/3_PTSD_CheckList_and_Scoring.pdf

Organizations/Associations

Health Resources Services Administration: Health Center Program. https://bphc.hrsa.gov
National Association of Community Health Centers. www.nachc.org
National Institute on Minority Health and Health Disparities. https://www.nimhd.nih.gov
RCHN Community Health Foundation. http://www.rchnfoundation.org
The Community Health Center Story. http://www.chcchronicles.org

References[1]

Aamar, R., Lamson, A., & Smith, D. (2015). Qualitative trends in psychosocial treatment for underserved patients with type 2 diabetes. *Contemporary Family Therapy, 37*, 33–44. https://doi.org/10.1007/s10591-015-9326-x
Agency for Healthcare Research and Quality. (2003). *The role of community-based participatory research: Creating partnerships, improving health*. Retrieved from https://archive.ahrq.gov/research/cbprrole.htm
Ahmedani, B. K. (2015). Racial/ethnic differences in health care visits made before suicide attempt across the United States. *Medical Care, 53*, 430–435. https://doi.org/10.1097/MLR.0000000000000335

---

[1] Note: References that are prefaced with an asterisk are recommended readings.

American Psychiatric Association. (2013). *Diagnostic and statistical manual of mental disorders* (5th ed.). Arlington, VA: Author.

Avery, L., Flynn, D., Van Wersch, A., Sniehotta, F. F., & Trenell, M. I. (2012). Changing physical activity behavior in type 2 diabetes: A systematic review and meta-analysis of behavioral interventions. *Diabetes Care, 35*, 2681–2689. https://doi.org/10.2337/dc11-2452

Babor, T. F., Higgins-Biddle, J. C., Saunders, J. B., & Monteiro, M. G. (2001). *The alcohol use disorders identification test: Guidelines for use in primary care*. Geneva, Switzerland: World Health Organization.

Berg, I. K., & De Jong, P. (1996). Solution-building conversations: Co-constructing a sense of competence with clients. *Families in Society, 77*, 376–391. https://doi.org/10.1606/1044-3894.934

Berge, J. M., Mendenhall, T. J., & Doherty, W. J. (2009). Using community-based participatory research (CBPR) to target health disparities in families. *Family Relations, 58*, 475–488. https://doi.org/10.1111/j.1741-3729.2009.00567.x

Bloom, B. L. (2001). Focused single-session psychotherapy: A review of the clinical and research literature. *Brief Treatment and Crisis Intervention, 1*, 75–86. https://doi.org/10.1093/brief-treatment/1.1.75

Blount, A. (2003). Integrated primary care: Organizing the evidence. *Families, Systems, & Health, 21*, 121–133. https://doi.org/10.1037/1091-7527.21.2.121

Brach, C., & Fraserirector, I. (2000). Can cultural competency reduce racial and ethnic health disparities? A review and conceptual model. *Medical Care Research and Review, 57*(1_suppl), 181–217. https://doi.org/10.1177/1077558700057001S09

Britt, E., Hudson, S. M., & Blampied, N. M. (2004). Motivational interviewing in health settings: A review. *Patient Education and Counseling, 53*, 147–155. https://doi.org/10.1016/S0738-3991(03)00141-1

Cabral, R. R., & Smith, T. B. (2011). Racial/ethnic matching of clients and therapists in mental health services: A meta-analytic review of preferences, perceptions, and outcomes. *Journal of Counseling Psychology, 58*, 537. https://doi.org/10.1037/a0025266

Cashman, S. B., & Seifer, S. D. (2008). Service-learning: An integral part of undergraduate public health. *American Journal of Preventive Medicine, 35*, 273–278. https://doi.org/10.1016/j.amepre.2008.06.012

Charon, R. (2001). Narrative medicine: A model for empathy, reflection, profession, and trust. *Journal of the American Medical Association, 286*, 1897–1902. https://doi.org/10.1001/jama.286.15.1897

Christie, D. (2008). Dancing with diabetes: Brief therapy conversations with children, young people and families living with diabetes. *European Diabetes Nursing, 5*, 28–32. https://doi.org/10.1002/edn.99

Classen, T. J., & Dunn, R. A. (2012). The effect of job loss and unemployment duration on suicide risk in the United States: A new look using mass-layoffs and unemployment duration. *Health Economics, 21*, 338–350. https://doi.org/10.1002/hec.1719

Connor, K. M., & Davidson, J. R. T. (2001). SPRINT: A brief global assessment of post-traumatic stress disorder. *International Clinical Psychopharmacology, 16*, 279–284. https://doi.org/10.1097/00004850-200109000-00005

Conwell, Y., Duberstein, P. R., & Caine, E. D. (2002). Risk factors for suicide in later life. *Biological Psychiatry, 52*, 193–204. https://doi.org/10.1016/S0006-3223(02)01347-1

Cooper, L. A., Roter, D. L., Carson, K. A., Bone, L. R., Larson, S. M., Miller, E. R., ... Levine, D. M. (2011). A randomized trial to improve patient-centered care and hypertension control in underserved primary care patients. *Journal of General Internal Medicine, 26*, 1297–1304. https://doi.org/10.1007/s11606-011-1794-6

Cowan, C. F. (2004). Teaching patients with low literacy skills. In A. Lowenstein and M. Bradshaw (Eds.), *Fuszard's innovative teaching strategies in nursing* (3rd ed.). Sudbury, MA: Jones and Bartlett Publishers.

Cully, J. A., Teten, A. L., Benge, J. F., Sorocco, K. H., & Kauth, M. R. (2010). Multidisciplinary cognitive-behavioral therapy training for the veteran's affairs primary care setting. *The Primary*

Care Companion to the Journal of Clinical Psychiatry, 12, e1–e8. https://doi.org/10.4088/PCC.09m00838blu

Derose, K. P., Escarce, J. J., & Lurie, N. (2007). Immigrants and health care: Sources of vulnerability. Health Affairs, 26, 1258–1268. https://doi.org/10.1377/hlthaff.26.5.1258

De Shazer, S., Dolan, Y., Korman, H., Trepper, T. S., McCollom, E., & Berg, I. K. (2007). More than miracles: The state of the art of solution-focused brief therapy. Binghamton, NY: Haworth Press. https://doi.org/10.1111/j.1467-6427.2008.00419_4.x

*DiClemente, C. C., & Prochaska, J. O. (1998). Toward a comprehensive, transtheoretical model of change: Stages of change and addictive behaviors. New York, NY: Plenum Press. https://doi.org/10.1007/978-1-4899-1934-2_1.

DiClemente, C. C., & Velasquez, M. M. (2002). Motivational interviewing and the stages of change. In W. R. Miller and S. Rollnick (Eds.), Motivational interviewing: Preparing people for change (pp. 201–216). New York, NY: Guilford Press.

Doherty, W., McDaniel, S., & Baird, M. (1996). Five levels of primary care/behavioral healthcare collaboration. Behavioral Healthcare Tomorrow, 5, 25–28. Retrieved from https://www.ncbi.nlm.nih.gov/pubmed/10161572

Doran, G. T. (1981). There's a S.M.A.R.T. way to write management's goals and objectives. Management Review, 70, 35–36. Retrieved from http://community.mis.temple.edu/mis-0855002fall2015/files/2015/10/S.M.A.R.T-Way-Management-Review.pdf

Dulmus, C. N., & Cristalli, M. E. (2012). A university–community partnership to advance research in practice settings: The HUB research model. Research on Social Work Practice, 22, 195–202. https://doi.org/10.1177/1049731511423026

Eat Smart, Move More NC (2005). Physical activity and nutrition behaviors monitoring form. Retrieved from http://www.eatsmartmovemorenc.com/BehaviorsForm/BehaviorsForm.html

Emmons, K. M., & Rollnick, S. (2001). Motivational interviewing in health care settings: Opportunities and limitations. American Journal of Preventive Medicine, 20, 68–74. https://doi.org/10.1016/S0749-3797(00)00254-3

Engel, G. L. (1977). The need for a new medical model: A challenge for biomedicine. Science, 196, 129–136. https://doi.org/10.1016/b978-0-409-95009-0.50006-1

*Engel, G. L. (1980). The clinical application of the biopsychosocial model. American Journal of Family Medicine, 137, 535–544. https://doi.org/10.1176/ajp.137.5.535.

*Engel, J. (2006). Poor people's medicine: Medicaid and American charity care since 1965. Durham, NC: Duke University Press.

Fagiolini, A., & Goracci, A. (2009). The effects of undertreated chronic medical illnesses in patients with severe mental disorders. Journal of Clinical Psychiatry, 3, 22–29. https://doi.org/10.4088/JCP.7075su1c.04.

Felitti, V. J., Anda, R. F., Nordenberg, D., Williamson, D. F., Spitz, A. M., Edwards, V., … Marks, J. S. (1998). Relationship of childhood abuse and household dysfunction to many of the leading causes of death in adults: The adverse childhood experiences (ACE) study. American Journal of Preventive Medicine, 14, 245–258. https://doi.org/10.1016/S0749-3797(98)00017-8

Fischer, M. S., Baucom, D. H., & Cohen, M. J. (2016). Cognitive-behavioral couple therapies: Review of the evidence for the treatment of relationship distress, psychopathology, and chronic health conditions. Family Process, 55, 423–442. https://doi.org/10.1111/famp.12227

*Geiger, H. J. (1984). Community health centers: Health care as an instrument of social change. In V. W. Sidel and R. Sidel (Eds.), Reforming medicine: Lessons of the last quarter century (pp. 11–32). New York, NY: Pantheon Books.

Gibson, C. D., Jr. (1968). The neighborhood health center: The primary unit of health care. American Journal of Public Health and the Nation's Health, 58, 1188–1191. https://doi.org/10.2105/AJPH.58.7.1188

Gingerich, W. J., & Peterson, L. T. (2013). Effectiveness of solution-focused brief therapy: A systematic qualitative review of controlled outcome studies. Research on Social Work Practice, 23, 266–283. https://doi.org/10.1177/1049731512470859

Gleason, M. M., Zeanah, C. H., & Dickstein, S. (2010). Recognizing young children in need of mental health assessment: Development and preliminary validity of the early childhood screening assessment. *Infant Mental Health Journal, 31,* 335–357. https://doi.org/10.1002/imhj.20259

Grant, A. M. (2012). Making positive change: A randomized study comparing solution-focused vs. problem-focused coaching questions. *Journal of Systemic Therapies, 31,* 21–35. https://doi.org/10.1521/jsyt.2012.31.2.21

Haas, A. P., Eliason, M., Mays, V. M., Mathy, R. M., Cochran, S. D., D'Augelli, A. R., ... Clayton, P. J. (2010). Suicide and suicide risk in lesbian, gay, bisexual, and transgender populations: Review and recommendations. *Journal of Homosexuality, 58,* 10–51. https://doi.org/10.1080/00918369.2011.534038

Hartmann, M., Bäzner, E., Wild, B., Eisler, I., & Herzog, W. (2010). Effects of interventions involving the family in the treatment of adult patients with chronic physical diseases: A metaanalysis. *Psychotherapy and Psychosomatics, 79,* 136–148. https://doi.org/10.1159/000286958

Hecht, J., Borrelli, B., Breger, R. K., DeFrancesco, C., Ernst, D., & Resnicow, K. (2005). Motivational interviewing in community-based research: Experiences from the field. *Annals of Behavioral Medicine, 29,* 29–34. https://doi.org/10.1207/s15324796abm2902s_6

Hirschfeld, R. M. A., Williams, J. B. W., Spitzer, R. L., Calabrese, J. R., Flynn, L., Keck, P. E., ... Zajecka, J. (2000). Development and validation of a screening instrument for bipolar spectrum disorder: The mood disorder questionnaire. *American Journal of Psychiatry, 157,* 1873–1875. https://doi.org/10.1176/appi.ajp.157.11.1873

Hodgson, J., Lamson, A., Mendenhall, T., & Crane, D. (Eds.). (2014). *Medical family therapy: Advanced applications.* New York, NY: Springer.

*Hodgson, J., Lamson, A., Mendenhall, T., & Tyndall, L. (2014). Introduction to medical family therapy: Advanced applications. In J. Hodgson, A. Lamson, T. Mendenhall, and D. Crane, (Eds.) *Medical family therapy: Advanced applications* (pp. 1-9). New York, NY: Springer.

*Hoffman, B. (2012). *Health care for some: Rights and rationing in the United States since 1930.* Chicago, IL: University of Chicago Press.

Horowitz, C., & Lawlor, E.F. (2008). *Challenges and successes in reducing health disparities: Workshop summary.* Washington, DC: The National Academies Press. https://doi.org/10.17226/12154

Hu, J., Amirehsani, K. A., Wallace, D. C., McCoy, T. P., & Silva, Z. (2016). A family-based, culturally tailored diabetes intervention for Hispanics and their family members. *Diabetes Educator, 42,* 299–314. https://doi.org/10.1177/0145721716636961

Israel, B. A., Parker, E. A., Rowe, Z., Salvatore, A., Minkler, M., López, J., ... Potito, P. A. (2005). Community-based participatory research: Lessons learned from the centers for Children's environmental health and disease prevention research. *Environmental Health Perspectives, 113,* 1463–1471. https://doi.org/10.1289/ehp.7675

Jellinek, M. S., Murphy, J. M., Robinson, J., Feins, A., Lamb, S., & Fenton, T. (1988). Pediatric symptom checklist: Screening school-age children for psychosocial dysfunction. *Journal of Pediatrics, 112,* 201–209. https://doi.org/10.1016/S0022-3476(88)80056-8

Johns, M. W. (1991). A new method for measuring daytime sleepiness: The Epworth sleepiness scale. *Sleep, 14,* 540–545. https://doi.org/10.1093/sleep/14.6.540

Katon, W. J., Lin, E. H., Von Korff, M., Ciechanowski, P., Ludman, E. J., Young, B., ... McCulloch, D. (2010). Collaborative care for patients with depression and chronic illnesses. *New England Journal of Medicine, 363,* 2611–2620. https://doi.org/10.1056/NEJMoa1003955

Keeton, V., Soleimanpour, S., & Brindis, C. D. (2012). School-based health centers in an era of health care reform: Building on history. *Current Problems in Pediatric and Adolescent Health Care, 42,* 132–156. https://doi.org/10.1016/j.cppeds.2012.03.002

Knight, J. R., Shrier, L. A., Bravender, T. D., Farrell, M., Vander Bilt, J., & Shaffer, H. J. (1999). A new brief screen for adolescent substance abuse. *Archives of Pediatrics & Adolescent Medicine, 153,* 591–596. https://doi.org/10.1001/archpedi.153.6.591

Kroenke, K., Spitzer, R. L., & Williams, J. B. (2001). The PHQ-9: Validity of a brief depression severity measure. *Journal of General Internal Medicine, 16*, 606–613. https://doi.org/10.1046/j.1525-1497.2001.016009606.x

Krupski, A., West, I. I., Scharf, D. M., Hopfenbeck, J., Andrus, G., Joesch, J. M., & Snowden, M. (2016). Integrating primary care into community mental health centers: Impact on utilization and costs of health care. *Psychiatric Services, 67*, 1233–1239. https://doi.org/10.1176/appi.ps.201500424

Lamprecht, H., Laydon, C., McQuillan, C., Wiseman, S., Williams, L., Gash, A., & Reilly, J. (2007). Single-session solution-focused brief therapy and self-harm: A pilot study. *Journal of Psychiatric and Mental Health Nursing, 14*, 601–602. https://doi.org/10.1111/j.1365-2850.2007.01105.x

*Lefkowitz, B. (2007). *Community health centers: A movement and the people who made it happen*. New Brunswick, NJ: Rutgers University Press.

Lundahl, B. W., Kunz, C., Brownell, C., Tollefson, D., & Burke, B. L. (2010). A meta-analysis of motivational interviewing: Twenty-five years of empirical studies. *Research on Social Work Practice, 20*, 137–160. https://doi.org/10.1177/1049731509347850

Marlowe, D., Hodgson, J., Lamson, A., White, M., & Irons, T. (2012). Medical family therapy in a primary care setting: A framework for integration. *Contemporary Family Therapy, 34*, 244–258. https://doi.org/10.1007/s10591-012-9195-5

Martire, L. M., Schulz, R., Helgeson, V. S., Small, B. J., & Saghafi, E. M. (2010). Review and meta-analysis of couple-oriented interventions for chronic illness. *Annals of Behavioral Medicine, 40*, 325–342. https://doi.org/10.1007/s12160-010-9216-2

*McDaniel, S. H., Doherty, W. J., & Hepworth, J. (2014). *Medical family therapy and integrated care (2nd ed.)*. Washington, DC: American Psychological Association.

*Mendenhall, T. J., Berge, J. M., Harper, P., GreenCrow, B., LittleWalker, N., WhiteEagle, S., & BrownOwl, S. (2010). The family education diabetes series (FEDS): Community-based participatory research with a Midwestern American Indian community. *Nursing Inquiry, 17*, 359–372. https://doi.org/10.1111/j.1440-1800.2010.00508.x.

Mendenhall, T., Seal, K., GreenCrow, B., LittleWalker, K., & BrownOwl, S. (2012). The family education diabetes series (FEDS): Improving health in an urban-dwelling American Indian community. *Qualitative Health Research, 22*, 1524–1534. https://doi.org/10.1177/1049732312457469

Middlebrook, D. L., LeMaster, P. L., Beals, J., Novins, D. K., & Manson, S. M. (2001). Suicide prevention in American Indian and Alaska native communities: A critical review of programs. *Suicide and Life-threatening Behavior, 31*, 132–149. https://doi.org/10.1521/suli.31.1.5.132.24225

Mignogna, J., Hundt, N. E., Kauth, M. R., Kunik, M. E., Sorocco, K. H., Naik, A. D., … Cully, J. A. (2014). Implementing brief cognitive behavioral therapy in primary care: A pilot study. *Translational Behavioral Medicine, 4*, 175–183. https://doi.org/10.1007/s13142-013-0248-6

Miller, W. R., & Rollnick, S. (2002). *Motivational interviewing: preparing people for change*. New York, NY: Guilford Press.

Miller, W. R., & Rollnick, S. (2009). Ten things that motivational interviewing is not. *Behavioral and Cognitive Psychotherapy, 37*, 129–140. https://doi.org/10.1017/S1352465809005128

Miller, W. R., & Rose, G. S. (2009). Toward a theory of motivational interviewing. *American Psychologist, 64*, 527–537. https://doi.org/10.1037/a0016830

*Minkler, M., & Wallerstein, N. (Eds.). (2011). *Community-based participatory research for health: From process to outcomes*. San Francisco, CA: Wiley.

Mukamel, D. B., White, L. M., Nocon, R. S., Huang, E. S., Sharma, R., Shi, L., & Ngo-Metzger, Q. (2016). Comparing the cost of caring for Medicare beneficiaries in federally funded health centers to other care settings. *Health Services Research, 51*, 625–644. https://doi.org/10.1111/1475-6773.12339

Murphy, J. W. (2015). Primary health care and narrative medicine. *The Permanente Journal, 19*, 90–94. https://doi.org/10.7812/TPP/14-206

Nam, S., Chesla, C., Stotts, N. A., Kroon, L., & Janson, S. L. (2011). Barriers to diabetes management: Patient and provider factors. *Diabetes Research and Clinical Practice, 93*, 1–9. https://doi.org/10.1016/j.diabres.2011.02.002

Nasreddine, Z. S., Phillips, N. A., Bédirian, V., Charbonneau, S., Whitehead, V., Collin, I., … Chertkow, H. (2005). The Montreal cognitive assessment, MoCA: A brief screening tool for mild cognitive impairment. *Journal of the American Geriatrics Society, 53*, 695–699. https://doi.org/10.1111/j.1532-5415.2005.53221.x

*National Associations of Community Health Centers. (2011). *So you want to start a health center…?: A practical guide for starting a federally qualified health center*. Retrieved from http://iweb.nachc.com/Downloads/Products/11_START_CHC.pdf

*National Associations of Community Health Centers. (2017a). *America's health centers: What are health centers and who do they serve*. Retrieved from http://www.nachc.org/wp-content/uploads/2017/03/Americas-Health-Centers_2017.pdf

*National Associations of Community Health Centers. (2017b). *Health centers expanding reach*. Retrieved from http://www.nachc.org/wp-content/uploads/2017/02/HCs-Expanding-Reach_Feb17.pdf

National Certification Board for Diabetes Educators. (2017). *Welcome to the National Certification Board for Diabetes Educators*. Retrieved from https://www.ncbde.org/

Norcross, J. C., Krebs, P. M., & Prochaska, J. O. (2011). Stages of change. *Journal of Clinical Psychology, 67*, 143–154. https://doi.org/10.1002/jclp.20758

Otte, C. (2011). Cognitive behavioral therapy in anxiety disorders: Current state of the evidence. *Dialogues of Clinical Neuroscience, 13*, 413–421. Retrieved from https://www.ncbi.nlm.nih.gov/pmc/articles/PMC3263389/pdf/DialoguesClinNeurosci-13-413.pdf

Owens, J. A., & Dalzell, V. (2005). Use of the "BEARS" sleep screening tool in a pediatric residents' continuity clinic: A pilot study. *Sleep Medicine, 6*, 63–69. https://doi.org/10.1016/j.sleep.2004.07.015

Parra-Medina, D., Wilcox, S., Salinas, J., Addy, C., Fore, E., Poston, M., & Wilson, D. K. (2011). Results of the heart healthy and ethnically relevant lifestyle trial: A cardiovascular risk reduction intervention for African American women attending community health centers. *American Journal of Public Health, 101*, 1914–1921. https://doi.org/10.2105/AJPH.2011.300151

Peek, C. J. (2008). Planning care in the clinical, operational, and financial worlds. In R. Kessler and D. Stafford (Eds.), *Collaborative medicine case studies* (pp. 25–38). New York, NY: Springer.

Perkins, R. (2006). The effectiveness of one session of therapy using a single-session therapy approach for children and adolescents with mental health problems. *Psychology and Psychotherapy: Theory, Research and Practice, 79*, 215–227. https://doi.org/10.1348/147608305X60523

*Phelps, K., Hodgson, J., Lamson, A., Swanson, M., & White, M. (2012). Satisfaction with life and psychosocial factors among underserved minorities with type 2 diabetes. *Social Indicators Research, 106*, 359–370. https://doi.org/10.1007/s11205-011-9811-z

*Phelps, K., Howell, C., Hill, S., Seeman, T., Lamson, A., Hodgson, J., & Smith, D. (2009). A collaborative care model for patients with type II diabetes. *Families, Systems, & Health, 27*, 131–140. doi: https://doi.org/10.1037/a0015027

Plosker, R., & Chang, J. (2014). A solution-focused therapy group designed for caregivers of stroke survivors. *Journal of Systemic Therapies, 33*, 35–49. https://doi.org/10.1521/jsyt.2014.33.2.35

Posner, K., Brown, G. K., Stanley, B., Brent, D. A., Yershova, K. V., Oquendo, M. A., … Mann, J. J. (2011). The Columbia–suicide severity rating scale: Initial validity and internal consistency findings from three multisite studies with adolescents and adults. *American Journal of Psychiatry, 168*, 1266–1277. https://doi.org/10.1176/appi.ajp.2011.10111704

Priebe, S., Kelley, L., Omer, S., Golden, E., Walsh, S., Khanom, H., … McCabe, R. (2015). The effectiveness of a patient-centered assessment with a solution-focused approach (DIALOG+) for patients with psychosis: A pragmatic cluster-randomized controlled trial in community care. *Psychotherapy and Psychosomatics, 84*, 304–313. https://doi.org/10.1159/000430991

Prochaska, J. O., DiClemente, C. C., & Norcross, J. C. (1992). In search of how people change: Applications to the addictive behaviors. *American Psychologist, 47*, 1102–1114. https://doi.org/10.1037/0003-066X.47.9.1102

Ramezani, S., Khosravi, A., Motaghi, Z., Hamidzadeh, A., & Mousavi, S. A. (2017). The effect of cognitive-behavioural and solution-focused counselling on prevention of postpartum depression in nulliparous pregnant women. *Journal of Reproductive and Infant Psychology, 35*, 172–182. https://doi.org/10.1080/02646838.2016.1266470

Rao, J. K., Anderson, L. A., Inui, T. S., & Frankel, R. M. (2007). Communication interventions make a difference in conversations between physicians and patients: A systematic review of the evidence. *Medical Care, 45*, 340–349. https://doi.org/10.1097/01.mlr.0000254516.04961.d5

Rhodes, S. D., Malow, R. M., & Jolly, C. (2010). Community-based participatory research: A new and not-so-new approach to HIV/AIDS prevention, care, and treatment. *AIDS Education and Prevention, 22*, 173–183. https://doi.org/10.1521/aeap.2010.22.3.173

Rolland, J. S., Emanuel, L. L., & Torke, A. M. (2017). Applying a family systems lens to proxy decision making in clinical practice and research. *Families, Systems, & Health, 35*, 7–17. https://doi.org/10.1037/fsh0000250

*Rollnick, S., Miller, W. R., & Butler, C. (2007). *Motivational interviewing in health care: Helping patients change behavior*. New York, NY: Guilford Press.

Rosenthal, E. L., Brownstein, J. N., Rush, C. H., Hirsch, G. R., Willaert, A. M., Scott, J. R., ... Fox, D. J. (2010). Community health workers: Part of the solution. *Health Affairs, 29*, 1338–1342. https://doi.org/10.1377/hlthaff.2010.0081

Rudolf, M. C. J., Hunt, C., George, J., Hajibagheri, K., & Blair, M. (2010). HENRY: Development, pilot and long-term evaluation of a programme to help practitioners work more effectively with parents of babies and pre-school children to prevent childhood obesity. *Child: Care, Health and Development, 36*, 850–857. https://doi.org/10.1111/j.1365-2214.2010.01116.x

Safren, S. A., Sprich, S., Mimiaga, M. J., Surman, C., Knouse, L., Groves, M., & Otto, M. W. (2010). Cognitive behavioral therapy vs relaxation with educational support for medication-treated adults with ADHD and persistent symptoms: A randomized controlled trial. *Journal of the American Medical Association, 304*, 875–880. https://doi.org/10.1001/jama.2010.1192

Sakalys, J. A. (2003). Restoring the patient's voice: The therapeutics of illness narratives. *Journal of Holistic Nursing, 21*, 228–241. https://doi.org/10.1177/0898010103256204

Schoener, E. P., Madeja, C. L., Henderson, M. J., Ondersma, S. J., & Janisse, J. J. (2006). Effects of motivational interviewing training on mental health therapist behavior. *Drug and Alcohol Dependence, 82*, 269–275. https://doi.org/10.1016/j.drugalcdep.2005.10.003

Seal, K., Blum, M., Didericksen, K., Mendenhall, T., Gagner, N., GreenCrow, B., ... Benton, K. (2016). The east metro American Indian diabetes initiative: Engaging indigenous men in the reclaiming of health and spirituality through community-based participatory research. *Health Education Research & Development, 4*, 1–8. https://doi.org/10.4172/2380-5439.1000152

Seifer, S. D. (1998). Service-learning: Community-campus partnerships for health professions education. *Academic Medicine, 73*, 273–277. https://doi.org/10.1097/00001888-199803000-00015

Serfaty, M. A., Haworth, D., Blanchard, M., Buszewicz, M., Murad, S., & King, M. (2009). Clinical effectiveness of individual cognitive behavioral therapy for depressed older people in primary care: A randomized controlled trial. *Archives of General Psychiatry, 66*, 1332–1340. https://doi.org/10.1001/archgenpsychiatry.2009.165

Skinner, H. A. (1982). The drug abuse screening test. *Addictive Behaviors, 7*, 363–371. https://doi.org/10.1016/0306-4603(82)90005-3

Spencer, M. S., Rosland, A. M., Kieffer, E. C., Sinco, B. R., Valerio, M., Palmisano, G., ... Heisler, M. (2011). Effectiveness of a community health worker intervention among African American and Latino adults with type 2 diabetes: A randomized controlled trial. *American Journal of Public Health, 101*, 2253–2260. https://doi.org/10.2105/AJPH.2010.300106

Spitzer, R. L., Kroenke, K., Williams, J. B. W., & Lowe, B. (2006). A brief measure for assessing generalized anxiety disorder. *Archives of Internal Medicine, 166*, 1092–1097. https://doi.org/10.1001/archinte.166.10.1092

Squires, J., Bricker, D., & Potter, L. (1997). Revision of a parent-completed developmental screening tool: Ages and stages questionnaires. *Journal of Pediatric Psychology, 22*, 313–328. https://doi.org/10.1093/jpepsy/22.3.313

Street, R. L., Makoul, G., Arora, N. K., & Epstein, R. M. (2009). How does communication heal? Pathways linking clinician–patient communication to health outcomes. *Patient Education and Counseling, 74*, 295–301. https://doi.org/10.1016/j.pec.2008.11.015

Sudore, R. L., Mehta, K. M., Simonsick, E. M., Harris, T. B., Newman, A. B., Satterfield, S., ... Yaffe, K. (2006). Limited literacy in older people and disparities in health and healthcare access. *Journal of the American Geriatrics Society, 54*, 770–776. https://doi.org/10.1111/j.1532-5415.2006.00691.x

Sulmasy, D. P. (2002). A biopsychosocial-spiritual model for the care of patients at the end of life. *The Gerontologist, 42*, 24–33. https://doi.org/10.1093/geront/42.suppl_3.24

Tambling, R. B., & Johnson, L. N. (2008). The relationship between stages of change and outcome in couple therapy. *American Journal of Family Therapy, 36*, 229–241. https://doi.org/10.1080/01926180701290941

Taylor, J. (2014). The fundamentals of community health centers. In *National health policy forum: Background paper*. Washington, DC: George Washington University.

Tidemalm, D., Runeson, B., Waern, M., Frisell, T., Carlström, E., Lichtenstein, P., & Långström, N. (2011). Familial clustering of suicide risk: A total population study of 11.4 million individuals. *Psychological Medicine, 41*, 2527–2534. https://doi.org/10.1017/S0033291711000833

Topolski, T. D., LoGerfo, J., Patrick, D. L., Williams, B., Walwick, J., & Patrick, M. B. (2006). The rapid assessment of physical activity (RAPA) among older adults. *Preventing Chronic Disease, 3*, A118–A125. Retrieved from https://www.ncbi.nlm.nih.gov/pubmed/16978493

Trockel, M., Manber, R., Chang, V., Thurston, A., & Taylor, C. B. (2011). An e-mail delivered CBT for sleep-health program for college students: Effects on sleep quality and depression symptoms. *Journal of Clinical Sleep Medicine, 7*, 276–281. https://doi.org/10.5664/JCSM.1072

Valve, P., Lehtinen-Jacks, S., Eriksson, T., Lehtinen, M., Lindfors, P., Saha, M. T., ... Anglé, S. (2013). A solution-focused low-intensity intervention aimed at improving health behaviors of young females: A cluster-randomized controlled trial. *BMC Public Health, 13*, 1044–1056. https://doi.org/10.1186/1471-2458-13-1044

Viner, R. M., Christie, D., Taylor, V., & Hey, S. (2003). Motivational/solution-focused intervention improves HbA1c in adolescents with type 1 diabetes: A pilot study. *Diabetic Medicine, 20*, 739–742. https://doi.org/10.1046/j.1464-5491.2003.00995.x

*Wallerstein, N. B., & Duran, B. (2006). Using community-based participatory research to address health disparities. *Health Promotion Practice, 7*, 312–323. https://doi.org/10.1177/1524839906289376.

*Ward Jr, T. J., & Geiger, H. J. (2016). *Out in the rural: A Mississippi health center and its war on poverty*. New York, NY: Oxford University Press.

Weisberg, R. B., & Magidson, J. F. (2014). Integrating cognitive behavioral therapy into primary care settings. *Cognitive and Behavioral Practice, 21*, 247–251. https://doi.org/10.1016/j.cbpra.2014.04.002

Weiss, S. J., Ernst, A. A., Cham, E., & Nick, T. G. (2003). Development of a screen for ongoing intimate partner violence. *Violence and Victims, 18*, 131–141. https://doi.org/10.1891/vivi.2003.18.2.131

Weiss, B. D., & Palmer, R. (2004). Relationship between health care costs and very low literacy skills in a medically needy and indigent Medicaid population. *Journal of the American Board of Family Practice, 17*, 44–47. https://doi.org/10.3122/jabfm.17.1.44

Wissow, L. S., Gadomski, A., Roter, D., Larson, S., Brown, J., Zachary, C., ... Wang, M. C. (2008). Improving child and parent mental health in primary care: A cluster-randomized trial of communication skills training. *Pediatrics, 121*, 266–275. https://doi.org/10.1542/peds.2007-0418

Wolraich, M. L., Lambert, W., Doffing, M. A., Bickman, L., Simmons, T., & Worley, K. (2003). Psychometric properties of the Vanderbilt ADHD diagnostic parent rating scale in a referred population. *Journal of Pediatric Psychology, 28,* 559–568. https://doi.org/10.1093/jpepsy/jsg046

World Health Organization. (1992). *The ICD-10 classification of mental and behavioural disorders: Clinical descriptions and diagnostic guidelines.* Geneva, Switzerland: World Health Organization.

Wright, L. M., Watson, W. L., & Bell, J. M. (1996). *Beliefs: The heart of healing in families and illness.* New York, NY: Basic Books.

Wyder, M., Ward, P., & De Leo, D. (2009). Separation as a suicide risk factor. *Journal of Affective Disorders, 116,* 208–213. https://doi.org/10.1016/j.jad.2008.11.007

Wu, I. H., & Windle, C. (1980). Ethnic specificity in the relative minority use and staffing of community mental health centers. *Community Mental Health Journal, 16,* 156–168. https://doi.org/10.1007/BF00778587

Chapter 14
Medical Family Therapy in Community Engagement

Tai Mendenhall, William Doherty, Elizabeth "Nan" LittleWalker, and Jerica Berge

"Community engagement" has been defined in a variety of ways over the years, ranging from petition and protests by disenfranchised groups against powerful others (e.g., businesses, governments) who have hurt or neglected them to purposeful partnerships advanced by lay community members and professional organizations. In health care, we have seen community engagement evolve from early efforts in peer support that do not directly involve professionals (e.g., Alcoholics Anonymous, Al-Anon) to those that are positioned within communities—but are professionally led (e.g., community-oriented primary care). Today, cutting-edge efforts in community engagement are gaining ground through community-based participatory research (CBPR); this manner of partnering communities and professionals is driven by the wisdom that everyone involved—patients, family members, community leaders, healthcare providers, administrators, etc.—has something to contribute. Collectively, this mosaic of expertise and energy is far more powerful than the sum of its parts.

Medical family therapists (MedFTs) represent an active and visible contributor to the advancement of community engagement and CBPR in healthcare. They bring an orientation comfortable with the complexities of multiple and overlapping human systems (biological, psychological, family/social, spiritual) and readily connect these dots within and across the communities of care provision (e.g., clinics, hospitals) and the patient populations that they are positioned within or oriented to (e.g., geographic

---

T. Mendenhall (✉) · W. Doherty
Department of Family Social Science, University of Minnesota, Saint Paul, MN, USA
e-mail: mend0009@umn.edu

E. LittleWalker
Department of Indian Work, Family Education Diabetes Series, Interfaith Action of Greater Saint Paul, St. Paul, MN, USA

J. Berge
Department of Family Medicine and Community Health,
University of Minnesota Medical School, Minneapolis, MN, USA

locales, groups united through a shared disease or experience). To set the stage for our discussion of the practice of MedFT in community engagement, we begin by sharing the following story of Kadin (a MedFT) and Teresa (an American Indian elder).

> **Clinical Vignette**
> [Note: This vignette is a compilation of cases that represent MedFT in community engagement. All patients' names and/or identifying information have been changed to maintain confidentiality.]
> "You have diabetes," the attending physician said. Teresa was lying on a hospital bed in the emergency department, surrounded by loved ones. She had been feeling very sick while at a powwow a couple of hours away from her home.
> "No I don't," she said. "I've always been healthy."
> "Yes, you do," the physician countered. "I recommend when you get home that you follow up with your primary care physician right away. There are a lot of lifestyle things that you are going to need to do to." He seemed like he was in a hurry.
> Teresa started to cry. She knew many people in her American Indian community who had been diagnosed with diabetes. Most had lost toes, feet, or even whole limbs. Some had lost their eyesight. Many had died.
> "I can't have diabetes," she said to her partner, Henry. He was holding her hand. "I've always been healthy. How did I get diabetes?"
> When she came home, Teresa followed up with her primary care physician. Dr. Roth—Teresa called him "Dr. Scott"—had known her for a long time.
> "I'm so sorry, Teresa. I know that this is scary for you," he said.
> "Is this going to kill me?," Teresa asked.
> "People can live long lives with diabetes. But it takes a fair amount of attention and care."
> Scott and his diabetes nurse educator worked hard with Teresa over the next several months to control her new disease. Changes in diet and physical activity represented most of the work. Integrating blood sugar monitoring and tracking was a big deal, as well. Over time, Teresa's health improved. She lost more than 50 pounds. Her metabolic control (A1c) was good. She was feeling better.
> In synchrony with this, Teresa became increasingly aware of how diabetes was impacting her community. She began to learn about how much more common the disease is with American Indian (AI) patients than as compared with other ethnic groups. She talked extensively with friends, relatives, and other AI community members about their commonplace sense of doom about it (i.e., that diabetes is an "expected" health problem that will eventually claim everyone). She was very familiar with how so many Native people did not (do not) trust Western medicine providers to care for them. Generations of colonization and historical trauma by Western institutions (healthcare, education, government) had, understandably, done that.
> "Diabetes is decimating my people," she said during a peer support and mentoring program (called Partners in Diabetes) meeting at the clinic. Dr. Roth and Kadin, along with others, had helped to create the group.

"How do you think other members of your community would feel about coming here?," Kadin asked.

"Most won't come here. They don't feel safe. Or they don't have insurance," Teresa explained.

Then she got an idea. "Kadin? Dr. Scott? Would you two be willing to talk with me and my sister, who directs our local Department of Indian Work, about creating a program for Native people?"

For the next 2 years, they met. Considerable effort was spent in designing a partnership that differed from conventional top-down models of Western healthcare. Multiple community members worked to sensitize care providers (Kadin, Dr. Scott, and others) to the process(es), pace, and importance of building trust within American Indian circles. They talked about AI culture, the diversity of cultures and tribes within this larger frame (e.g., Dakota, Ojibwe), spirituality and belief systems, and Indigenous conceptualizations of health. In turn, community members gained more insight about how Western healthcare is oriented; they learned about providers' habits, workloads and administrative expectations, and perspectives in care delivery.

Culminating from these efforts, the Family Education Diabetes Series (FEDS) was launched. Situated in a local AI community center, the program engages patients, their families (spouses, parents, children, and other relatives/friends), and providers (physicians and physician extenders, nurses, dieticians, behavioral health personnel, and other professionals) every 2 weeks for an evening of fellowship, education, and support. The group shares meals that are consistent with traditional Native diets. They learn about disease-related topics identified by the community through a variety of lively activities consistent with AI cultures (e.g., talking circles, Native games, creative arts). Health data (e.g., weight, BMI, blood pressure, random blood glucose, A1c) was also collected and tracked.

"I think that this is working," Teresa whispered to Kadin as he sat down next to her one evening at a FEDS meeting. He had just shared with the group how their collective metabolic control had improved significantly over the previous 6 months, alongside an average weight loss of 20 pounds. Kadin and Teresa then turned to Dr. Scott and another AI elder who were beginning a copresentation about diabetes and foot care. All of the presentations were (are) done this way: one person with professional expertise and one community member with personal expertise and/or experience.

"Most of these folks don't see a doctor for their diabetes," Teresa said. It was not clear if she was talking to Kadin or to herself. "This is their 'doctor,' this is their 'healthcare'."

"Outside of the clinic's walls," Kadin said.

Teresa looked over at Kadin and then back at Dr. Scott and his copresenter. "Absolutely. And we're all in this together."

What Is Community-Based Participatory Research?

Contemporary efforts in integrated behavioral healthcare are making great strides to facilitate collaboration between providers representing multiple disciplines. However, we still tend to miss two things: (a) attention to the active roles that our patients and their families can play in cocreating health and (b) attention to the potential collective power of broader patient communities to advance health. Instead, most healthcare ("integrated," "collaborative," or otherwise) continues to frame professionals as the sources of knowledge, wisdom, and services vis-à-vis patients and families who are relatively passive. Further, most care that is provided to patients/families is delivered in a single patient/family at a timely manner, with no ways of connecting patients with each other along the way. Instead, patients and families sit straightforward in waiting rooms, reading outdated magazines and not talking with each other.

As large national and international organizations like the Agency for Healthcare Research and Quality (AHRQ), National Institutes for Health (NIH), and the World Health Organization (WHO) have called for collaborative efforts to address complex health and social problems that are ill-suited for conventional service delivery and/or research endeavors, community-based participatory research (CBPR) has become an increasingly visible way for us to partner with patient communities. Many are now working to extend these collaborative emphases of integrated behavioral healthcare to include collaboration with the patients and families we serve.

CBPR evolved from *action research* in the 1940s and has been framed in a number of ways since this time (see Figure 14.1). It is characterized by efforts in which

> Action Learning
> > (e.g., Pedler, 2011; Revans, 2011)
> Action Research
> > (e.g., Brydon-Miller, Greenwood, & Maguire, 2003; Stringer, 2013)
> Action Science
> > (e.g., Friedman, Razer, & Sykes, 2004; Rudolph, Taylor, & Foldy, 2005)
> Classroom Action Research
> > (e.g., Mettetal, 2012; Schmidt, 2002)
> Community-based Participatory Action Research
> > (e.g., Giachello et al., 2003; Maiter, Simich, Jacobson, & Wise, 2008)
> Community-based Research
> > (e.g., Minkler, 2005; Strand, Cutforth, Stoecker, Marullo, & Donohue, 2003)
> Critical Action Research
> > (e.g., DePoy, Hartman, & Haslett, 1999; Huzzard & Johansson, 2014)
> Industrial Action Research
> > (e.g., Goodnough, 2003; Richter & Koch, 2004)
> Participatory Action Development
> > (e.g., Lammerink, Bury, & Bolt, 1999; Okomoda & Alamu, 2002)
> Participatory Action Learning
> > (e.g., King, Gaffiiey, & Gunton, 2001; Mayoux, 2005)
> Participatory Action Research
> > (e.g., Kemmis & McTaggart, 2005; McIntyre, 2007)
> Participatory Research
> > (e.g., Cornwall & Jewkes, 1995; Macaulay, Commanda, Freeman, & Gibson, 1999)

Figure 14.1 Alternative Terms in Professional Literature for CBPR

professional researchers partner with communities to generate new knowledge and solve local problems (AHRQ, 2004; Lewin, 1946). Several key assumptions permeate these projects; they include:

1. Partnerships between all project members (e.g., patients, families, care providers, researchers) are collaborative, equitable, and democratic through every stage of knowledge and intervention development.
2. Projects are built upon the strengths and resources that already exist within the community (i.e., not seeking new resources from elsewhere).
3. Reciprocal learning and capacity building strengthen contributions between engaged participants.
4. Deep investment in improving community members' health and well-being is recognizable by joining participants.
5. Iterative processes in which problems are co-identified, solutions are codeveloped within the context(s) of a community's existing resources, interventions are advanced, outcomes are evaluated in accord with what participants collectively see as important, and interventions are adapted and refined in response to outcome data.
6. Project members are humble and flexible in making changes to their interventions.
7. Dissemination of findings and new understandings is shared across both professional and lay audiences and arenas.
8. Recognition that CBPR can be slow and messy, particularly during early phases of a new initiative's development.
9. Participants recognize long-term engagement and commitment to the effort (Bradbury & Reason, 2003; LaVeaux & Christopher, 2009; Mendenhall, Pratt, Phelps, Baird, & Yonkin, 2014; Montoya & Kent, 2011; Scharff & Mathews, 2008; Strickland, 2006).

Citizen Health Care

Citizen Health Care (CHC) is a model that was designed purposefully in the spirit of CBPR as a framework for biomedical and behavioral healthcare professionals who engage with families in community settings (Berge, Mendenhall, & Doherty, 2009; Doherty and Mendenhall, 2006). It begins with the notion that all personal health problems can also be seen as public problems. For example, ethnic disparities in diabetes—like the ones that Teresa observed in our vignette, above—can be viewed in terms of their implications for a minority community's sense of dignity and social pride. It views providers as citizens with knowledge and skills who work actively with other citizens (patients, families) who also possess important knowledge and skills. The following represents this approach's principal tenets (for in-depth description of these tenets and key strategies for their implementation, see Doherty, Mendenhall, & Berge, 2010):

The greatest untapped resource for improving healthcare is the knowledge, wisdom, and energy of individuals, families, and communities who face chal-

lenging health issues in their everyday lives. Conventional healthcare renders patients and families as passive recipients of professionals' services. CHC works to integrate providers' expertise with the wisdom and resources of a local community. For example, Dr. Scott's and Kadin's disease-related knowledge about diabetes management (e.g., what constitutes a healthy diet; indicated ranges of blood sugar, body mass index (BMI), and blood pressure; ways to engage family members as active participators in co-owing new lifestyles related to exercise and disease management) is good on its own—but partnered with Teresa's and others' wisdom about Native foods, Indigenous games, physical activities, and traditional conceptualizations of health through Medicine Wheel models (Dapice, 2006; Garrett & Garrett, 1994) and habitudes of "walking in balance" to connect mind, body, spirit, and community well-being, this knowledge is made infinitely more engaging, personalized, and effective (Muehlenkamp, Marrone, Gray, & Brown, 2009; Robbins, Hong, Engler, & King, 2016; Rybak & Decker-Fitts, 2009).

People must be engaged as coproducers of healthcare for themselves and their communities, not just as patients or consumers of services. Alongside the passive roles of patients and families within conventional healthcare is the expectation that care's focus is on one patient at a time. After all, this is how insurance billing, electronic medical records, and healthcare training are generally framed. In CHC, patients and families take active roles in reclaiming their own health (e.g., exercising or changing their diets together vs. expecting identified patients to improve solely through prescribed medications) and the health of others in their broader community, however defined (e.g., those belonging to a particular geographic area, others who live with a similar health condition). Patients and family members think about—and care about—how those beyond their immediate circles are doing. They support each other's efforts toward collective healing and growth.

Professionals can play a catalytic role in fostering citizen initiatives when they develop their public skills as citizen professionals in groups with flattened hierarchies. At the same time that patients and families are socialized to be passive in healthcare, providers are socialized to lead. Community engagement initiatives can be challenging for providers until they develop skills related to working "with" people (not just "for" them or "on" them). These skills encompass a variety of proficiencies, including how to plan and facilitate community meetings and conversations, collaboratively problem-solve, cooperatively collect and analyze data, disseminate findings across lay and professional arenas, and engage—all the while—as a learner (not just a leader or expert).

If you begin with an established program, you will not end up with an initiative that is "owned and operated" by citizens. Although learnings and elements from CHC projects can spread to other communities, each project must be created or adapted in light of the unique challenges and resources within each community. To simply replicate (off-the-shelf) something that worked in a different community could miss some of these unique elements and thereby fail to elicit a sense of co-ownership and investment by the patients, family members, and other community participants who are involved. Along the way, outside resources (e.g., a local food shelf that holds weekly cooking demonstrations) could be integrated into a larger whole—but only through active and collective agreement by its members.

Local communities must retrieve their own historical, cultural, and religious traditions of health and healing and bring these into dialogue with contemporary healthcare systems. Western healthcare strives to be "value neutral" and empirically driven. If providers' efforts are not oriented to "best practices" (i.e., care strategies that are supported by objective research data), like-minded colleagues can challenge whatever is being done as less than ideal (at best) or even unsafe and irresponsible. And while there are benefits to empirical approaches (e.g., prescribing a treatment with the confidence that randomized controlled trials have shown that it works), there is also considerable richness in local communities' health and healing traditions. Integrating both viewpoints and care models can serve to bolster confidence in any treatment. Further, it can sensitize Western providers to core belief systems that patients and families hold dear. For example, contemporary notions of "integrated behavioral healthcare" that are guided by the biopsychosocial-spiritual (BPSS) model (Engel, 1977, 1980; Wright, Watson & Bell, 1996) endeavor to integrate biomedical care with behavioral health and other social services. Indigenous conceptualizations of the Medicine Wheel have viewed health in such a manner for millennia. In the FEDS project, described above, Dr. Scott and Kadin could have advanced education about diabetes in a frame consistent with the BPSS model. Instead, in partnership with the wisdom of Teresa and other community elders, they advanced conversations about "walking in balance." This served to connect effective disease management with respective components of the medicine wheel.

Citizen health initiatives should have a bold vision (a BHAG—a big, hairy, audacious goal) while working pragmatically on focused, specific projects. Projects advanced in CHC are purposefully ambitious in their vision and ultimate goals. In the FEDS, members are working toward eliminating (not just reducing) diabetes in the AI community. Along the way, pragmatic steps are identified, pursued, and completed (Mendenhall, Seal, GreenCrow, LittleWalker, & BrownOwl, 2012; Seal et al., 2016). These specific steps have included arranging community events and powwows oriented to health education, community 5-K walks, the authoring of diabetes-friendly cookbooks that feature Native ingredients, public listings of local farmers' markets, and the creation of an American Indian Men's Group that engages Native men in a variety of physical activities that are consistent with their culture (e.g., canoe building, lacrosse, sugar bushing, harvesting wild rice, fishing). The accomplishment of any and all of these smaller steps is, in itself, motivating and energizing to its participants as they, all the while, strive toward a larger vision of eradicating diabetes altogether.

Teams in Community Engagement

In contrast to other chapters in this book (wherein respective members of healthcare teams are described with specificity), teams engaged in CBPR can arguably include professional representatives from any discipline or institutional position. In partnership with them, these teams include patients, families, and other community members (elders, leaders, etc.) who are affected by any myriad of health presentations or social issues.

Community members. By definition (i.e., the "C" in CBPR), community members' participation in health initiatives facilitates the inclusion of healthcare's most commonly untapped resource: the knowledge, wisdom, and energy of the very patients and families that Western healthcare endeavors to engage. These include persons who live with a targeted health condition (e.g., alcoholism, diabetes), alongside their spouses, family members, friends, and other loved ones. They include Indigenous leaders and community elders (like Teresa), who oftentimes maintain key positions to educate providers about local cultures, customs, and habitudes that are essential for professional/community partnerships to work.

Biomedical healthcare providers. Providers whose primary training is focused on caring for patients' physical health include medical technicians, nurses, nurse practitioners, family physicians and physician extenders, specialty care physicians (e.g., endocrinologists, nephrologists), and others. Respective representation of these fields in community engagement varies in accord with the focus of the health initiative (e.g., pediatricians involved in a teen-based initiative targeting adolescent health, primary care nurses involved in an adult-based initiative targeting chronic pain).

Care coordinators/community health workers/promotoras. These providers go between healthcare clinics and patients' homes to provide care directly to patients in the environments wherein they need the most support. They provide education and social support for patients struggling with physical, behavioral, or social problems. They collaborate with healthcare providers to coordinate care for the patient both in the clinic and at home. They bridge the typical disconnect between what happens in the clinic and the home environment. They are keys to developing care plans and in supporting patients and providers to successfully carry out treatment plans for managing biomedical and/or behavioral health conditions.

Health educators. Providers whose primary training is focused on the provision of psychoeducation and/or skills-based instruction for patients (usually carried out in synchrony or coordination with biomedical treatment) include educators who specialize in nutrition and diabetes management, alcohol/drug use treatment, tobacco cessation, safe sex practices, family planning, disaster preparedness, life skills, and others. Respective representation of these fields in community engagement varies in accord with the focus of the community initiative (e.g., tobacco cessation specialists involved in a school initiative to reduce smoking, nutritionists involved in a diabetes program).

Behavioral health providers. Providers whose primary training is focused on caring for patients' mental/behavioral health include couple/marriage and family therapists (MFTs), MedFTs, social workers, counselors, psychologists, and others.

Respective representation of these fields in CBPR can vary widely. School counselors, for example, are readily positioned to participate in school-based initiatives targeting a broad range of adolescent concerns (e.g., pregnancy prevention, smoking cessation). MedFTs are readily positioned to participate in health initiatives that partner with clinics and healthcare sites oriented to any of the primary, secondary, tertiary, and other contexts highlighted in this text.

Community professionals. CBPR can include professionals whose primary training is not specifically focused in healthcare but who are nevertheless positioned to offer a great deal to a larger mosaic of specialized wisdom. These can include persons who maintain administrative power and influence within involved organizations (e.g., school principals, business owners, church and/or religious leaders), employees of such organizations (e.g., elementary- and secondary-school teachers, coaches, youth mentors), and/or highly respected Indigenous/Native healers or consultants within select communities (e.g., curanderos, shamans).

Fundamentals of Community Engagement

A provider's knowledge and skills in community-engaged work begin with his or her professional identity and extend from there into the care and/or research-related activities that he or she ultimately advances. For MFTs and MedFTs in particular, this process is informed by the systems thinking that permeates everything that we do across clinical practice and integrated behavioral healthcare.

Identity as a Citizen Professional

A MedFT working in community engagement should carry with him/herself a professional identity as a citizen with special skills and expertise (e.g., as a therapist) who works collaboratively with colleagues and other citizens who have special skills and expertise (e.g., as a primary care provider or nurse, a community elder, a patient with a particular condition, a spouse or family member related to a patient with a particular condition). This "citizen professional" mind frame is an essential grounding from which to advance authentic community engagement.

Citizen professionals maintain content knowledge about health topics for which they have been formally trained. Extending beyond this knowledge, they are also sensitive to the complex connections between the personal and public dimensions of unique health topics. A MedFT or family medicine provider who works with patients living with diabetes, for example, is conversant with the biomechanics and treatment of the disease—alongside the connections between it and the fast food industry, costs of healthy foods versus unhealthy foods, cultural practices regarding diet and exercise, and larger social forces like insurance companies that cover diabetes management (e.g., testing supplies, health visits) but not diabetes prevention (e.g., dietary education, access to fitness facilities).

Systems Thinking

Systems thinking is an advantage for MedFTs in community engagement by nature of the experience and comfort that they bring with working in groups (versus only one-on-one). MedFTs are skilled in connecting multiple people together who often begin conversations with different—and even conflicting—goals and agendas. They can facilitate processes whereby every person is heard and in so doing give voice to minority opinions and curb others from dominating a dialogue. These skills are essential in cocreating new ideas and solutions within families and other groups who were heretofore at an impasse. MedFTs understand how to pose questions to a group and allow the ensuing interactions to evolve dynamically. As they do this, MedFTs know how to function centrally so as to lead a conversation in a productive direction and when to be peripheral so as to not get in the way. This continuity between baseline MFT training and community engagement sets the stage for the public conversations and collective actions that are so central to CBPR.

Facilitating Public Conversations and Mobilizing Public Action

MedFTs functioning as citizen professionals must develop skills in facilitating public conversations and catalyzing collective—public—action. In the contexts of their "day jobs," they skillfully interweave the "personal" and "public" dimensions of the issues that they and their patients face. They are sensitive to timing, as well, in bringing together other project participants (patients, families, providers, etc.) for public conversations. A MedFT working with Teresa, for example, has the skills to engage her and other patients in a discussion that connects the importance of physical activity to personal safety in relatively unsafe neighborhoods, to encourage patients to become active in their communities around issues of safety, and to create responses where patients can meet with each other and community leaders to effect change.

Competence in Mixed-Methods Approaches

When MedFTs function as citizen professionals in research roles, they must be methodologically flexible in order to best match data collection efforts with what is going on in the CBPR process (McNicoll, 1999; Mendenhall & Doherty, 2005). In order to be sensitive to the perspectives and needs of multiple participants, careful use of methods and measures that have high face validity and practical (and immediate) utility is indicated. For this reason, community-engaged scholars often gravitate toward qualitative methods of data collection and analysis during early phases of the work. Exploring, for example, participants' personal experiences and viewpoints about a health issue can engage communities in identifying concerns that lead them to collective action. Qualitative inquiry can also serve to track inter-member and inter-group processes as interventions are democratically and collaboratively developed, as action is taken, and/or in assessing satisfaction with the results of new interventions. While objective (read: quantitative) measures of "success" can be created to assess a program's impact on a particular dependent variable (e.g., changes weight or metabolic control in FEDS participants), most projects do not do this until after a project is comparatively underway.

Consistent with this frame, a myriad of qualitative data in CBPR have been described in the literature, including in-depth interviews (Allen, Culhane-Pera, Pergament, & Call, 2010; Lindsey & McGuinness, 1998; Mendenhall & Doherty, 2003; Mendenhall et al., 2012; Razum, Gorgen, & Diesfeld, 1997), naturalistic case studies (Casswell, 2000; Holkup, Tripp-Reimer, Salois, & Weinert, 2004), reflexive journaling and meeting minutes (Hampshire, Blair, Crown, Avery, & Williams, 1999; Mosavel, Ahmed, Daniels, & Simon, 2011), focus groups (Seal et al., 2016; Small, 1995), participant observation (Lindsey & McGuinness, 1998; Maxwell, 1993; Rhodes, Malow, & Jolly, 2010), social network mapping (Bradbury & Reason, 2003; Ramanadhan et al., 2012), and oral histories and open-ended stories (Madsen, McNicol, & O'Mullan, 2015; Sieber, 2010). Access to many of these types of data is generally easy for investigators in CBPR, because the very nature of the work requires that they be active participators in the research that is being evaluated (Coughlin, Smith, & Fernandez, 2017; Israel, Eng, Schulz, & Parker, 2012).

Whereas qualitative analyses are especially useful in helping investigators to understand participants' contexts, cultures, beliefs, attitudes, community practices, and subjective experiences related to CBPR processes, quantitative measures are most usually and most usefully employed to evaluate an intervention's efficacy (Israel et al., 2012; Mendenhall & Doherty, 2005; Reese et al., 1999). These efforts are also important on "political" grounds, insofar as formally testing for objective change in tangible measures (whatever measures these may be) helps to advance confidence by the broader scientific community that the work is rigorous and credible (Minkler & Wallerstein, 2011; National Institutes of Health, 2009). For example, it was not until the authors had quantitative data confirming effectiveness in the above-referenced FEDS project that our team was able to secure ongoing external grant funding to support the work.

Consistent with basic tenets of CBPR, however, it is important to involve participants in selecting what to quantitatively evaluate, test, or measure. For example, in a CBPR initiative designed to reduce on-campus smoking, participants (researchers and community members) discussed how students' smoking prevalence was—and was not—an important measure of "success." Students saw the number of available after-school activities (delivered to target stress and boredom) as a more important quantitative measure of success than the straightforward number of students who reported that they smoke. Put simply, they saw after-school activities as a stage setter for the improved self-efficacy and social support that students needed to eventually quit smoking—and they were right (Mendenhall, Harper, Stephenson, & Haas, 2011; Mendenhall, Whipple, Harper, & Haas, 2008).

In another project, providers involved in a diabetes CBPR initiative for adolescents saw metabolic control as the most important dependent variable of success, whereas adolescent patients wanted to track school policies regarding whether students with diabetes were allowed to go on fieldtrips with their peers (Mendenhall & Doherty, 2007). As the MedFT facilitator of this initiative worked to align these very different foci within the group, a collective sense of ownership in action items and outcome data evolved; school policies regarding fieldtrips were altered, and teens' disease management and physical health improved.

A project aimed at childhood obesity prevention identified increased physical activity as an important outcome, alongside increasing social capital (connectedness), as a key outcome in its neighborhood community (Berge et al., 2016). In this and other CBPR projects, what was (is) tested quantitatively is up to the whole group to decide. It is important to note, too, that these quantitative analyses tend to remain "local"—i.e., for, by, and within the community in which a project is positioned (Mendenhall & Doherty, 2005; Minkler & Wallerstein, 2011). Efforts to test widespread generalizability (e.g., a randomized control trial) are less indicated than efforts to test local impact (e.g., a single-group repeated-measures trial) because CBPR projects are designed purposefully to tap and reflect the unique resources and challenges of their immediate contexts.

Ultimately, participants in CBPR tend to combine both qualitative and quantitative methods. Using multiple methods over the course of a project enables researchers to triangulate different sources of data, and this increases confidence in conclusions that are drawn (Blumenthal, & DiClemente, 2013; Israel et al., 2012). Throughout this and the cyclical processes of CBPR, all data that are collected and analyzed are presented back to the initiative's participants (Hambridge, 2000; Mendenhall & Doherty, 2005; Meyer, 2000; Nichols, 1995; Seal et al., 2016). This facilitates an active and purposeful dialogue between providers, researchers, and community participants about the meaning and usefulness of data—which then informs the generation of ensuing action steps to further improve and/or maintain success in the work.

Competence in Research Ethics and Human Subjects' Protection

Anyone engaged in social science and/or biomedical research must be trained in and familiar with the culture, rules, and practices of human-subjects protection. Protecting and promoting the rights and interests of all research participants—including those who are vulnerable and susceptible to diminished or coerced consent and/or who lack (or may come to lack) the capacity to consent to or decline continued participation in investigative pursuits—is essential to the conduct of ethical research. Work that involves protected health information further necessitates familiarity with Health Insurance Portability and Accountability Act (HIPAA) standards. In CBPR, it is especially important to maintain close collaboration (and frequent consultation) with universities'—and/or health systems'—institutional review boards (IRBs) regarding the fast-paced and ever-changing nature of community-engaged efforts. Unlike conventional research projects that may only require annual renewals after receiving an IRB's initial approval to begin, CBPR projects frequently require change-of-protocol requests/procedures, articulations (and rearticulations) of "public" versus "private" study data, and adding/removing study personnel (alongside ensuring the successful completion of indicated Collaborative Institutional Training Initiative (CITI) and HIPAA training of said personnel). In the authors' experience, monthly interactions with IRBs are commonplace.

Disseminating Scholarship Across Lay and Professional Forums

Disseminating research findings is essential when sharing scholarship and newfound wisdom with academic researchers, providers, administrators—and with patients, families, and communities—who are involved in the work. Results communicate success of the project, changes brought about by its labors, and the ongoing efforts that providers/researchers/families/community members are doing to sustain the initiative. CBPR teams, then, collaborate fully in writing and disseminate study findings to professional/scientific communities, community-specific organizations, and the general public. To share knowledge with the scientific community, they target refereed journals and local, national, and international conferences and forums. To share knowledge with community-specific organizations, the local community itself, and the general public, team members connect with community service-providing sites and resources, e.g., targeting local and state-wide public print and electronic media and community events/celebrations (Berge et al., 2009; Mendenhall, Doherty, Berge, Fauth, & Tremblay, 2013; Minkler & Wallerstein, 2008).

Community Engagement Across the MedFT Healthcare Continuum

Medical family therapy serves as a useful framework for the integration of community energies and expertise with conventional professional knowledge and contributions to program development and care services. Specific training and collaborative, teaching/mentoring, and research competencies represent important facets of this work as professionals engage in what they can feel very different than what they were trained to do in graduate school (i.e., deliver care or education in professionally led ways). Tables 14.1 and 14.2 highlight specific skills that characterize MedFTs'

Table 14.1 Medical Family Therapy in Community Engagement: Basic Knowledge and Skills

MedFT Healthcare Continuum Level	Level 1	Level 2	Level 3
Knowledge	Basic knowledge about BPSS approaches to working with highly distressed individuals, couples, families, and communities. Basic knowledge regarding local community issues (e.g., common and/or highly prevalent health or social concerns of patient populations served).	Familiar with benefits of patient and family engagement with others in the community (e.g., benefits of receiving and offering support to/from others who share similar struggles). Basic knowledge about local community resources, including structures, leadership, and key groups and individuals.	Basic knowledge regarding CBPR and its value in cocreating new knowledge and interventions that are clinically useful. Understanding regarding interrelationships of BPSS elements in patients/families/communities' experiences in health. Understanding regarding the difference(s) between conventional professional roles and identity and those of a citizen professional.
Skills	Can discuss (and psycho-educate) basic relationships between biological, psychological, and behavioral foci vis-à-vis common health issues. Collaborative skills within standard healthcare professional networks.	Can coordinate care with local community agency personnel inside and outside of healthcare.	Coordinate and integrate respective community members' expertise and counsel into the creation of an interconnected "map" of professional and lay resources and outreach initiatives.

involvement in community engagement through CBPR across Hodgson, Lamson, Mendenhall, and Tyndall's (2014) MedFT Healthcare Continuum. As we move along the continuum, we carry different expectations regarding the appropriately matched roles, knowledge, and overall contributions to the creation of new knowledge through the iterative designing, evaluating, and refining of interventions that reflect the collective wisdom, efforts, and participation of both professional and lay team members.

At the beginning of the continuum, MedFTs at *Level 1* should possess a general understanding about BPSS approaches to working with highly distressed persons (individuals, couples, families, and communities) and be able to provide psycho-education about the ways that multiple human systems can influence and impact each other. While minimally involved in community engagement activities, they are familiar with the local cultures and concerns within the populations that their prac-

Table 14.2 Medical Family Therapy in Community Engagement: Advanced Knowledge and Skills

MedFT Healthcare Continuum Level	Level 4	Level 5
Knowledge	Adept understanding of CBPR and CHC strategies (see Appendixes 1 and 2). Understands common lessons learned from a wide range of CBPR projects regarding initiative development, processes, timing, etc.	Conversant with evidence-based ways of evaluating CBPR processes and outcomes; indicated methodologies include both quantitative and qualitative traditions. Knowledgeable regarding CBPR project "scaffolding," which enables new partnerships between professional and lay community members to create new initiatives with some facilitative structure and guidance (but not in a manner that undermines their natural growth and evolution).
Skills	Adept in the facilitation of community member/professional provider conversations regarding shared pressure points. Able to deliver seminars and workshops about CBPR, articulating methodological tenets and strategies. Can apply for and secure external grant funding by effectively communicating CBPR tenets, strategies, and processes; can negotiate adequate flexibility in grant-related timelines and deliverables so as to not sabotage the natural evolution of professional/community partnership(s). Consistently collaborates with key team members, working democratically through every step of CBPR's iterative processes.	Able to conduct qualitative research regarding community members' and professionals' collaborative efforts in CBPR; foci include (but are not limited to) shared pressure points, project development, and perspectives regarding intervention components' contributions to objective outcomes; methods include (but are not limited to) individual and group key informant interviews, observational analysis, and ethnography. Can conduct quantitative research that informs evaluation of a CBPR project; this can range from (but is not limited to) pilot testing of a new initiative (e.g., single group, repeated measures) to cross-group comparisons of an established program (via randomized or quasi-experimental methods). Teach and mentor professional and lay community members in the creation, conduct, evaluation, and refinement(s) of CBPR initiatives. Disseminate new knowledge, lessons learned, etc. through both professional (e.g., peer-reviewed journals, guild conferences) and lay (e.g., local news, powwows, community health fairs) arenas.

tices are positioned in, such as common and/or highly prevalent health challenges (like obesity, diabetes, chronic pain, etc.) or social worries (like poverty, poor access to high-quality education, etc.)—and evidence collaborative skills within standard health professional networks (e.g., referring patients to indicated specialist sites) to address particular presenting problems.

MedFTs functioning at *Level 2* demonstrate basic community engagement by nature of their familiarity with—and encouragement regarding—the utility of peer-support processes for their patients. They maintain important knowledge about local community resources, including organizations' structures, leadership, and key individuals and groups with whom to coordinate care. While still delivering most of their services within the context of a local practice, MedFTs at this level are able to—and often do—coordinate referrals and collaborative efforts with local community agencies that are both inside (e.g., specialist sites) and outside (e.g., faith-based groups, community-led education/support initiatives) of standard healthcare.

MedFTs equipped with knowledge and skills outlined in *Level 3* are functioning as community-oriented practitioners. They are able to articulate the manners in which combining professional wisdom with patients' and communities' "lived experience" can inform the creation of new knowledge and, potentially, interventions. They understand their professional contributions to care as existing within a mosaic of collaborative assets that can combine together into a whole amounting to more than the sum of its parts. These MedFTs see themselves as citizens of the community (versus providers for it). They may or may not be actively engaged in CBPR that partners with professional and lay community members and groups but are nevertheless conceptualizing care efforts with this mindset in place. A MedFT working with Teresa, for example, could facilitate her loved ones' co-ownership of disease management within the family (e.g., shared routines in diet and exercise) and contextualize these efforts within the larger American Indian community through discussions about health disparities and/or collective efforts to engage community members in supportive forums. He or she could offer care that is consciously delivered in a manner that is mapped and integrated into a complex and interconnected milieu of professional (e.g., local American Indian serving organizations) and lay (e.g., local powwows, health fairs) resources available to Teresa and her family.

MedFTs at *Level 4* maintain high skill and knowledge in the conduct of CBPR. They have generally gained these competencies through both textbook and real-life applications of such collaborative work. As experts in community engagement, they are familiar with common lessons learned (e.g., those regarding the often messy and unpredictable pace of CBPR projects, the importance of administrative support through institution champions; see Appendix 1) in this work and are able to advance strategies in collaborative leadership and team efforts that are essential to project development and sustainability (e.g., democratic planning at every step, folding new learning back into the community; see Appendix 2). Equipped with these understandings and skill sets, MedFTs at this level are able to construct compelling proposals for external monies to support the work. A MedFT working with Teresa and the FEDS project, for example, could effectively collect and integrate pilot data into the construction of a proposal to fund more extensive evaluation of a community's participation in the work. This grant writing would be carried out in a manner that carefully honors researchers' wants for objective outcome data, community participants' voices in identifying what data are most relevant to collect (and how to collect said data), and funders' wants for clear timelines and deliverables (vis-à-vis the comparative ambiguities of CBPR's natural evolution). These efforts would be carried out with purposeful timing so as to not sabotage a project's evolution (e.g., applying for funding to formally evaluate the FEDS project after it has been created and achieved initial stability versus during its early planning stages).

MedFTs who function at *Level 5* are leaders in community engagement. They maintain in-depth familiarity with CBPR literature relevant to their field(s) of practice, alongside extensive experience in the conduct and iterative processes of evaluating and refining CBPR programs that demonstrate both clinical utility and temporal sustainability. They are well positioned to teach (usually via observational and consultative mentoring over 1–2 years' time) professional and lay community members in how to conduct CBPR of their own. Their knowledge regarding the theoretical and methodological underpinnings and tactics in CBPR equips this teaching with ready "scaffolding" for community projects. These MedFTs are thereby able to foster and grow new partnerships between professional and lay team members in manners that are more efficient as compared to beginning an initiative "from scratch" while at the same time not bypassing important steps in a unique project's evolution or dishonor (or miss) the unique needs, challenges, resources, and strengths of the community in which novel efforts are positioned. Their investigative competencies include both qualitative and quantitative methods, as a broad range of evaluative methodologies are indicated over the course of any CBPR project's lifespan. A MedFT at this level is able to, for example, conduct key informant interviews with Teresa and other community members to assess (via thematic analyses) common and shared viewpoints regarding which components of a complex intervention are most influential to positive health outcomes that have already been quantitatively confirmed through single-group, repeated-measures assessments during a project's pilot phases (and/or later via experimental or quasi-experimental comparisons of intervention and control/wait-list participants). He or she disseminates new knowledge and lessons learned across both professional (e.g., referred journals, guild conferences) and lay (e.g., local health fairs, news stories) arenas.

Research-Informed Practices

Since the early 1990s, CBPR has evolved from a fringe science of sorts to one of established credibility across the helping professions (e.g., primary care, nursing, public health, behavioral health). It has served to increase understanding of patients' and their loved ones' experiences with a wide variety of health struggles, inform the design and/or improvement of healthcare services, facilitate community outreach and participation in health activities, and improve health-related education

(Coughlin, Smith, & Fernandez, 2017; Seal et al., 2016; Tobin, 2000; Ward & Trigler, 2001).

More healthcare providers and researchers—many of whom identify as MedFTs—are engaging in CBPR projects nowadays than ever before (Dombrowski, 2016; Ivankova, 2015; Mendenhall, Pratt, Phelps, Baird, & Younkin, 2014). As they do this, rigorous expert-driven investigatory methods aimed at widespread generalizability are losing ground to comparatively small but locally relevant and meaningful efforts that are cocreated by patient and provider communities working collaboratively toward shared goals. This evolution is advancing in synchrony with our increased emphases on patient/family-centered healthcare homes (Abdouch, 2017; Stange et al., 2010), wherein comprehensive approaches for children, youth, and adults are attended to within settings that facilitate partnerships between individuals/families and respective (and collaborating) members of interdisciplinary care teams (Minkler & Wallerstein, 2008; Peek, 2011; Wallerstein & Duran, 2010). Through CBPR methods, the patient/family community partnerships with providers are held up as an essential foundation to create care that is high quality, culturally competent, strengths based, and effective (Chavez, Duran, Baker, Avila, & Wallerstein, 2003; Doherty et al., 2010; Israel et al., 2012).

Exhaustively reviewing or presenting all outcome studies in CBPR is beyond the scope of this chapter, insofar as the approach has been employed across dozens of professional fields targeting innumerable topics and challenges. Echoing this widespread visibility and scope, CBPR within healthcare professions has been advanced and evaluated across a range of health foci, including (but not limited to) obesity (Berge et al., 2016; Davison, Jurkowski, Li, Kranz, & Lawson, 2013), diabetes (Doherty et al., 2010; Mendenhall & Doherty, 2005), healthy diet (DeHaven et al., 2011; Smith, Mateo, Morita, Hutchinson, & Cohall, 2015), smoking cessation (Mendenhall et al., 2011; Mendenhall et al., 2008), asthma (Brugge et al., 2010; Garwick & Auger, 2003), dental and mouth-care practices (Park et al., 2017; Walker et al., 2017), accident reduction (Brunette & Ibarra, 2009; Gallagher & Scott, 1997), safe sexual practices (Stevens & Hall, 1998; Rhodes et al., 2011), midwifery (Barrett, 2011; Foster, Chiang, Hillard, Hall, & Heath, 2010), living with disabilities (Hassouneh, Alcala-Moss, & McNeff, 2011; Ravesloot, 2016), child and adolescent mental illness (Breland-Noble, Bell, & Nicolas, 2006; Gewirtz, 2007; Novins et al., 2012), and overall physical well-being (Davis & Reid, 1999; Ferrera et al., 2015; Hampshire et al., 1999; Kondrat & Julia, 1998; Lewis, Sallee, Trumbo, & Janousek, 2010; Lindsey & McGuinness, 1998; Meyer, 2000; Schulz et al., 2003).

The inclusion and engagement of family members and/or close friends across this work is visible—and arguably essential—because many health-related foci are situated in the everyday lifestyles, routines, and habitudes carried out within the social systems that patients inhabit. Indeed, it is easier for patients—like Teresa—to adopt new healthy habits (e.g., diet, exercise) and/or to discontinue old unhealthy habits (e.g., smoking, sedentariness) if the people they are most close to change their behaviors in synchrony. Doing this in a broader community context of other engaged patients, families, and friends—like in the FEDS project—further supports a collective energy and investment facilitative of beneficent change. It is upon these grounds that MFTs and MedFTs—as systems thinkers, practitioners, scholars, and citizens—are uniquely equipped to learn and advance CBPR (Doherty et al., 2010; Mendenhall & Doherty, 2005; Mendenhall et al., 2013, 2014).

Conclusion

The greater vision for community-engaged care and scholarship is to create models of healthcare, education, and outreach as work that is by and for its citizens, with all stakeholders—including patients, families, healthcare providers, and other community members—working together. MedFTs—equipped with behavioral and relational skills in care provision and scholarship—represent a valuable addition to these teams. Emerging evidence supports their contributions (specifically) and CBPR (generally). As this type of work continues to advance across both depth and scope, professional providers/researchers and lay communities will increasingly create effective interventions that neither could create alone. Working within the contexts of flattened hierarchies and with a mindset that values everyone's respective wisdom and contributions, we will ultimately advance better care and improved health.

Reflection Questions
1. How can you, as a MedFT, incorporate CBPR values of tapping community members' lived experience and wisdom into the work that you do in everyday practice?
2. What are the pressure points (i.e., concerns shared by both professional service providers and the communities that they serve) in the context(s) of your own practice?
3. What type of CBPR initiative could you potentially engage in via professional/community partnerships through your university, workplace, or practice? How could you begin conversations and steps toward doing this?

Additional Resources

Literature

Blumenthal, D. S., & DiClemente, R. J. (Eds.). (2013). *Community-based participatory health research: Issues, methods, and translation to practice*. New York, NY: Springer.

Coughlin, S., Smith, S., & Fernandez, M. (Eds.) (2017). *Handbook of community-based participatory research*. New York, NY: Oxford University Press.

Hacker, K. (2013). *Community-based participatory research*. Los Angeles, CA: Sage.

Ivankova, N. V. (2014). *Mixed methods applications in action research.* Los Angeles, CA: Sage.

Minkler, M., & Wallerstein, N. (Eds.). (2011). *Community-based participatory research for health: From process to outcomes.* Hoboken, NJ: Wiley.

Organizations/Associations

Colorado School of Public Health's Rocky Mountain Prevention Research Center. http://www.ucdenver.edu/academics/colleges/PublicHealth/research/centers/RMPRC/training/Pages/CBPR.aspx

Detroit Community-Academic Urban Research Center. http://detroitcenter.umich.edu/projects/detroit-community-academic-urbanresearch-center

University of Chicago's Institute for Translational Medicine. http://itm.uchicago.edu/community-based-participatory-research/

University of Minnesota's (UMN) Citizen Professional Center. www.citizenprofessional.org

University of New Mexico's (UNM) Center for Participatory Research. http://cpr.unm.edu/

Appendix 1: Strategies for CBPR and Citizen Health Care[1]

1. *Get buy-in from key professional leaders and administrators.*

    These are the gatekeepers who must support the initiation of a project based on its potential to meet one of the goals of the healthcare setting. However, we have found it best to request little or no budget, aside from a small amount of staff time, in order to allow the project enough incubation time before being expected to justify its outcomes.

2. *Identify a health issue that is of great concern to both professionals and members of a specific community (clinic, neighborhood, cultural group in a geographical location).*

    Stated differently, the issue must be one that a community of citizens actually cares about—not just something that we think they should care about. The professionals initiating the project must have enough passion for the issue to sustain their efforts over time.

3. *Identify potential community leaders who have personal experience with the health issue and who have relationships with the professional team.*

---

[1] Source: Doherty, W., Mendenhall, T., & Berge, J. (2010). The families & democracy and citizen healthcare project. *Journal of Marital and Family Therapy, 36,* 389–402. https://doi.org/10.1111/j.1752-0606.2009.00142.x

These leaders should generally be ordinary members of the community who in some way have mastered the health issue in their own lives and who have a desire to give back to their community. "Positional" leaders who head community agencies are generally not the best group to engage at this stage, because they bring institutional priorities and constraints.

4. *Invite a small group of community leaders (3 to 4 people) to meet several times with the professional team to explore the issue and see if there is a consensus to proceed with a larger community project.*

    These are preliminary discussions to see if a Citizen Health Care project is feasible and to begin creating a professional/citizen leadership group.

5. *This group decides on how to invite a larger group of community leaders (10–15) to begin the process of generating the project.*

    One invitational strategy we have used is for providers to nominate patients and family members who have lived expertise with a health issue and who appear to have leadership potential.

6. *Over the next 6 months of biweekly meetings, implement the following steps of community organizing:*
    (a) *Exploring the community and citizen dimensions of the issue in depth*
    (b) *Creating a name and mission*
    (c) *Doing one-to-one interviews with a range of stakeholders*
    (d) *Generating potential action initiatives, processing them in terms of the Citizen Health Care model and their feasibility with existing community resources*
    (e) *Deciding on a specific action initiative and implementing it*

7. *Employ the following key Citizen Health Care processes:*
    (a) *Democratic planning and decision-making at every step.* As mentioned before, this requires training of the professionals who bring a disciplined process model and a vision of collective action that does not lapse back into the conventional provider/consumer model, but who do not control the outcome or action steps the group decides to take.
    (b) *Mutual teaching and learning among community members.* Action initiatives consistent with the model first call upon the lived experience of community members, with the support of professionals, rather than recruiting community members to support a professionally created initiative.
    (c) *Creating ways to fold new learnings back into the community.* All learnings can become "community property" if there is a way for them to be passed on. Currently we have vehicles for professionals to become "learning communities," but few vehicles outside of Internet chat rooms for patients and families to become learning communities.
    (d) *Identifying and developing leaders.* The heart of community organizing is finding and nurturing people who have leadership ability but who are not necessarily heads of organizations with turfs to protect.

(e) *Using professional expertise selectively—"on tap," not "on top."* In this way of working, all knowledge is public knowledge, democratically held and shared when it can be useful. Professionals bring a unique font of knowledge and experience—and access to current research—to Citizen Health Care initiatives. But everyone else around the table also brings unique knowledge and expertise. Because of the powerful draw of the provider/consumer way of operating, professionals must learn to share their unique expertise when it fits the moment, and to be quiet when someone else can just as readily speak to the issue. A community organizing axiom applies here: Never say what someone in the community could say, and never do what someone else in the community could do.

(f) *Forging a sense of larger purpose beyond helping immediate participants.* Keep the Big, Hairy, Audacious Goal (BHAG) in mind as you act in a local community. Citizen Health Care is not just about people helping people; it is about social change toward more activated citizens in the healthcare system and larger culture. This understanding inspires members of the Citizen Health Care project about the larger significance of their work. It also attracts media and other prominent community members to seek to understand, publicize, and disseminate Citizen Health Care projects.

Appendix 2: Lessons Learned in CBPR and Citizen Health Care[2]

1. This work is about identity transformation as a citizen professional, not just about learning a new set of skills.
2. It is about identifying and developing leaders in the community more than about a specific issue or action.
3. It is about sustained initiatives, not onetime events.
4. Citizen initiatives are often slow and messy, especially during the gestation period.
5. You need a champion with influence in the institution.
6. Until grounded in an institution's culture and practices, these initiatives are quite vulnerable to shifts in the organizational context.
7. A professional who is putting too much time into a project is over-functioning and not using the model. We have found that the average time commitment to be on the order of 6–8 hours/month, but over a number of years.
8. External funding at the outset can be a trap because of timelines and deliverables, but funding can be useful for capacity building to learn the model and for expanding the scope of citizen projects once they are developed.

---

[2] Source: Doherty, W., & Mendenhall, T. (2006). Citizen health care: A model for engaging patients, families, and communities as co-producers of health. *Families, Systems, & Health, 24*, 357–362. https://doi.org/10.1037/1091-7527.24.3.251

9. The pull of the traditional provider/consumer model is very strong on all sides; democratic decision-making requires eternal vigilance.
10. You cannot learn this approach without mentoring, and it takes 2 years to get good at it.

References[3]

Abdouch, I. (2017). Patient-centered medical home. In P. Paulman, R. Taylor, A. Paulman, and L. Nasir (Eds.), *Family medicine: Principles and practice* (pp. 1793–1804). London, England: Springer.

Agency for Healthcare Research and Quality. (2004). *Community-based participatory research: Assessing the Evidence* (Research Report No. 99). Retrieved from https://archive.ahrq.gov/downloads/pub/evidence/pdf/cbpr/cbpr.pdf

*Allen, M. L., Culhane-Pera, K. A., Pergament, S. L., & Call, K. T. (2010). Facilitating research faculty participation in CBPR: Development of a model based on key informant interviews. *Clinical and Translational Science, 3*, 233–238. https://doi.org/10.1111/j.1752-8062.2010.00231.x.

Barrett, P. (2011). The Early Mothering Project: What happened when the words 'action research' came to life for a group of midwives. In P. Reason and H. Bradbury (Eds.), *Handbook of action research: Participative inquiry and practice* (pp. 294–300). London, England: Sage.

Berge, J., Jin, S., Hanson, C., Doty, J., Jagaraj, K., Braaten, K., & Doherty, W. (2016). Play it forward! A community-based participatory research approach to childhood obesity prevention. *Families, Systems, & Health, 34*, 15–30. https://doi.org/10.1037/fsh0000116

*Berge, J., Mendenhall, T., & Doherty, W. (2009). Using community-based participatory research (CBPR) to target health disparities in families. *Family Relations, 58*, 475–488. https://doi.org/10.1111/j.1741-3729.2009.00567.x.

*Blumenthal, D. S., & DiClemente, R. J. (Eds.). (2013). *Community-based participatory health research: Issues, methods, and translation to practice*. New York, NY: Springer.

Bradbury, H., & Reason, P. (2003). Action research: An opportunity for revitalizing research purpose and practices. *Qualitative Social Work, 2*, 155–175. https://doi.org/10.1177/1473325003002002003

Breland-Noble, A. M., Bell, C., & Nicolas, G. (2006). Family first: The development of an evidence-based family intervention for increasing participation in psychiatric clinical care and research in depressed African American adolescents. *Family Process, 45*, 153–169. https://doi.org/10.1111/j.1545-5300.2006.00088.x

Brugge, D., Rivera-Carrasco, E., Zotter, J., & Leung, A. (2010). Community-based participatory research in Boston's neighborhoods: A review of asthma case examples. *Archives of Environmental & Occupational Health, 12*, 70–76. https://doi.org/10.1080/19338240903390214

Brunette, M. J., & Ibarra, M. T. S. A. (2009). Ergonomics, safety, and health in industrially developing countries: A needed multilevel interdisciplinary approach. In P. Scott (Ed.), *Ergonomics in developing regions: Needs and applications* (pp. 29–38). New York, NY: CRC Press.

Brydon-Miller, M., Greenwood, D., & Maguire, P. (2003). Why action research? *Action Research, 1*, 9–28. https://doi.org/10.1177/14767503030011002

Casswell, S. (2000). A decade of community action research. *Substance Use and Abuse, 35*, 55–74. https://doi.org/10.3109/10826080009147686

Chavez, V., Duran, B., Baker, Q., Avila, M., & Wallerstein, N. (2003). The dance of race and privilege in community based participatory research. In M. Minkler and N. Wallerstein

---

[3] Note: References that are prefaced with an asterisk are recommended readings.

(Eds.), *Community based participatory research in health* (pp. 81–97). San Francisco, CA: Jossey-Bass.

Cornwall, A., & Jewkes, R. (1995). What is participatory research? *Social Science & Medicine, 41*(12), 1667–1676. https://doi.org/10.1016/0277-9536(95)00127-s

*Coughlin, S., Smith, S., & Fernandez, M. (Eds.) (2017). *Handbook of community-based participatory research.* New York, NY: Oxford University Press.

Dapice, A. N. (2006). The medicine wheel. *Journal of Transcultural Nursing, 17*, 251–260. https://doi.org/10.1177/1043659606288383

Davison, K. K., Jurkowski, J. M., Li, K., Kranz, S., & Lawson, H. A. (2013). A childhood obesity intervention developed by families for families: Results from a pilot study. *International Journal of Behavioral Nutrition and Physical Activity, 10*, 3–14. https://doi.org/10.1186/1479-5868-10-3

Davis, S. M., & Reid, R. (1999). Practicing participatory research in American Indian communities. *American Journal of Clinical Nutrition, 69*, 755S–759S. Retrieved from http://ajcn.nutrition.org/

DeHaven, M. J., Ramos-Roman, M. A., Gimpel, N., Carson, J., DeLemos, J., Pickens, S., ... Duval, J. (2011). The GoodNEWS (genes, nutrition, exercise, wellness, and spiritual growth) trial: A community-based participatory research (CBPR) trial with African-American church congregations for reducing cardiovascular disease risk factors—Recruitment, measurement, and randomization. *Contemporary Clinical Trials, 32*, 630–640. https://doi.org/10.1016/j.cct.2011.05.017

DePoy, E., Hartman, A., & Haslett, D. (1999). Critical action research: A model of social work knowing. *Social Work, 44*, 560–569. https://doi.org/10.1093/sw/44.6.560

Doherty, W., & Mendenhall, T. (2006). Citizen health care: A model for engaging patients, families, and communities as co-producers of health. *Families, Systems, & Health, 24*, 357–362. https://doi.org/10.1037/1091-7527.24.3.251

*Doherty, W., Mendenhall, T., & Berge, J. (2010). The families & democracy and citizen healthcare project. *Journal of Marital and Family Therapy, 36*, 389–402. https://doi.org/10.1111/j.1752-0606.2009.00142.x.

Dombrowski, K. (Ed.). (2016). *Reducing health disparities: Research updates from the field.* Lincoln, NE: Syron Design Academic Publishing.

Engel, G. L. (1977). The need for a new medical model: A challenge for biomedicine. *Science, 196*, 129–136. https://doi.org/10.1016/b978-0-409-95009-0.50006-1

Engel, G. L. (1980). The clinical application of the biopsychosocial model. *American Journal of Family Medicine, 137*, 535–544. https://doi.org/10.1176/ajp.137.5.535

Ferrera, M. J., Sacks, T. K., Perez, M., Nixon, J. P., Asis, D., & Coleman, R. W. L. (2015). Empowering immigrant youth in Chicago: Utilizing CBPR to document the impact of a youth health service corps program. *Family & Community Health, 38*, 12–21. https://doi.org/10.1097/FCH.0000000000000058

Foster, J., Chiang, F., Hillard, R. C., Hall, P., & Heath, A. (2010). Team process in community-based participatory research on maternity care in the Dominican Republic. *Nursing Inquiry, 17*, 309–316. https://doi.org/10.1111/j.1440-1800.2010.00514.x

Friedman, V., Razer, M., & Sykes, I. (2004). Towards a theory of inclusive practice: An action science approach. *Action Research, 2*, 167–189. https://doi.org/10.1177/1476750304043729

Gallagher, E., & Scott, V. (1997). The STEPS project: Participatory action research to reduce falls in public places among seniors and persons with disabilities. *Canadian Journal of Public Health, 88*, 129–133. Retrieved from http://journal.cpha.ca/index.php/cjph

Garrett, J. T., & Garrett, M. W. (1994). The path of good medicine: Understanding and counseling Native American Indians. *Journal of Multicultural Counseling and Development, 22*, 134–144. https://doi.org/10.1002/j.2161-1912.1994.tb00459.x

Garwick, A. W., & Auger, S. (2003). Participatory action research: The Indian Family Stories Project. *Nursing Outlook, 51*, 261–266. https://doi.org/10.1016/j.outlook.2003.09.006

Gewirtz, A. H. (2007). Promoting children's mental health in family supportive housing: A community–university partnership for formerly homeless children and families. *Journal of Primary Prevention, 28,* 359–374. https://doi.org/10.1007/s10935-007-0102-z

Giachello, A. L., Arrom, J. O., Davis, M., Sayad, J. V., Ramirez, D., Nandi, C., & Ramos, C. (2003). Reducing diabetes health disparities through community-based participatory action research: The Chicago Southeast Diabetes Community Action Coalition. *Public Health Reports, 118,* 309–323. https://doi.org/10.1016/s0033-3549(04)50255-8

Goodnough, K. (2003). Facilitating action research in the context of science education: Reflections of a university researcher. *Educational Action Research, 11,* 41–64. https://doi.org/10.1080/09650790300200203

*Hacker, K. (2013). *Community-based participatory research.* Los Angeles, CA: Sage.

Hambridge, K. (2000). Action research. *Journal of Professional Nursing, 15,* 598–601. Retrieved from http://www.professionalnursing.org/

Hampshire, A., Blair, M., Crown, N., Avery, A., & Williams, I. (1999). Action research: A useful method of promoting change in primary care? *Family Practice, 16,* 305–311. https://doi.org/10.1093/fampra/16.3.305

Hassouneh, D., Alcala-Moss, A., & McNeff, E. (2011). Practical strategies for promoting full inclusion of individuals with disabilities in community-based participatory intervention research. *Research in Nursing & Health, 34,* 253–265. https://doi.org/10.1002/nur.20434

Hodgson, J., Lamson, A., Mendenhall, T., & Tyndall, L. (2014). Introduction to medical family therapy: Advanced applications. In J. Hodgson, A. Lamson, T. Mendenhall, and R. Crane (Eds.), *Medical family therapy: Advanced applications* (pp. 1–9). New York, NY: Springer.

Holkup, P. A., Tripp-Reimer, T., Salois, E. M., & Weinert, C. (2004). Community-based participatory research: An approach to intervention research with a native American community. *Advances in Nursing Science, 27,* 162–175. Retrieved from http://journals.lww.com/advancesinnursingscience/Pages/default.aspx

*Huzzard, T., & Johansson, Y. (2014). Critical action research. In E. Jeanes and T. Huzzard (Eds.), *Critical management research: Reflections from the field* (pp. 81–100). London, England: Sage.

Israel, B., Eng, E., Schulz, A., & Parker, E. (Eds. (2012). *Methods in community-based participatory research for health.* San Fransisco, CA: Jossey-Bass.

*Ivankova, N. (2015). *Mixed methods applications in action research: From methods to community action.* Los Angeles, CA: Sage.

Kemmis, S., & McTaggart, R. (2005). Participatory action research: Communicative action and the public sphere. In N. Denzin and Y. Lincoln (Eds.), *The Sage handbook of qualitative research* (3rd ed., pp. 559–604). Thousand Oaks, CA: Sage.

King, C., Gaffney, J., & Gunton, J. (2001). Does participatory action learning make a difference? Perspectives of effective learning tools and indicators from the conservation cropping group in North Queensland, Australia. *Journal of Agricultural Education & Extension, 7,* 133–146. https://doi.org/10.1080/13892240108438821

Kondrat, M., & Julia, M. (1998). Democratizing knowledge for human social development: Case studies in the use of participatory action research to enhance people's choice and well-being. *Social Development Issues, 20,* 1–20. Retrieved from http://www.ingentaconnect.com/content/icsd/sdi

Lammerink, M., Bury, P., & Bolt, E. (1999). An introduction to participatory action development (PAD). *Participatory Learning Action Notes, 35,* 29–33. Retrieved from http://www.iied.org/participatory-learning-action

*LaVeaux, D., & Christopher, S. (2009). Contextualizing CBPR: Key principles of CBPR meet the Indigenous research context. *Pimatisiwin, 7,* 1–16. Retrieved from http://www.pimatisiwin.com/online/

Lewin, K. (1946). Action research and minority problems. *Journal of Social Issues, 2,* 34–46. https://doi.org/10.1111/j.1540-4560.1946.tb02295.x

Lewis, K., Sallee, D., Trumbo, J., & Janousek, K. (2010). Use of community-based participatory research methods in adults' health assessment. *Journal of Applied Psychology, 40*, 195–211. https://doi.org/10.1111/j.1559-1816.2009.00570.x

Lindsey, E., & McGuinness, L. (1998). Significant elements of community involvement in participatory action research: Evidence from a community project. *Journal of Advanced Nursing, 28*, 1106–1114. https://doi.org/10.1046/j.1365-2648.1998.00816.x

Macaulay, A. C., Commanda, L. E., Freeman, W. L., & Gibson, N. (1999). Participatory research maximises community and lay involvement. *British Medical Journal, 319*, 774–778. Retrieved from http://www.bmj.com/

Madsen, W., McNicol, S., & O'Mullan, C. (2015). Engaging with the past: Reflecting on resilience from community oral history projects. In W. Madsen, L. Costigan, S. McNicol, and R. Turner (Eds.), *Community resilience, universities and engaged research for today's world* (pp. 32–43). London, UK: Palgrave Macmillan.

Maiter, S., Simich, L., Jacobson, N., & Wise, J. (2008). Reciprocity: An ethic for community-based participatory action research. *Action Research, 6*, 305–325. https://doi.org/10.1177/1476750307083720

Maxwell, L. (1993). Action research: A useful strategy for combining action and research in nursing? *Canadian Journal of Cardiovascular Nursing, 4*, 19–20. Retrieved from http://pappin.com/journals/cjcn.php

Mayoux, L. (2005). Participatory action learning system (PALS): Impact assessment for civil society development and grassroots-based advocacy in Anandi, India. *Journal of International Development, 17*, 211–242. https://doi.org/10.1002/jid.1211

McIntyre, A. (2008). *Participatory action research* (Vol. 52). Thousand Oaks, CA: Sage.

McNicoll, P. (1999). Issues in teaching participatory action research. *Journal of Social Work Education, 35*, 51–62. https://doi.org/10.1080/10437797.1999.10778946

Mendenhall, T. J., & Doherty, W. J. (2005). Action research methods in family therapy. In D. H. Sprenkle and F. P. Piercy (Eds.), *Research methods in family therapy* (2nd ed., pp. 100–118). New York, NY: Guilford Press.

Mendenhall, T., & Doherty, W. J. (2003). Partners in diabetes: A collaborative, democratic initiative in primary care. *Families, Systems & Health, 21*, 329–335. https://doi.org/10.1037/1091-7527.21.3.329

Mendenhall, T., & Doherty, W. (2007). Partners in diabetes: Action research in a primary care setting. *Action Research, 4*, 378–406. https://doi.org/10.1177/1476750307083722

Mendenhall, T., Doherty, W., Berge, J., Fauth, J., & Tremblay, G. (2013). Community-based participatory research: Advancing collaborative care through novel partnerships. In L. Ronan and M. Tehan (Eds.), *The landscape of collaborative care: Evaluating the evidence, identifying the essentials* (pp. 99–130). Philadelphia, PA: Springer.

Mendenhall, T., Harper, P., Stephenson, H., & Haas, S. (2011). The SANTA project (students against nicotine and tobacco addiction): Using community-based participatory research to improve health in a high-risk young adult population. *Action Research, 9*, 199–213. https://doi.org/10.1177/1476750310388051

Mendenhall, T., Pratt, K., Phelps, K., Baird, M., & Younkin, F. (2014). Advancing medical family therapy through qualitative, quantitative, and mixed-methods research. In J. Hodgson, A. Lamson, T. Mendenhall, and D. Crane (Eds.), *Medical family therapy: Advanced applications* (pp. 241–258). New York, NY: Springer.

Mendenhall, T., Seal, K., GreenCrow, B., LittleWalker, K., & BrownOwl, S. (2012). The Family Education Diabetes Series (FEDS): Improving health in an urban-dwelling American Indian community. *Qualitative Health Research, 22*, 1524–1534. https://doi.org/10.1177/1049732312457469

Mendenhall, T., Whipple, H., Harper, P., & Haas, S. (2008). Students against nicotine and tobacco addiction (SANTA): Community-based participatory research in a high-risk young adult population. *Families, Systems & Health, 26*, 225–231. https://doi.org/10.1037/1091-7527.26.2.225

Mettetal, G. (2012). The what, why and how of classroom action research. *Journal of the Scholarship of Teaching and Learning, 2*, 6–13. Retrieved from http://josotl.indiana.edu/

Meyer, J. (2000). Using qualitative methods in health related action research. *British Medical Journal, 320*, 178–181. Retrieved from www.bmj.com

Minkler, M. (2005). Community-based research partnerships: Challenges and opportunities. *Journal of Urban Health, 82*, ii3–ii12. https://doi.org/10.1093/jurban/jti034

*Minkler, M., & Wallerstein, N. (Eds.). (2011). *Community-based participatory research for health: From process to outcomes* (3rd ed.). Hoboken, NJ: Wiley.

Minkler, M., & Wallerstein, N. (Eds.). (2008). *Community based participatory research for health: From process to outcomes* (2nd ed.). San Francisco, CA: Jossey-Bass.

Montoya, M. J., & Kent, E. E. (2011). Dialogical action: Moving from community-based to community-driven participatory research. *Qualitative Health Research, 21*, 1000–1011. https://doi.org/10.1177/1049732311403500

Mosavel, M., Ahmed, R., Daniels, D., & Simon, C. (2011). Community researchers conducting health disparities research: Ethical and other insights from fieldwork journaling. *Social Science & Medicine, 73*, 145–152. https://doi.org/10.1016/j.socscimed.2011.04.029

Muehlenkamp, J., Marrone, S., Gray, J. S., & Brown, D. (2009). A college suicide prevention model for American Indian students. *Professional Psychology, 40*, 134–240. Retrieved from https://ssrn.com/abstract=2118676

National Institutes of Health (2009). *Community-based particpatory research program*. Retrieved from https://www.nimhd.nih.gov/programs/extramural/community-based-participatory.html

Nichols, B. (1995). Action research: A method for practitioners. *Nursing Connections, 8*, 5–11. http://www.ncbi.nlm.nih.gov/pubmed/7777076

Novins, D. K., Boyd, M. L., Brotherton, D. T., Fickenscher, A., Moore, L., & Spicer, P. (2012). Walking on: Celebrating the journeys of Native American adolescents with substance use problems on the winding road to healing. *Journal of Psychoactive Drugs, 44*, 153–159. https://doi.org/10.1080/02791072.2012.684628

Okomoda, J. K., & Alamu, S. O. (2002). Participatory action development as a strategy within a community-based approach to aquatic resource management for Nigeria inland waters. *National Institute for Freshwater Fisheries Research, 159–164*. Retrieved from http://aquaticcommons.org/951/1/WH_159-164.pdf

Park, S. K., Lee, G. Y., Kim, Y. J., Lee, M. Y., Byun, D. H., Kim, K. H., … Kim, N. H. (2017). Evaluation of a community-based participatory professional periodontal care program for hypertension and diabetes patients. *Journal of the Korean Academy of Oral Health, 41*, 56–64. 10.11149/jkaoh.2017.41.1.56

Pedler, M. (2011). *Action learning in practice*. Surrey, England: Gower.

Peek, C. (2011). A collaborative care lexicon for asking practice and research development questions: A national agenda for research in collaborative care. *Agency for Healthcare Research and Quality*. Retrieved from http://www.ahrq.gov/

Ramanadhan, S., Salhi, C., Achille, E., Baril, N., D'Entremont, K., Grullon, M., … Viswanath, K. (2012). Addressing cancer disparities via community network mobilization and intersectoral partnerships: A social network analysis. *PloS One, 7*, 1–9. https://doi.org/10.1371/journal.pone.0032130

Ravesloot, C. (2016). Living well with a disability: A self-management program. *Morbidity and Mortality Weekly Report/Supplements, 65*, 61–67. Retrieved from https://www.cdc.gov/mmwr/volumes/65/su/su6501a10.htm

Razum, O., Gorgen, R., & Diesfeld, H. (1997). Action research in health programs. *World Health Forum, 18*, 54–55. Retrieved from http://apps.who.int/iris/handle/10665/54647

Reese, D., Ahern, R., Nair, S., O'Faire, J., & Warren, C. (1999). Hospice access and use by African Americans: Addressing cultural and institutional barriers through participatory action research. *Social Work, 44*, 549–559. https://doi.org/10.1093/sw/44.6.549

Revans, R. (2011). *ABC of action learning*. Surrey, England: Gower.

Rhodes, S. D., Hergenrather, K. C., Vissman, A. T., Stowers, J., Davis, A. B., Hannah, A., ... Marsiglia, F. F. (2011). Boys must be men, and men must have sex with women: A qualitative CBPR study to explore sexual risk among African American, Latino, and white gay men and MSM. *American Journal of Men's Health, 5*, 140–151. https://doi.org/10.1177/1557988310366298

Rhodes, S. D., Malow, R. M., & Jolly, C. (2010). Community-based participatory research (CBPR): A new and not-so-new approach to HIV/AIDS prevention, care, and treatment. *AIDS Education and Prevention, 22*, 173–183. https://doi.org/10.1521/aeap.2010.22.3.173

Richter, A., & Koch, C. (2004). Integration, differentiation and ambiguity in safety cultures. *Safety Science, 42*, 703–722. https://doi.org/10.1016/j.ssci.2003.12.003

Robbins, R., Hong, J., Engler, C., & King, C. (2016). A study of the effectiveness of the gifts of the seven directions alcohol prevention model for Native Americans: Culturally sustaining education for Native American adolescents. *Contemporary Educational Psychology, 47*, 24–31. https://doi.org/10.1016/j.cedpsych.2016.04.004

Rudolph, J. W., Taylor, S. S., & Foldy, E. G. (2005). Collaborative off-line reflection: A way to develop skill in action science and action inquiry. In P. Reason and H. Bradbury (Eds.), *Handbook of action research* (pp. 405–412). Thousand Oaks, CA: Sage.

Rybak, C., & Decker-Fitts, A. (2009). Understanding Native American healing practices. *Counseling Psychology Quarterly, 22*, 333–342. https://doi.org/10.1080/09515070903270900

Scharff, D., & Mathews, K. (2008). Working with communities to translate research into practice. *Journal of Public Health Management and Practice, 14*, 94–98. https://doi.org/10.1097/01.PHH.0000311885.60509.61

Schmidt, K. (2002). Classroom action research: A case study assessing students' perceptions and learning outcomes of classroom teaching versus on-line teaching. *Journal of Industrial Teacher Education, 40*(1), 45–59. Retrieved from http://scholar.lib.vt.edu/ejournals/JITE/v40n1/schmidt.html

Schulz, A., Israel, B., Parker, E., Lockett, M., Hill, Y., & Wills, R. (2003). Engaging women in community-based participatory research for health: The East Side Village Health Worker Partnership. In M. Minkler and N. Wallerstein (Eds.), *Community-based participatory research for health* (pp. 293–315). San Francisco, CA: Jossey-Bass.

Seal, K., Blum, M., Didericksen, K., Mendenhall, T., Gagner, N., GreenCrow, B., ... Benton, K. (2016). The East Metro American Indian Diabetes Initiative: Engaging indigenous men in the reclaiming of health and spirituality through community-based participatory research. *Health Education Research and Development, 4*, 1–8. https://doi.org/10.4172/2380-5439.1000152

Sieber, J. E. (2010). New research domains create new ethical challenges. *Journal of Empirical Research on Human Research Ethics, 5*, 1–2. https://doi.org/10.1525/jer.2010.5.1.1

Small, S. (1995). Action-oriented research: Models and methods. *Journal of Marriage and the Family, 57*, 941–955. Retrieved from https://www.ncfr.org/jmf

Smith, M., Mateo, K. F., Morita, H., Hutchinson, C., & Cohall, A. T. (2015). Effectiveness of a multifaceted community-based promotion strategy on use of GetHealthyHarlem.org, a local community health education website. *Health Promotion Practice, 16*, 480–491. https://doi.org/10.1177/1524839915571632

Strand, K. J., Cutforth, N., Stoecker, R., Marullo, S., & Donohue, P. (2003). *Community-based research and higher education: Principles and practices*. San Francisco, CA: Wiley.

Stange, K. C., Nutting, P. A., Miller, W. L., Jaén, C. R., Crabtree, B. F., Flocke, S. A., & Gill, J. M. (2010). Defining and measuring the patient-centered medical home. *Journal of General Internal Medicine, 25*, 601–612. https://doi.org/10.1007/s11606-010-1291-3

Stevens, P. E., & Hall, J. (1998). Participatory action research for sustaining individual and community change: A model of HIV prevention education. *AIDS Education and Prevention, 10*, 387–402. Retrieved from http://guilfordjournals.com/loi/aeap

Strickland, C. (2006). Challenges in community-based participatory research implementation: Experiences in cancer prevention with Pacific Northwest American Indian tribes. *Cancer Control, 13*, 230–236. Retrieved from https://moffitt.org/publications/cancer-control-journal/

Stringer, E. T. (2013). *Action research*. Thousand Oaks, CA: Sage.

Tobin, M. (2000). Developing mental health rehabilitation services in a culturally appropriate context: An action research project involving Arabic-speaking clients. *Australian Health Review, 23*, 177–184. https://doi.org/10.1071/ah000177.

Walker, K. K., Martínez-Mier, E. A., Soto-Rojas, A. E., Jackson, R. D., Stelzner, S. M., Galvez, L. C., ... Vega, D. (2017). Midwestern Latino caregivers' knowledge, attitudes and sense making of the oral health etiology, prevention and barriers that inhibit their children's oral health: A CBPR approach. *BMC Oral Health, 17*, 1–11. https://doi.org/10.1186/s12903-017-0354-9

*Wallerstein, N., & Duran, B. (2010). Community-based participatory research contributions to intervention research: The intersection of science and practice to improve health equity. *American Journal of Public Health, 100*, S40-S46. https://doi.org/10.2105/ajph.2009.184036.

Ward, K., & Trigler, J. S. (2001). Reflections on participatory action research with people who have developmental disabilities. *Mental Retardation, 39*, 57–59. https://doi.org/10.1352/00476765(2001)039<0057:roparw>2.0.co;2

Wright, L. M., Watson, W. L., & Bell, J. M. (1996). *Beliefs: The heart of healing in families and illness*. New York, NY: Basic Books.

Chapter 15
Medical Family Therapy in Disaster Preparedness and Trauma-Response Teams

Tai Mendenhall, Jonathan Bundt, and Cigdem Yumbul

Attention to mental health in disaster preparedness and trauma-response teams has increased considerably over the last decade. From the formal development and expansion of stand-alone teams and those positioned within existing care structures to the integration of Psychological First Aid (PFA) as part of standard education and preparation for first responders (e.g., police officers, firefighters), behavioral health clinicians (e.g., psychology, social work), and biomedical providers (e.g., emergency medicine, family medicine), it is clear that what once was a subspecialty advanced by a small collection of practitioners has now evolved to a mainstream standing within the broader arenas of the helping professions.

Family therapists (generally) and medical family therapists (specifically) represent a comparatively new discipline to join this larger movement. They bring an orientation comfortable with the complexities of overlapping human and relationship systems and thereby add value to the nature in which fieldwork is conducted and the manners in which interdisciplinary teams function on the ground (Boss, 2006; Mendenhall & Berge, 2010). As disaster response teams evolve to most effectively engage the communities they serve, integrated groups that include a wide variety of professionals are becoming more standard. To set the stage for our discussion of this as it relates to the practice of medical family therapy (MedFT) in disaster response, we begin by sharing the story of a young graduate student, Lisa. After first working as a behavioral health responder for several incidents, she was deployed as a team leader within days of a large-scale flooding.

T. Mendenhall (✉) · C. Yumbul
Department of Family Social Science, University of Minnesota, Saint Paul, MN, USA
e-mail: mend0009@umn.edu

J. Bundt
Masa Consulting, Minnetonka, MN, USA

© Springer International Publishing AG, part of Springer Nature 2018
T. Mendenhall et al. (eds.), *Clinical Methods in Medical Family Therapy*,
Focused Issues in Family Therapy, https://doi.org/10.1007/978-3-319-68834-3_15

Clinical Vignette
[Note: This vignette is a compilation of cases that represent a disaster response effort. All patients' names and/or identifying information have been changed to maintain confidentiality.]

Lisa first got involved in disaster response work as a graduate student when one of her professors encouraged her to take part in a University-sponsored workshop regarding PFA. Over the next 2 years of her doctoral program, she was deployed to one large event (tornado) and several smaller-scale crises (e.g., student suicide at a local school, neighborhood shooting). When she was called in this morning to help at a multiagency disaster recovery center (DRC) set up in a school gymnasium in response to flooding in a rural community several miles away, Lisa was designated by the site lead, Bill Jones, as the behavioral health team's lead. This role would include efforts in providing psychological support for surviving victims and responders, alongside coordinating the efforts of four other behavioral health volunteers.

"Finally. You're here," said Mr. Jones. He sounded huffy and rushed. "Name's Bill. I'm in charge of this DRC. Your counselor colleagues are already here. I've set you all up over there."

He pointed to a corner of a large room with a table that said "mental health" on an attached poster board. "We'll send folks over if and when they need you."

Earlier in her training, this would have frustrated Lisa more than it did nowadays. She had come to understand that DRC and incident command personnel were primarily focused on saving lives and property. Mental health was (is) important to them, but not the most important.

"Bill, my experience is that providing psychosocial support is better done if it's integrated throughout the whole center. I can coordinate folks to help with the lines and registration, and we can use the space over there for more intense conversations—with survivors and/or your other staff, if they need it," Lisa said.

"Whatever," Bill said. "Just be sure we can find you. We're opening up the doors in 20 minutes."

Lisa continued to reach out. "I have a couple more thoughts about preparing our staff who will work with the impacted community members and your other staff. We will be wearing purple vests; that way folks can see us easily." Bill responded affirmatively and then ran off.

Lisa directed two of the mental health volunteers to the registration lines at the front door and instructed the others to "float" as community members quickly filled the gym looking for answers about local resources and seeking information about when and how they could return to their homes. For the next several hours, she and her colleagues worked with other team members to direct, connect with, and support dozens of highly distressed people. They also encouraged staff members to take breaks and spend time with youth so that parents could have discussions with different agency providers, checked

> in with people as they registered, and assessed if/when there was more that they could do to help. In some cases, Lisa and her other mental health volunteers helped with de-escalating especially angry and/or grieving people. At other times, they helped to refer people to local resources.
>
> Many community members had lost their homes, cars, and prized personal possessions, their businesses, and even their very livelihoods. Some had lost pets, like the inconsolable teen who one of Lisa's volunteers had been sitting with on and off now for most of the afternoon. Some had witnessed dead bodies in the water when they had been airlifted by helicopters from houses' rooftops.
>
> "I can't do this," a volunteer—who had been staffing an information station about insurance services—said. He walked past Lisa, tearing up his nametag and wiping away tears. "If I hear one more story about a family losing everything, I'm going to lose my mind." He was visibly shaken and looked exhausted.
>
> "I don't care about filling out your stupid forms!" someone raised their voice from the registration area. "I just need answers! Look at all these pictures! Look what happened to my home! I thought you said that you would be able to help us with money to fix these things!" The child in her arms was crying now.
>
> "Lisa! Do something!" Bill seethed, coming up behind her.

This case is illustrative of how a medical family therapist may function on a disaster response team. Instead of sitting on the sidelines (literally) and attending only to extremely upset survivors or volunteers who need behavioral health interventions, care is purposively integrated into all facets of a response. This can look like "crowd control" vis-à-vis long lines of anxious people, helping to connect community members to other professionals and/or information sources aligning with specific needs, or offering a compassionate presence to those for whom no comforting words will "fix" the losses or trauma that they have sustained. It also includes attention to our own and other team members' functioning, driving indicated attention to ethical mandates that we maintain our own physical and emotional well-being. Lisa's immersion within the complex processes of a disaster response is illustrative of this.

In this chapter, we further describe disaster response teams and fieldwork as a care setting type. We characterize common makeup(s) of our interdisciplinary teams and outline key knowledge and skill areas for MedFTs within these teams. We describe the practice of MedFT in disaster response in accord with Hodgson, Lamson, Mendenhall, and Tyndall's (2014) five-level continuum. We present common terminology, reflection questions, recommended readings, and resources in the conclusion.

What Is Disaster Response?

The principal aims of a disaster response include the preservation of life and property and restoration of normal services to the affected population. Secondary (but as Lisa knew in the above vignette, a close second) to this mission is to support the morale and psychosocial health of the said population. Elements of disaster response are varied and personalized to the needs of a specific group or event; these include the provision of healthcare services, food and water, temporary shelter, indicated transport, reunification of family members, information regarding community resources, and connections to short- and long-term services and support.

Within this work, it is essential to integrate providers of care from diverse areas of expertise to address biopsychosocial-spiritual (BPSS) needs of survivors, their families, and communities (Engel, 1977, 1980; Mendenhall & Berge, 2010, Walsh, 2007; Wright, Watson & Bell, 1996). At such times, multiple local, national, and international agencies, personnel, policies, facilities, and jurisdictions desire to be involved in responding to trauma. However, emergency response operations need to be performed by a flexible yet well-defined structure within an organization in which people from diverse disciplines can work collaboratively. The National Incident Management System (NIMS) is a systemic and proactive management process that integrates all levels of government to work together in managing any size of disaster event (Department of Homeland Security [DHS], 2016a). The NIMS program was established in 2004 and continues to be a foundational response structure that all levels of government are required to utilize (DHS, 2016b) in times of human-caused and natural disasters.

It is important to note, too, that "disasters" can encompass foci that are both diverse and far-reaching. Responders involved in this work can face any variety of localized, small-scale incidents (that only impact a limited number of persons and families) to large-scale events (that can impact tens of thousands of—or even more—people). Events can be human-caused (e.g., school shootings, terrorist attacks, structural collapses) or natural in their geneses (e.g., pandemics, hurricanes, tsunamis, tornados, floods). They can occur across rural, suburban, and urban contexts. They can impact groups representing any ethnicity and/or socioeconomic stratum. Because teams engaged in disaster response must be equipped to handle whatever occurs within the areas that they serve, baseline training and preparation that they advance are "general" in nature; the content presented in this chapter echoes this frame. MedFTs focused on specific types of disaster response (only) are encouraged to pursue specialized training that is so oriented (for more information, see International Critical Stress Incident Stress Foundation [ICISF], 2016).

Teams in Disaster Response

Teams within disaster response are comprised of a broad range of disciplinary backgrounds and training. There is a common slogan in disaster response: "It's better to exchange business cards during training than in a real disaster." This motto pertains to the critical importance of understanding and knowing personally the different responders that come forward to respond to a disaster. Each team's leader holds primary responsibilities to (a) maintain flow of information to the team about the rapidly changing events in the field, (b) make successful decisions in facilitating team activities, and (c) help the team plan and work efficiently toward aiding individuals, families, and communities within their scope of expertise. Team members (responders), who work under the team leader, help to carry out the team's goals and functions. The following highlight key professionals who are involved in delivering disaster response services on the ground.

Incident command. The Incident Command System (ICS) is a widely used standard management system that incorporates procedures of selecting and assigning funds, personnel, facilities, and equipment at the time of the incident (Bigley & Roberts, 2001; DHS, 2016c). ICS—which can be advanced by local, state, federal, or military organizations—is the "first-on-scene" system to organize the structure of care and support in a disaster area (Buck, Trainor & Aguirre, 2006). As a hierarchical model, ICS identifies a clear chain of command, assigns emergency management team leaders and responders, and clearly defines the responsibility and role of each team member when participating in a response (PHS Commissioned Officers Foundation, 2010). Incident command is responsible for building the following major functions: (a) command (to appoint team leaders and members), (b) information/planning (to keep all team members informed and communicating), (c) needs assessment (to identify short- and long-term needs for the affected population), (d) operations (to develop objectives to carry out plans related to care and resource provision and response), (e) logistics (to receive, store, and distribute resources like food, water, shelter, clothing, etc.), and (f) finance/administration (to track financial activities related to funding/purchasing/securing necessary resources and/or services) (Bigley & Roberts, 2001; DHS, 2016c).

Emergency management. Understanding the discipline of emergency management can best be understood through the emergency management cycle, which includes mitigation, preparedness, response, and recovery (DHS, 2016d). Initial efforts in mitigation and preparation relate to preventing disaster and crisis events from happening altogether or to minimizing the scope or intensity of events when they occur. For example, to mitigate flooding, protective barriers may be built or people's homes may be relocated away from high-risk areas. Emergency managers may also oversee the placement and functioning of notification sirens, emergency broadcast messages, and/or planned locations for DRCs if/when they are needed. Their scope in these preparedness efforts can range from an individual city to a county, a state, or even the nation as a whole—and they thereby coordinate and support other government and public safety personnel as needed. Efforts during response phases of a disaster include those designed to limit any further loss of life, personal injury, and/or damage to property. These may include the coordination of search-and-rescue teams, mass vaccinations and/or evacuations, food and water distribution, and/or emergency shelters. Efforts in the recovery phases of a disaster response (which can sometimes take months or years to complete) include early attention to things like neighborhood cleanup, restoration of power and water facilities, and/or the construction of temporary housing or schools. Longer-term work in recovery overlaps with newfound mitigation and preparedness efforts and includes things like the relocation of personal and public buildings (and to construct these in ways that are resistant to earthquakes, flooding, or fire), restoring local economies and businesses, etc. (Baird, 2010; DHS, 2016d; Rubin, 2012).

Healthcare providers. Any disaster carries with it the potential for people to be physically injured or killed; nearby hospitals and clinics are consequently treated as secondary sites for the provision of emergency/critical care (Reily & Markenson, 2010; U.S. Fire Administration, 2016). Core providers and staff include emergency physicians, physician assistants and physician extenders, medical residents, nurses, medical assistants, pharmacists, trauma surgeons, emergency medical technicians, emergency room technicians, radiologists, radiological technicians, police and other security personnel, chaplains, social workers, behavioral health providers, emergency medicine clerks, health unit coordinators, and scribes (see chapter "Medical Family Therapy in Emergency Medicine" in this text for a detailed description of these teams and team members). Such sites can range from small community clinics to large metropolitan hospitals—and any of these can become quickly overwhelmed with the surge of patients (and/or loved ones who are looking for said patients). Many hospitals carry formal accreditations that require them to be prepared to respond to disasters dealing with these types of influxes of people—patients and loved ones alike—to their facilities (Agency for Healthcare Research and Quality, 2011; Joint Commission on the Accreditation of Healthcare Organizations, 2016). Oftentimes, however, the human elements of these influxes are not well rehearsed and can thereby punctuate gaps in training, resources, and protocols. These experiences, when assessed and evaluated, can assist in future preparedness exercises.

Public health. Public health personnel in disaster response tend to be positioned within emergency management roles (see description above). These professionals take on the responsibility of preventing, protecting against, and quickly responding to and assisting with recovery efforts from multiple types of large-scale emergencies—from infectious diseases; foodborne illnesses; chemical radiological accidents or intentional events; natural disasters like hurricanes, tornadoes, or pandemics; and even acts of human violence (Centers for Disease Control and Prevention [CDC], 2016). All public health jurisdictions are responsible for preparedness in these types of events; they are thereby an important discipline to coordinate with in relation to disaster response efforts (U.S. Department of Health and Human Services, 2016).

Volunteer agencies. A common and encouraging element of many communities' response to disastrous events centers on the strong and commonplace human desire to help each other. Churches, schools, local aid organizations, and even individual people will often arrive at disaster sites, recovery centers, healthcare facilities, and other locations to offer assistance. However, not all volunteers are created alike. While most are well intentioned, many impromptu volunteers can actually be disruptive to the efforts of a formal response. In disaster preparedness work, Incident

Command and DRC Systems are set up to work with agencies that have extensive experience with disaster response training—like those formally recognized by nationwide networks such as Voluntary Organizations Active in Disaster (VOAD, 2016). Groups mobilized by the American Red Cross, The Salvation Army, and the International Critical Incident Stress Foundation are some of the most consistently active of these organizations. Other organizations—many of which are faith-based—focus on providing cleanup of debris, dissemination of food and clothing, and a wide range of human service support systems (e.g., case management).

Community representatives. Local community members and representatives are often utilized to provide basic information and physical/behavioral healthcare services within a disaster response (Federal Emergency Management Administration, 2011; Lichterman, 2000). These team members are generally trained through aforementioned VOAD agencies beforehand; others who receive just-in-time (JIT) training are integrated into targeted facets of a formal response as necessary. Some may serve as cultural translators (e.g., when working with refugee or other minority populations). Community representatives can include schoolteachers, village resources (e.g., the village headman), spiritual leaders, elders, governmental and nongovernmental organizations (NGOs), volunteers and survivor camp workers, and media workers (TV, radio, newspaper).

Chaplains. Chaplains are important to differentiate from clergy (Association of Professional Chaplains, 2016; Joyner, 2016). A member of a clergy maintains a specific faith-based ideology and practice (e.g., Catholic, Lutheran). His or her orientation is to work within that faith-based system. Secondary to the vulnerability that people tend to have in the midst of a disaster event and recovery, it is considered unethical for members of a clergy to impress their faith-based system onto individuals who have not identified themselves as followers of that specific religion. Conversely, a chaplain brings a nondenominational (read: spiritual) perspective; his/her goal is to meet individuals where they are. Chaplains do not bring forward any particular religion's perspective unless the individual(s) they are supporting ask for this. Chaplains who have experience and training with public safety or hospital care are preferred during disaster events (National Disaster Interfaiths Network, 2007; North American Mission Board, 2016). Their skill sets offer a wide range of personal and spiritual resources for individuals and families who are coping with traumatic events, ambiguities about the future, and losses of property and/or of loved ones through death.

Fundamentals of Disaster Response

MedFTs working in disaster response must be familiar with, and skilled in, a myriad of contents. Principal foci include the following.

Psychological First Aid

PFA is an evidence-informed approach that builds upon core concepts of human resilience (National Child Traumatic Stress Network, 2006; Ruzek et al., 2007). At its core is the recognition of signs and symptoms of stress, alongside providing a safe environment, facilitating a sense of calm, and empowering recipients toward healthy action. Many disaster response organizations have developed their own versions of PFA training, e.g., the Federal Emergency Management Agency (FEMA), National Child Traumatic Stress Network (NCTS), and International Critical Incident Stress Foundation (ICISF). These trainings range in time and intensity, from single introductory courses (e.g., half-day, online) to in-depth and extensive course collections and foci (FEMA, 2013; ICISF, 2016; NCTS, 2006).

Common elements in PFA include, but are not limited to, the following: (a) engaging distressed persons through composed safe self-introductions (e.g., assuring confidentiality) and attention to immediate needs (e.g., offering food or water); (b) providing safety and comfort (e.g., offering blankets for warmth, offering information about events/responses/resources); (c) stabilizing survivors who are emotionally overwhelmed (e.g., offering a compassionate presence and good listening skills, relaxation, and calming sequence); (d) gathering information regarding needs and concerns about separations from loved ones, worries about property, potential suicidality, etc.; (e) offering practical assistance (e.g., accessing childcare resources); (f) promoting social connections and other support systems (e.g., friends, faith communities); (g) psychoeducation about common stress reactions and coping sequences; and (h) linking people to collaborative services for follow-up and/or longer-term needs. PFA can be used when working with individuals, couples, and families (Fox et al., 2012; Pynoos & Nader, 1988; Vernberg et al., 2008). It can also inform the design of support centers, e.g., attending to the physical layout of DRC facilities and resource/information desks so that those needing services are effectively identified and promptly cared for (University of Minnesota Academic Health Center, 2017).

Team Coordination

As discussed earlier, a formal disaster response is embedded within a structured management system. Behavioral health providers within this system focus their principal energies on and across two teams. The first team is the team of behavioral responders, themselves. These teams tend to be comprised of multiple disciplines and are organized in a 2 × 2 "buddy system" fashion. These sub-teams of two professionals each are best advanced with purposeful attention to the diverse nature of their members, e.g., pairing a MedFT with a psychologist and pairing a social worker with a chaplain. Doing this equips each team with a rich interdisciplinary mixture of wisdom and expertise (Mendenhall, 2006). Pairing the teams in groups of two (regardless of which disciplinary backgrounds are represented therein) is also purposeful because it enables team members to check in with each other, process difficult stories, and encourage breaks and other self-care sequences (Mendenhall, 2006; Mendenhall & Berge, 2010).

The second team that MedFTs and other behavioral health providers function within is the larger, overarching team that is responding to the incident. Members within this frame include other care providers of all types (behavioral health and physical health), law enforcement, police officers, firefighters, public health officials, community leaders, and government officials. It is important to conduct one's self with persistent attention to the manner in which these multiple team members (and the respective constituents they represent) function. Doing this effectively is facilitated by a priori efforts to learn about and get to know each other (e.g., meeting with and/or shadowing members of local law enforcement, participating in local training and simulation exercises that include multiple response agencies), becoming conversant in common terms and phrases/acronyms employed by ICS and others (see Figure 15.1 and Glossary), and being flexible and responsive to lead agencies' efforts in managing personnel and related resources (Kaji, Langford, & Lewis, 2008; Larkin, 2010).

Figure 15.1 Common Abbreviations in Disaster Response

ACS	Alternate Care Site
ARC	American Red Cross
CBRNE	Chemical Biological Radiological Nuclear Explosive
CDC	Centers for Disaster Control and Prevention
CFLOP	Command Finance Logistics Operations and Planning
CIKR	Critical Infrastructure and Key Resources
COOP	Continuity of Operations
DA	Disaster Assistance
DBH	Disaster Behavioral Health
DHS	Department of Homeland Security
DMAT	Disaster Medical Assistance Team
DRC	Disaster Recovery Center
EEG	Exercise Evaluation Guide
ESF	Emergency Support Function
FEMA	Federal Emergency Management Agency
HHS	Department of Health and Human Services
HICS	Hospital Incident Command System
HSEEP	Homeland Security Exercise and Evaluation Program
IC	Incident Commander
LTCR	Long-term Community Recovery
MRC	Medical Reserve Corps
NDMS	National Disaster Medical System
NICS	National Incident Management System
NTSB	National Transportation Safety Board
PFA	Psychological First Aid
PIO	Public Information Officer
PPE	Personal Protective Equipment
RDD	Radiological Dispersion Device
SOP	Standard Operating Procedure
SME	Subject Matter Expert
VOAD	Voluntary Organizations Active in Disasters
WMD	Weapons of Mass Destruction

Timing of Mental Health Services

Most individuals who are exposed to a disaster event will present with some degree of BPSS stress (e.g., insomnia, racing thoughts, interpersonal conflict, poor work performance, spiritual crisis). These responses are both common and expected, and it is thereby important to normalize them in the contexts of providing early support. Research has shown that the majority of those impacted by a disaster will experience a reduction and/or dissipation of symptoms over the next few weeks and that more than two thirds of surviving victims do not manifest long-term psychological disorders (e.g., PTSD) that would indicate formal mental health treatment (American Red Cross, 2016; Butler, Panzer, & Goldfrank, 2003).

During the early stages of a disaster response, then, PFA interventions are most indicated. On some (usually rare) occasions, providers may need to advance care that prioritizes personal safety above all else (e.g., when a person is suicidal). For individuals who have pre-existing mental health challenges (e.g., major depression, anxiety) or significant life stressors leading up to an event (e.g., unemployment, marital distress), MedFTs are well equipped to assess for such concerns and provide care in a manner that simultaneously honors immediate needs for stability and longer-term needs for psychological healing, adaptation, and growth. Once the initial phases of response have concluded (i.e., as an immediate disaster response moves into a recovery phase), the most common interventions that survivors benefit from include group and/or responder support (formal or informal). Aforementioned long-term interventions—e.g., those that either target stressor build-ups now overwhelmed by trauma or those that promote adaptation to lasting effects of trauma per se—are described in more detail below. These efforts are most indicated for individuals who are still presenting with problematic symptomology 1–2 months after a disaster event (Foa, Stein, & McFarlane, 2006; North & Pfefferbaum, 2013).

Working with the Media

In the current age of social media, the desire to communicate information in a timely and accurate manner can be complicated. Initial information during disasters may, indeed, be timely—but oftentimes it is not very accurate. Developing the capability and capacity to respond through social media is important for any organization. Part of this preparedness activity includes establishing relationships with reputable media outlets (Mangeri, 2015). Oftentimes this responsibility rests in the hands of an organization's public information officer (PIO). The PIO is responsible for the interaction between the general public and the media. He or she reports to the incident commander to assure that the information that is being communicated to the general public is accurate (Hughes & Palen, 2012). A MedFT's role in all of this—unless serving in the formal capacity of a PIO—is to purposefully not engage with the media and to encourage and support colleagues and community members to do the same. And while the MedFT may be asked to help craft messages that a PIO delivers (e.g., for content that speaks to human resilience), he or she—not the university, care site, or professional organization that the MedFT is primarily affiliated with—should be formally identified.

Compassionate Presence

One of the greatest needs that individuals have during times of crisis is knowing that there are people who are trying to assist them—even if and when there are not clear ways to solve the struggles that they face. Many trainees and young professionals worry about what to say when working with those who are hurting, but oftentimes the best way to respond is to not say anything (at least not verbally). A core element of PFA is providing this compassionate presence; providers work to meet people where they are (not where they believe they "should" be). Aligning with the adages that God gave us two ears and a mouth for a reason and that the word "listen" and "silent" contain the exact same letters, there are times in disaster response that the most helpful thing to offer a surviving victim is one's undivided attention. Listening—indeed, being wholly present (without waiting to jump in and say something "helpful" or "supportive")—is sometimes difficult for providers who are trained to ask questions, assess for diagnoses, and/or advance interventions to "help" (Engel, Zarconi, Pethtel, & Missimi, 2008; Gehart & McCollum, 2007; Puchalski, 2001). But just as "common factors" in baseline clinical work go further than any one particular clinical approach, so too does compassionately walking alongside (not leading) someone who is figuring out his/her own path (Lambert & Barley, 2001; Morse, Bottorff, Anderson, O'Brien, & Solberg, 2006).

Active Listening Skills

In conjunction with compassionate presence, the effective conduct of behavioral health support in disaster response includes skill sets in active listening. While the execution of specific skills in active listening varies in accord with the personal attributes, cultures, and contexts in which the work is carried out, common nonverbal sequences include eye contact, pleasant or smiling facial expressions, concerned or empathic facial expressions, and posturing one's body to lean forward. Common verbal sequences include asking questions for further information or clarification, recalling details (e.g., bringing them back up in conversation) within the context of loved ones and/or others with whom survivors have safe and ongoing relationships, and paraphrasing or summarizing what speakers have said so as to demonstrate comprehension (Fassaert, van Dulmen, Schellevis, & Bensing, 2007; Levitt, 2002; Roberston, 2005).

Suicide Ideation Assessment

While relatively uncommon, suicidality is nevertheless a real danger encountered by MedFTs engaged in disaster response. Any team deployed in this work must maintain a general skill set in doing suicide screenings and have at least one team member qualified to make these types of formal assessments (for a list of recommended assessment tools, see Additional Resources section at the conclusion of this chapter). An effective assessment targets verbal ques that are direct (e.g., "I want to kill myself.") and indirect (e.g., "My life isn't worth living anymore."). It includes attention to a person's psychological functioning (e.g., feeling overwhelmed or hopeless) and behaviors (e.g., giving away prized possessions, marked withdrawal from family or friends). Providers ask questions directly about whether a person is thinking about hurting or killing himself/herself and if he or she has a plan and/or means to carry out this intent. If and when the provider determines that a person is at risk, then he or she must work to ensure the person's safety. Indicated methods for doing this vary in accord with each situation and include interventions that range from less intense (e.g., no-harm contract) to more intense (e.g., hospitalization) (Berman, Jobes, & Silverman, 2006; Simon & Hales, 2012). Having referral resources within the team or at a healthcare facility to conduct assessments and follow through with, especially, more intense responses is essential within a disaster response.

Sensitivity to Diversity

Communities display diverse responses in the face of trauma and death. Assessment of risks, vulnerabilities, resources, and capacities of a trauma-impacted population is substantial in developing and implementing effective PFA models for these populations (Buckle, Marsh, & Smale, 2003). Studies have long demonstrated the need to focus on transnational and ethno-cultural issues while responding to mental health of mass trauma-affected populations (Green, 1996). Disasters can have severe consequences, especially on communities of ethnic minorities and developing countries, such as populations affected by Hurricane Katrina or the East-Asian tsunami of 2004 (Masella & Christopher, 2004). In the face of disasters, trauma response and recovery should incorporate cultural and ecological factors associated with resilience and resources of individuals, families, and communities. This standpoint has challenged individualized, Western, medical approaches to trauma recovery, which often lack consideration for contextual elements (Summerfield, 2004). And indeed, some people from different cultural backgrounds may react poorly to Western intervention models (Shah, 2007). Incorporating indigenous healing methods and values into Western evidence-based models, for example, may facilitate a more rapid and drastic change in individuals and families exposed to trauma (Brave Heart, Chase, Elkins, & Altschul, 2011; Mock, 2004; Mollica, 1988). This does not mean that Western models should not be used in non-Western populations; with appropriate cultural adaptations and by paying careful attention to local cultures' authentic ways of reacting to and coping with trauma, these models can be effectively adapted for communities affected by disasters (Hoshmand, 2007).

Disaster Response Across the MedFT Healthcare Continuum

Medical family therapy is an important field in the integration of behavioral health, disaster preparedness, and trauma-response team efforts. Specific training, practice, research, and policy competencies represent important facets of this work as professionals engage in this often chaotic and unpredictable work. Tables 15.1 and 15.2 highlight specific skills that characterize MedFTs' involvement in trauma-response contexts across Hodgson et al.'s (2014) MedFT Healthcare Continuum. As we move along the continuum, we carry greater expectations regarding roles, knowledge, and overall contributions to care.

At the beginning of the continuum, MedFTs at *Levels 1* and *2* should possess general understanding(s) of BPSS approaches to working with highly distressed persons (individuals, couples, families). They are familiar with normative stress reactions to acute situations versus longer-term sequences (e.g., posttraumatic stress disorder) and are familiar with PFA as a basic intervention. They do not likely engage with trauma teams regularly, but maintain a basic understanding of their structure when volunteering in this kind of effort. While clinical knowledge and skills in balancing active listening and compassionate presence are arguably manifest within any competent clinician, maintaining this balance is more difficult for practitioners situated within the fast-paced and potentially high-intensity contexts of a disaster response. MedFTs are adept in maintaining such balance when they need to (e.g., during times that they are deployed). As they perform in-the-field assessments for suicidality and homicidality, they are knowledgeable about and highly capable of coordinating the services of other providers and institutional resources if and when indicated. Lisa and her supervisees (in our vignette above), for example, would need to be vigilant about doing such assessments for survivors of the flood. Adults who had lost their homes and livelihoods—or the teen who had lost his beloved pet—could very well experience such emotional and/or behavioral instability during acute phases of a disaster recovery.

A clinician equipped with knowledge and skills outlined in *Level 3* is able to collaborate with and/or function within a trauma-response team without considerable orientation and/or just-in-time preparation. He or she is thereby readily able to integrate family therapy interventions with PFA principles in the conduct of care. For example, Lisa could work to promote baseline safety (a PFA goal) through facilitating discussions and collaboratively problem-solving with a couple who had recently lost their home to secure temporary housing. MedFTs at this level are also familiar with multiple constituents (e.g., incident command, volunteer organizations, community leaders) and their respective roles, missions, and work foci; equipped with this fluency and a comfort for working with groups of people (versus

Table 15.1 MedFTs in Disaster Preparedness and Trauma-response Teams: Basic Knowledge and Skills

MedFT Healthcare Continuum Level	Level 1	Level 2	Level 3
Knowledge	Basic knowledge about BPSS approaches to working with highly distressed individuals, couples, and families; sensitive to how acute stress responses, mood, and behaviors are mutually influential. Familiar with Psychological First Aid as a baseline trauma intervention. Limited understanding of trauma-team structure(s).	Can differentiate between types of trauma reactions (e.g., normative stress responses to acute situations, PTSD). Familiar with benefits of couple and family engagement in acute fieldwork processes and follow-up recovery (accomplished on survivors' own and/or with clinical support). Basic knowledge about trauma-team structures (e.g., incident command, buddy systems).	Working knowledge of specific team members (e.g., incident commander, public information officer, first responder, chaplain) and terms in trauma response (e.g., family reunification center, PFA, JIT, ICS, NIMS). Basic knowledge of team coordination (e.g., behavioral response teams, law enforcement, community leaders) and timing of mental health services within a response (psychoeducation, PFA, long-term interventions). Familiar with the family therapy interventions as applied to trauma contexts and informed by BPSS and systems training.
Skills	Can discuss (and psychoeducate) basic relationships between biological, psychological, and behavioral foci vis-à-vis acute stress. Can effectively balance active listening and compassionate presence with highly distressed individuals, couples, and families. Minimal collaborative skills with other providers; generally works in an individual practitioner model, but occasionally volunteers in trauma-response teams.	Able to apply systemic PFA interventions in practice; assess survivors for potential suicidality/homicidality. Adequate collaborative skills; works with trauma-team personnel with some regularity; can coordinate referrals and follow-up with indicated specialists if longer-term care is indicated.	Coordinate and integrate respective team members' expertise and counsel into immediate response sequences and follow-up planning. Able to conduct family therapy interventions in a manner that effectively integrates key elements of PFA; advances these efforts in a manner sensitive to short- versus long-term treatment goals and sequences. Can effectively work with the media (if designated to do so) or encourage and support PIO colleagues who do.

one on one), they are able to coordinate and integrate behavioral health providers into the moving parts of a coordinated response without undue disruption. Within a leadership role (as with Lisa in our vignette), this MedFT competently organizes and directs (and redirects) behavioral health providers' efforts in synchrony with the changing needs and evolution of larger response efforts.

A MedFT functioning at *Level 4* maintains high skill and knowledge in the range of human reactions to stress (acute and long-term) and can readily bridge his/her efforts in fieldwork to follow-up care provided for individuals, couples, and families for whom this is necessary. Being capable with core content and terms essential to trauma therapies enables him/her to effectively translate and track respective team members' efforts over the course of a referral (when this is possible)—and it is at this level that such efforts are most likely to occur within the

Table 15.2 MedFTs in Disaster Preparedness and Trauma-response Teams: Advanced Knowledge and Skills

MedFT Healthcare Continuum Level	Level 4	Level 5
Knowledge	Adept understanding of acute trauma reactions (e.g., normative responses, triggered responses vis-à-vis high-risk psychosocial histories) and related clinical behaviors and presentations. Conversant in a range of trauma-focused treatments and terminologies. Conversant in nearly all terms, measures, and facets of disaster preparedness and behavioral health response. Basic knowledge of emergency management phases and the manners in which behavioral health is (or can be) effectively integrated into them.	Understand treatment and care sequences for unique and/or challenging topics in trauma response (e.g., suicidality, intimate partner violence, alcohol and/or drug abuse); can consult effectively with diverse healthcare professionals. Conversant with evidence-based treatments regarding most follow-up trauma-related therapies; has background to provide psychoeducation to patients about a variety of symptoms, medications, and stress management leading up to indicated referrals. High content knowledge in clinical topics, research practice, policy, and administrative areas of disaster response; proficient in developing a curriculum on PFA, behavioral health roles, and other supportive sequences to provide other professionals involved in all phases of emergency management response cycle(s). Experienced and well informed regarding common symptoms of (and ways to mitigate) compassion fatigue.

(continued)

MedFT Healthcare Continuum Level	Level 4	Level 5
Skills	Able to deliver seminars and workshops about the BPSS complexities of disaster preparedness and trauma-response work to a variety of professional types (e.g., mental health, biomedical).	Proficient in nearly all aspects of trauma-response efforts; able to synthesize and conduct research; engages in collaborative efforts to organize and advance team preparedness.
	Can apply several BPSS interventions in trauma response (e.g., greeter and reunification roles, assisting medical examiners with death notifications) and follow-up care.	Routinely engages in team-based approaches to trauma-response work, with consistent communication through patient introductions, curbside-consultations, and team debriefing meetings and visits.
	Consistently collaborates with key team members (e.g., incident commander, public health, volunteer agencies, primary care provider, chaplain); coordinates behavioral providers within larger team of multiple providers engaged in a response.	Proficiently integrates research-informed practices (across multiple system levels) with trainees, alongside vigilant attention to compassion fatigue assessment (and, when necessary, intervention and support).
		Proficiently coordinates, directs, and leads disaster response teams within larger ICS deployments.
		Engaged in advocacy efforts to integrate behavioral health foci into mitigation, preparation, and response phases of emergency management.

arenas of trauma response. If or as a MedFT's work overlaps with the provision of such longer-term care (albeit not with persons originally encountered during fieldwork), he or she would evidence working familiarity and competence with multiple treatment modalities—e.g., cognitive behavioral therapy (CBT) and eye movement desensitization and reprocessing—performed in family-based contexts. For example, a clinician's work with individuals and families over the weeks and months following a traumatic event (e.g., the flood that Lisa and her team initially responded to) could be toward repairing attachment injuries that were acutely brought forth or exacerbated. Alongside this, MedFTs at this level will work purposefully to build relationships with other members of an integrated behavioral healthcare team (e.g., primary care provider, social worker) so that they are ready and able to either serve in immediate response efforts (like Lisa) or as a resource for those who need assistance later on.

MedFTs who function at *Level 5* generally have practiced at all levels of care and work in various roles within a trauma-response team (e.g., behavioral health team member, team lead, team coordinator). As a baseline clinician, proficiency in acute interventions and BPSS approaches includes competence and knowledge regarding other providers' contributions (e.g., healthcare, food assistance). This is evidenced in active and effective participation in—and leading of—team-based collaboration, which by default extends beyond the acute incident's time frame. As an educator and mentor, the MedFT is proficient in the didactic and supervisory instruction of these skill sets and knowledge—evidenced across live classroom and fieldwork sequences and professional development workshops and/or in the construction of instructional materials (e.g., refereed journal articles, texts, conference workshops). Further, professionals at this level tend to be involved in research (e.g., testing and/or comparing interdisciplinary team-based methodologies, evaluating care efficiency across different team-based models), policymaking (e.g., advocacy for the integration of behavioral health foci into all phases of emergency management), and other administrative duties (e.g., overseeing behavioral health internships that include training for and experience in disaster preparedness and trauma-response team work).

Level 5 clinical efforts following the vignette provided in this chapter could engage MedFT trainees in how to coordinate the presence of behavioral health providers throughout the geography of a response (e.g., from check-in lines to behind-the-scenes break rooms for staff), alongside how to deliver PFA to a range of surviving victims (e.g., from the angry person wanting insurance information to the despondent teenager whose pet died). As a supervisor, the MedFT is likely to also see and attend to symptoms of compassion fatigue or burnout for any team member or trainee under his or her watch and to—when needed—support said team member or trainee in steps toward self-care, recovery, and healing. As a researcher, a MedFT could seek in-depth understandings about survivors' and responders' experiences in the acute phases of a response (e.g., a qualitative case study targeting what community members found most helpful in stabilizing their psychosocial disruptions, a quantitative study tracking first responders' depressive and anxiety symptoms over the course of the deployment vis-à-vis their engagement—or not—in supportive sequences of team debriefing and related self-care). As an educator, the MedFT could use survivors' or responders' stories (either with their permission or in a manner appropriately disguised and potentially even with their coauthorship) as case examples in training manuals and/or professional presentations. As an advocate, he or she could present patients' and families' stories in preventative and/or reparative efforts as examples to persuade and/or guide indicated policy and administrative sequences that facilitate the purposeful integration of behavioral health foci in larger emergency management efforts.

Research-Informed Practices

In this section, we briefly review what is known about preventing posttraumatic symptoms and treating early symptoms of posttraumatic stress and other potential sequelae of traumatic events. We highlight ecologically oriented approaches (or the lack thereof) within the immediate and acute phases of post-incident care. Attention to PTSD-related measures in our review reflects the major focus of literature in the area of trauma, and this is not meant to give the impression that PTSD is necessarily the primary or sole focus of PFA.

Litz (2008) defines "immediate" interventions as those occurring within 48 hours of the potentially traumatic event(s) and "acute" as taking place a few weeks later. Following the acute phase, treatment of chronic symptomology is the focus of most formal interventions. For the purposes of this account, then, we focus this review on immediate and acute time frames.

Immediate Interventions

At the present time, there is no empirical support for any behavioral health intervention that is advanced during the first few hours after a traumatic event (e.g., as a way to prevent PTSD) and only some support for cognitive behavioral interventions in the hours and days that follow (Agorastos, Marmar, & Otte, 2011; Fox et al., 2012; Watson, 2015). It is also important to note that research regarding immediate interventions has largely focused on psychological debriefing and multicomponent interventions, such as critical incident stress management (CISM) (Everly, Flannery, & Eyler, 2002; Everly, Flannery, & Mitchell, 2000; Peltier & Peltier, 2016). Most of these efforts have been conducted with individuals (not couples or families) across 1:1 or group therapy formats. And while MedFT in disaster response should build on the current knowledge that is available, we must endeavor to advance methods and understandings that are sensitive to the BPSS complexities of the patients and families we treat. The following is a summary of what we know so far.

Psychological Debriefing

A great deal of research attention to lessening negative effects post disaster—often measured by preventing PTSD—has been given to a group of interventions known as psychological debriefing (PD). The mostly widely known form of PD is critical incident stress debriefing (CISD) (Campfield & Hills, 2001; Fantini-Hauwel, Dovi, & Antoine, 2015). PD is generally understood as a single individual or group (not couple/family) session occurring soon after a traumatic event in which the event is collectively recounted and debriefed. This is an area surrounded by considerable controversy (Rabstejnek, 2014; Robinson, 2007; Wagner, 2005) and thus warrants attention here.

A number of randomized control trials (RCTs) have yielded mixed results regarding the effectiveness of PD (e.g., Adler et al., 2008; Rose, Brewin, Andrews, & Kirk, 1999; Sijbrandij, Olff, Reitsma, Carlier, & Gersons, 2006). Some studies have found no significant effects of PD over no-treatment control groups (e.g., Bisson, McFarlane, Rose, Ruzek, & Watson, 2009). Others have advanced support for the approach (e.g., Adler, Bliese, McGurk, Hoge, & Castro, 2009; Campfield & Hills, 2001), while others still have found that PD as a stand-alone intervention may actually increase posttraumatic symptomology (Bisson, Jenkins, Alexander, & Bannister, 1997; Deahl et al., 2000; Mayou, Ehlers, & Hobbs, 2000; Sijbrandij et al., 2006).

To make sense of these conflicting findings, researchers have argued that many studies evaluating PD have used the intervention incorrectly. Hawker, Durkin, & Hawker (2011), for example, maintain that PD is intended for groups of people who have ongoing relationships with each other (e.g., family, friends, co-workers) and that studies that have found harmful effects with individuals (especially those that treated strangers together) should thereby not be generalized. Robinson (2008) adds to this discussion in claiming that CISD is not meant to be a stand-alone or individual intervention, anyway. Instead, it should be integrated as a component to other, more complex, approaches.

Multicomponent and Multisession Interventions

One common multicomponent intervention is critical incident stress management (CISM), which utilizes PD as one of its facets. In a similar manner to PD literature described above, researchers have found mixed and contradictory findings (e.g., Everly et al., 2002; Roberts, Kitchiner, Kenardy, & Bisson, 2010; Wei et al., 2010). For example, Everly et al. (2002) conducted a statistical review of CISM and concluded that it is effective at reducing psychological distress (Cohen's $d = 3.11, p < 0.0001$). It is important to note, however, that the studies they reviewed included a variety of outcome measures and were not all immediate interventions or identified as being RCTs.

In a Cochrane Review of multisession interventions (which did not include CISM) for preventing PTSD, Roberts et al. (2010) concluded that—at the time of the review—there was (is) "little evidence to support the use of psychological interventions for routine use following traumatic events and that some multiple session interventions, like single session interventions, may have an adverse effect on some individuals" (p. 12). They further recommend that researchers continue to evaluate areas that show promise with caution because of the evidence that some interventions appear to be harmful at times. The studies included in this review represented a range of interventions (e.g., adapted PD, group counseling, integrated CBT and family counseling, and individual counseling).

No studies of such multicomponent/multisession interventions to date have purposefully evaluated BPSS outcomes; future research should investigate the effects of relational interventions (advanced in the immediate aftermath of disasters) on such health factors so as to better inform MedFT practice and related clinical methods.

Acute Interventions

MedFT can readily integrate with efforts to address negative effects of traumatic events during acute phases of treatment. The interventions with the most support during these phases are forms of cognitive behavioral therapy (CBT). Other interventions, such as eye movement desensitization and reprocessing (EMDR) and school-based interventions, are also being used—but empirical support for these is less developed.

Cognitive Behavioral Therapy

CBT is used in various forms for treating acute stress disorder (ASD) and for preventing chronic PTSD. These studies have generally been carried out with people who have ASD or PTSD symptoms weeks or months after a traumatic event and have generally yielded positive results. In a thorough review of the literature in this area, Litz and Bryant (2009) conclude that early CBT "should be employed routinely as an early intervention for survivors of relatively discrete accidents who endorse significant, enduring posttraumatic difficulties" (p. 128). Because of the resources involved with administering most forms of CBT, it is recommended that CBT only be used once time has elapsed so that those who continue to experience posttraumatic symptomology can be identified and receive treatment. While the use of CBT to prevent chronic PTSD following non-interpersonal accidents has strong support (Bryant, Harvey, Dang, Sackville, & Basten, 1998; Ehlers et al., 2003; Litz and Bryant, 2009), the support for CBT for PTSD resulting from interpersonal traumatic events is less definitive—with both positive results (e.g., Bryant, Moulds, & Nixon, 2006) and neutral results (e.g., Foa, Zoellner, & Feeny, 2006).

Eye Movement Desensitization and Reprocessing

EMDR is an integrative therapy method that employs a number of standard protocols that reflect several unique treatment approaches. It targets past memories of trauma, present disturbances and struggles, and future/planned actions and behaviors. The goal of this therapy is equip patients with the emotions, insights/understandings, and perspectives/life approaches that they need to lead to healthy and satisfying lives (for more information, see EMDR International Association, 2017). A number of protocols for the early application of EMDR have emerged (e.g., Shapiro, 2009; Shapiro & Laub, 2008). Early support for EMDR in the relief of posttraumatic symptoms during acute phases of care (and in the prevention of future symptoms) is promising—whether the intervention occurs weeks after the event (Jarero, Artigas, & Luber, 2011; Silver, Rogers, Knipe, & Colelli, 2005) or months after the event (Grainger, Levin, Allen-Byrd, Doctor, & Lee, 1997). More comprehensive research is needed in this area, however, especially as it relates to couple and family therapy interventions and physical health outcomes.

Family and/or Ecologically Oriented Interventions

Most researched interventions during the acute stages of trauma work have focused on individual therapies. While some focus on the community is seen in the literature, little attention has been paid to the effects of trauma on the family. The importance of understanding the relationship between trauma and the family has been addressed (Gewirtz, Forgatch, & Wieling, 2008); however, this has not yet significantly translated into clinical models for or application to disaster relief. Early calls to address this gap in knowledge are only beginning to be answered. For example, Salloum and Overstreet (2012) found trauma narration with children combined with coping skills training to be more effective than unimodal approaches. Boyd-Franklin and Bry (2012) have shown how family therapy interventions can extend and overlap into school and community foci. As with other approaches, more comprehensive research is needed regarding couple and family therapy interventions—especially—and their respective impact(s) on BPSS outcomes.

Interventions for Chronic Symptoms

There is strong empirical support for many interventions that address trauma-related symptoms and disorders for chronic symptoms; the majority—as already described—are individual treatments for PTSD (Cohen, Mannarino, & Deblinger, 2016; Haagen, Smid, Knipscheer, & Kleber, 2015; Najavits & Hein, 2013; Niles et al., 2012). MedFT strategies can draw on the knowledge gained from these interventions, alongside recognizing that we must maintain vigilance in identifying those potentially in need of long-term treatment, make appropriate referrals when/as necessary, and/or honor patients' BPSS systemic complexities in care. In this section we briefly review systems-oriented interventions for addressing chronic trauma-related symptoms and grief and loss. These treatments are recognized across couple/family therapy, psychoeducation, and school-based interventions.

Couple/Family Therapy Approaches

A few small studies have introduced the use of conjoint treatments for couples to address PTSD, such as cognitive behavioral conjoint therapy (Monson et al., 2011) and structured approach therapy (Sautter, Armelie, Glynn, & Wielt, 2011). Other interventions have directly targeted the family or partner of someone affected by trauma, such as support and family education (Sherman, 2003). Trauma interventions with the most strong theoretical bases that focus on both couples and families, such as emotion-focused therapy (EFT; Johnson, 2012; Johnson, 2002), are demonstrating especially promising results (Agnus, 2012; Ehlers et al., 2014). Specifically, EFT is an approach to therapy that purposefully integrates the science on adult attachment and bonding to couple's functioning in their relationships. Clinicians work with patients and partners to (a) expand and reorganize key emotional responses to attachment- and other trauma-related foci, (b) promote changes in partners' respective interaction patterns, and (c) build secure relational bonds. Figley and Figley (2009) articulate further support for such systemic thinking in the treatment of trauma, too; they maintain that collaborative meaning-making processes in couples and families are a primary component of healing from trauma upon which all other growth evolves.

Psychoeducation Approaches

While psychoeducation can arguably be a part of any intervention type, some evidence exists for its utility as a stand-alone approach with couples, families, and groups in addressing trauma. A lifestyle management course described by Devilly (2002), for example, showed improvement in measures of anxiety, stress, depression, and PTSD. The *Linking Human Systems* approach has been used with a wide range of populations, including those affected by trauma, and highlights the importance of family and community connections (Landau, Mittal, & Wieling, 2008) in healing from traumatic events. For a thorough review, Makin-Byrd et al. (2011) have described these and other couple and family interventions and guidelines in depth.

School-Based Interventions

While many may not be familiar with the notion that family therapists and MedFTs are well equipped to function within school environments, emerging evidence supports this (Alexander, Waldron, Robbins, & Neeb, 2013; Kennedy, 2008; Laundy, 2015). Treatment of PTSD for youth in these environments is becoming increasingly recognized and supported. In a review of school-based interventions and protocols, for example, Kataoka et al. (2012) highlighted *Multimodality Trauma Treatment* (Amaya-Jackson et al., 2003), the University of California's *Trauma Grief Component Treatment Program* (Saltzman, Pynoos, Layne, Steinberg, & Aisenberg, 2001), and *Cognitive-Behavioral Intervention for Trauma in Schools* (Stein et al., 2003) as effective evidence-based approaches. Rolfsnes and Idsoe (2011) conducted a meta-analysis of school-based interventions for PTSD; they concluded that those employing CBT strategies had the most support (with others demonstrating promising results as well).

Conclusion

Disaster preparedness and trauma-response teams represent an increasingly visible and important presence across local, state, federal, and international agencies. MedFTs—equipped with behavioral and relational skills in working with individuals, couples, and families (alongside BPSS understandings of trauma per se)—are well equipped to engage in this work. Emerging evidence supports their systems-informed contributions, and—as behavioral health foci are progressively more valued in response and recovery efforts—MedFTs' participation across multiple and overlapping foci in disaster preparedness and response will continue to grow.

Reflection Questions
1. As a MedFT who is already busy with clinical, teaching, and/or research commitments, how can you effectively plan so that you are ready and able to deploy on a disaster response team?
2. Efforts in self-care and compassion fatigue prevention are especially important for providers engaged in disaster relief efforts. What are some strategies and methods that would be especially important and/or helpful for you to do so as to best maintain your own BPSS health?
3. How would you most appropriately respond to a request to do an interview with a local news station after returning from a deployment? How about a request from your boss, department head, major professor, or colleague to do a presentation in your academic department or clinical site?

Glossary of Important Terms in Disaster Response

After action report (AAR) A retrospective analysis regarding a simulated or actual disaster response sequence. Key content generally includes a summary and overview of the response, major strengths and successes of the effort, key weaknesses and lessons learned, and recommendations for improvement.
Family Assistance Center (FAC) A site set up to provide resources and support for families affected by a disaster. Principal goals include facilitating effective communication about evolving events, exchanging information with appropriate personnel to assist in identifying missing or deceased loved ones, providing death notifications (and discussions with medical examiners regarding the release of human remains), providing private spaces for families to grieve, protection from media and/or curiosity seekers, and offering medical, psychological, and/or logistical support.
Just-in-time training (JIT) A collection of online or app-based resources designed to train (or refresh knowledge of) responders rapidly. These resources are generally employed immediately after a disaster has occurred, during which time responders are preparing for—or awaiting directions relevant to—deployment.
Nongovernmental organization (NGO) A nonprofit organization involved in a disaster response that is independent from state, federal, or international governance. NGOs are usually funded by donations and run by volunteers.
Point of contact (POC) Identified supervisor to whom a person involved in a disaster response reports with relevant updates, field reports, troubleshooting, and questions. The POC directs personnel under his or her watch regarding indicated tasks, duties, and responsibilities.
Tabletop exercise (TTX) During trainings and/or simulations, TTXs involve key and indicated personnel discussing how to best respond to hypothetical scenarios. These sequences facilitate understanding regarding the viability and adequacy of plans and procedures vis-à-vis extant resources. They also serve to establish and promote collaborative relationships and agreements between agency leads that can be utilized during an actual incident.

Additional Resources

Literature

Beach, M. (2010). *Disaster preparedness and management*. Philadelphia, PA: F.A. Davis Co.

Jacobs, G. (2016). *Community-based psychological first aid: A practical guide to helping individuals and communities during difficult times*. Cambridge, MA: Butterworth-Heinemann.

U.S. Department of Veterans Affairs. (2006). *Psychological first aid: Field operations guide* (2nd ed.). National Child Traumatic Stress Network and National Center for PTSD. Retrieved from http://www.ptsd.va.gov/professional/manuals/psych-first-aid.asp

World Health Organization. (2011). *Psychological first aid: Guide for field workers*. Geneva, Switzerland: United Nations.

Measures/Instruments

Columbia-Suicide Severity Rating Scale (C-SSRS). http://www.integration.samhsa.gov/clinical-practice/Columbia_Suicide_Severity_Rating_Scale.pdf

Life Events Checklist (LEC). http://www.integration.samhsa.gov/clinical-practice/life-event-checklist-lec.pdf

Professional Quality of Life Measure (Version 5). http://www.proqol.org/uploads/ProQOL5_English.pdf

Suicide Assessment Five-step Evaluation and Triage (SAFE-T). http://www.integration.samhsa.gov/images/res/SAFE_T.pdf

Trauma-informed Care in Behavioral Health Service. http://www.integration.samhsa.gov/clinical-practice/SAMSA_TIP_Trauma.pdf

UCLA Child/Adolescent PTSD Reaction Index for DSM-5. https://www.ptsd.va.gov/professional/assessment/child/ucla_child_reaction_dsm-5.asp

Organizations/Associations

American Red Cross. http://www.redcross.org/
Department of Homeland Security. https://www.dhs.gov/
Federal Emergency Management Administration. www.fema.gov
Green Cross Academy of Traumatology. http://greencross.org/
International Committee of the Red Cross. https://www.icrc.org/
International Critical Incident Stress Foundation. https://www.icisf.org/
National Child Traumatic Stress Network. http://www.nctsn.org/
National Incident Management System. http://www.fema.gov/national-incident-management-system

References[1]

Adler, A., Bliese, P., McGurk, D., Hoge, C., & Castro, C. (2009). Battlemind debriefing and battlemind training as early interventions with soldiers returning from Iraq: Randomization by platoon. *Journal of Consulting and Clinical Psychology, 77*, 928–940. https://doi.org/10.1037/a0016877

Adler, A., Litz, B., Castro, C., Suvak, M., Thomas, J., Burrell, L, ... Bliese, P. (2008). A group randomized trial of critical incident stress debriefing provided to U.S. peacekeepers. *Journal of Traumatic Stress, 21*, 253–263. https://doi.org/10.1002/jts.20342.

*Agency for Healthcare Research and Quality. (2011). *Disaster response tools and resources*. Retrieved from http://archive.ahrq.gov/path/katrina.htm

Agorastos, A., Marmar, C., & Otte, C. (2011). Immediate and early behavioral interventions for the prevention of acute and posttraumatic stress disorder. *Current Opinion in Psychiatry, 24*, 526–532. https://doi.org/10.1097/YCO.0b013e32834cdde2

Angus, L. (2012). Toward an integrative understanding of narrative and emotion processes in emotion-focused therapy of depression: Implications for theory, research and practice. *Psychotherapy Research, 22*, 367–380. https://doi.org/10.1080/10503307.2012.683988

Alexander, J. F., Waldron, H. B., Robbins, M. S., & Neeb, A. A. (2013). *Functional family therapy for adolescent behavior problems*. Washington, DC: American Psychological Association.

Amaya-Jackson, L., Reynolds, V., Murray, M., McCarthy, G., Nelson, A., Cherney, M ... March, J. (2003) Cognitive-behavioral treatment for pediatric posttraumatic stress disorder: Protocol and application in school and community settings. *Cognitive and Behavioral Practice, 10*, 204–213. https://doi.org/10.1016/S1077-7229(03)80032-9.

American Red Cross. (2016). *Recovering emotionally*. Retrieved from http://www.redcross.org/find-help/disaster-recovery/recovering-emotionally

Association of Professional Chaplains. (2016). *Healing through spiritual care*. Retrieved from http://www.professionalchaplains.org/content.asp

Baird, M. (2010). *The "phases" of emergency management*. Paper prepared for the Intermodal Freight Transportation Institute. University of Memphis. Retrieved from http://www.vanderbilt.edu/vector/research/emmgtphases.pdf

*Beach, M. (2010). *Disaster preparedness and management*. Philadelphia, PA: F.A. Davis Co.

Berman, A., Jobes, D., & Silverman, M. (2006). *Adolescent suicide: Assessment and intervention*. Washington, DC: American Psychological Association.

Bigley, G. A., & Roberts, K. H. (2001). The incident command system: High reliability of organizing for complex and volatile task environments. *Academy of Management Journal, 44*, 1281–1300. https://doi.org/10.2307/3069401

Bisson, J., Jenkins, P., Alexander, J., & Bannister, C. (1997). Randomised controlled trial of psychological debriefing for victims of acute burn trauma. *British Journal of Psychiatry, 171*, 78–81. https://doi.org/10.1192/bjp.171.1.78

Bisson, J., McFarlane, A., Rose, S., Ruzek, J., & Watson, P. (2009). Psychological debriefing for adults. In E. Foa, T. Keane, M. Friedman, and J. Cohen (Eds.), *Effective treatments for PTSD* (pp. 83–105). New York, NY: Guilford Press.

*Boss, P. (2006). *Loss, trauma, and resilience: Therapeutic work with ambiguous loss*. New York, NY: WW Norton & Company.

Boyd-Franklin, N., & Bry, B. (2012). *Reaching out in family therapy: Home-based, school, and community interventions*. New York, NY: Guilford Press.

Brave Heart, M. Y. H., Chase, J., Elkins, J., & Altschul, D. B. (2011). Historical trauma among indigenous peoples of the Americas: Concepts, research, and clinical considerations. *Journal of Psychoactive Drugs, 43*, 282–290. https://doi.org/10.1080/02791072.2011.628913

Bryant, R., Harvey, A., Dang, S., Sackville, T., & Basten, C. (1998). Treatment of acute stress disorder: A comparison of cognitive-behavioral therapy and supportive counseling. *Journal of Consulting and Clinical Psychology, 66*, 862–866. https://doi.org/10.1037/0022-006X.66.5.862

---

[1] [Note: References that are prefaced with an asterisk are recommended readings.]

Bryant, R., Moulds, M., & Nixon, R. (2006). Hypnotherapy and cognitive behavior therapy of acute stress disorder: A three year follow-up. *Behaviour Research and Therapy, 44*, 1331–1335. https://doi.org/10.1016/j.brat.2005.04.007

Buck, D. A., Trainor, J. E., & Aguirre, B. E. (2006). A critical evaluation of the incident command system and NIMS. *Journal of Homeland Security and Emergency Management, 3*, 1–29. https://doi.org/10.2202/1547-7355.1252

Buckle, P., Marsh, G., & Smale, S. (2003). Reframing risk, hazards, disasters, and daily life: A report of research into local appreciation of risks and threats. *Australian Journal of Emergency Management, 18*, 81–87. Retrieved from http://www.ijmed.org/articles/579/download/

Butler, A. S., Panzer, A. M., & Goldfrank, L. R. (Eds.). (2003). *Preparing for the psychological consequences of terrorism: A public health strategy*. Washington, DC: National Academies Press.

Campfield, K., & Hills, A. (2001). Effect of timing of critical incident stress debriefing (CISD) on posttraumatic symptoms. *Journal of Traumatic Stress, 14*, 327–340. https://doi.org/10.1023/A:1011117018705

Centers for Disease Control and Prevention. (2016). *About CDC and the US public health system*. Retrieved from http://www.cdc.gov/stltpublichealth/about/index.html

*Cohen, J. A., Mannarino, A. P., & Deblinger, E. (2016). *Treating trauma and traumatic grief in children and adolescents*. New York, NY: Guilford Press.

Deahl, M., Srinivasan, M., Jones, N., Thomas, J., Neblett, C., & Jolly, A. (2000). Preventing psychological trauma in soldiers: The role of operational stress training and psychological debriefing. *British Journal of Medical Psychology, 73*, 77–85. https://doi.org/10.1348/000711200160318

Department of Homeland Security. (2016a). *NIMS: Frequently asked questions*. Retrieved from https://www.fema.gov/pdf/emergency/nims/nimsfaqs.pdf

Department of Homeland Security. (2016b). *What is NIMS?* Retrieved from https://www.nh.gov/safety/divisions/hsem/documents/NIMSQA1305.pdf

Department of Homeland Security. (2016c). *National Incident Management System*. Retrieved from http://www.fema.gov/national-incident-management-system

Department of Homeland Security. (2016d). *Plan and prepare for disasters*. Retrieved from https://www.dhs.gov/topic/plan-and-prepare-disasters

Devilly, G. (2002). The psychological effects of a lifestyle management course on war veterans and their spouses. *Journal of Clinical Psychology, 58*, 1119–1134. https://doi.org/10.1002/jclp.10041

Ehlers, A., Clark, D., Hackmann, A., McManus, F., Fennell, M., Herbert, C., & Mayou, R. (2003). A randomized controlled trial of cognitive therapy, a self-help booklet, and repeated assessments as early interventions for posttraumatic stress disorder. *Archives of General Psychiatry, 60*, 1024–1032. https://doi.org/10.1001/archpsyc.60.10.1024

Ehlers, A., Hackmann, A., Grey, N., Wild, J., Liness, S., Albert, I., … & Clark, D. M. (2014). A randomized controlled trial of 7-day intensive and standard weekly cognitive therapy for PTSD and emotion-focused supportive therapy. *American Journal of Psychiatry, 171*, 294–304. https://doi.org/10.1176/appi.ajp.2013.13040552.

EMDR International Association. (2017). *Frequently asked questions*. Retrieved from https://emdria.site-ym.com/?page=5

Engel, J. D., Zarconi, J., Pethtel, L. L., & Missimi, S. A. (2008). *Narrative in health care: Healing patients, practitioners, profession, and community*. Oxon, UK: Radcliffe Publishing.

Engel, G. L. (1977). The need for a new medical model: A challenge for biomedicine. *Science, 196*, 129–136. https://doi.org/10.1016/b978-0-409-95009-0.50006-1

Engel, G. L. (1980). The clinical application of the biopsychosocial model. *American Journal of Family Medicine, 137*, 535–544. https://doi.org/10.1176/ajp.137.5.535

Everly, G., Flannery, R., & Eyler, V. (2002). Critical incident stress management: A statistical review of the literature. *Psychiatric Quarterly, 73*, 171–182. https://doi.org/10.1023/A:1016068003615

Everly, G. S., Flannery, R. B., & Mitchell, J. T. (2000). Critical incident stress management (CISM): A review of the literature. *Aggression and Violent Behavior*, *5*, 23–40. https://doi.org/10.1016/S1359-1789(98)00026-3

Fantini-Hauwel, C., Dovi, E., & Antoine, P. (2015). Validation of the short-cognitive inventory of subjective distress (S-CISD). *International Psychogeriatrics*, *27*, 261–266. https://doi.org/10.1017/S104161021400194X

Fassaert, T., van Dulmen, S., Schellevis, F., & Bensing, J. (2007). Active listening in medical consultations: Development of the Active Listening Observation Scale (ALOS-global). *Patient Education and Counseling*, *68*, 258–264. https://doi.org/10.1016/j.pec.2007.06.011

Federal Emergency Management Administration. (2011). *A whole community approach to emergency management: Principles, themes, and pathways for action*. Retrieved from https://www.fema.gov/media-library-data/20130726-1813-25045-0649/whole_community_dec2011__2_.pdf

Federal Emergency Management Administration. (2013). *Crisis counseling: Psychological first aid*. Retrieved from http://www.fema.gov/disaster/4085/updates/crisis-counseling-psychological-first-aid

Figley, C., & Figley, K. (2009). Stemming the tide of trauma systemically: The role of family therapy. *Australian and New Zealand Journal of Family Therapy*, *30*, 173–183. http://dx.doi.org.ezp1.lib.umn.edu/10.1375/anft.30.3.173

Foa, E. B., Stein, D. J., & McFarlane, A. C. (2006). Symptomatology and psychopathology of mental health problems after disaster. *Journal of Clinical Psychiatry*, *67*, 15–25.

Foa, E., Zoellner, L., & Feeny, N. (2006). An evaluation of three brief programs for facilitating recovery after assault. *Journal of Traumatic Stress*, *19*, 29–43. https://doi.org/10.1002/jts.20096

Fox, J. H., Burkle, F. M., Bass, J., Pia, F. A., Epstein, J. L., & Markenson, D. (2012). The effectiveness of psychological first aid as a disaster intervention tool: Research analysis of peer-reviewed literature from 1990–2010. *Disaster Medicine and Public Health Preparedness*, *6*, 247–252. https://doi.org/10.1001/dmp.2012.39

Gehart, D. R., & McCollum, E. E. (2007). Engaging suffering: Towards a mindful re-visioning of family therapy practice. *Journal of Marital and Family Therapy*, *33*, 214–226. https://doi.org/10.1111/j.1752-0606.2007.00017.x

Gewirtz, A., Forgatch, M., & Wieling, E. (2008). Parenting practices as potential mechanisms for child adjustment following mass trauma. *Journal of Marital and Family Therapy*, *34*, 177–192. https://doi.org/10.1111/j.1752-0606.2008.00063.x

Grainger, R., Levin, C., Allen-Byrd, L., Doctor, R., & Lee, H. (1997). An empirical evaluation of eye movement desensitization and reprocessing (EMDR) with survivors of a natural disaster. *Journal of Traumatic Stress*, *10*, 665–671. https://doi.org/10.1023/A:1024806105473

Green, B. L. (1996). Cross-national and ethnocultural issues in disaster research. In A. J. Marsella, M. J. Friedman, E. Gerrity, and R. M. Scurfield (Eds.), *Ethnocultural aspects of posttraumatic stress disorder: Issues, research and applications* (pp. 341–361). Washington, DC: American Psychological Association Press.

Haagen, J. F., Smid, G. E., Knipscheer, J. W., & Kleber, R. J. (2015). The efficacy of recommended treatments for veterans with PTSD: A metaregression analysis. *Clinical Psychology Review*, *40*, 184–194. https://doi.org/10.1016/j.cpr.2015.06.008

Hawker, D., Durkin, J., & Hawker, D. (2011). To debrief or not to debrief our heroes: That is the question. *Clinical Psychology & Psychotherapy*, *18*, 453–463. https://doi.org/10.1002/cpp.730

Hodgson, J., Lamson, A., Mendenhall, T., & Tyndall, L. (2014). Introduction to Medical family therapy: Advanced applications. In J. Hodgson, A. Lamson, T. Mendenhall., and D. Crane, (Eds.). *Medical family therapy: Advanced applications* (pp. 1–9). New York, NY: Springer.

Hoshmand, L. (2007). Cross-cultural assessment of psychological trauma and PTSD. *International and Cultural Psychology*, *1*, 31–50. https://doi.org/10.1007/978-0-387-70990-1_2

Hughes, A. L., & Palen, L. (2012). The evolving role of the public information officer: An examination of social media in emergency management. *Journal of Homeland Security and Emergency Management*, *9*, 1–20. https://doi.org/10.1515/1547-7355.1976

International Critical Incident Stress Foundation. (2016). *ICISF, Inc.: Helping save the heroes.* Retrieved from https://www.icisf.org/

*Jacobs, G. (2016). *Community-based psychological first aid: A practical guide to helping individuals and communities during difficult times.* Cambridge, MA: Butterworth-Heinemann.

Jarero, I., Artigas, L., & Luber, M. (2011). The EMDR protocol for recent critical incidents: Application in a disaster mental health continuum of care context. *Journal of EMDR Practice and Research, 5,* 82–94. https://doi.org/10.1891/1933-3196.5.3.82

Joint Commission on the Accreditation of Healthcare Organizations. (2016). *The joint commission.* Retrieved from https://www.jointcommission.org/

Johnson, S. (2002). *Emotionally focused couple therapy with trauma survivors: Strengthening attachment bonds.* New York, NY: Guilford Press.

*Johnson, S. (2012). *The practice of emotionally focused couple therapy: Creating connection.* New York, NY: Routledge.

Joyner, J. (2016). *What is the difference between a chaplain and a pastor?* Retrieved from http://work.chron.com/difference-between-chaplain-pastor-5956.html

Kaji, A. H., Langford, V., & Lewis, R. J. (2008). Assessing hospital disaster preparedness: A comparison of an on-site survey, directly observed drill performance, and video analysis of teamwork. *Annals of Emergency Medicine, 52,* 195–201. https://doi.org/10.1016/j.annemergmed.2007.10.026

Kataoka, S., Langley, A., Wong, M., Baweja, S., & Stein, B. (2012). Responding to students with posttraumatic stress disorder in schools. *Child and Adolescent Psychiatric Clinics of North America, 21,* 119–133. https://doi.org/10.1016/j.chc.2011.08.009

Kennedy, A. (2008). *Opening school doors to MFTs. Counseling Today (on-line article).* Retrieved from https://ct.counseling.org/2008/01/opening-school-doors-to-mfts/

Lambert, M. J., & Barley, D. E. (2001). Research summary on the therapeutic relationship and psychotherapy outcome. *Psychotherapy, 38,* 357–361. https://doi.org/10.1037/0033-3204.38.4.357

Landau, J., Mittal, M., & Wieling, E. (2008). Linking human systems: Strengthening individuals, families and communities in the wake of mass trauma. *Journal of Marital and Family Therapy, 34,* 193–209. https://doi.org/10.1111/j.1752-0606.2008.00064.x

Larkin, G. L. (2010). The ethics of teamwork in disaster management. *Virtual Mentor, 12,* 495–501. Retrieved from http://journalofethics.ama-assn.org/2010/06/oped1-1006.html

Laundy, K. (2015). Family therapy in schools. *Family Therapy Magazine, 14,* 52–27. Retrieved from https://www.aamft.org/imis15/Documents/JFFTMSINGLEPAGEreduce.pdf

Levitt, D. H. (2002). Active listening and counselor self-efficacy: Emphasis on one microskill in beginning counselor training. *The Clinical Supervisor, 20,* 101–115. https://doi.org/10.1300/J001v20n02_09

Lichterman, J. D. (2000). A "community as resource" strategy for disaster response. *Public Health Reports, 115,* 262–265. Retrieved from file:///C:/Users/mend0009/Downloads/pubhealthrep00022-0160.pdf

Litz, B. (2008). Early intervention for trauma: Where are we and where do we need to go? A commentary. *Journal of Traumatic Stress, 21,* 503–506. https://doi.org/10.1002/jts.20373

Litz, B., & Bryant, R. (2009). Early cognitive-behavior interventions for adults. In E. Foa, T. Keane, M. Friedman, and J. Cohen (Eds.), *Effective treatments for PTSD* (pp. 117–135). New York, NY: Guilford Press.

Makin-Byrd, K., Gifford, E., McCutcheon, S., & Glynn, S. (2011). Family and couples treatment for newly returning veterans. *Professional Psychology: Research and Practice, 42,* 47–55. https://doi.org/10.1037/a0022292

Mangeri, A. (2015). Defining and working with 21st century mass media. *Domestic Preparedness* (May Issue). Retrieved from http://www.domesticpreparedness.com/First_Responder/Emergency_Management/Defining_%26_Working_With_21st_Century_Mass_Media/

Marsella, A. J., & Christopher, M. A. (2004). Ethnocultural considerations in disasters: An overview of research issues and directions. *Psychiatric Clinics of North America, 27,* 521–539. https://doi.org/10.1016/j.psc.2004.03.011

Mayou, R., Ehlers, A., & Hobbs, M. (2000). Psychological debriefing for road traffic accident victims: Three-year follow-up of a randomised controlled trial. *British Journal of Psychiatry, 176*, 589–593. https://doi.org/10.1192/bjp.176.6.589

*Mendenhall, T. (2006). Trauma-response teams: Inherent challenges and practical strategies in interdisciplinary fieldwork. *Families, Systems & Health, 24*, 357–362. https://doi.org/10.1037/1091-7527.24.3.357.

*Mendenhall, T., & Berge, J. (2010). Family therapists in trauma-response teams: Bringing systems thinking into interdisciplinary fieldwork. *Journal of Family Therapy, 32*, 43–57. https://doi.org/10.1111/j.1467-6427.2009.00482.x.

Mock, C. (Ed.). (2004). *Guidelines for essential trauma care*. Geneva, Switzerland: World Health Organization.

Monson, C., Fredman, S., Adair, K., Stevens, S., Resick, P., Schnurr, P. ... Macdonald, A. (2011). Cognitive–behavioral conjoint therapy for PTSD: Pilot results from a community sample, *Journal of Traumatic Stress, 24*, 97–101. https://doi.org/10.1002/jts.20604.

Mollica, R. F. (1988). The trauma story: The psychiatric care of refugee survivors of violence and torture. In F. Ochberg (Ed.), *Post-traumatic therapy and victims of violence* (pp. 295–314). New York, NY: Brunner/Mazel.

Morse, J. M., Bottorff, J., Anderson, G., O'Brien, B., & Solberg, S. (2006). Beyond empathy: Expanding expressions of caring. *Journal of Advanced Nursing, 53*, 75–87. https://doi.org/10.1111/j.1365-2648.2006.03677.x

Najavits, L. M., & Hien, D. (2013). Helping vulnerable populations: A comprehensive review of the treatment outcome literature on substance use disorder and PTSD. *Journal of Clinical Psychology, 69*, 433–479. https://doi.org/10.1002/jclp.21980

*National Child Traumatic Stress Network. (2006). *Psychological first aid: Field operations guide* (2nd ed.). Retrieved from http://www.nctsn.org/sites/default/files/pfa/english/1-psyfirstaid:final_complete_manual.pdf

National Disaster Interfaiths Network. (2007). *NDIN: Connect with a network of experienced trainers, disaster human services, & IT consultants*. Retrieved from http://www.n-din.org/

Niles, B. L., Klunk-Gillis, J., Ryngala, D. J., Silberbogen, A. K., Paysnick, A., & Wolf, E. J. (2012). Comparing mindfulness and psychoeducation treatments for combat-related PTSD using a telehealth approach. *Psychological Trauma: Theory, Research, Practice, and Policy, 4*, 538–547. https://doi.org/10.1037/a0026161

North American Mission Board. (2016). *Chaplaincy: Do you have a heart of compassion?* Retrieved from https://www.namb.net/chaplaincy/index

North, C., & Pfefferbaum, B. (2013). Mental health response to community disasters: A systematic review. *Journal of the American Medical Association, 310*, 507–518. https://doi.org/10.1001/jama.2013.107799

Peltier, T. R., & Peltier, J. (2016). *Complete guide to CISM certification*. New York, NY: Auerbach Publications.

PHS Commissioned Officers Foundation. (2010). *Public health emergency preparedness & response: Principles & practice*. Landover, MD: PHS Commissioned Officers Foundation for the Advancement of Public Health.

Puchalski, C. M. (2001). The role of spirituality in health care. *Baylor University Medical Center Proceedings, 14*, 352–357. Retrieved from http://crawl.prod.proquest.com.s3.amazonaws.com/fpcache/8c6be7a4148f50f9ecc424cee948b167.pdf?AWSAccessKeyId=AKIAJF7V7KNV2KKY2NUQ&Expires=1474573911&Signature=Ka2UbJWLRUqC%2BglN5nyZaCaywQU%3D

Pynoos, R. S., & Nader, K. (1988). Psychological first aid and treatment approach to children exposed to community violence: Research implications. *Journal of Traumatic Stress, 1*, 445–473. https://doi.org/10.1002/jts.2490010406

Rabstejnek, C. V. (2014). *Evaluating the efficacy of critical incident stress debriefing: A look at the evidence*. Retrieved from http://www.houd.info/CISD.pdf

Reilly, M. J., & Markenson, D. S. (2010). *Health care emergency management: Principles and practice*. Sudbury, MA: Jones & Bartlett Publishers.

Roberts, N., Kitchiner, N., Kenardy, J., & Bisson, J. (2010). Multiple session early psychological interventions for the prevention of post-traumatic stress disorder (Review). *Cochrane Database of Systematic Reviews, 2009*. Hoboken, NJ: Wiley.

Roberston, K. (2005). Active listening: More than just paying attention. *Australian Family Physician, 34*, 1053–1055. Retrieved from http://www.ncbi.nlm.nih.gov/pubmed/16333490

Robinson, R. (2007). Commentary on Issues in the debriefing debate for the emergency services: Moving research outcomes rorward. *Clinical Psychology: Science and Practice 14*, 121–123. https://doi.org/10.1111/j.1468-2850.2007.00071.x

Robinson, R. (2008). Reflections on the debriefing debate. *International Journal of Emergency Mental Health, 10*, 253–259. Retrieved from http://www.omicsonline.com/open-access/from-controversy-to-confirmation-crisis-support-services-for-the-twentyfirst-century.pdf#page=13

Rolfsnes, E., & Idsoe, T. (2011). School-based intervention program for PTSD symptoms: A review and meta-analysis. *Journal of Traumatic Stress, 24*, 155–165. https://doi.org/10.1002/jts.20622

Rose, S., Brewin, C., Andrews, A., & Kirk, M. (1999). A randomized controlled trial of psychological debriefing for victims of violent crime. *Psychological Medicine, 29*, 793–799. Retrieved from http://www.ncbi.nlm.nih.gov/pubmed/10473306

Rubin, C. B. (Ed.). (2012). *Emergency management: The American experience 1900–2010* (2nd ed.). New York, NY: CRC Press.

Ruzek, J. I., Brymer, M. J., Jacobs, A. K., Layne, C. M., Vernberg, E. M., & Watson, P. J. (2007). Psychological first aid. *Journal of Mental Health Counseling, 29*, 17–49. 10.17744/mehc.29.1.5racqxjueafabgwp

Salloum, A., & Overstreet, S. (2012). Grief and trauma intervention for children after disaster: Exploring coping skills versus trauma narration. *Behaviour Research and Therapy, 50*, 169–179. https://doi.org/10.1016/j.brat.2012.01.001

Saltzman, W., Pynoos, R., Layne, C., Steinberg, A., & Aisenberg, E. (2001). Trauma and grief-focused intervention for adolescents exposed to community violence: Results of a school-based screening and group treatment protocol. *Group Dynamics: Theory, Research, and Practice, 5*, 291–303. https://doi.org/10.1037/1089-2699.5.4.291

Sautter, F., Armelie, A., Glynn, S., & Wielt, D. (2011). The development of a couple-based treatment for PTSD in returning veterans. *Professional Psychology: Research and Practice, 42*, 63–69. https://doi.org/10.1037/a0022323

Shah, S. (2007). Ethnomedical best practices for international psychosocial efforts in disaster and trauma. *Cross-Cultural Assessment of Psychological Trauma and PTSD International and Cultural Psychology, 1*, 51–64. https://doi.org/10.1007/978-0-387-70990-1_3

Shapiro, E. (2009). EMDR treatment of recent trauma. *Journal of EMDR Practice and Research, 3*, 141–151. https://doi.org/10.1891/1933-3196.3.3.141

Shapiro, E., & Laub, B. (2008). Early EMDR intervention (EEI): A summary, a theoretical model, and the recent traumatic episode protocol (R-TEP). *Journal of EMDR Practice and Research, 2*, 79–96. https://doi.org/10.1891/1933-3196.2.2.79

Sherman, M. (2003). The SAFE program: A family psychoeducational curriculum developed in a Veterans Affairs medical center. *Professional Psychology: Research and Practice, 34*, 42–48. https://doi.org/10.1037/0735-7028.34.1.42

Sijbrandij, M., Olff, M., Reitsma, J., Carlier, I., & Gersons, B. (2006). Emotional or educational debriefing after psychological trauma: Randomised controlled trial. *British Journal of Psychiatry, 189*, 150–155. https://doi.org/10.1192/bjp.bp.105.021121

Silver, S., Rogers, S., Knipe, J., & Colelli, G. (2005). EMDR therapy following the 9/11 terrorist attacks: A community-based intervention project in New York City. *International Journal of Stress Management, 12*, 29–42. https://doi.org/10.1037/1072-5245.12.1.29

Simon, R. I., & Hales, R. E. (Eds.). (2012). *Textbook of suicide assessment and management* (2nd ed.). Washington, DC: American Psychiatric Publishing.

Stein, B., Jaycox, L., Kataoka, S., Wong, M., Tu, W., Elliott, M., & Fink, A. (2003). A mental health intervention for schoolchildren exposed to violence: A randomized controlled trial. *Journal of the American Medical Association, 290*, 603–611. https://doi.org/10.1001/jama.290.5.603

Summerfield, D. (2004). Cross-cultural perspectives on the medicalization of human suffering. In G. M. Rosen (Ed.), *Posttraumatic stress disorder: Issues and controversies* (pp. 233–245). New York, NY: Wiley.
University of Minnesota Academic Health Center. (2017). *Reunification and family assistance center training exercise: After action report*. Minneapolis, MN: UMN/AHC Office of Emergency Response.
U.S. Department of Health and Human Services. (2016). *Commissioned corps of the US Public Health Service: America's health responders*. Retrieved from http://usphs.gov/aboutus/agencies/hhs.aspx
*U.S. Department of Veterans Affairs. (2006). *Psychological first aid: Field operations guide* (2nd ed.). National Child Traumatic Stress Network and National Center for PTSD. Retrieved from http://www.ptsd.va.gov/professional/manuals/psych-first-aid.asp
U.S. Fire Administration. (2016). *Working for a fire-safe America*. Retrieved from https://www.usfa.fema.gov/
Vernberg, E. M., Steinberg, A. M., Jacobs, A. K., Brymer, M. J., Watson, P. J., Osofsky, J. D., … Ruzek, J. I. (2008). Innovations in disaster mental health: Psychological first aid. *Professional Psychology: Research and Practice, 39*, 381–388. https://doi.org/10.1037/a0012663
Voluntary Organizations Active in Disaster. (2016). *Who we are*. Retrieved from http://www.nvoad.org/about-us/
Wagner, S. L. (2005). Emergency response service personnel and the critical incident stress debriefing debate. *International Journal of Emergency Mental Health, 7*, 33–41. Retrieved from http://psycnet.apa.org/psycinfo/2005-04527-006
*Walsh, F. (2007). Traumatic loss and major disasters: Strengthening family and community resilience. *Family Process, 46*, 207–227. https://doi.org/10.1111/j.1545-5300.2007.00205.x
*Watson, P. J. (2015). How different is psychological first aid from other psychotherapeutic modalities? In G. Quitangon and M. Evces (Eds.), *Vicarious trauma and disaster mental health: Understanding risks and promoting resilience* (pp. 61–72). New York, NY: Routledge.
Wei, Y., Szumilas, M., & Kutcher, S. (2010). Effectiveness on mental health of psychological debriefing for crisis intervention in schools. *Educational Psychology Review, 22*, 339–347. https://doi.org/10.1007/s10648-010-9139-2
*World Health Organization. (2011). *Psychological first aid: Guide for field workers*. Geneva, Switzerland: United Nations.
Wright, L. M., Watson, W. L., & Bell, J. M. (1996). *Beliefs: The heart of healing in families and illness*. New York, NY: Basic Books.

Chapter 16
Medical Family Therapy in Spiritual Care

Jonathan Wilson, Jennifer Hodgson, Eunicia Jones, and Grace Wilson

Religious and spiritual concerns often play an important role in patients' and their families' healthcare decisions. As a whole, Americans are a highly religious people; 89% report believing in God, with 75% indicating that religion is "fairly" or "very" important in their lives. Almost as many (73%) say that they try hard to incorporate their faith into all areas of life (Curlin, Lantos, Roach, Sellergren, & Chin, 2005; Gallup, 2017). Medical and behavioral communities are increasingly recognizing religion and spirituality as fundamental components of health and well-being (Oh & Kim, 2014; Yanez et al., 2009). Multiple research teams have demonstrated positive effects of each on physical and mental health (e.g., George, Ellison, & Larson, 2002; Hill & Pargament, 2003; Thorensen, Harris, & Onan, 2001). And while the terms "religion" and "spirituality" share some overlapping components, and are often used interchangeably, they are formally defined in different ways (see Glossary). In healthcare, as throughout this chapter, the term "spirituality" is preferred because it better encapsulates personal experiences of faith.

Medical family therapists (MedFTs) who will be assessing for and/or providing spiritual care must acquire specialized areas of knowledge and skills to be effective in their work. The purpose of this chapter is to examine the role of MedFTs and spiri-

---

J. Wilson (✉)
Department of Behavioral and Social Sciences, Oklahoma Baptist University, Shawnee, OK, USA
e-mail: jonathan.wilson@okbu.edu

J. Hodgson · E. Jones
Department of Human Development and Family Science, East Carolina University, Greenville, NC, USA

G. Wilson
Great Plains Family Medicine Residency Program, Oklahoma City, OK, USA

tual care within the healthcare system, including opportunities for collaboration with chaplains (described below) and other key members of the treatment team. The following vignette is provided to illustrate a typical patient encounter involving a chaplain, surgeon, and MedFT who work together in a large metropolitan hospital setting.

Clinical Vignette
[Note: This vignette is a compilation of cases that represent treatment in spiritual care. All patients' names and/or identifying information have been changed to maintain confidentiality.]

Mark begins his day as any other—completing case notes while drinking coffee and planning out his patient encounter schedule for the day. A chaplain for 23 years, he typically spends his mornings at a local suburban hospice and his afternoons visiting hospital patients and their providers.

A self-identified Christian, Mark is prepared to assist with the spiritual needs of patients from a variety of faith-belief systems. At the hospice facility, he regularly delivers the Lord's Prayer with Catholic patients and their families and is able to consult with a priest to deliver the Eucharist if requested. With Muslim families, he routinely reads passages from the Qur'an and is mindful of the cultural preference of Muslim men and women for Muslim women to meet with male providers only in the presence of their husbands. With Christian families, though very familiar with beliefs and practices of the Christian faith, Mark does not assume that the religious/spiritual experiences of his patients are the same as his own. During times of unfamiliarity with patients' spiritual beliefs and practices, Mark allows patients and families to educate him about their belief systems. He also requests guidance from the family about how to best support their spiritual needs and preferences.

While on rounds at the hospital, Mark meets with David and his wife Carol. David is a 56-year-old Caucasian, Christian male. He is a recent below-the-knee amputee (BKA) admitted for wound healing challenges that could not be successfully managed with outpatient treatment. He has not been caring for his post-op wounds as directed, which is further complicating the healing process. David's surgeon, Dr. Harris, informs Mark that since his operation 6 weeks ago (due to complications resulting from diabetes), David has been depressed and unwilling to eat. Although David had met with Christine, the MedFT on staff, Dr. Harris indicates that many of David's concerns are spiritual in nature. Specifically, David keeps engaging in self-deprecating thought patterns centered around his previous lifestyle choices—particularly his poor diet and lack of exercise. He (David) believes that his diabetes is a "punishment from God" for his unhealthy lifestyle despite being warned by his family and medical providers that such a lifestyle would eventually catch up to him.

Dr. Harris seems frustrated with David's "noncompliance" and requests Mark's assistance. During their encounter, David requests that Mark pray

> with him as he struggles with the imminent realities of living without his lower left leg. Furthermore, David considers his own refusal of food to be "punishment" for his self-perceived life choices that led to the eventual decline of his health and loss of his leg. Before praying with David and Carol, Mark gently and empathically reminds David of the power of forgiveness that is offered through his faith in Jesus and encourages David to consider moving toward self-forgiveness. Additionally, Mark encourages Carol to express her own forgiveness to David.
>
> Later that day, Dr. Harris and Mark schedule a family meeting to collaborate with Christine. As a team, Dr. Harris, Mark, and Christine work with the Harris family to make sure that David's multiple needs are being met. A comprehensive biopsychosocial-spiritual (BPSS) plan is established, including (a) routine individual and family therapy sessions with Christine; (b) a medication regimen involving a selective serotonin reuptake inhibitor (SSRI) if symptoms persist; (c) spiritual consults, prayer, and/or scripture reading with Mark and Carol and their local pastor as needed; and (d) a referral to an online support group for adults living with physical disabilities. With this plan in place, David expresses hope and optimism about his future for the first time since his surgery. He also agrees to begin eating again. He communicates, too, that he is looking forward to the mobility that his prosthesis will provide once his wound heals.

What Is Spiritual Care?

Social trends suggest that the recognition and valuing of spirituality in modern healthcare is growing, even in the absence of concomitant increases in institutional religious participation (Vanderwerker et al., 2008). Healthcare teams are working to address—or at least be prepared to address—the spiritual needs and concerns of patients across multiple system levels (McClung, Grossoehme, & Jacobson, 2006). Chaplains and other providers sensitive to these needs are thereby visible across a variety of settings, including hospitals (McClung et al., 2006), hospices (Williams, Wright, Cobb, & Shields, 2004), primary care clinics (Kevern & Hill, 2015), and other sites. Responsibilities encompassed in this work include meeting with patients and families (Flannelly, Galek, Tannenbaum, & Handzo, 2007), attending to the spiritual care of both patients and staff (Williams, Meltzer, Arora, Chung, & Curlin, 2011), bereavement support for relatives (Williams et al., 2011), and coordinating interdisciplinary meetings (Williams et al., 2011).

Treatment Teams in Spiritual Care

The following are key contributors to work in caring for patients' and families' spiritual needs as part of a guiding biopsychosocial-spiritual (BPSS) framework (Engel, 1977, 1980; Wright, Watson & Bell, 1996). Depending on the care context wherein spiritual services are offered, this list of said contributors may vary or differ.

Chaplains. Chaplaincy is a profession devoted to addressing the intersection(s) of spirituality and healthcare. Chaplains are trained to provide their services in a nondenominational manner and are thereby uniquely situated to serve patients' religious and spiritual concerns by addressing these needs across the patient/family, provider/staff, and healthcare system levels (McClung, Grossoehme, & Jacobson, 2006). They are typically not credentialed as behavioral health professionals and can—as a result—practice with expectations regarding confidentiality that are more broad (Waynick, Frederich, Schneider, Thomas, & Bloomstrom, 2006).

Behavioral health providers. Behavioral health providers may include MedFTs, psychiatrists, social workers, substance abuse counselors, and psychologists. They may be found in primary, secondary, and tertiary care settings, as well as schools, churches, employee assistance programs, etc. They are trained to work collaboratively with each other, as well as other members of the treatment team. Their focus is to help integrate psychosocial assessment and services wherever people are receiving healthcare services. While each may be trained differently about how to assess and address patients' and families' spiritual needs, they are also often referral sources for it. MedFTs, especially, work to engage families as active members of the care team and are trained to coordinate and lead said teams in designing BPSS treatment plans.

Attending physicians, residents, and physician assistants. Physicians, residents, and physician assistants are trained across a wide variety of medical specialties (e.g., family medicine, emergency medicine, neurology, palliative care). Attending physicians are physicians who have completed residency training in a specialty area of medicine, passed all board and certification exams, and practice in an outpatient or inpatient setting. They oftentimes lead treatment teams, which may include trainees (e.g., residents, medical students) and other healthcare discipline members. Residents are physicians who completed medical school and are still in the graduate medical training phase of their selected specialization. They are under the direct or indirect supervision of an attending physician. Physician assistants (PA) have completed their training and are board certified to practice in primary, secondary, and/or tertiary care. They practice medicine in healthcare teams with physicians and other providers. PAs can also prescribe medication in all 50 states, the District of Columbia, the U.S. territories, and the uniformed services. All of the above may be the designated provider for a patient and thereby a potential referral source for spiritual care and consultation as needed.

Hospital administrators. Hospital administrators may include directors of pastoral care, nursing, social services, and healthcare (medical and/or behavioral) services. They make sure that hospitals run efficiently and that care is provided in accordance with state and federal government rules and regulations—alongside the mission and tenets of their board of trustees, the institution's strategic plan, and other (many) accrediting bodies that oversee care and services provided on-site. They may serve as liaisons with governing boards, medical staff, and department leadership. Administrators create and maintain policies and procedures, oversee budgets, and possibly set rates for health services. They recruit, hire, evaluate, and may train employees. They may also oversee programs/departments for research, training, fund-raising, public relations, quality assurance, patient services, and community engagement. Regarding spiritual care, they will oftentimes be the ones to allocate resources to ensure that there are such services in place. Their endorsement for these services (and prioritization of them) in budget and programming is critical to ensuring that patients' and families' spiritual needs are met.

Nurses. Nursing represents a profession in the healthcare industry focused on caring for individuals, families, and communities toward attaining, maintaining, and recovering health. They may include registered nurses (RN), licensed practical nurses (LPN), and advanced practice registered nurses (APRN). APRNs hold graduate degrees in nursing with additional qualifications in specialty areas such as nurse midwifery, anesthesiology, or behavioral health. They may practice in many specialty areas across primary, secondary, and tertiary care contexts, as well as in other settings like schools, camps, group homes, and employee assistance programs. Nurses are critical collaborators on hospital units where chaplaincy services are recognized and requested. They observe patients and families with greater frequency than other interdisciplinary team members throughout their shifts because of their proximity and job duties. Nurses refer to chaplains more than any other discipline or hospital staff member (Vanderwerker et al., 2008); most common times for this include during end-of-life (EOL) decisions, grief, and when patients/families report needing emotional support (Weinberger-Litman, Muncie, Flannelly, & Flannelly, 2010).

Fundamentals of Spiritual Care

MedFTs are uniquely positioned to address religious and spiritual concerns with patients and thus have the capacity to bolster the systemic impact of interdisciplinary treatment teams. The Joint Commission on Accreditation of Healthcare Organization (JCAHO) has maintained that "physicians, therapists, nurses, and clinical pastoral staff should receive training on the value of spiritual assessment and the tools that should be used to assess a patient's spirituality" (2005, p. 6). Furthermore, JCAHO requires spiritual assessment to be part of the overall patient assessment process. Researchers found up to 94% of patients want their spirituality addressed by healthcare providers (Williams et al., 2011). Some settings may not have a chaplain, which establishes rationale for MedFTs to secure training in order to help attend to patients' and families' spiritual needs. However, if chaplains are on-site, they are critical collaborators and members of the treatment team. MedFTs should work closely with them and on a consistent basis.

Religious and spiritual concerns become especially necessary during times of illness, suffering, and death (Balboni, Vanderwerker, & Block, 2007; Daaleman & Frey, 1998; Ellis, & Campbell, 2004; MacLean et al., 2003). Spiritual or religious beliefs may help end-of-life (EOL) patients and their families cope by offering a way to grieve impending death, find meaning and purpose, and adjust to problems associated with dying, such as the impact of a patient's death on friends and family (Oh & Kim, 2014; Tarakeshwar et al., 2006). Spiritual well-being is related to better quality of life (QOL; Frost et al., 2012), lower anxiety and depression (Gaston-Johansson, Haisfield-Wolfe, Reddick, Goldstein, & Lawal, 2013; Oh & Kim, 2014; Rawdin, Evans, & Rabow, 2013), and protection against psychological morbidity (Noble & Jones, 2010).

MedFTs must be prepared to care for patients who espouse a myriad of spiritual beliefs, especially with modern-day trends in religious globalization (Beyer & Beaman, 2007). According to Delbridge et al. (2014), the collaborative and systemic philosophy of MedFT, along with its emphasis on relationships and the self of the therapist, offers a beneficial setup for cultivating spiritually sensitive professionals. With proper training, then, MedFTs are specially poised to fill this gap in the healthcare team. Therefore, it is important that they attend to several important fundamentals of assessing and providing spiritual support and care. Important basics regarding education about spirituality and world religions, the assessment of spirituality, and the need for competencies for BHPs (particularly MedFTs) are presented below.

Education about Spirituality and World Religions

Knowing how to address spirituality is something that has received growing attention in professional literature. It is a foundational skill for MedFTs who work to promote the BPSS framework; however, not all MedFTs have in-depth training in this area of health. Many healthcare providers feel uncomfortable addressing patients' spirituality, citing unfamiliarity with varying belief systems and a lack of time during encounters as primary issues (Balboni et al., 2014; Edwards, Pang, Shiu, & Chan, 2010). Healthcare providers also report ethical concerns about competently addressing patients whose belief systems differ from their own (Casarez & Engebretson, 2012; Considine, 2007).

MedFTs should seek to gain familiarity with a variety of religious tenets as a starting point for working with patients of different faiths. They should self-evaluate their respective levels of knowledge about each of these religions and then seek to gain further information if they have gaps in understanding. Beyond baseline familiarity with the world's five most common religions (Hinduism, Judaism, Buddhism, Christianity, and Islam), MedFTs should be aware of cultural demographics unique to the area(s) in which they practice and seek to gain understanding about any other locally prevalent belief systems. Some specific constructs to understand include the religion's beliefs about deity(ies), good and evil, the afterlife, clergy and/or other leaders, major goals for living, and sacred texts.

Additionally, the MedFT's attitude in working with patients with an unfamiliar religion is as important as his or her knowledge about various spiritual belief systems. Patients should be approached with a curious stance and an attitude of cultural humility. Cultural humility is a skill that promotes awareness of the provider's self and limitations in perspective while maintaining a focus on others and their perspectives in any relationship (Hook, Davis, Owen, Worthington, & Utsey, 2013). Engaging in self-of-the-therapist work is an opportunity for MedFTs to examine their own identity, values, and attitudes surrounding their beliefs. This self-knowledge should inform the MedFT's work with patients and help to reduce bias-based interventions and decision-making. For example, if a behavioral health provider has a positive or negative sentiment about prayer, he or she should avoid projecting that onto a patient. While the MedFT should maintain a curious and patient-led stance to approaching unfamiliar religions, he or she should balance this attitude with a willingness to seek out information and build competence in understanding the unfamiliar so that the burden is not entirely on the patient or family to educate the MedFT. The knowledge base that the MedFT has developed can serve as a launching point for further conversation and assessment of the patient's specific spiritual needs.

Assessment of Spiritual Needs

Sometimes the challenge in working with patients and families around their spirituality is in opening the assessment. There is no universally accepted definition of spirituality, so an open-ended tool can be helpful to provide structure for the conversation while leaving space for the family's definition of spirituality to emerge. Hodgson, Lamson, and Reese (2007) designed a BPSS interview method for helping MedFTs to engage patients and families in conversations about their whole health, including spirituality. Open-ended questions offer clinicians a way to tap into the beliefs and meanings that patients and families attribute to their current health status (Wright et al., 1996). Advocated for use in busy medical settings, other options for spiritual assessment and history taking have been designed around an easy-to-remember pneumonic (see Table 16.1).

Additionally, there are assessment tools that may assist in gathering more detailed and robust data useful for tracking symptoms over time and research. Table 16.2 includes examples of self-report spiritual assessment tools that MedFT researchers and clinicians may use in healthcare settings.

Table 16.1 Tools for Conducting a Spiritual History

Instrument	Developer	Description
FICA Spiritual History Tool©	Puchalski (2014)	Brief open- and closed-ended questions eliciting information about patients' *f*aith and belief, *i*mportance, *c*ommunity, and *a*ccess in care.
HOPE Questions	Anandarajah & Hight (2001)	Brief open- and closed-ended questions designed to ask about patients' sources of *h*ope and meaning, whether they belong to an *o*rganized religion, their *p*ersonal spirituality and practices, and what *e*ffect their spirituality may have on medical care and end-of-life decisions.
Open Invite Mnemonic	Saguil & Phelps (2012)	Brief open- and closed-ended questions designed to *o*pen the door to conversation about faith background and spiritual preferences and *i*nvite the patient to discuss their spiritual needs.

Table 16.2 Instruments for Spiritual Assessment

Instrument	Developer	Description
Spiritual Well-Being Scale (SWBS)	Ellison (2006)	A 20-item scale that assesses both spiritual well-being (relationship with God) and existential well-being (sense of life purpose and satisfaction). Available in English or Spanish; takes 10–15 minutes to complete.
Daily Spiritual Experience Scale (DSES)	Underwood & Teresi (2002)	A 16-item scale that assesses experiences with the divine in everyday life via constructs such as awe, gratitude, mercy, sense of connection with the transcendent, and compassionate love. Available in 20 languages and validated across cultures.
Spiritual Involvement and Beliefs Scale (SIBS)	Hatch, Burg, Naberhaus, & Hellmich (1998)	A 26-item measure that was validated in primary care settings to assess actions as well as beliefs applicable across religious traditions.
Spirituality Index of Well-Being (SIWB)	Daaleman & Frey (2004)	A 12-item scale with two domains: self-efficacy and life scheme. Specifically designed to be inclusive with no mention of deity or Higher Power.

Competencies in Spiritual Care

Although all behavioral health provider disciplines maintain codes of ethics that mention respect for diversity across cultures, specific competencies in spiritual care are generally not stated. Instead, working with patients' and families' spirituality is typically combined in sections about treating various cultures (e.g., in the core competencies for BHPs working in primary care prepared through the Colorado Consensus Conference; Miller, Gilchrist, Ross, Wong, Blount, & Peek, 2016). Other times they are not mentioned at all (e.g., in the competencies for integrated behavioral health and primary care published by SAMHSA-HRSA Center for Health Solutions (Hoge, Morris, Laraia, Pomerantz, & Farley, 2014) or the review of provider-practice level competencies for integrated behavioral health in primary care (Kinman, Gilchrist, Payne-Murphy, & Miller, 2015).

According to Vieten et al. (2016), there remains a need for established spiritual competencies for BHPs. They conducted a survey where 16 competencies for BHPs providing spiritual care were identified. The BHPs who participated, all psychologists, reported the following to be critical:

1. Showing empathy, respect, and appreciation for patients from diverse spiritual, religious, or secular backgrounds and affiliations.
2. Ability to conduct empathic and effective psychotherapy with patients from diverse spiritual and religious backgrounds.
3. Cultivating an awareness of how clinicians' own spiritual and/or religious background and beliefs may influence their clinical practice, attitudes, perceptions, and assumptions about the nature of psychological processes.

Participants identified the attitudes dimension (regarding empathy, respect, and appreciation) as most important. This is the area where one's own ethnic and cultural attitudes and beliefs are explored and understood. The reason why this is so important rests in how shortcomings in one's knowledge about a specific culture, spiritual belief, etc., can be overlooked or overemphasized based on religious and/or spiritual biases (or even in the belief that spiritualty does not have a place in healthcare). While this study was done with psychologists, it applies to all BHPs.

Spiritual Care Across the MedFT Healthcare Continuum

The MedFT Healthcare Continuum (Hodgson, Lamson, Mendenhall, & Tyndall, 2014) offers a way for multiple healthcare disciplines to apply knowledge and skills common to the practice of MedFT. The continuum was developed to showcase how care providers (e.g., chaplains, nurses, social workers, psychologists) may showcase MedFT knowledge and skills at initial levels and how those who identify as a MedFT expand on that knowledge and those skills in their clinical, research, training/supervision, policy, and administrative duties. Many of these skills were demonstrated in the case vignette that opened this chapter; Mark is an experienced chaplain who advances skills that fall in various places along the MedFT Healthcare Continuum. However, when the case exceeds his skill level, he integrates Christine, a MedFT, to help care for the patient. The following describes how MedFTs collaborate with patients, family members and support persons, chaplains, and other team members to attend to spiritual issues in healthcare.

MedFTs at *Levels 1* and *2* really function at a similar level, but *Level 2* practitioners perform the skills more often in their work. These MedFTs may be somewhat to occasionally familiar with addressing spiritual health (e.g., importance of prayer or asking about a patient's and family's spirituality), but they do not engage patients regularly about it. MedFTs may have limited knowledge about how to help others with the spiritual component of a balanced BPSS lifestyle or interest in collaborating with other professionals. As a result, they may rarely to occasionally discuss spiritual issues and/or concerns with patients and their families unless initiated by the patients themselves or if they are in a health situation where it seems socially and/or culturally appropriate (e.g., end-of-life, uncertain survival). Researchers at this level may consider including a measure regarding spiritualty, but oftentimes leave it out due to time constraints or a belief that it is not a central component of health. Mark (the chaplain), Dr. Harris (the surgeon), and Christine (the MedFT) demonstrate some of the skills noted at these two levels. Mark and Christine even move past these levels into one or more of the following (Table 16.3).

MedFTs functioning at a *Level 3* stand out with their application of a BPSS framework as clinical interventionists, researchers, educators, supervisors, policy makers, and administrators. They are well informed about the current best practices in addressing patients' and family members' spiritual needs and make efforts to include such practices whenever possible. This includes providing research-informed family therapy and BPSS interventions relevant to the patient's and family's cultural and health-related needs. The *Level 3* MedFT will also actively engage and collaborate with different BPSS disciplines to ensure that the patient's care plan, policies, and/or research studies are complete and respectful of all health domains. Policy and advocacy work engaged at this level identifies and intervenes on behalf of individuals, couples, families, and healthcare teams toward advancing BPSS health and well-being. *Level 3* MedFTs routinely screen and assess for BPSS aspects of injuries/conditions and/or comorbid diseases and ask about resources within the family. They make sure to incorporate spiritual needs and resources into patients' treatment plans and engage with other disciplines, on- and off-site. MedFTs share any spiritual information acquired during the BPSS assessment process with the overall goal to codesign a comprehensive BPSS treatment plan. Mark is functioning at this level with his intent to address the spiritual needs of all patients and his willingness to learn from patients and families about their unique spiritual belief systems. He clearly is BPSS attentive as he has consulted with Christine, the MedFT, to help address David's psychosocial issues related to his biological illness, diabetes. Mark is also collaborating with David's surgeon and is bringing David's wife into the conversations as he sees her to be a crucial member of the team.

At *Level 4*, MedFTs are knowledgeable about evidence-based and emerging literature regarding spiritual interventions beneficial for the biological and behavioral health conditions commonly diagnosed and treated in one's setting. They identify as a MedFT with expertise in assessing and/or treating patients and family members with spiritual health concerns, utilizing the electronic health record (EHR) to prepare for and document patient care encounters. They competently demonstrate knowledge of commonly treated health conditions and BPSS impacts and consistently collaborate with other disciplines to implement evidence-based BPSS and family therapy protocols in colocated and integrated behavioral healthcare settings. With regard to policy and training, they design and advocate for policies that govern BPSS-oriented healthcare services and deliver seminars and workshops about the BPSS complexities about context-relevant health concerns to a variety of professional types. At this level, they can independently and collaboratively construct research and program evaluation studies that study the impact of BPSS interventions with a variety of diagnoses and patient/family units of care. Since Christine is

Table 16.3 MedFTs and Spiritual Care: Basic Knowledge and Skills

MedFT Healthcare Continuum Level	Level 1	Level 2	Level 3
Knowledge	Somewhat familiar with addressing spiritual needs in a healthcare system and the care team's overall structure and purpose. Limited knowledge about BPSS impacts on a few common illnesses, injuries, diseases, traumas, and/or other events (e.g., births) seen in one's occupational and/or healthcare setting. Basic understanding regarding strategies for a healthy lifestyle when managing a health condition or event but little application of strategies to BPSS health. Limited knowledge about the benefits of collaboration with other healthcare professionals; rarely seeks out opportunities to do so and consults the electronic health record system only when necessary. Able to recognize at a basic level the BPSS dimensions of health events and conditions and apply a BPSS lens to practice, research, and/or policy/advocacy work.	Moderately familiar with benefits of addressing the spiritual needs of patients and family members and comfortable doing so when spiritual needs are obvious. Knowledgeable about how to apply systemic interventions in practice and does it occasionally; capable of assessing patients' BPSS health and invite support system members to be present for background health issues such as family history and risk-related factors, as well as treatment planning inclusive of spiritual health. Is an occasional contributor to discussions about research design and policy/advocacy work that include relational and/or BPSS aspects of health events and/or conditions.	Well informed about the current best practices in addressing spiritual needs of patients and family members and values the inclusion of such practices with every patient, when possible. Broad range of knowledge about research-informed family therapy and BPSS interventions relevant to clinical practice. Understands the importance of and actively engages different disciplines on the treatment team in the patient's care plan. When work permits, is knowledgeable and usually committed to conducting research and constructing policy/advocacy work that identifies and intervenes on behalf of individuals, couples, families, and healthcare teams toward the advancement of BPSS health and well-being.

(continued)

Table 16.3 (continued)

MedFT Healthcare Continuum Level	Level 1	Level 2	Level 3
Skills	Although capable of doing so, rarely discusses spiritual issues and/or concerns with patients and their families unless initiated by the patients themselves. Can discuss (and psychoeducate) basic relationships between biological processes, personal and spiritual well-being, and interpersonal functioning. Demonstrates minimal collaborative skills with healthcare providers; prefers to work independently, but when care is complex enough, will contact/collaborate with other providers about additional services. Rarely engages other professional members, patients, and support system members collaboratively. If conducting research and/or policy/advocacy work, on rare occasions will collaborate with other disciplines and consider relational and/or BPSS aspects of health and well-being.	Occasionally incorporates spirituality into treatment, particularly when patients clearly identify spiritual concerns. Capable of discussing spiritual concerns from multiple faith practices. Will occasionally explain to patients, support system members, and other members of the treatment team how each of the BPSS systems plays a part in supporting a patient's journey to health and wellness. Demonstrates occasional collaborative skills through (a) written and verbal communication mediums that are understandable to all team members, (b) coordination of referrals to other professionals (e.g., specialty behavioral health providers, hospital chaplains), and (c) communication with the patient's healthcare team around BPSS treatment planning. Competent in basic collaboration with other disciplines when conducting research and/or policy work as long as the need for collaboration is clearly indicated.	Routinely and actively utilizes various screening tools and resources to assess for spiritual health and incorporates spiritual goals into patient treatment plans. Can successfully conduct a systemic assessment of a patient and family with competencies in assessing for BPSS aspects of the injury/condition and/or comorbid disease and resources within the family. Usually engages multidisciplinary team members in a discussion about the patient and what skills each person has that could contribute to the best patient outcome. Usually engages other professionals within and outside of the practice/hospital setting who are actively involved in the patient's care (e.g., specialists, clergy). Skilled with standardized measures to track patients' individual and relational strengths and challenges (e.g., depression, anxiety, pain, social support, spiritual health) and capable of conducting research using such data. Will actively collaborate with other disciplines for advocacy/policy work.

the only healthcare team member that identifies at a MedFT, this level is easily recognizable for her. Her attention to the importance of the BPSS framework, participation in the integrated behavioral healthcare team, recognition of David and his wife playing critical roles in the treatment plan, and her respect for the spiritual domain, in particular, showcase her knowledge and skills at this level. While her role in the system at a *Level 5* is not evident, what could be observed in this setting is described below (Table 16.4).

Table 16.4 MedFTs and Spiritual Care: Advanced Knowledge and Skills

MedFT Healthcare Continuum Level	Level 4	Level 5
Knowledge	Knowledgeable about evidence-based and emerging literature regarding spiritual interventions beneficial for the biological and mental health conditions commonly diagnosed and treated in one's setting. Identifies self as a MedFT with expertise in assessing and/or treating patients and family members with spiritual health concerns. Competently demonstrates knowledge of commonly treated health conditions and BPSS impacts. Understands how to collaborate with other disciplines to implement evidence-based BPSS and family therapy protocols in colocated and integrated behavioral healthcare contexts. Thoroughly competent understanding of the benefits of engaging multiple healthcare professionals in integrated BPSS treatment teams. Knowledgeable about designing and advocating for policies that govern BPSS-oriented healthcare services.	Understands and educates others about treatment and spiritual health strengths and challenges unique and/or common to the healthcare context; can consult proficiently with professionals about BPSS topics from other fields. Proficient at explaining evidence-based BPSS treatments regarding injuries/conditions and their role(s) in the workplace and family systems; has background to provide psychoeducation to patients and families about a variety of symptoms, medications, spiritual, and behavioral health management techniques. Understands leadership and supervision strategies for building integrated healthcare teams inclusive of spiritual health providers. Knowledgeable about BPSS research designs and execution, policies, and advocacy need for attention to spiritual health as relevant to colocated and integrated behavioral healthcare; proficient in developing a curriculum on integrated behavioral healthcare, BPSS applications, MedFT, etc. to mental health, chaplains, and other health professionals employed in a healthcare setting.

(continued)

Table 16.4 (continued)

MedFT Healthcare Continuum Level	Level 4	Level 5
Skills	Seeks opportunities to train others about the benefits of incorporating spirituality into treatment planning; is keenly familiar with a variety of faith-belief systems and is comfortable discussing spiritual concerns from each. Able to deliver seminars and workshops about the BPSS complexities about context-relevant health concerns to a variety of professional types (e.g., mental health, biomedical); can apply several BPSS interventions in care (including most types of brief interventions); can administer mood, spiritual, and disease-specific assessment tools as the healthcare context requires. Consistently collaborates with key healthcare team members (e.g., treating providers, workers' compensation case manager, nurse manager, physical therapist, dietician); initiates and facilitates team visits with multiple providers when working with patients and families. Frequently utilizes electronic health record systems and contributes to discussions of how to do so more efficiently and effectively. Can independently and collaboratively construct research and program evaluation studies that study the impact of BPSS interventions with a variety of diagnoses and patient/family units of care.	Proficient in assessing and obtaining support for nearly all aspects of commonly seen spiritual health matters common to one's setting; able to synthesize and conduct research and clinical work; engages in community-oriented projects outside of the healthcare setting to help improve overall BPSS health and well-being. Goes beyond interventions routine for this population; can integrate specific models of BPSS integrated behavioral healthcare (e.g., patient-centered behavioral health, chronic care model), with spiritual health enhancements, into healthcare settings. Leads, supervises, and/or studies success of the implementation and dissemination of BPSS curriculum on spiritual health, routinely engages as an administrator/leader and supervisor in a team-based BPSS approach to inpatient and/or outpatient care, with consistent communication through electronic health records, "patient introductions," "curb-side consultations," and team meetings and visits. Works proficiently as a MedFT and collaborates with other providers from a variety of disciples. Explains at a high level of skill evidence-based treatments regarding most spiritual health concerns and their role(s) in the care of patients and family members; has background to provide psychoeducation to patients and families about a variety of symptoms, medications, and behavioral and spiritual health techniques that facilitate returning to optimal BPSS health.

MedFTs working at a *Level 5* typically have developed all the skills at the prior four levels and are now in a position of leadership or generators of new and innovative applications of MedFT. They go beyond interventions unique to their fields and can integrate specific models of BPSS-integrated behavioral healthcare with spiritual health enhancements, into healthcare settings. They are proficient at explaining evidence-based BPSS treatments regarding injuries/conditions and their role(s) in the workplace and family systems. They have training to provide psychoeducation to patients and families about a variety of symptoms, medications, spirituality(ies), and behavioral health management techniques. Additionally, they understand and apply leadership and supervision strategies for building integrated behavioral healthcare (IBHC) teams inclusive of spiritual health providers, as well as synthesizing and conducting research/program evaluation studies that advance the BPSS framework.

Research-Informed Practices

Over the years, interventions focused on spirituality have gained more attention (e.g., Razali, Hasanah, Aminah, & Subramaniam, 1998; Rosmarin, Auerbach, Bigda-Peyton, Björgvinsson, & Levendusky, 2011). However, O'Connor (2002) made the argument that spiritual care needs to become more evidence-based, and several studies grounded in theory followed this call to guide the process and explain outcomes for those receiving spiritual interventions (Hook et al., 2010; Jafari et al., 2013). Several of these interventions are described below, along with the conditions under which MedFTs may use them in clinical care.

Individual Approaches

Prayer

The use of prayer as an intervention is popular because it fits within the framework of many religions and spiritual practices. Theoretically speaking, prayer is communication with the divine (Dein & Littlewood, 2008). Through that communication, a relationship is formed, which then promotes biological and psychosocial well-being (Poloma & Hoelter, 1998). At its root, prayer is considered a mindful practice; it is an opportunity to reflect on the present moment and accept one's current thoughts and feelings (Germer, 2009; Monroe & Jankowski, 2016). Research findings about prayer are mixed: while some studies demonstrate small measureable effects (see the systematic review by Hodge, 2007), other meta-analyses describe conflicting results and methodological problems (e.g., Andrade & Radhakrishnan, 2009; Masters & Spielmans, 2007). Qualitative findings, however, show that people who identify as religious tend to report positive health outcomes with prayer (Esperandio & Ladd, 2015; Jors, Büssing, Hvidt, & Baumann, 2015).

Receptive prayer consists of dialogue with a Higher Power that comes through visions, hearing a message, or some other type of sensory experience (Poloma & Lee, 2011). *Meditative prayer*, on the other hand, consists of quiet reflection while thinking about a Higher Power or element of one's spirituality (Ai, Tice, Huang, Rodgers, & Bolling 2008). A third type of prayer, *petitionary prayer*, involves requesting divine help on behalf of oneself or another person. According to a study of patients who underwent open-heart surgery, the use of petitionary prayer before surgery was associated with lower levels of depression when patients were reassessed 30 months after surgery (Ai et al., 2010). While these are only a few examples of the health benefits of certain types of prayer, it is clear that it can be used in a variety of ways in accord with patients' and families' preferences.

It is important to note, too, that who one prays to (and how) may differ between and among different religious and spiritual dispositions. For example, when working within certain Christian belief systems, inviting the patient to pray may be appropriate (Poloma & Lee, 2011). However, to whom the patient prays (e.g., God, Jesus, the Holy Trinity, a specific saint) may depend upon the type of Christianity practiced (e.g., Catholic, Episcopal, Lutheran, Baptist, Methodist, Unitarian/Universalist). Patients who identify as Buddhist may prefer the opportunity to meditate and recite a favorite sutra (Fan & Wu, 2007). Alternatively, a Muslim could be most comfortable being able to physically move into different positions while engaging in Salat, which is a prayer ritual observed at five specific times per day (Doufesh, Ibrahim, Ismail, & Ahmad, 2014).

Similar to diversity within Christian faiths, people across a variety of different belief systems may not all ascribe to the same ideas and viewpoints about prayer. Careful attention must thereby be given to asking patients about what works for them. Additionally, although many spiritual and religious practices include prayer, it is imperative that MedFTs not assume that patients who identify as being spiritual or religious automatically use prayer as a resource. By remaining curious and listening to patients, one may better comprehend if prayer is viewed as a useful and positive coping sequence or intervention. Patients may, indeed, engage in prayer—and/or they may respond preferentially to other spiritually and/or religiously integrated psychotherapy interventions.

Religiously Integrated Cognitive Behavioral Therapy

Several studies have focused on the benefits of integrating spiritual and religious practices into the well-researched practice of cognitive behavioral therapy (CBT); these integrated practices are called religious CBT (RCBT; Berk et al., 2015; Koenig, Pearce, Nelson, & Daher, 2015; Pearce et al., 2015). Like traditional CBT, RCBT focuses on challenging cognitions that increase—and supporting thoughts and behaviors that decrease—depressive and anxious symptoms. The approach involves incorporating patients' and families' spiritual beliefs into their treatment plans and care (Koenig et al., 2015).

Common RCBT interventions include mindful meditation through prayer, expressing gratitude, and confronting problematic cognitions through the lens of the patient's spiritual practices. In addition, the memorization of scripture by patients is important as a strategy to oppose cognitive distortions (Pearce et al., 2015). RCBT can be used for a variety of religious backgrounds to allow for broad usage by healthcare professionals, such as MedFTs. RCBT has been adapted to accommodate patients from Christian, Buddhist, Hindu, Islamic, and Jewish backgrounds (Koenig et al., 2015; Pearce et al., 2015).

As of yet, there is no strong evidence that RCBT significantly decreases these symptoms in patients more than traditional CBT. Researchers have provided evidence that it is just as effective as traditional CBT (Koenig et al., 2015; Pearce et al., 2015) in increasing optimism and generosity in patients with both major depressive disorder and a chronic medical illness (Koenig et al., 2015; Pearce et al., 2015). Most of the participants in this scholarship were Christian, White, and considered spirituality to be somewhat important, which could have potentially skewed the results. It is important to note, too, that not all patients who endorse being spiritual are religious and not all patients who identify as being religious describe themselves as being spiritual. Utilizing RCBT may prove to be a promising intervention with more research and clinical application to diverse populations and belief systems.

Mindfulness-Based Interventions

Researchers have found that patients with cancer have better coping and health outcomes (Jim et al., 2015; Mollica, Underwood, Homish, Homish, & Orom, 2016; Peteet & Balboni, 2013) when they have strong spiritual beliefs. A meta-analysis conducted by Oh and Kim (2014) found that patients with cancer who receive spiritual interventions had moderate but significant effects on spiritual well-being, meaning of life, and depression. This is especially so with interventions based on mindfulness.

According to a randomized clinical study by Cole et al. (2011), spiritually based mindfulness is associated with reduced depression and increased positive affect—particularly among patients who reported decreases in perceived social support. An example of such a spiritually based mindfulness intervention is *Re-Creating Your Life: During and After Cancer* (Cole & Pargament, 1999). This program uses spiritual psychotherapeutic interventions to make the coping process smoother and more meaningful for patients with cancer. Interventions include relaxation/meditation and receptive and petitionary prayer. Jafari et al. (2013) implemented this program for women who had been diagnosed with breast cancer within the previous 12 months; they found that the intervention significantly increased patients' quality of life.

While Cole and Pargament's (1999) program is only one example of how a spiritually based mindfulness intervention is used in patient coping strategies with cancer, other variations studied with other health conditions exist. For example, a randomized control trial of mindfulness-based interventions for the treatment of fibromyalgia syndrome (FMS) demonstrated significant and sustained improvements over control group participants in disease symptomatology, pain perception, sleep quality, psychological distress, nonattachment (to self, symptoms, and environment), and civic engagement (Van Gordon, Shonin, Dunn, Garcia-Campayo, & Griffiths, 2017). Other health conditions where such interventions have shown positive outcomes include cardiovascular health (Prazak et al. 2012), reducing risk for drug relapse (Bowen et al., 2014), inflammation (Rosenkranz et al., 2013), and reductions in stress reactivity (Taren et al., 2015). There is even recent expansion to family-based mindfulness interventions that demonstrate symptom reductions in young children diagnosed with attention deficit hyperactivity disorder and stress reduction for their parents (Lo, Wong, Wong, Wong, & Yeung, 2016).

Family Approaches

There is a pronounced gap in research regarding evidence-based interventions specifically designed to strengthen spirituality (or utilize it as a part of treatment) at the family level. However, some authors have proposed several ways to incorporate spirituality into such care: Tanyi (2006) argued that the majority of published guidelines on spiritual assessment and interventions are written for individually oriented care and that these fail to differentiate between individual and family spirituality. She suggested to clinicians and researchers that the goals of spiritual assessment should be to (a) support and enhance families' spiritual well-being and development, (b) discern spiritual distress and its effect(s) on overall family health, and (c) incorporate family spirituality when providing treatment. Tanyi recommended specific assessment questions that fall into the categories of meaning and purpose, strengths, relationships, beliefs, individual family member spirituality, and the family's preferences for spiritual care. While her work was not in the area of developing interventions, she touched on the importance of using spiritual interventions that are designed for families specifically (i.e., not simply individual approaches that are adapted to fit families).

Hodge and colleagues recommended the use of spiritual ecomaps and lifemaps as tools to both assess and treat families with regard to spirituality (Hodge, 2000, 2005; Limb, Hodge, Leckie, & Ward, 2013). Spiritual ecomaps provide rich assessment data for healthcare providers about families' spirituality; they can be used to uncover places where there might be conflicts in family members' beliefs or values that could affect both relationships and health decision-making. These tools also serve as an intervention to help families visualize disconnects in their spiritual lives and areas where they may need to reconnect with each other, faith communities and culture, and/or a Higher Power. For example, in a study by Limb and Hodge (2011) with Native American families, spiritual ecomaps were found to be consistent with indigenous cultures and spiritual conversations between therapists and patients. Spiritual ecomaps are most effective when driven by the family's unique culture and language. Hodge and Limb (2011) also found that clinicians' respective levels of cultural and spiritual competence are essential to ensuring that clinical conversations are therapeutically effective.

Hodge (2005) also endorsed lifemaps as a way to help patients who value spirituality and religion and who want to make sense out of current life situations. Lifemaps provide the clinician with a retrospective understanding of a presenting concern, alongside an understanding for where the family wants to go as a result of care. When studied with patients and families aligned with the Mormon Church of Latter-Day Saints (LDS), Limb, Hodge, Leckie, and Ward (2013) found that this particular assessment tool was consistent with LDS communities' beliefs, lifestyle, and culture. This work was done with the LDS population exclusively; Limb et al. (2013) thereby advocated that spiritual assessments be validated across a wide variety of spiritual beliefs and religions before implementing them broadly with families.

Some research teams have advocated for assessment of patients' religious and spiritual functioning prior to and after a traumatic/significant life event, because some experience spiritual ambivalence later on (Walker, Reid, O'Neill, & Brown, 2009). The spiritually oriented trauma-focused CBT approach (Walker, Reese, Hughes, & Troskie, 2010) grew from the trauma-focused CBT approach (Cohen, Mannarino, & Deblinger, 2006). It is a conjoint treatment for both children and parents or caregivers (when available) wherein the child is supported in talking to his or her parent about the trauma in a manner that allows for mutual support and healing to be addressed. In one known study regarding this approach, researchers reported outcomes related to lower post-traumatic stress disorder (PTSD) symptoms and deceased spiritual struggles among child survivors of restavek (i.e., modern-day slavery in Haiti; Wang et al., 2016). More research is needed to understand the effectiveness and efficacy of this approach with children and parents/caregivers.

While there are not many known couples therapy approaches that integrate spiritualty, the strategic hope-focused couples approach (HFCA) is one empirically supported therapy and enrichment intervention (Worthington, 2005). It is based in Christian theology (denomination not defined) but is purported to be adaptable to non-Christian couples as well. Jakubowski, Milne, Brunner, and Miller (2004) found in their review of comparable couples' approaches that HFCS was efficacious in helping couples advance beneficent change. It has been shown to improve marital satisfaction (Worthington et al., 1997), marital communication (Ripley & Worthington, 2002), and overall quality of life (Burchard et al., 2003). Unfortunately, recent literature in this area is scarce.

Community Approaches

As spiritual interventions and spiritually oriented treatments for couples and families are still developing a more robust research base, community approaches have also emerged as an alternative form of treatment (Cornish & Wade, 2010).

Psychoeducation Groups

Psychoeducation groups, also known as group therapy, can be beneficial for several presenting problems—ranging from anxiety and depression to the struggles of chronic illness for patients and their families. The American Psychological Association (APA, 2017) has noted that benefits of group therapy include building social support and a sounding board for concerns. Group members can help each other find solutions to ideas and hold each other accountable for decisions they make.

Benefits of psychoeducation groups have also been explored in literature. Incorporating spirituality into such groups has provided evidence that it decreases anxiety and increases overall quality of life (McCorkle, Bohn, Hughes, & Kim, 2005). For example, Rye and Pargament (2002) found that implementing religious interventions focused on forgiveness in a psychotherapy group setting for recently uncoupled college-age women was just as effective as using a similar, yet secular, approach (group leaders did not refer to religion or spirituality with participants). They used a modified version of the REACH model for forgiveness (Worthington, Sandage, & Berry, 2000), which included five steps for forgiveness: (a) *r*ecalling the hurt, (b) developing *e*mpathy toward the offender, (c) *a*ltruistic gifting, (d) *c*ommitment to forgive, and (e) *h*olding onto the forgiveness. Each session is focused on addressing a portion of the model through interventions, such as letter writing to the offender, exploring coping mechanisms, examining grudges, practicing with vignettes surrounding forgiveness, and considering reconciliation. The modification was made to encourage group members to talk about the impact(s) of their religious/spiritual beliefs on each of these processes. The study found significant increases in forgiveness, anticipation for the future, and existential well-being, while depression and anxiety symptoms decreased. A similar investigation was done for women who had been through a divorce, looking at forgiveness of an ex-spouse instead; it yielded similar results (Rye et al., 2005).

One spiritually oriented psychotherapy group in healthcare specifically focused on HIV-positive adults and changes in symptoms before and after the intervention (Tarakeshwar, Pearce, & Sikkema, 2005). Using the cognitive theory of stress and coping along with a spiritual coping, an eight-session group was conducted that used a mixture of psychoeducation about HIV, mindfulness, and discussion that was focused on helping participants utilize their spiritual beliefs for positive coping skills. At the conclusion of the group, participants exhibited significantly higher levels of positive spiritual coping and reported significantly decreased depression symptoms.

Currently, there are only a few studies on the utilization of community-based psychoeducation groups with a spiritual focus to address health issues. This paucity of empirical research may be due to the fact that most are designed to be layperson-led groups (i.e., professionals are not allowed in or included). One organization that is worldwide and offers a mutual-help recovery method is Alcoholics Anonymous (Bill, 1976). A recent review of 25 years of research (Kelly, 2017) reported that spirituality is a significant mediator of AA's beneficial effects, particularly among those with significant addiction issues. It has even found to be equally effective for atheists and agnostics (Kelly, Stout, Zywiak, & Schneider, 2006; Rolland & Kaskutas, 2002; Tonigan, Miller, & Schermer, 2002), although they are less likely to sustain involvement over time (Bogenschutz, 2008; Tonigan et al., 2002). For most other participants with less severe forms of addition, Kelly (2017) found that the primary drivers of abstinence were cognitive changes, improved social networks, self-efficacy, healthier coping skills, and recovery motivation. This is important as secular alternatives to AA (e.g., Women for Sobriety, LifeRing, and SMART Recovery) are growing in popularity as care alternatives (Zemore, Kaskutas, Mericle, & Hemberg, 2016). See *Chapter 12* in this text for more information about community-based interventions with these populations.

Population Health Measures Designed for Spiritual Participants

MedFTs and chaplains may intervene in a community setting, thereby expanding the integration of biomedical health and spirituality to other places outside of the healthcare setting. One 6-month intervention was piloted to target health behavior change in the lower Mississippi Delta region (Tussing-Humphreys, Tomson, & Onufrak, 2015). This intervention, specifically designed to be conducted in a church setting by trained church members, showed high rates of retention and adherence. Patients in the program experienced improved dietary quality and improved metabolic control. These findings illustrate the power of uniting with spiritual stakeholders to effect health behavior change in a community. A model for a similar intervention, known as the Disconnected Values Model, centers on acknowledging that negative health behaviors are often at odds with faith values. It advocates for the utilization of sacred texts and teachings to enhance behavior change among religious parishioners (Anshel, 2010).

In another population health measure, spirituality can also be integrated into health promotion literature. In a systematic review of 14 faith-based studies, researchers identified faith-based organizations as promising avenues for delivering diabetes self-management education to Black Americans with type 2 diabetes (Newlin, Dyess, Allard, Chase, & Melkus, 2012). Although most of the studies reviewed used similar recruitment methods and pre-experimental designs, participants appeared to benefit from the use of culturally sensitive, behaviorally oriented interventions that incorporate spirituality and social support within religious organizations.

Conclusion

The privilege of working alongside patients, families, healthcare providers, and chaplains is something that MedFTs are doing with greater frequency. Researchers have demonstrated the power of spiritual interventions and impacts that one's belief systems can have on the healing process. While nondenominational spiritual interventions are something that not all healthcare providers specifically are trained to do, they represent an important area for MedFTs to gain competence in. Through purposefully engaging in spiritual assessments, interventions, research, and collaborations, MedFTs play an important role in enhancing the BPSS care experience for patients and families who view spirituality as a vital component to their health and well-being.

Reflection Questions
1. How do you think spirituality plays a role in healthcare? Who should address it?
2. What are some potential ways that MedFTs and chaplains can work together to ensure that patients' spiritual health is addressed in light of the clinical, operational, and financial challenges that may be present in the healthcare system?
3. If you were Christine, the MedFT in the case vignette, how would you bring what was raised in the patient/family meeting to the chaplain and surgeon? How would you integrate this content into the patient's/family's treatment plan?

Glossary of Important Terms in Spiritual Care

Agnostic One who believes that nothing is known, or can be known, about a Higher Power. This person neither believes nor disbelieves in a Higher Power.

Atheist One who does not believe in a Higher Power. Some atheists may consider themselves to be spiritual, but they do not subscribe to any specific deity or organized religion.

Buddhism A spiritual practice based on the teachings of the Buddha. Buddhism originated in India, and, currently, around 7% of the global population follows this faith. Its clergy consist of monks and the Dalai Lama. Key concepts in Buddhism include mindfulness, loving-kindness, and compassion. They have no rituals, gods, or priests. Enlightenment comes through meditation.

Cao Dai Originating in Vietnam in 1926, this practice has over 6.7 million followers who believe in the existence of one Supreme Being. Cao Dai places a great deal of stress on universal concepts, such as justice, love, peace, and tolerance. It draws from other major world religions, including Christianity, Buddhism, Hinduism, Judaism, Islam, and Taoism.

Chaplain A nondenominational ordained member of the clergy who may work within a variety of contexts—such as hospitals, prisons, and the armed forces—to provide services focused on spiritual well-being.

Christianity A religion that is focused on the life and teachings of Jesus Christ. It originated in the Middle East. Its clergy may include priests, preachers, ministers, pastors, bishops, and the Pope. Key concepts include a belief in God, his Son (Jesus Christ), and the Holy Ghost as divine sources of guidance for daily living. There are many sects of Christianity, including Catholic, Protestant,

Methodist, Lutheran, Episcopal, Unitarian/Universalist, and hundreds of other groups and denominations.

Daoism Also known as Taoism, this philosophy originated in China about 2000 years ago. The majority of its followers live in China, Japan, South Korea, and Vietnam. It is associated with a belief in the supernatural and mystical and values knowledge of the paranormal (as opposed to the knowledge of the measureable). Devotees do not support political interference and/or imposition of regulations and economic restrictions. They see their diet as critical to psychological and physical well-being and encourage the practices of fasting and veganism (abstaining from animal products).

Eucharist A Christian ceremony done in commemoration of the Last Supper, in which bread and wine are consecrated and consumed to symbolize the body and blood of Jesus Christ.

Forgiveness The process by which one party pardons the negative actions of another party. Forgiveness is an act encouraged by many religions and spiritual practices, and it is believed to lead to improved relationships with oneself and others.

God In many religions, God (uppercase) is the creator of all life on earth. Depending on the religion, God may be all-knowing, ever-present, and/or the sustainer of life. In polytheistic religions, god (lowercase) is a term referring to a divine being. Religions such as Hinduism, for example, include several gods that believers may worship for different causes or occasions.

Grace An understanding of Christian faith and life defined as love and mercy given by God freely.

Higher Power A term that has been credited to Alcoholics Anonymous; it refers to something that is greater than ourselves. Some refer to this as God, the universe, or life forces.

Hinduism A religion that predates several major world religions, including Christianity. It originated and is most widely practiced in India. Hinduism is one of the world's largest religions, with over 1 billion followers. Its clergy are called Brahmins. Its four principal goals of life include ethics, prosperity, desires, and liberation.

Islam A religion that professes that there is only one and incomparable God (Allah) and that Muhammad is the last messenger of God. Muslims consider the Qur'an to be the unaltered and final revelation of God. Islam originated in the Middle East. Its clergy are called prophets. Its key doctrine includes the ideas that sin is caused by forgetfulness, human weakness, and the spirit of rebellion—whereas salvation is work-oriented and achieved by submitting to the will of Allah and living a good life.

Jesus Christ The being on whom Christianity is based. During his life, Christ's teachings focused on the importance of repenting past wrongs and implementing values such as faith, hope, and charity in order to live peacefully on earth and after death.

Judaism An ancient religion that focuses on the teachings of God as given in the sacred text, the Torah. Originating in Mesopotamia, Judaism is one of the largest religions in the world, along with Islam and Christianity. Its clergy are called Rabbi. Its key tenet is to lead a moral life through obedience to God's law.

Muism Also known as Sinism or Shingyo, this religion is rooted in Korean culture. It is most commonly practiced in South Korea. Key concepts of this faith include belief in the existence of ghosts, spirits, and gods in the spirit world. Followers believe that when a person is sick, it is actually his or her soul that is sick. For example, when a person has a mental illness, he or she is beheld as a lost, possessed, or transitioned soul. There is no specific religious text or theology associated with this faith. Spiritual leaders are called "Mudangs"; they are typically females who serve as intermediaries between the gods and humans.

Muslim A person who follows the teachings of Islam.

Prayer A way in which one communicates with God or a Higher Power. Different types of prayers exist for various religious and spiritual practices.

Qur'an The central sacred text of Islam, which contains revelations from Allah, Islam's God. It is divided into chapters and verses, much like the Christian Bible.

Religion An oftentimes structured and dogmatic way of living that occurs within established institutions designed to facilitate spirituality. It involves rules, moral guidelines, principles, and philosophies that guide beliefs and behaviors. Often, a God or Higher Power is involved in religions, from where the rules and principles originate.

Scripture Either a portion or an entire work of religious text that is considered to be sacred. Several religions have works that are considered scripture to them.

Shintoism An estimated 80% of people living in Japan practice this faith. Its beginnings are thought to date back to the eighth century. Followers believe in the existence of many gods. Key concepts include impurity and purification, and rituals are performed on a regular basis to cleanse followers of sin, guilt, and bad luck.

Sikhism This relatively new faith, founded during the fifteenth century, began in India. It has over 28 million followers. Key concepts include sewa (community service) and simran (remembrance of God). Sikhs think religion should be practiced by living in the world and coping with life's everyday problems. In India, followers have included major political influencers, particularly during the Partition of India in 1947.

Spirituality The dimension of a person that treats how one is making meaning or sense of his or her life experiences. Religion may comprise part of one's spirituality, but spirituality does not necessarily have to include religious beliefs.

Sutra An ancient or medieval Indian text that teaches an idea, philosophy, or rule to consider.

The Lord's Prayer A prayer that Jesus Christ taught to his followers; it is still used today by many Christians for a variety of reasons.

Additional Resources

Literature

Bulling, D., DeKraai, M., Abdel-Monem, T., Nieuwsma, J. A., Cantrell, W. C., Ethridge, K., & Meador, K. (2013). Confidentiality and mental health/chaplaincy collaboration. *Military Psychology, 25*, 557–567. https://doi.org/10.1037/mil0000019

Cabot, R. C., & Dicks, D. L. (1953). *The art of ministering to the sick.* New York, NY: MacMillan Company.

Dell, M. L. (2004). Religious professionals and institutions: Untapped resources for clinical care. *Child and Adolescent Psychiatric Clinics of North America, 13*, 85–110. https://doi.org/10.1016/S1056-4993(03)00098-1

Flannelly, K. J., Galek, K., Bucchino, J., & Vane, A. (2006). The relative prevalence of various spiritual needs. *Scottish Journal of Healthcare Chaplaincy, 9*, 25–30. Retrieved from https://www.researchgate.net/publication/237138829_The_Relative_Prevalence_of_Various_Spiritual_Needs

Galek, K., Flannelly, K. J., Koenig, H. G., & Fogg, S. L. (2007). Referrals to chaplains: The role of religion and spirituality in healthcare settings. *Mental Health, Religion & Culture, 10*, 363–377. https://doi.org/10.1080/13674670600757064

Handzo, G. F., Cobb, M., Holmes, C., Kelly, E., & Sinclair, S. (2014). Outcomes for professional health care chaplaincy: An international call to action. *Journal of Health Care Chaplaincy, 20*, 43–53. https://doi.org/10.1080/08854726.2014.902713

Joint Commission on the Accreditation of Healthcare Organizations. (2005). *Evaluating your spiritual assessment process,* February. Retrieved from http://www.professionalchaplains.org/files/resources/reading_room/evaluating_your_spiritual_assessment_process.pdf

Taylor, J. J., Hodgson, J. L., Kolobova, I., Lamson, A. L., Sira, N., & Musick, D. (2015). Exploring the phenomenon of spiritual care between hospital chaplains and hospital based healthcare providers. *Journal of Health Care Chaplaincy, 21*, 91–107. https://doi.org/10.1080/08854726.2015.1015302

Vanderwerker, L. C., Flannelly, K. J., Galek, K., Harding, S. R., Handzo, G. F., Oettinger, M., & Bauman, J. P. (2008). What do chaplains really do? Referrals in the New York Chaplaincy Study. *Journal of Health Care Chaplaincy, 14*, 57–73. https://doi.org/10.1080/08854720802053861

Electronic Resources

Association for Clinical Pastoral Education (ACPE) Research Network. http://acperesearch.net

Australian Journal of Pastoral Care and Health. http://www.pastoraljournal.findaus.com/index.php

Health and Social Care Chaplaincy Journal. https://journals.equinoxpub.com/index.php/HSCC
Journal of Health Care Chaplaincy. http://www.tandf.co.uk/journals/WHCC
Plainviews E-Newsletter. https://plainviews.healthcarechaplaincy.org/

Measures/Instruments

FICA Spiritual History Tool. http://hces-online.net/miscellaneous/Isabel_Quinn/End_of_Life_Summit_FICA_ References.pdf
HOPE Approach to Spiritual Assessment. http://wps.prenhall.com/wps/media/objects/2791/2858109/toolbox/Table5_1.pdf
Open Invite Mnemonic Assessment. http://www.faithandhealthconnection.org/wp-content/uploads/Spiritual-Assessments-for-Health-Practitioners.pdf

Organizations/Associations

American Association of Pastoral Counselors. http://aapc.org
Association for Clinical Pastoral Education. http://acpe.edu
Canadian Association for Spiritual Care. http://spiritualcare.ca

References[1]

Ai, A. L., Ladd, K. L., Peterson, C., Cook, C. A., Shearer, M., & Koenig, H. G. (2010). Long-term adjustment after surviving open heart surgery: The effect of using prayer for coping replicated in a prospective design. *The Gerontologist, 50*, 798–809. https://doi.org/10.1093/geront/gnq046

Ai, A. L., Tice, T. N., Huang, B., Rodgers, W., & Bolling, S. F. (2008). Types of prayer, optimism, and well-being of middle-aged and older patients undergoing open-heart surgery. *Mental Health, Religion and Culture, 11*, 131–150. https://doi.org/10.1080/13674670701324798

American Psychological Association. (2017). *Psychotherapy: Understanding group therapy.* Retrieved from http://www.apa.org/helpcenter/group-therapy.aspx

Anandarajah, G., & Hight, E. (2001). Spirituality and medical practice: Using the HOPE questions as a practical tool for spiritual assessment. *American Family Physician, 63*, 81–89. https://doi.org/10.1016/S1443-8461(01)80044-7

Andrade, C., & Radhakrishnan, R. (2009). Prayer and healing: A medical and scientific perspective on randomized controlled trials. *Indian Journal of Psychiatry, 51*, 247–253. https://doi.org/10.4103/0019-5545.58288

Anshel, M. (2010). The Disconnected Values (Intervention) Model for promoting healthy habits in religious institutions. *Journal of Religion & Health, 49*, 32–49. https://doi.org/10.1007/s10943-008-9230-x

---

[1] Note: References that are prefaced with an asterisk are recommended readings.

Balboni, M. J., Sullivan, A., Enzinger, A. C., Epstein-Peterson, Z. D., Tseng, Y. D., Mitchell, C., ... Balboni, T. A. (2014). Nurse and physician barriers to spiritual care provision at the end of life. *Journal of Pain and Symptom Management, 48*, 400–410. https://doi.org/10.1016/j.jpainsymman.2013.09.020

Balboni, T. A., Vanderwerker, L. C., & Block, S. D. (2007). Religiousness and spiritual support among advanced cancer patients and associations with end-of-life treatment preferences and quality of life. *Journal of Clinical Oncology, 25*, 555–560. https://doi.org/10.1200/JCO.2006.07.9046

Berk, L. S., Bellinger, D. L., Koenig, H. G., Daher, N., Pearce, M. J., Robins, C. J., ... King, M. B. (2015). Effects of religious vs. conventional cognitive-behavioral therapy on inflammatory markers and stress hormones in major depression and chronic medical illness: A randomized clinical trial. *Open Journal of Psychiatry, 5*, 238–259. https://doi.org/10.4236/ojpsych.2015.53028

Beyer, P., & Beaman, L. (2007). *Religion, globalization, and culture (international studies in religion and society)*. Leiden, Netherlands: Brill Publishers.

Bill, W. (1976). *Alcoholics anonymous: The story of how many thousands of men and women have recovered from alcoholism* (3d ed.). New York, NY: Alcoholics Anonymous World Services.

Bogenschutz, M. P. (2008). Individual and contextual factors that influence AA affiliation and outcomes. In M. Galanter, L. Kaskutas, T. Borkman, S. Zemore, and J. Tonigan (Eds.), *Recent developments in alcoholism: Research on Alcoholics Anonymous and spirituality in addiction recovery* (Vol. 18, pp. 413–433). New York, NY: Springer.

Bowen, S., Witkiewitz, K., Clifasefi, S. L., Grow, J., Chawla, N., Hsu, S. H., ... Larimer, M. E. (2014). Relative efficacy of mindfulness-based relapse prevention, standard relapse prevention, and treatment as usual for substance use disorders: A randomized clinical trial. *JAMA Psychiatry, 71*, 547–556. https://doi.org/10.1001/jamapsychiatry.2013.4546

*Bulling, D., DeKraai, M., Abdel-Monem, T., Nieuwsma, J. A., Cantrell, W. C., Ethridge, K., & Meador, K. (2013). Confidentiality and mental health/chaplaincy collaboration. *Military Psychology, 25*, 557–567. https://doi.org/10.1037/mil0000019.

Burchard, G. A., Yarthouse, M. A., Kilian, M. E., Worthington, E. L., Jr., Berry, J. W., & Canter, D. E. (2003). A study of two marital enrichment programs and couples' quality of life. *Journal of Psychology and Theology, 31*, 240–252. Retrieved from http://search.proquest.com.jproxy.lib.ecu.edu/docview/223669829?accountid=10639

*Cabot, R. C., & Dicks, D. L. (1953). *The art of ministering to the sick*. New York, NY: MacMillan Company.

Casarez, R. L. P., & Engebretson, J. C. (2012). Ethical issues of incorporating spiritual care into clinical practice. *Journal of Clinical Nursing, 21*, 2099–2107. https://doi.org/10.1111/j.1365-2702.2012.04168.x

Cohen, J. A., Mannarino, A. P., & Deblinger, E. (2006). *Treating trauma and traumatic grief in children and adolescents*. New York, NY: Guilford Press.

Cole, B. S., Hopkins, C. M., Spiegel, J., Tisak, J., Agarwala, S., & Kirkwood, J. M. (2011). A randomised clinical trial of the effects of spiritually focused meditation for people with metastatic melanoma. *Mental Health, Religion & Culture, 15*, 161–14. https://doi.org/10.1080/13674676.2011.562492

Cole, B., & Pargament, K. (1999). Re-creating your life: A spiritual/psychotherapeutic intervention for people diagnosed with cancer. *Psycho-Oncology, 8*, 395–407. https://doi.org/10.1002/(SICI)1099-1611(199909/10)8:5<395::AID-PON408>3.0.CO;2-B

Considine, J. R. (2007). The dilemmas of spirituality in the caring professions: Care-provider spiritual orientation and the communication of care. *Communication Studies, 58*, 227–242. https://doi.org/10.1080/10510970701518330

Cornish, M. A., & Wade, N. G. (2010). Spirituality and religion in group counseling: A literature review with practice guidelines. *Professional Psychology: Research and Practice, 41*, 398–404. https://doi.org/10.1037/a0020179

Curlin, F. A., Lantos, J. D., Roach, C. J., Sellergren, S. A., & Chin, M. H. (2005). Religious characteristics of US physicians: A national survey. *Journal of General Internal Medicine, 20*, 629–634. https://doi.org/10.1111/j.1525-1497.2005.0119.x

Daaleman, T. P., & Frey, B. (1998). Prevalence and patterns of physician referral to clergy and pastoral care providers. *Archives of Family Medicine, 7*, 548–553. https://doi.org/10.1001/archfami.7.6.548

Daaleman, T. P., & Frey, B. B. (2004). The spirituality index of well-being: A new instrument for health-related quality-of-life research. *Annals of Family Medicine, 2*, 499–503. https://doi.org/10.1370/afm.89

Dein, S., & Littlewood, R. (2008). The psychology of prayer and the development of the Prayer Experience Questionnaire. *Mental Health, Religion and Culture, 11*, 39–52. https://doi.org/10.1080/13674670701384396

Delbridge, E., Taylor, J., & Hanson, C. (2014). Honoring the "spiritual" in biopsychosocial-spiritual health care: Medical family therapists on the front lines of graduate education, clinical practice, and research. In J. Hodgson, A. Lamson, T. Mendenhall, and D. Crane (Eds.), *Medical family therapy: Advanced applications* (pp. 197–216). New York, NY: Springer.

*Dell, M. L. (2004). Religious professionals and institutions: Untapped resources for clinical care. *Child and Adolescent Psychiatric Clinics of North America, 13*, 85–110. https://doi.org/10.1016/S1056-4993(03)00098-1.

Doufesh, H., Ibrahim, F., Ismail, N. A., & Ahmad, W. A. W. (2014). Effect of Muslim prayer (Salat) on α electroencephalography and its relationship with autonomic nervous system activity. *Journal of Alternative and Complementary Medicine, 20*, 558–562. https://doi.org/10.1089/acm.2013.0426

Edwards, A., Pang, N., Shiu, V., & Chan, C. (2010). The understanding of spirituality and the potential role of spiritual care in end-of-life and palliative care: A meta-study of qualitative research. *Palliative Medicine, 24*, 753–770. https://doi.org/10.1177/0269216310375860

Ellis, M. R., & Campbell, J. D. (2004). Patients' views about discussing spiritual issues with primary care physicians. *Southern Medical Journal, 97*, 1158–1164. https://doi.org/10.1097/01.SMJ.0000146486.69217.EE

Ellison, L. L. (2006). *The spiritual well-being scale*. Retrieved from http://mds.marshall.edu/cgi/viewcontent.cgi?article=1008&context=co_faculty

Engel, G. L. (1977). The need for a new medical model: A challenge for biomedicine. *Science, 196*, 129–136. https://doi.org/10.1016/b978-0-409-95009-0.50006-1

Engel, G. L. (1980). The clinical application of the biopsychosocial model. *American Journal of Family Medicine, 137*, 535–544. https://doi.org/10.1176/ajp.137.5.535

Esperandio, M. R. G., & Ladd, K. L. (2015). "I heard the voice. I felt the presence:" Prayer, health, and implications for clinical practice. *Religions, 6*, 670–685. https://doi.org/10.3390/rel6020670

Fan, Y., & Wu, J. J. (2007). Journey of my mind: A story of recovery. *Psychiatric Rehabilitation Journal, 30*, 313–314. https://doi.org/10.2975/30.4.2007.313.314

*Flannelly, K. J., Galek, K., Bucchino, J., & Vane, A. (2006). The relative prevalence of various spiritual needs. *Scottish Journal of Healthcare Chaplaincy, 9*, 25–30. https://doi.org/10.1558/hscc.v9i2.25.

Flannelly, K. J., Galek, K., Tannenbaum, H. P., & Handzo, G. F. (2007). A preliminary proposal for a scale to measure the effectiveness of pastoral care with family members of hospitalized patients. *Journal of Pastoral Care and Counseling, 62*, 19–29. https://doi.org/10.1177/154230500706100103

Frost, M. H., Johnson, M. E., Atherton, P. J., Petersen, W. O., Dose, A. M., Kasner, M. J., … Pipe, T. B. (2012). Spiritual well-being and quality of life of women with ovarian cancer and their spouses. *Journal of Supportive Oncology, 10*, 72–80. https://doi.org/10.1016/j.suponc.2011.09.001

*Galek, K., Flannelly, K. J., Koenig, H. G., & Fogg, S. L. (2007). Referrals to chaplains: The role of religion and spirituality in healthcare settings. *Mental Health, Religion & Culture, 10*, 363–377. https://doi.org/10.1080/13674670600757064.

Gaston-Johansson, F., Haisfield-Wolfe, M. E., Reddick, B., Goldstein, N., & Lawal, T. A. (2013). The relationships among coping strategies, religious coping, and spirituality in African American women with breast cancer receiving chemotherapy. *Oncology Nursing Forum, 40*, 120–131. https://doi.org/10.1188/13.ONF.120-131

Gallup (2017). *Religion.* Retrieved from http://www.gallup.com/poll/1690/religion.aspx
George, L. K., Ellison, C. G., & Larson, D. B. (2002). Explaining the relationships between religious involvement and health. *Psychological Inquiry, 13,* 190–200. https://doi.org/10.1207/S15327965PLI1303_04
Germer, C. K. (2009). *The mindful path to self-compassion: Freeing yourself from destructive thoughts and emotions.* New York, NY: Guilford Press.
*Handzo, G. F., Cobb, M., Holmes, C., Kelly, E., & Sinclair, S. (2014). Outcomes for professional health care chaplaincy: An international call to action. *Journal of Health Care Chaplaincy, 20,* 43–53. https://doi.org/10.1080/08854726.2014.902713.
Hatch, R. L., Burg, M. A., Naberhaus, D. S., & Hellmich, L. K. (1998). The spiritual involvement and beliefs scale. *Journal of Family Practice, 46,* 476–486. https://doi.org/10.1037/t06493-000
Hill, P. C., & Pargament, K. I. (2003). Advances in the conceptualization and measurement of religion and spirituality: Implications for physical and mental health research. *American Psychologist, 58,* 64–74. https://doi.org/10.1037/0003-066X.58.1.64
*Hodge, D. R. (2000). Spiritual ecomaps: A new diagrammatic tool for assessing marital and family spirituality. *Journal of Marital and Family Therapy, 26,* 217–228. https://doi.org/10.1111/j.1752-0606.2000.tb00291.x.
*Hodge, D. R. (2005). Spiritual lifemaps: A client-centered pictorial instrument for spiritual assessment, planning, and intervention. *Social Work, 50,* 77–87. https://doi.org/10.1093/sw/50.1.77.
Hodge, D. R. (2007). A systematic review of the empirical literature on intercessory prayer. *Research on Social Work Practice, 17,* 174–187. https://doi.org/10.1177/1049731506296170
Hodge, D. R., & Limb, G. E. (2011). Spiritual assessment and Native Americans: Establishing the social validity of a complementary set of assessment tools. *Social Work, 56,* 213–223. https://doi.org/10.1093/sw/56.3.213
Hodgson, J., Lamson, A. L., & Reese, L. (2007). The Biopsychosocial-Spiritual Interview method. In D. Linville, K. M. Hertlein, and Associates (Eds.), *The therapist's notebook for family health care: Homework, handouts, and activities for individuals, couples, and families coping with illness, loss, and disability* (pp. 3–12). New York, NY: Haworth Press.
Hodgson, J., Lamson, A., Mendenhall, T., & Tyndall, L. (2014). Introduction to Medical Family Therapy: Advanced Applications. In J. Hodgson, A. Lamson, T. Mendenhall, and D. Crane (Eds.), *Medical family therapy: Advanced applications* (pp. 1–9). New York, NY: Springer.
Hoge, M. A., Morris, J. A., Laraia, M., Pomerantz, A., & Farley, T. (2014). *Core competencies for integrated behavioral health and primary care.* Washington, DC: SAMHSA—HRSA Center for Integrated Health Solutions.
Hook, J. N., Davis, D. E., Owen, J., Worthington, E. L., Jr., & Utsey, S. O. (2013). Cultural humility: Measuring openness to culturally diverse clients. *Journal of Counseling Psychology, 60,* 353–366. https://doi.org/10.1037/a0032595
*Hook, J. N., Worthington, E. L. J., Davis, D. E., Jennings, D. J. I., Gartner, A. L., & Hook, J. P. (2010). Empirically supported religious and spiritual therapies. *Journal of Clinical Psychology, 66,* 46–72. https://doi.org/10.1002/jclp.20626.
Jafari, N., Zamani, A., Farajzadegan, Z., Bahrami, F., Emami, H., & Loghmani, A. (2013). The effect of spiritual therapy for improving the quality of life of women with breast cancer: A randomized controlled trial. *Psychology, Health & Medicine, 18,* 56–69. https://doi.org/10.1080/13548506.2012.679738
Jakubowski, S. F., Milne, E. P., Brunner, H., & Miller, R. B. (2004). A review of empirically supported marital enrichment programs. *Family Relations, 53,* 528–536. https://doi.org/10.1111/j.0197-6664.2004.00062.x
Jim, H. S. L., Pustejovsky, J. E., Park, C. L., Danhauer, S. C., Sherman, A. C., Fitchett, G., … Salsman, J. M. (2015). Religion, spirituality, and physical health in cancer patients: A meta-analysis. *Cancer, 121,* 3760–3768. https://doi.org/10.1002/cncr.29353
*Joint Commission on the Accreditation of Healthcare Organizations. (2005). *Evaluating your spiritual assessment process.* Retrieved from http://www.professionalchaplains.org/files/resources/reading_room/evaluating_your_spiritual_assessment_process.pdf

Jors, K., Büssing, A., Hvidt, N. C., & Baumann, K. (2015). Personal prayer in patients dealing with chronic illness: A review of the research literature. *Evidence-Based Complementary & Alternative Medicine, 2015*, 1–12. https://doi.org/10.1155/2015/927973

Kelly, J. F. (2017). Is alcoholics anonymous religious, spiritual, neither? Findings from 25 years of mechanisms of behavior change research. *Addiction, 112*, 929–936. https://doi.org/10.1111/add.13590

Kelly, J. F., Stout, R., Zywiak, W., & Schneider, R. (2006). A 3-year study of addiction mutual-help group participation following intensive outpatient treatment. *Alcoholism Clinical and Experimental Research, 30*, 1381–1392. https://doi.org/10.1111/j.1530-0277.2006.00165.x

Kevern, P., & Hill, L. (2015). Chaplains for well-being' in primary care: Analysis of the results of a retrospective study. *Primary Health Care Research & Development (Cambridge University Press/UK), 16*, 87–99. https://doi.org/10.1017/S1463423613000492

Kinman, C. R., Gilchrist, E. C., Payne-Murphy, J. C., & Miller, B. F. (2015). *Provider- and practice-level competencies for integrated behavioral health in primary care: A literature review*. Rockville, MD: Agency for Healthcare Research and Quality.

Koenig, H. G., Pearce, M. J., Nelson, B., & Daher, N. (2015). Effects of religious versus standard cognitive-behavioral therapy on optimism in persons with major depression and chronic medical illness. *Depression and Anxiety, 32*, 835–842. https://doi.org/10.1002/da.22398

Limb, G. E., & Hodge, D. R. (2011). Utilizing spiritual ecograms with Native American families and children to promote cultural competence in family therapy. *Journal of Marital and Family Therapy, 37*, 81–94. https://doi.org/10.1111/j.1752-0606.2009.00163.x

Limb, G. E., Hodge, D. R., Leckie, R., & Ward, P. (2013). Utilizing spiritual lifemaps with LDS clients: Enhancing cultural competence in social work practice. *Clinical Social Work Journal, 41*, 395–405. https://doi.org/10.1007/s10615-012-0404-3

Lo, H. H. M., Wong, S. Y. S., Wong, J. Y. H., Wong, S. W. L., & Yeung, J. W. K. (2016). The effect of a family-based mindfulness intervention on children with attention deficit and hyperactivity symptoms and their parents: Design and rationale for a randomized, controlled clinical trial (study protocol). *BMC Psychiatry, 16*, 65–74. https://doi.org/10.1186/s12888-016-0773-1

MacLean, C. D., Susi, B., Phifer, N., Schultz, L., Bynum, L., Franco, M., ... Cykert, S. (2003). Patient preference for physician discussion and practice of spirituality. *Journal of General Internal Medicine, 18*, 38–43. https://doi.org/10.1046/j.1525-1497.2003.20403.x

Masters, K., & Spielmans, G. (2007). Prayer and health: Review, meta-analysis, and research agenda. *Journal of Behavioral Medicine, 30*, 329–338. https://doi.org/10.1007/s10865-007-9106-7

McClung, E., Grossoehme, D. H., & Jacobson, A. F. (2006). Collaborating with chaplains to meet spiritual needs. *Medsurg Nursing, 15*, 147–156. Retrieved from http://search.proquest.com.jproxy.lib.ecu.edu/docview/230524645?accountid=10639

McCorkle, B. H., Bohn, C., Hughes, T., & Kim, D. (2005). "Sacred moments": Social anxiety in a larger perspective. *Mental Health, Religion and Culture, 8*, 227–238. https://doi.org/10.1080/13694670500138874

Miller, B.F., Gilchrist, E.C., Ross, K.M., Wong, S.L., Blount, A., & Peek, C.J. (2016). *Core competencies for behavioral health providers working in primary care*. Eugene S. Farley, Jr. Health Policy Center. Retrieved from http://farleyhealthpolicycenter.org/wp-content/uploads/2016/02/Core-Competencies-for-Behavioral-Health-Providers-Working-in-Primary-Care.pdf

Mollica, M. A., Underwood, W., Homish, G. G., Homish, D. L., & Orom, H. (2016). Spirituality is associated with better prostate cancer treatment decision making experiences. *Journal of Behavioral Medicine, 39*, 161–169. https://doi.org/10.1007/s10865-015-9662-1

Monroe, N., & Jankowski, P. J. (2016). The effectiveness of a prayer intervention in promoting change in perceived attachment to God, positive affect, and psychological distress. *Spirituality in Clinical Practice, 3*, 237–249. https://doi.org/10.1037/scp0000117

Newlin, K., Dyess, S. M., Allard, E., Chase, S., & Melkus, G. D. (2012). A methodological review of faith-based health promotion literature: Advancing the science to expand delivery of diabetes education to Black Americans. *Journal of Religion and Health, 51*, 1075–1097. https://doi.org/10.1007/s10943-011-9481-9

Noble, A., & Jones, C. (2010). Getting it right: Oncology nurses' understanding of spirituality. *International Journal of Palliative Nursing, 16*, 565–569. 10.12968/ijpn.2010.16.11.80022

O'Connor, T. S. (2002). The search for truth: The care for evidence-based chaplaincy. *Journal of Health Care Chaplaincy, 13*, 185–194. https://doi.org/10.1300/J080v13n01_03

Oh, P., & Kim, S. H. (2014). The effects of spiritual interventions in patients with cancer: A meta-analysis. *Oncology Nursing Forum, 41*, E290–E301. https://doi.org/10.1188/14.ONF.E290

Pearce, M. J., Koenig, H. G., Robins, C. J., Daher, N., Shaw, S. F., Nelson, B., … King, M. B. (2015). Effects of religious versus conventional cognitive-behavioral therapy on generosity in major depression and chronic medical illness: A randomized clinical trial. *Spirituality in Clinical Practice, 2*, 202–215. https://doi.org/10.1037/scp0000076

Peteet, J. R., & Balboni, M. J. (2013). Spirituality and religion in oncology. *CA: a Cancer Journal for Clinicians, 63*, 280–289. https://doi.org/10.3322/caac.21187

Poloma, M. M., & Hoelter, L. F. (1998). The "Toronto blessing": A holistic model of healing. *Journal for the Scientific Study of Religion, 37*, 257–272. https://doi.org/10.2307/1387526

Poloma, M. M., & Lee, M. T. (2011). From prayer activities to receptive prayer: Godly love and the knowledge that surpasses understanding. *Journal of Psychology and Theology, 39*, 143–154. Retrieved from http://search.proquest.com.jproxy.lib.ecu.edu/docview/882399952?accountid=10639

Prazak, M., Critelli, J., Martin, L., Miranda, V., Purdum, M., & Powers, C. (2012). Mindfulness and its role in physical and psychological health. *Applied Psychology: Health and Well-Being, 4*, 91–105. https://doi.org/10.1111/j.1758-0854.2011.01063.x

Puchalski, C. M. (2014). The FICA spiritual history tool #274. *Journal of Palliative Medicine, 17*, 105–106. https://doi.org/10.1089/jpm.2013.9458

Rawdin, B., Evans, C., & Rabow, M. W. (2013). The relationships among hope, pain, psychological distress, and spiritual well-being in oncology outpatients. *Journal of Palliative Medicine, 16*, 167–172. https://doi.org/10.1089/jpm.2012.0223

Razali, S. M., Hasanah, C. I., Aminah, K., & Subramaniam, M. (1998). Religious-sociocultural psychotherapy in patients with anxiety and depression. *Australian and New Zealand Journal of Psychiatry, 32*, 867–872. https://doi.org/10.3109/00048679809073877

Ripley, J. S., & Worthington, E. L., Jr. (2002). Hope-focused and forgiveness-based group interventions to promote marital enrichment. *Journal of Counseling and Development, 80*, 452–463. https://doi.org/10.1002/j.1556-6678.2002.tb00212.x

Rolland, E. J., & Kaskutas, L. A. (2002). Alcoholics anonymous and church involvement as predictors of sobriety among three ethnic treatment populations. *Alcoholism Treatment Quarterly, 20*, 61–77. https://doi.org/10.1300/j020v20n01_04

Rosenkranz, M. A., Davidson, R. J., MacCoon, D. G., Sheridan, J. F., Kalin, N. H., & Lutz, A. (2013). A comparison of mindfulness-based stress reduction and an active control in modulation of neurogenic inflammation. *Brain, Behavior, and Immunity, 27*, 174–184. https://doi.org/10.1016/j.bbi.2012.10.013

Rosmarin, D. H., Auerbach, R. P., Bigda-Peyton, J. S., Björgvinsson, T., & Levendusky, P. G. (2011). Integrating spirituality into cognitive behavioral therapy in an acute psychiatric setting: A pilot study. *Journal of Cognitive Psychotherapy, 25*, 287–303. https://doi.org/10.1891/0889-8391.25.4.287

Rye, M. S., & Pargament, K. I. (2002). Forgiveness and romantic relationships in college: Can it heal the wounded heart? *Journal of Clinical Psychology, 58*, 419–441. https://doi.org/10.1002/jclp.1153

Rye, M. S., Pargament, K. I., Pan, W., Yingling, D. W., Shogren, K. A., & Ito, M. (2005). Can group interventions facilitate forgiveness of an ex-spouse? A randomized clinical trial. *Journal of Consulting and Clinical Psychology, 73*, 880–892. https://doi.org/10.1037/0022-006X.73.5.880

Saguil, A., & Phelps, K. (2012). The spiritual assessment. *American Family Physician, 86*, 546–550. Retrieved from http://www.aafp.org/afp/2012/0915/p546.html

Tanyi, R. A. (2006). Spirituality and family nursing: Spiritual assessment and interventions for families. *Journal of Advanced Nursing, 53*, 287–294. https://doi.org/10.1111/j.1365-2648.2006.03731.x

Tarakeshwar, N., Pearce, M. J., & Sikkema, K. J. (2005). Development and implementation of a spiritual coping group intervention for adults living with HIV/AIDS: A pilot study. *Mental Health, Religion and Culture, 8*, 179–190. https://doi.org/10.1080/13694670500138908

Tarakeshwar, N., Vanderwerker, L. C., Paulk, E., Pearce, M. J., Kasl, S. V., & Prigerson, H. G. (2006). Religious coping is associated with the quality of life of patients with advanced cancer. *Journal of Palliative Medicine, 9*, 646–657. https://doi.org/10.1089/jpm.2006.9.646

Taren, A., Gianaros, P. J., Greco, C. M., Lindsay, E. K., Fairgrieve, A., Brown, K. W., … Creswell, J. D. (2015). Mindfulness meditation training alters stress-related amygdala resting state functional connectivity: A randomized controlled trial. *Social Cognitive Affective Neuroscience, 12*, 1758–1768. https://doi.org/10.1093/scan/nsv066

*Taylor, J. J., Hodgson, J. L., Kolobova, I., Lamson, A. L., Sira, N., & Musick, D. (2015). Exploring the phenomenon of spiritual care between hospital chaplains and hospital based healthcare providers. *Journal of Health Care Chaplaincy, 21*, 91–107. https://doi.org/10.1080/08854726.2015.1015302.

Thorensen, C. E., Harris, A. H., & Onan, D. (2001). Spirituality, religion, and health: Evidence, issues, and concerns. In T. G. Plante and A. C. Sherman (Eds.), *Faith and health: Psychological perspectives*. New York, NY: Guilford Press.

Tonigan, J. S., Miller, W. R., & Schermer, C. (2002). Atheists, agnostics and alcoholics anonymous. *Journal of Studies on Alcohol, 63*, 534–541. 10.15288/jsa.2002.63.534

Tussing-Humphreys, L. M., Tomson, J. L., & Onufrak, S. J. (2015). A church-based pilot study designed to improve dietary quality for rural, Lower Mississippi Delta, African American adults. *Journal of Religion and Health, 54*, 455–469. https://doi.org/10.1007/s10943-104-9823-5

Underwood, L. G., & Teresi, J. A. (2002). The daily spiritual experience scale: Development, theoretical description, reliability, exploratory factor analysis, and preliminary construct validity using health-related data. *Annals of Family Medicine, 24*, 22–33. https://doi.org/10.1207/S15324796ABM2401_04

*Vanderwerker, L. C., Flannelly, K. J., Galek, K., Harding, S. R., Handzo, G. F., Oettinger, M., & Bauman, J. P. (2008). What do chaplains really do? III. Referrals in the New York Chaplaincy Study. *Journal of Health Care Chaplaincy, 14*, 57–73. https://doi.org/10.1080/08854720802053861.

Van Gordon, W., Shonin, E., Dunn, T. J., Garcia-Campayo, J., & Griffiths, M. D. (2017). Meditation awareness training for the treatment of fibromyalgia syndrome: A randomized controlled trial. *British Journal of Health Psychology, 22*, 186–206. https://doi.org/10.1111/bjhp.12224

Vieten, C., Scammell, S., Pierce, A., Pilato, R., Ammondson, I., Pargament, K. I., & Lukoff, D. (2016). Competencies for psychologists in the domains of religion and spirituality. *Spirituality in Clinical Practice, 3*, 92–114. https://doi.org/10.1037/scp0000078

Walker, D. F., Reese, J. B., Hughes, J. P., & Troskie, M. J. (2010). Addressing religious and spiritual issues in trauma-focused cognitive behavior therapy with children and adolescents. *Professional Psychology: Research and Practice, 41*, 174–180. https://doi.org/10.1037/a0017782

Walker, D. F., Reid, H. W., O'Neill, T., & Brown, L. (2009). Changes in personal religion/spirituality during and after childhood abuse: A review and synthesis. *Psychological Trauma: Theory, Research, Practice, and Policy, 1*, 130–145. https://doi.org/10.1037/a0016211

Wang, D. C., Aten, J. D., Boan, D., Jean-Charles, W., Griff, K. P., Valcin, V. C., … Wang, A. (2016). Culturally adapted spiritually oriented trauma-focused cognitive–behavioral therapy for child survivors of restavek. *Spirituality in Clinical Practice, 3*, 224–236. https://doi.org/10.1037/scp0000120

Waynick, T., Frederich, P., Schneider, D., Thomas, R., & Bloomstrom, G. (2006). Human spirituality, resilience, and the role of military chaplains. In A. Adler, C. Castro, and T. Britt (Eds.), *Military life: The psychology of serving in peace and combat* (pp. 173–191). Westport, CT: Praeger Security International.

Weinberger-Litman, S. L., Muncie, M. A., Flannelly, L. T., & Flannelly, K. J. (2010). When do nurses refer patients to professional chaplains? *Holistic Nursing Practice, 24,* 44–48. https://doi.org/10.1097/HNP.0b013e3181c8e491

Williams, J. A., Meltzer, D., Arora, V., Chung, G., & Curlin, F. A. (2011). Attention to inpatients' religious and spiritual concerns: Predictors and association with patient satisfaction. *Journal of General Internal Medicine, 26,* 1265–1271. https://doi.org/10.1007/s11606-011-1781-y

Williams, M. L., Wright, M., Cobb, M., & Shields, C. (2004). A prospective study of the roles, responsibilities, and stresses of chaplains working within a hospice. *Palliative Medicine, 18,* 638–645. https://doi.org/10.1191/0269216304pm929oa

Worthington, E. L. (2005). *Hope-focused marriage counseling: A guide to brief therapy* (2nd ed.). Westmont, IL: IVP Academic.

Worthington, E. L., Jr., Might, T. L., Ripley, J. S., Perrone, K. M., Kurusu, T. A., & Jones, D. J. (1997). Strategic hope-focused relationship-enrichment counseling with individuals. *Journal of Counseling Psychology, 44,* 381–389. https://doi.org/10.1037/0022-0167.44.4.381

Worthington, E. L., Sandage, S. J., & Berry, J. W. (2000). Group interventions to promote forgiveness: What researchers and clinicians ought to know. In M. McCullough, K. Pargament, and C. Thoresen (Eds.), *Forgiveness: Theory, research, and practice* (pp. 228–253). New York, NY: Guilford Press.

*Wright, L. M., Watson, W. L., & Bell, J. M. (1996). *Beliefs: The heart of healing in families and illness.* New York, NY: Basic Books.

Yanez, B., Edmondson, D., Stanton, A. L., Park, C. L., Kwan, L., Gans, P. A., & Blank, T. O. (2009). Facets of spirituality as predictors of adjustment to cancer: Relative contributions of having faith and finding meaning. *Journal of Consulting and Clinical Psychology, 77,* 730–741. https://doi.org/10.1037/a0015820

Zemore, S., Kaskutas, L. A., Mericle, A., & Hemberg, J. (2016). Comparison of 12-Step groups to mutual help alternatives for AUD in a large, national study: Differences in membership characteristics and group participation, cohesion, and satisfaction. *Journal of Substance Abuse Treatment, 73,* 16–26. https://doi.org/10.1016/j.jsat.2016.10.004

Chapter 17
Medical Family Therapy in Employee Assistance Programs

Calvin Paries, Angela Lamson, Jennifer Hodgson, Amelia Muse, and Glenda Mutinda

Companies and industries influence a considerable number of policy changes in the United States, especially when it comes to healthcare. Their influence is grounded in the large number of employees hired and concomitant budget lines that are directed toward employees' healthcare coverage. Businesses often pay partial or full health insurance on behalf of both the employee and his/her family. Healthcare costs for individuals, families, and employers continue to rise on a yearly basis; these have a "pocketbook impact" on both ordinary families and U.S. businesses alike (National Conference of State Legislators [NCSL], 2017).

Healthcare costs shape employers' bottom line; thus, businesses and organizations must look for alternative strategies to control those costs (Marsh, 2014). They are forced to look at alternative solutions in their healthcare strategies to keep health-related expenses low or at a reasonable level. Willis Towers Watson (WTW), an international broker and actuarial firm, conducts annual assessments with U.S. businesses. They found that 84% of respondents reported that health and productivity are core components of organizations' health strategies and that most organizations are looking beyond the scope of direct benefits for employees (e.g., health insurance plans) by seeking ways that enhance employees' emotional, social, and financial well-being (WTW, 2017).

C. Paries (✉)
Profile EAP, Colorado Springs, CO, USA
e-mail: cparies@msn.com

A. Lamson · J. Hodgson · G. Mutinda
Department of Human Development and Family Science, East Carolina University, Greenville, NC, USA

A. Muse
Center of Excellence for Integrated Care, Cary, NC, USA

A longitudinal study was conducted to investigate the association between modifiable well-being risks and productivity (Shi, Sears, Coberley, Pope, 2013). Researches found that poor emotional health (e.g., stress, depression, and physiological distress) and inadequate exercise impacted productivity greater than other health risks. These results support the need for employers to provide both direct (i.e., health insurance plans) and indirect (i.e., wellness programs) forms of healthcare. And several organizations are now taking the lead in such wellness efforts. For example, Fitbit advances direction in this arena for both consumers and employees (see https://www.fitbit.com/content/assets/group-health/FitbitWellness_InfoSheet.pdf). Google provides educational and mindfulness programs for its workers (see https://careers.google.com/how-we-care-for-googlers). Zappos works to make their employees' environments better for overall health (see http://www.healthyworksofpa.com/wellness-case-study-zappos).

Employers are increasingly looking to employee assistance programs (EAP) and Wellness Services as a way to improve productivity and overall employee health. EAP services are seen as way to address the chasm between behavioral or physical health concerns and performance. Successful EAPs are embedded in an organization (workforce), understand the workplace system's culture, and facilitate success through service(s) utilization. EAP utilization has been attributed to a variety of workforce improvements, including lowering unscheduled absences, lowing absenteeism, increasing productivity, shortening disability stay, and impacting workers' compensation claims (Attridge, 2016; Attridge et al., 2007; Attridge & Wallace, 2010; Dewa, Hoch, Carmen, Guscott, & Anderson, 2009; Goldner et al., 2004; Morneau Shepell, 2014; Sharar & DeLapp, 2016). This is a positive step away from traditional EAP care models that focused on a particular incident or injury that precipitated care.

Advanced and nontraditional EAPs are repositioning themselves to better impact employee health by providing on-site healthcare. Situating EAPs into contexts such as primary care clinics allows employees to be served through integrated behavioral healthcare (IBHC) models that work to better address physical health concerns in tandem with behavioral health needs. All providers within the IBHC model work with the intent of increasing employees' well-being and decreasing employees' time away from work. IBHC visits are prime opportunities for medical family therapists (MedFTs) to function as collaborators and part of the patient's healthcare team at point of care, particularly when 70% of primary care visits have a psychosocial component (Fries, Coop, & Beadle, 1993; Gatchel & Oordt, 2003). MedFTs may also be an important addition to the EAP collaborative care team because family therapy (especially when compared to individual treatment) is more effective and less expensive—particularly when it is embedded in primary care (Crane & Christianson, 2014; Crane & Payne, 2011). Historically, family therapy has had some presence within industry (Skidmore, & Skidmore, 1975), organizations as human systems consultants (Boverie, 1991), the workplace (Korner, 1986), and employee assistance programs (Bayer, 1995; Shumway, Wampler, Dersch, & Arredondo, 2004; Smith, Salts, & Smith, 1989). In fact, Wynne, Weber, and McDaniel (1986) were early supporters of the need for family therapists and systems-oriented healthcare professionals to serve as consultants in diverse contexts; they were foundational to the development of MedFT.

MedFTs within EAPs deal with multiple and complex macro-, micro-, and subsystems within the workplace. An employee with a family problem who is working within a dysfunctional working environment and reporting to an administrator pressured to reduce costs, for example, is a common scenario. One minor shift in a complex system (e.g., new financial officer) can offset another system (e.g., demands on work productivity), which can influence other systems' positivity (e.g., an employee receives a merit raise) or negativity (e.g., an employee becomes more irritable with his/her partner and children at home). MedFTs trained in systems theory have wise insights and keen perceptions into such workplace situations, which help them and others better navigate these nonlinear, multilayered, and complex systemic issues. A MedFT's robust systemic training benefits patients, alongside offering the capacity for influencing workplace dynamics at large (e.g., maximizing collaborative relationships between colleagues or enhancing communication between an employee and employer)—thereby making MedFTs a great addition to any business or organization's EAP team.

Recognizing the advantages of being embedded in a company's culture, and understanding an organization's complex systems and subsystems, positions EAPs to be a strategic partner for any employee-based organization. Traditional EAPs provide therapy for employees and their families, as well as organizational help for struggling managers or workplaces needing worksite crisis interventions. In this chapter, we discuss how a nontraditional EAP model, strategically repositioned and embedded within primary care, occupational health, workers' compensation, wellness, disability, and/or organizational development, can improve EAPs' leverage for change that results in program's increased organizational value.

The following clinical vignette is about an injured employee who received workers' compensation (WC) healthcare services at an occupational health center organized through an EAP as an integrated behavioral health clinic. The clinic has access to both traditional and nontraditional EAP services. Nontraditional services include an on-site presence of MedFTs who serve under the EAP but are part of the health-

Clinical Vignette
Note: This vignette is a compilation of cases that represent treatment in an EAP context. All patients' names and/or identifying information have been changed to maintain confidentiality.]
The MedFT first met Jose, a twenty-something behavioral health technician, when he was attending a follow-up appointment at the occupational health clinic for work-related injuries. The occupational health department administrator was under pressure by corporate to better control the workers' compensation and disability costs, which were on the rise. Dr. Christenson, the workers' compensation doctor and medical director, was looking for solutions. He recently saw a patient for a second time that he expected to be fully functional and back on the job. He came into the MedFT's office to discuss his concerns.

"This is the second time I have seen Jose in the last four months," Dr. Christenson said. "Three months ago he came in after being assaulted by a patient on the unit [this employee worked for an in-patient department]. He had some minor bruising and scratches, but nothing significant. I referred him to our traditional EAP services, but he declined. He has a new physical injury, but also shows a laundry list of behavioral issues. I can't get him to go; since you are here now, can you talk to him? Do your magic?"

Dr. Christenson and the MedFT then reviewed Jose's chart together. Jose was brought into the occupational health center by his supervisor after a visit to the emergency room (ER). This was Jose's second injury from a patient assault. This time, he received minor head trauma, a broken arm, and a bruised eye socket. He was knocked unconscious and was hospitalized for one night.

The MedFT entered Jose's exam room and introduced herself. "Jose, it is great to meet with you today. I am part of the healthcare team that is working with you on your Workers Compensation treatment. I work closely with Dr. Christenson and the team here in Workers Comp."

The MedFT did not introduce herself as being with EAP, as that could have been perceived as a separate, more focused, behavioral health intervention. The MedFT wanted Jose to see her as more than only EAP, i.e., as part of his healthcare team.

The MedFT then explained her purpose for being there. "Jose, my role today is to gain information about biological, psychological, social, and spiritual factors that may have an impact on your health, your recovery from your injuries, and returning to work. I can assist with approaches for pain management, sleep management, as well as talk with you about how you are doing emotionally since the incident."

For all patients seen on-site, the protocol was to assess for depression and anxiety at the first integrated behavioral healthcare visit, but in this case the MedFT felt as though she also needed to assess for symptoms of post-traumatic stress.

Jose quickly responded, "So they sent in the shrink to make sure my head is okay?"

The MedFT responded in a way that normalized her presence. "I am part of the healthcare team and meet with all patients—regardless of whether they have behavioral needs or not. We have a holistic approach to how we treat everyone here."

Jose nodded and told the MedFT more about his health. "The doc told me my blood pressure is high, 170/99, and I have gained some weight. I was honest and told him I don't really exercise, and I eat fast food during every shift. I just don't have the energy to exercise, but I wish I did."

Hearing Jose's desire to change, the MedFT then asked for permission to use an assessment instrument. She asked him questions from the Patient Health Questionnaire (PHQ-9; Kroenke, Spitzer, Williams, 2001). Jose's depression score indicated that he was experiencing moderately severe depression symptoms. He and the MedFT discussed the score, and the MedFT provided a brief intervention focused on mindfulness techniques to improve Jose's specific depression symptoms. After using some motivational interviewing questions, Jose agreed to meeting with a wellness coach, who was available to him for free through the EAP program, to discuss beginning an exercise routine. After the consult, the MedFT spoke with the wellness coach about Jose's goals and noted a follow-up in the integrated chart.

As care proceeded, the MedFT continued to assess for depression and post-traumatic stress. Additionally, the MedFT and Jose discussed Jose's plan for returning to work. He expressed his aversion to doing this following the second patient assault. Jose explained that each time he thinks about going back, he gets sweaty palms and a dry throat and has racing thoughts and feelings of fear.

"I don't think I can ever walk down that hallway again," Jose said. "I think it's time for me to look at finding another, less stressful job."

During this brief consult, the MedFT used a heart rate variability monitor, a device used to detect a patient's heart rate and respiration, for a brief biofeedback intervention. The output let the MedFT know that Jose had a higher pulse and respiration rate than someone who is typically at rest. When the MedFT asked Jose to think about returning to work, his heart and respiration rate increased significantly. While he was visualizing walking into work and starting his duties, the MedFT coached him on diaphragmatic breathing and helped Jose to focus on positive work experiences and interactions. The heart rate variability monitor registered changes that showed he was returning to a more relaxed state. The intervention lasted approximately 15 minutes.

At the end of the biofeedback session, Jose stated, "I don't know what you've done to me, but I feel calmer than I have in years."

Jose and the MedFT then went to the nurse's station together to check his blood pressure; it had dropped to 132/89. Before the end of the appointment, Jose and the MedFT met with Dr. Christensen to discuss Jose's return to work. Jose said that after the intervention, he felt that he could return to work the next day. They discussed indicated next steps for doing this; these included a formal evaluation at occupational health/EAP. Dr. Christensen scheduled one more appointment for Jose later in the week. The MedFT consulted with the occupational health/EAP team to inform them about the positive behavioral and physical steps Jose had made.

Jose showed up for his final appointment before his return-to-work assessment. The occupational health nurse checked his vitals and Dr. Christensen followed up with him. After reviewing his vitals and talking with Dr. Christensen,

> the MedFT met with him. He presented as less anxious and more excited about returning to work. The MedFT did some mindfulness exercises with Jose, making sure he was not using avoidance techniques to cope, and further discussed some of Jose's anxious thoughts.
> The MedFT updated the integrated chart and consulted with EAP about Jose being ready to return to work. The EAP called and consulted with Dr. Christensen and the MedFT about this. Dr. Christensen agreed to release Jose to go back to work with a follow-up appointment at the clinic in 2 weeks.
> Two weeks later, Jose's PHQ-9 results showed that he was experiencing only mild depression symptoms. He shared, too, how he had taught his coworkers a diaphragmatic breathing technique during a recent staff meeting. After each of Jose's appointments, the MedFT entered the data from his vitals (blood pressure, weight, pain score) and behavioral health screenings into the clinical outcomes' tracking system. At each monthly team meeting, the MedFT presented the de-identified outcomes data to the team and senior administrators from the occupational health system.

care team in the clinic. The injured employee, Jose, received integrated behavioral healthcare services from a MedFT during an appointment pertaining to a new injury.

As evidenced in this vignette, EAPs are different from most behavioral health services because of the high likelihood for—and inevitably of—dual roles. Dual roles, in this situation, revealed that the employee is both (a) the identified patient and (b) a worker for the company. This results in a twofold "customer" scenario for the MedFT, being both the employee and employer. As previously mentioned, system-trained therapists such as MedFTs can be a company's best asset in understanding complex relationships and incorporating this knowledge to solve problems.

In this chapter, we explore the history of EAPs, their evolution, and their need for continued growth to remain relevant as a workplace benefit. We discuss the roles that MedFTs play in an EAP environment and how these roles play out across the MedFT Healthcare Continuum. The chapter concludes with research-supported findings that demonstrate the need for EAP/MedFTs in an IBHC environment to facilitate early behavioral change demonstrated by positive health outcomes (e.g., improvement in chronic medical conditions and reduction in workers' compensation consequences for organizations) .

What Are Employee Assistance Programs?

Beginning in the 1940s, alcohol use and abuse were on the rise; these trends influenced employers to start addressing industrial (or occupational) alcoholism in the workplace (Henderson & Bacon, 1953). In the 1950s and 1960s, companies such as

Consolidated Edison, Standard Oil of New Jersey, and American Cyanamid extended alcoholism programs to include some mental health services for employees, due to presenting symptoms, reported diagnoses, and increasing severity of concerns. In the 1960s, companies started seeing success with these internal company-run industrial alcohol treatment programs, and, as a result, workplace employee assistance programs (EAP) were born (Presnall, 1981; Roman, 1988; Steele & Trice, 1995).

The term "EAP" did not make its way into the workplace until the 1970s. This was the result of companies wanting more than in-house programs focused on alcohol use for their employees. Additionally, a position paper was published stating that workplace interventions should not be solely focused on alcoholism but also on a broad spectrum of behavioral health problems. In 1971, the Association of Labor Management Administrators and Consultants on Alcoholism (ALMACA) was formed. Its mission was highly influenced by the first occupational program consultants (OPCs) who moved industrial alcoholism programs throughout the United States and into the world of "broad-brush" EAPs (Roman, 1988; Wrich, 1974, 1980).

By 1979, 59% of Fortune 500 companies had an established and functional EAP (Milgram & McCrady, 1986; Roman, 1988). During the 1980s, EAPs continued to grow and change. The number of EAP programs expanded from between 2,500 and 4,000 companies in the 1970s to appropriately 12,000 by 1985 (Blum, Roman, & Tootle, 1988). Many companies were developing their own EAP programs, but the costs of providing these services were challenging for most. In response, community-based agencies and proprietor-owned organizations developed contractual third-party EAP services (York, 1985). Third-party EAP programs assisted companies by helping them to implement policies toward a drug-free workplace through random substance abuse testing, mandatory referrals for mental illness or substance abuse, critical incident response training, management consultation for interactions with difficult employees, and procedures to reduce workplace violence (Bennet, Blum, & Roman, 1994; Oss & Clary, 1998).

The years of growth in the EAP field from 1980 through the 1990s were fueled by an expansion of programs and services that were specific to the needs of American businesses. Open Minds (2000), a research and consulting firm, observed that EAPs had a 245% increase in the use of their services from the early 1990s to 2000. As EAPs moved into the year 2000, competition in the field increased as insurance companies, counseling centers, free-standing psychiatric hospitals, medical hospitals, and private entrepreneurs got into the EAP market. EAPs started to leverage technology, too, through telephonic and web-based tools that both addressed needs and cut costs (Pompe & Sharar, 2014). For EAPs to survive in the twenty-first century, they needed to continue to seek out ways to meet the contemporary demands of workplaces. This meant that they must be robust in their service offerings and do so at lower costs within a competitive market. Services such as work-life needs (e.g., finding child or elder care, financial counseling, and legal consultation) and work-life balance tools for employees (e.g., stress management and depression screening) needed to become standard EAP services (Macy, Watkins, Lartey, & Golla, 2017). Programs specific for managers and leaders have existed since the early days of ALMACA (i.e., 1970s). However, starting in the year 2000, EAP vendors also began to develop specialized teams of professionals who handle the concerns of administrators and management (Joseph & Walker, 2016).

Since 2010, the strength of the EAP profession has been its ability to focus on companies' ongoing and evolving needs. EAP services must stay on the front lines of a company's needs at all times. They concentrate on current essentials via (a) consulting with organizations in assessing leadership requirements, (b) monitoring employees' biopsychosocial concerns, (c) seeking ways to enhance work environments and improve job performance, (d) improving pathways to better access medical and behavioral assistance, and (e) decreasing risks in the workforce and workplace. EAPs have evolved from seeing companies as two-dimensional objects (e.g., company handles an injured employee as needing treatment with a goal to return to work) to seeing them as complex multidimensional systems. As such, the needs described above encourage EAPs to become as familiar as possible with (a) turnover rates (and collaborating with human resources (HR)), (b) records of any poor hospital consumer assessments of healthcare provider scores (HCAP), (c) patient experience (PE) surveys, (d) logged safety policy violations, and (e) patient screens for depression—all in order to maximize a contextual appreciation for what employees may be encountering in their work contexts.

The more involved an EAP is with key decision makers in an organization, the better the EAP will be seen by the organization as an asset. MedFTs' strengths in EAPs include their relational and collaborative natures when working with diverse treatment team members, alongside their capacities to use a range of systemic knowledge and skills in their clinical work with patients. They do this while addressing employees' biopsychosocial-spiritual health (Engel, 1977, 1980; Wright, Watson, & Bell, 1996) across individual, family, and larger system levels. MedFTs working in EAP settings are also trained to work within interdisciplinary teams and to understand how to prioritize services and collaborate in the provision of optimal care.

Treatment Teams in Employee Assistance Programs

In traditional EAPs, the term "treatment team" is not typically used. We use it here to describe potential key collaborators in EAP contexts. As EAPs move into more IBHC models within wellness, disease management, employee clinics, and occupational health, working with a treatment team is a key strength that must be utilized. Typically, the EAP professional will work with two teams or groups to provide services: clinical and organizational. The clinical team, in an IBHC model, typically consists of a medical director, EAP director, MedFT, workers' compensation nurse manager, workers' compensation case manager, corporate safety officer, ergonomist, and director of occupational health. These individuals are influential in assessing policy and procedures, as well as managing care in the IBHC context. The organizational team includes key individuals that the EAP partners with to provide organizational support. This is often comprised of managers, benefits brokers, and administrators. These individuals are human resource officers, compensation and benefit managers, leave and disability managers, employee health medical directors, occupational health directors, organizational development directors, directors of nursing (healthcare), training managers, police/security chiefs, and emergency planning coordinators. Each of the key partners for clinical and organizational support is described below. They are listed in no certain order of importance. These descriptions align with those cited within the U.S. Department of Labor's *Occupational Outlook Handbook* (2015).

Case managers. The role of the case manager in an EAP is to oversee the coordination, monitoring, discharge, and return-to-work planning. The case manager also ensures that treatment gains are realized and that the employee makes the most benefit of each resource available for employees.

Compensation and benefits personnel. Compensation managers plan, develop, and oversee programs to determine how much an organization pays its employees and how employees are paid. Benefits managers plan, direct, and coordinate retirement plans, health insurance, and other benefits that an organization offers its employees.

Corporate safety officers. Safety officers review, evaluate, and analyze work environments. Furthermore, they design programs and procedures to control, eliminate, and prevent disease or injury caused by chemical, physical, and biological agents or ergonomic factors. A safety officer may conduct inspections and enforce adherence to laws and regulations governing the health and safety of individuals.

Directors of occupational health. Occupational health and safety programs are either a contracted entity through an occupational health service or provided by the company itself. The director oversees many types of specialists; he or she also conducts, interprets, and/or directs changes based on analyses of work environments and procedures. These professionals inspect workplaces for adherence to regulations on safety, health, and the environment. Occupational health directors also design programs to prevent disease or injury to workers and damage to the environment.

EAP directors. The EAP director (or manager) develops, organizes, directs, and controls operations of employee assistance programs. Administratively, this leader hires, supervises, and evaluates employees, determines program priorities, and oversees the fiscal budget. Clinically, he or she oversees the direct clinical service to patients, including but not limited to assessment, counseling, referral, and case management. The EAP director also participates in strategic planning, serves as a consultant as requested on organizational and personnel issues, and develops new programs as needed by corporate clients, including marketing and sales planning and efforts.

Emergency planning coordinators. Planning coordinators typically manage the organization's emergency management (preparation) team. They prepare plans and procedures for responding to natural disasters or other emergencies. They also help lead the response during and after emergencies, often in coordination with public safety officials, elected officials, nonprofit organizations, and government agencies.

Medical directors. A medical director can be an employee of the organization or a contracted entity through an occupational health or workers' compensation service. Typically, these professionals are responsible for giving complete and comprehensive preemployment physical examinations and to document findings in a systematic manner on a problem-oriented medical record. They help to ensure that patient privacy and medical record confidentiality are maintained. In a healthcare setting, the medical director oversees the Infection Control Committee (ICC), which is responsible for immunizations as recommended by the Centers for Disease Control and Prevention (CDC). The director must be able to accurately assess those employees who require treatment and initiate appropriate diagnostic and therapeutic measures according to protocol. He or she is also responsible for directing and assigning work to clinicians and staff and provides managerial responsibilities such as personnel counseling, recruitment or discipline/dismissal, and general performance reviews for these people.

Ergonomists. The ergonomist job title and responsibilities typically fall under the occupational health department. The job description focuses around applying information about human behavior, abilities and limitations, and other characteristics to the design of tools, machines, tasks, jobs, and environments for productive, safe, comfortable, and effective human use.

Human resources managers. Human resources managers plan, direct, and coordinate the administrative functions of an organization. They oversee the recruiting, interviewing, and hiring of new staff, consult with top executives on strategic planning, and serve as a link between an organization's management and its employees.

Leave and disability managers. These managers typically oversee the monitoring of all types of leaves, including those under the Family and Medical Leave Act, intermittent, and employer-sponsored leaves. They coordinate access to benefits such as short-term disability, long-term disability, and workers' compensation. Leave and disability managers help implement the documentation of workflows, define responsibilities, set program expectations, identify program gaps, manage human resources policy compliance, complete audit trails, and track leave history. They work closely with human resources managers and employees receiving services.

Nurse managers. The role of a nurse manager in an EAP is to assist the injured employee and facilitate his or her return to work through identifying medical services that are needed, coordinating those services, and functioning as an advocate, educator, and navigator for the employee's medical needs and solutions throughout the recovery process.

Organizational development (OD) directors. The OD director (manager) administers the design, planning, and implementation of various corporate organizational development programs, policies, and procedures. Typical responsibilities include approving change management initiatives, suggesting enhancements to existing OD programs, and demonstrating and championing the concept of human capital as being a critical component of an organization. They are familiar with a variety of EAP-based concepts, practices, and procedures.

Security chiefs. Chiefs of security for companies are either employees of a company or leaders of a contracted firm. A chief oversees information systems and company security for the organization. This person is expected to evaluate, report on, and suggest new ideas related to any security threats that the company currently faces, helping protect vital information and strategies. The chief information security officer typically works with a team that he or she has appointed to effectively develop the steps necessary to protect the company's interests. This person must provide advice and leadership related to existing administrative security policies; this can include auditing the current systems in place, as well as directing and implementing new standards.

Training managers. These managers plan, direct, and coordinate programs to enhance the knowledge and skills of an organization's employees. They also oversee a staff of training and development specialists.

Fundamentals of Employee Assistance Programs

Medical family therapists who work, or plan to work, in an EAP setting are encouraged to have specific knowledge and skills above and beyond those typically taught in behavioral health training programs. It is important that MedFTs are aware that executing these skills is different than what is commonly done in a specialty behavioral health or other IBHC setting. Their role may start off by consulting with a company and learning about its needs (e.g., via needs analysis) and requests for EAP services. MedFTs may then use that knowledge to strategically position EAP programs and services to meet those needs. The role may include marketing, strategic development, and business practices by selling the company on how EAPs can advance MedFT services to help (a) promote employee wellness, (b) increase employee productivity, and (c) show faster rates of returning injured employees to work.

The following is an example of how MedFTs, as members of an EAP team, may use their knowledge and skill sets. A company could request EAP services because its leaders are interested in finding ways to minimize absenteeism among workers. The EAP is brought to the table to deliver a solution to reduce sick days, tardiness, and turnover. The MedFT, in this case, would need to learn about the complexities of issues resulting in absenteeism (e.g., employee burnout, caregiving needs at home). Questions such as "What is the average number of sick days taken per employee each month?" or "What are the most concerning work related stressors experienced by employees?" are important to consider. MedFTs can work to assess burnout through a variety of research-informed screeners (von Kanel, van Nuffel, & Fuchs, 2016), as well as learn more about any themes among workers that may result in tardiness or turnover (e.g., long and inflexible work hours). Outcomes from these scenarios may be treated differently by the company, because each scenario can have positive or negative effects to the employee and employer (e.g., the financial cost of training to the employer may encourage the company to offer more flextime to employees in order to reduce turnover).

Other complex scenarios that MedFTs may engage in as part of an EAP system are those associated with workers' compensation and the likelihood for coverage of an injury or condition. MedFTs may become part of circumstances whereby they assess whether a behavioral health condition is pre-existing or newly developed, and if it is newly developed, then if it was related to a workplace injury. A mental illness deemed to be a result of a workplace accident would likely be covered and treated under workers' compensation benefits. A mental illness deemed to be a pre-existing condition and not a result of a workplace accident may not be covered under workers' compensation benefits; the patient may then be referred to a private behavioral health or traditional therapy for specialty behavioral health services (e.g., detox, eating disorders, complex mental illnesses). MedFTs working as part of an EAP or in collaboration with an EAP will find that each situation is in fact complex multilayered; they must thereby work to make sure to assess and treat employees in accord with appropriate ethical and best clinical practice guidelines (e.g., not be swayed by an employer to underdiagnose or undertreat employees). The following are a variety of knowledge- and skill- related foci that are essential to the success of MedFTs working in EAP settings.

Clinical Knowledge and Skills

The International Employee Assistance Professionals Association (IEAPA, 2011, para 4) has put forth key definitions referred to as EAP core technologies, which are central to the knowledge and skills of those who work within the field of EAP:

1. Consultation with, training of, and assistance to work with organization leadership (managers, supervisors, and union stewards) seeking to manage the troubled employee, enhance the work environment, and improve employee job performance.
2. Active promotion of the availability of EA [employee assistance] services to employees, their family members, and the work organization.
3. Confidential and timely problem identification/assessment services for employee patients with personal concerns that may affect job performance.

4. Use of constructive confrontation, motivation, and short-term intervention with employee patients to address problems that affect job performance.
5. Referral of employee patients for diagnosis, treatment, and assistance plus case monitoring and follow-up services, organizations, and insurers.
6. Assisting work organizations in establishing and maintaining effective relations with treatment and other service providers and in managing provider contracts.
7. Consultation to work organizations to encourage availability of and employee access to health benefits covering medical and behavioral problems including, but not limited to, alcoholism, drug abuse, and mental and emotional disorders.
8. Evaluation of the effects of EA services on the work organization and individual job performance.

The aforementioned EAP core technology list provides MedFTs with an understanding of the foundational clinical skills needed to function effectively in this complex and challenging role. MedFTs can benefit from administration and leadership style training to increase their confidence in the inevitable dual roles that occur in the EAP context (serving the patient and the employer simultaneously). For example, the MedFT may be assigned to assess and treat a patient, but he or she is also helping to determine an employee's readiness to return to work.

EAP-centric clinical skills also include referral navigation for patients (e.g., providing a patient with a referral to specialty care) (Cagney, 2012), proactive case management, on-site crisis counseling (Attridge & Vanderpol, 2010), and consultations with management teams (Harris, 2011). An EAP/MedFT professional should be prepared to provide continuity care services as well. These services may include behavioral health assessment, diagnosis, and extension of brief interventions. Because they may refer for specialty services when necessary (e.g., detox), they should be aware of what is available in the employee's community. The EAP/MedFT's diverse set of skills helps the organization (workplace safety and performance) be better equipped to meet employees' needs.

Training skills and public speaking abilities are also vital skill sets. EAP professionals are often doing behavioral wellness trainings, EAP orientations (educating employees about the service), and supervisory and management trainings with high-level administrators. Supervisory and management trainings require an understanding of human resource (HR) laws, awareness of Americans with Disabilities Act (ADA) regulations, alcohol and drug treatment knowledge, and management referral processes (Cagney, 2012). Knowledge and training in on-site crisis counseling are also key. Clinically, the MedFT should understand the concepts of resilience, solution-oriented treatment, psychological first aid (PFA), and management engagement. These are all key clinical skills that can be gained through MedFT courses and/or specific EAP critical incident response trainings (Attridge & Vanderpol, 2010; Gorter, Jacobsen, & O'Brien, 2015; Intveld, 2013; Slawinski, 2005a, 2005b; 2012).

Human Resource Knowledge and Clinical Business Skills

Key human resource knowledge and clinical business skills are important for MedFTs working in EAPs. Regarding HR knowledge, it is important to learn and be aware of various HR policies on such issues as progressive discipline, the ADA, the Family and Medical Leave Act (FMLA), long-term and short-term disability, company policy, procedure development, risk management, and workplace safety. Important clinical business skills are also important to learn and develop. These skills include conducting a needs assessment and then the organizational implementation of relevant assessment outcomes. Furthermore, the assessment can help strategic business plans to align with operational and financial goals central to the organization's needs. Typically, companies have a strong need for demonstrating cost savings. These outcomes come from obtaining data that demonstrates the EAP's impact. It is beneficial to demonstrate savings through claims data, leave and disability management savings, and pharmacy costs.

EAPs are working more closely than ever with brokers and insurance providers, as well as information technology professionals in order to provide outcomes in the way of cost-offset, healthcare utilization, and cost-effectiveness for EAP interventions. These needs are growing among organizations who have learned that psychosocial variables are greatly influencing performance and productivity. Terms such as data warehouses, data mining, and claims management are all outcome and data collection terms that MedFTs will need to understand in order to review and produce reports. These reports are vital to an EAP program's sustainability and, quite possibly, that of the company or organization.

There are several skills that a MedFT may need to adopt on location based on the organization's unique needs. The greater the need, the more knowledge and skills MedFTs should possess regarding how to design and implement various EAP programs. Sumiec (2016) argued that EAPs that only focus on individual patients and their needs instead of how each patient functions within the workplace system and culture are missing out on truly helping the organization. Sumiec's article can be used to support the need for a relationally and systemically trained behavioral health provider (BHP), such as a MedFT. This knowledge can be used to help MedFTs when designing programs at an organizational level instead of exclusively at the individual-employee level. Through this source, MedFTs can strengthen their opportunities via the delivery of training or services in leadership development and coaching, organizational awareness, collaborative communication, team building, survey development, and data collection of clinical, organizational, and financial variables.

One particular area that is missing from nearly all behavioral health programs is training in the area of billing and reimbursement. As such, MedFTs must gain knowledge in the ability to navigate third-party companies, particularly when EAPs do not service a single account (company) but instead service multiple companies with many different processes and cultures. An EAP company can literally have thousands of accounts (company contracts) that they manage. As a MedFT working in an EAP world, one's knowledge and skills must extend to understand multiple companies' contexts and workplace cultures, healthcare providers, human resource managers, and benefits structures. Without an understanding of the billing structure and process, the MedFT will not likely remain a viable resource to the system. Also, a lack of understanding in this area means that the MedFT is unaware of their own return on investment (ROI; measures gain or loss generated on an investment relative to the amount invested). MedFTs need to understand the operational indicators that their services are viable and making a difference for the organization.

Operational Knowledge and Skills

Overall, MedFTs need to be astute and carefully monitor any political and cultural ripples in the work environment. Being a MedFT within an EAP context means staying politically neutral to the environment. Not advocating for the patient (e.g., to get legal support in relation to his injury or encouraging his wife to do so on his behalf) but also not being the company's or organization's advocate (e.g., to push the employee back into the workplace prematurely) is important. This is a delicate balance between reducing future health and financial risks and providing services that are not perceived as adversarial for EAP contexts or the employee.

As a MedFT in EAP contexts, understanding workplace resources, important committees, key leaders, and protocols is important in aiding and influencing the organization as a whole. MedFTs collaborate with the EAP team and are often key professionals who break down unnecessary silos, by including voices from medical, behavioral, safety, leadership development, and training arenas. Making sure that a sometimes silo-ed organization or company talks and communicates with others is a masterful skill set of relationally trained MedFTs. In committee meetings, administrative meetings, and leadership orientations, a well-trained MedFT typically knows how to put forward useful solutions for common or sticky workplace problems. The importance of modeling good conflict resolution skills, mediation skills, and empathetic and reflective listening skills in meetings is also an invaluable skill among MedFTs. It is important to use these abilities to empower and enhance communication, not to enable dysfunctional communication, blame, shame, or find fault. The operational knowledge and skills of MedFTs are essential particularly for those who must maintain a strong ethical and legal stance in the healthiest or most tumultuous of atmospheres.

Sales and Marketing Skills

MedFTs will not be successful in the field of EAP unless they know the basics in sales and marketing (Lund, 2016). Performing sales presentations and developing professional marketing pieces are all important skills to learn and maintain. For example, prior to the implementation of an EAP-sponsored service into an IBHC context (e.g., a primary care site or workers' compensation clinic), the organization typically needs to be sold on an approach to solve their rising healthcare costs and how an IBHC option is an affordable solution. Educating, listening, understanding, and presenting solutions that could address the needs of the organization all fall under this skill set.

Once the MedFT has been successful in selling a program or service to a company, they must then continue to market the program internally to the company. If the company buys the service and nobody uses it, the service will either be discontinued or quickly go to some other EAP option. Being able to show service utilization and tying that utilization to successful outcomes is important to receive continued buy-in from the company paying for the service.

Reporting Outcome Knowledge and Skills

Another important skill set that MedFTs should know when initiating or sustaining EAP programs includes the ability to work with data. Producing quarterly utilization reports (QRs) and reports that pertain to clinical, operational, or financial outcomes is vital for an EAP to remain vital to the system. QRs are reports that are typically sent to "client companies" on a quarterly basis. These reports typically are broken down into different categories showing nonpersonal healthcare information (PHI) such as numbers of EAP therapy cases, types of therapy cases, consultations and types of consultations, trainings provided, on-site crisis responses, management referrals and reasons for referral, etc. Depending on the type of services, more integrated reports can show the role of wellness coaching, primary issues assessed during appointments, community resource recommendations, and website hits for employee assistance needs. These brief reports are used to show trends within a system. These reports may assist senior leaders in planning interventions and deciding upon the need for additional services.

Annual reports are typically based on showing how the benefits of a program outweigh the costs. These are a key factor in demonstrating the success (e.g., return on investment (ROI), patient satisfaction) of MedFT, IBHC, and/or EAP services to companies who could have been paying more for these services via more expensive and silo-ed programs (e.g., referring patients out to a variety of specialists). Annual reports that may offer compelling results include data about (a) reductions in absenteeism and risks associated with presenteeism, (b) return-to-work assessments (leave management), (c) reduction in workers' compensation costs, (d) reduction of behavioral health risks due to health coach utilization, and (e) cost savings in comparison to employees who did not request or receive IBHC services.

Through claims data analysis and health risk assessment, these reports should chronicle company health risk factors such as diet, exercise, smoking, high blood pressure, depression, stress, etc. and how those risk factors impact short-term disability, presenteeism, absenteeism, and paramedical costs associated with chronic conditions. Results on a report should calculate a ROI score, not typically found in organizational budget reports (e.g., cost savings by having on-site EAP services, as well as reductions in returning to work delays, legal settlements, and pain medication use). Reports should also show indirect and direct savings to the company when EAPs manage behavioral factors (psychosocial-spiritual and wellness) with employees who have chronic conditions. The presence of untreated psychosocial variables (e.g., depressed, anxious, traumatized) with an employee could have far-reaching implications on any company (Lerner & Henke, 2008). These impacts include using greater amounts of unscheduled absence, being less productive while at work, and, also, including a higher likelihood for risks of accidents when on the job compared to a healthy employee.

The goals for a MedFT in relation to the provision of a quality report are somewhat unique compared to other types of providers. MedFTs have the skills and knowledge to show the correlation between work-life factors and the likely interdependence on estimated costs and benefits to health (e.g., data that show what happens when considering positive or negative support from family or others in relation to symptom management and return-to-work outcomes). Typically, reports by an EAP compare outcomes from pre-baseline (prior to EAP intervention) to current operations. Their goal is to show the success of a new program's implementation on workforce performance. So, MedFTs need to be comfortable with obtaining and using data (e.g., claims data) to best support their contributions to the context. They also need to be aware of national trends in costs and variables associated with absenteeism and presenteeism. This information can then assist MedFTs in knowing what variables or outcomes should be tracked to analyze the cost savings, cost-offset, and reduction in costs associated with missed work, fewer injuries/accidents, or comparisons in types of treatment interventions that may be needed for the employees or employers.

Beyond having skills in report development and program evaluation, MedFTs who work in large health systems with multiple vendors (e.g., medical, wellness, EAP, workers' comp, disability) could benefit from periodically attending each vendor's business meetings in order to stay connected to all of the internal workings and programs. This is essential in order for the MedFT to stay connected to all levels of engagement, particularly as individuals at these meetings are typically the deciders on services provided to the system. MedFTs who work for large EAP firms that provide traditional services (rather than IBHC services) will likely be assigned multiple accounts (companies) and would be expected to attend these vendor meetings for their large (over 10,000 employee) accounts. A MedFT in an EAP context, whether providing traditional or IBHC services, would be wise to attend or present at "vendor summits" in which key vendors are brought in to learn how to work together holistically on ways to best treat diverse populations in the workplace.

MedFTs, as part of EAP teams, may function differently based on the needs of the context, collaborative team(s) involved, and relevance of BPSS or relational health to the environment. They may function across any one of five levels within Hodgson, Lamson, Mendenhall, and Tyndall's (2014) MedFT Healthcare Continuum—ranging from rarely using a BPSS framework or relational lens to functioning with a high level of proficiency in integrating systemic and BPSS practice, research, and policy-related efforts.

EAPs Across the MedFT Healthcare Continuum

The integration of MedFTs in EAPs is a new opportunity for both fields. The execution of skills by the MedFT depends on one's job and classification within an employer's system. Whether it is to clinically assist with employees' wellness, health concerns, injuries incurred on the job, etc. or designing program evaluation, planning, and implementing policies and studies, MedFTs have the potential to play a significant leadership role(s). It is important, though, that MedFTs investigate the benefits for obtaining a Certified Employee Assistance Professional (CEAP) certification when working on-site and/or the Employee Assistance Specialist Clinical (EAS-C) Certificate of Recognition when providing EAP assessment and short-term counseling services through their private practices. MedFTs interested in seeking these types of certifications should investigate the benefits further by visiting the International Employee Assistance Professionals Association website (see www.eapassn.com). While the benefits of such certifications may be advantageous to demonstrating command of contextual factors relevant to EAP services, this section will help illustrate how MedFTs function within an EAP setting. Tables 17.1 and 17.2 highlight specific knowledge and skills that characterize their involvement across Hodgson et al.'s (2014) MedFT Healthcare Continuum.

The vignette posed at the beginning of this chapter illustrates a sophisticated level of MedFT integration into an EAP and workplace setting. Depending on one's job duties, MedFTs functioning at *Levels 1* and *2* of the continuum may have the rare ability to function as an EAP clinician, researcher, and/or policy advocate who executes components of a relational and BPSS framework. At these levels, the MedFT may have the knowledge and skills to practice at a more advanced level, but may nevertheless not have a "green light" from the system to do so. The EAP system referenced in the vignette clearly has strong leadership and policies that engage the MedFT as an active and consistent member of the healthcare team versus a referral-based and/or colocated service determined for use at the provider's discretion. The MedFT focused on the employee and his workplace due to functioning in a workers' compensation environment. The MedFT did not engage in couple or family therapy with the patient. This approach is an artifact of the setting more than anything else. Typically, patients come to an EAP for individual care, not expecting the expertise of a relational approach to treatment. This expertise is often sought out for "special cases" or situations rather than as a routine service. There is an important distinction, though, as the MedFT can work relationally without having other members of the patient's family or support system present; he or she is mindful of the impact(s) that an injury event can have on the family system of an employee who depends on that income.

Table 17.1 MedFTs in Employee Assistance Programs: Basic Knowledge and Skills

MedFT Healthcare Continuum Level	Level 1	Level 2	Level 3
Knowledge	Somewhat familiar with EAP role in a healthcare system and the care team's overall structure and purpose. Limited knowledge about BPSS impacts on a few common injuries and/or conditions seen at EAP clinics. Rarely engages other professional members, patients, and support system members collaboratively. Basic understanding regarding strategies for a healthy lifestyle when managing with an EAP-related health condition or event. If conducting research and/or policy/advocacy work, on rare occasions will collaborate with other disciplines who could be helpful to the work of an EAP and consider relational and/or BPSS aspects of health and well-being.	Has some understanding and will occasionally explain to patients, support system members, and other members of the treatment team how each of the BPSS systems plays a part in supporting a patient's journey to wellness. Familiar with benefits of couple and family engagement in adjustment to EAP concerns but tends to refer more than provide this service. Knowledgeable about how to use the electronic health record system or other forms of secured communication to collaborate with various team members. Is an occasional contributor to discussions about research design and policy/advocacy work that include relational and/or BPSS aspects of EAP health events and/or conditions.	Understands the importance of and actively engages different disciplines on the treatment team in the patient's care plan. Broad range of knowledge about research-informed family therapy and BPSS interventions relevant to EAP practice; able to and usually will conduct couple and family meetings and incorporate BPSS health factors into treatment with minimal need to refer out. When work permits, is knowledgeable and usually committed to conducting research and constructing policy/advocacy work that identifies and intervenes on behalf of individuals, couples, families, and healthcare teams toward the advancement of BPSS health and well-being.

(continued)

Table 17.1 (continued)

MedFT Healthcare Continuum Level	Level 1	Level 2	Level 3
Skills	Able to recognize at a basic level the BPSS dimensions of health events and conditions and apply a BPSS lens to practice, research, and/or policy/advocacy work. Can discuss (and psycho-educate) basic relationships between biological processes, personal well-being, and interpersonal functioning. Demonstrates minimal collaborative skills with EAP and other related healthcare providers; prefers to work independently, but when care is complex enough, will contact/refer to other providers about additional services.	Knowledgeable about how to apply systemic interventions in practice but does it occasionally; capable of assessing patients BPSS and invite support system members to be present for background health issues such as family history and risk-related factors, as well as treatment planning. Demonstrates occasional collaborative skills through (a) written and verbal communication mediums that are understandable to all team members and (b) coordination of referrals to specialty behavioral health providers and communication with the patient's primary care provider. Can recognize the role of BPSS systems on one another and identify comorbid BPSS health conditions and impacts.	Usually engages multidisciplinary team members in a discussion about the patient and what skills each person has that could contribute to the best patient outcome. Can successfully conduct a systemic assessment of a patient and family with competencies in assessing for BPSS aspects of the EAP injury/condition and/ or comorbid disease and resources within the family. Usually engages other professionals within and outside of the practice who are actively involved in the patient's care. Skilled with standardized measures to track patients' individual and relational strengths and challenges (e.g., depression, anxiety, pain, social support). Attends and contributes to team meetings to help shape BPSS treatment plans for patients.

In our vignette, the MedFT did capture some relational data (e.g., patient was divorced 5 years ago), and hopefully this will be further addressed once the patient engages in specialty behavioral healthcare through the EAP therapy referral. For EAP systems that are less familiar with the research-informed practice of integrated behavioral healthcare, many *Level 1* and *2* engagements end at the initial consultation phase. With encounters ending at the consultation phrase, opportunities for coordination of services or treatment plans are minimal, and the likelihood for providing BPSS interventions at *Level 1* and *2* is few and far between.

At *Level 3*, MedFTs must be cautious to not perpetuate fragmented and pathocentric healthcare models, as even colocated providers use different documentation systems limiting providers' abilities to coordinate care. This may be just as inefficient as recommending that all workers' compensation patients attend psychoeducation groups with fixed topics while overlooking individual patients' unique BPSS needs. IBHC services allow the MedFT to assess for patients' BPSS needs efficiently, reducing length of time out of work (as noted earlier in the vignette) and ensuring a more evidence-based triaging of BPSS needs.

In the vignette, the MedFT functioned initially at a *Level 3* and then transitioned to a *Level 4* when she applied her knowledge and skills through BPSS interventions and a relational assessment. While not all MedFTs will have relational and BPSS research or policy/advocacy opportunities in EAP settings, this MedFT had the skills and experience necessary for conducting family therapy sessions. For example, if the MedFT found that the patient has a caregiver who was struggling to understand the patient's pain, psychosocial distress, and/or reluctance to be back to work, she could invite the caregiver to meet with the patient to help provide psychoeducation and intervention around these topics. In this case vignette, however, doing so was not indicated.

A *Level 4* MedFT is adept at collecting BPSS data to track patient- and program-level outcomes. She was responsive to the provider's concerns and reported that she attended the healthcare team meetings, which contributed to patient-care discus-

Table 17.2 MedFTs in Employee Assistance Programs: Advanced Knowledge and Skills

MedFT Healthcare Continuum Level	Level 4	Level 5
Knowledge	Understands the more commonly treated health conditions and BPSS impacts in EAP settings. Knowledgeable about benefits and risks of associated treatments of the more commonly seen biological and mental health conditions in EAP setting (e.g., pain, musculoskeletal injuries, depression, anxiety). Understands how to collaborate with other disciplines to implement evidence-based BPSS and family therapy protocols in traditional and integrated behavioral healthcare EAP contexts. Identifies self as a MedFT. Knowledgeable about designing and advocating for policies that govern BPSS-oriented EAP services.	Understands and educates others about treatment and care sequences for unique and/or challenging topics in EAP practice (e.g., pain management, workplace reintegration dynamics, comorbidities); can consult proficiently with professionals about BPSS topics from other fields. Knowledgeable about BPSS research designs and execution, policies, and advocacy needs as relevant to EAP care. Proficient in developing a curriculum on integrated behavioral healthcare, BPSS applications, MedFT, etc. to behavioral health and other health professionals employed in an EAP setting. Understands leadership and supervision strategies for building integrated behavioral healthcare teams in EAP settings.

(continued)

Table 17.2 (continued)

MedFT Healthcare Continuum Level	Level 4	Level 5
Skills	Able to deliver seminars and workshops about the BPSS complexities of a variety of commonly reported EAP injuries to a variety of professional types (e.g., behavioral health, biomedical). Can apply several BPSS interventions in care (including most types of brief interventions); can administer mood- and disease-specific assessment tools as the EAP context requires. Consistently collaborates with key EAP team members (e.g., treating providers, workers' compensation case manager and nurse manager, physical therapist, dietician); initiates and facilitates team visits with multiple providers when working with patients and families. Can independently and collaboratively construct research and program evaluation studies that study the impact of BPSS interventions with a variety of diagnoses and patient/family units of care.	Proficient in nearly all aspects of commonly seen EAP presenting problems; able to synthesize and conduct research and clinical work; engages in community-oriented projects outside of the EAP clinic to help reduce recidivism and employee injuries. Goes beyond interventions routine for this population; can integrate specific models of integrated behavioral healthcare (e.g., PCBH, Chronic Care Model) into EAP settings. Leads, supervises, and/or studies success of the implementation and dissemination of BPSS curriculum on integrated behavioral healthcare, BPSS applications, MedFT, etc. for EAP contexts. Routinely engages as an administrator/leader and supervisor in a team-based EAP approach to inpatient and/or outpatient care, with consistent communication through electronic health records, patient introductions, curb-side consultations, and team meetings and visits. Works proficiently as a MedFT and collaborates with other providers from a variety of disciples. Explains at a high level of skill evidence-based treatments regarding most EAP injuries/conditions and their role(s) in the workplace and family systems; has background to provide psychoeducation to patients and families about a variety of symptoms, medications, and behavioral health management techniques that facilitate returning to work and reducing symptom distress.

sions and treatment planning. In some cases, a *Level 4* MedFT in an EAP setting will also provide specialty behavioral health services and continuity family therapy sessions, but the role of that person needs to be made clear to the patient, system, and EAP administrators. For example, if the MedFT is providing integrated behavioral healthcare to a workers' compensation patient, it is often optimal to have the specialty behavioral healthcare provided by a separate provider. This policy ultimately is protective in the event that the patient discloses details about the injury that could compromise his or her receipt of benefits.

MedFTs at *Level 5* evidence consistent and proficient application of BPSS and relational knowledge and skills. If the MedFT had indicated that he or she (a) supervised other BHPs in an EAP setting, as well as in other healthcare contexts; (b) trained health professionals in family therapy theories and interventions, research, and developing MedFT policies; and/or (c) assumed an administrative position, it would showcase a depth and breadth of *Level 5* MedFT knowledge and skills. However, when one is the lone MedFT in an EAP system, it is more difficult to display this skill set. As one's workforce and role expands, these skills can become more evident.

Research-Informed Practices

When it comes to EAP behavioral health interventions, it is important that MedFTs are aware of issues critical to employers and employees. The primary reasons for employees' missed work days (i.e., absenteesism), for example, include (a) work-life stress (e.g., bullying or harassment, disengagement due to difficult coworkers, heavy workloads, lack of child- or eldercare), (b) injury, and/or (c) chronic health conditions (e.g., asthma, depression, diabetes, high blood pressure, high cholesterol, obesity, substance use disorders) (Shumway, Wampler, & Arredondo, 2004; Stewart, Ricci, Chee, Morganstein, & Lipton, 2003). The top three issues for employees seeking EAP services, however, are (a) psychological problems, (b) family issues, and (c) work-related problems (Mulligan, 2007). Given the direct and indirect annual costs ($84 billion) associated with absenteeism and the fact that about 77% of all workers in the United States report having a chronic health condition (Bankert, Coberley, Pope, & Wells, 2014), MedFTs must be prepared for the provision of research-informed individual and family-based treatments in EAP contexts. They must also know how to minimize systemic costs.

Researchers have conducted analyses on behavioral health visits and costs related to healthcare benefits (Hodgkin, Merrick, Hiatt, Constance, & McGuire, 2010). They found that companies who have an EAP behavioral health provider on-site, and who offer 4 to 5 behavioral health visits to employees, actually reduce the use of the behavioral health benefits compared to employees who use external behavioral health services via their health insurance. These researchers also found that having more generous EAP allowances for on-site services reduced employers' payments for outpatient care. MedFTs have the capacity to serve as key players in this cost reduction for employers and employees, especially when considering the benefits of attending to psychosocial variables in tandem with physical health concerns through research-informed practices.

Understanding psychosocial variables and how they impact chronic conditions within EAP contexts is important for MedFTs, given the likelihood for increases in symptom severity if treatment is delayed or absent (Lamson, Hodgson, Goodman, & Lewis, 2017; Loisel et al., 2003). Best practice literature suggests that a biopsychosocial perspective on treatment and early intervention (i.e., day one of injury) is needed to effectively manage musculoskeletal injuries and reduce the likelihood toward any chronic health condition (Noonan & Wagner, 2010). The sections below provide research-informed techniques that MedFTs can implement to address work-life stress and chronic comorbid conditions using individual and family interventions, with additional details pertaining to screening, assessments, interventions, and cost-offsets by using MedFTs in EAP contexts.

Individual Approaches

As with any therapeutic relationship, MedFTs should be adept, first and foremost, at building rapport with patients in EAP systems. Both in the subacute stage of disability (4–12 weeks after injury) and throughout care, it is essential to establish and maintain a therapeutic alliance—which is one of the most effective interventions when working with patients (Duncan, Miller, & Sparks, 2011). Joining and rapport building are foundational constructs in nearly every theory and model taught to MedFTs in their family therapy training (Greif, 1990). One individually oriented approach, motivational interviewing (MI; Rollnick, Miller & Butler, 2008), has been shown to be an effective method of developing therapeutic alliances, particularly with pain patients. Cheing et al. (2014) reported that techniques such as MI help to establish a good therapeutic alliance with chronic pain patients and can increase patients' outcome expectancy and reduce subjective pain intensity. The desire for a healthy alliance may in part be due to employees who feel doubted by their employers that their injury was really work-related (e.g., Steenstra et al., 2015). For the MedFT, having characteristics of a good therapeutic alliance including genuineness, empathy, trustworthiness, and a nonjudgmental attitude is an important first step in developing a positive relationship with the EAP system and those it serves.

The next important step in engaging EAP patients in care is conducting an efficient yet thorough behavioral health assessment. Employees who seek assistance through their EAP often have a small number of allotted sessions; MedFTs should thereby be proficient in using brief, validated screening tools like the PHQ-9 (Patient Health Questionnaire-9 item scale; Kroenke, Spitzer, & Williams, 2001), GAD-7 (Generalized Anxiety Disorder 7-item scale; Spitzer, Kroenke, Williams, & Lowe, 2006), DAST-10 (Drug Abuse Screening Test; Skinner, 1982), and other commonly used instruments created for EAPs (e.g., Workplace Outcome Suite; Chestnut

Global Partners, 2013). All of these tools represent efficient ways to identify employees who are most at risk for serious mental health problems. Screening for substance use is also a high priority in EAP settings, and SBIRT (Screening, Brief Intervention, and Referral to Treatment) has been found to be effective in nonmedical settings such as the workplace (Mcpherson, Goplerud, Derr, Mickenberg, & Courtemanche, 2010). MedFTs must be prepared to deliver a variety of screeners and assessments for diverse mental health, behavioral health, and substance use disorders (such as those described above) in EAP contexts. Based on results from the screener or assessment, the MedFT must determine if he or she will proceed with psychoeducation, prevention techniques, or intervention.

Psychoeducation

Along with establishing a good therapeutic alliance and determining best assessments to implement in practice, MedFTs should be prepared to deliver psychoeducation about various treatment-related topics. For example, MedFTs can provide BPSS-focused psychoeducation and psychotherapy to help patients learn about the benefits of exercise in relation to pain management (Cole, 1998). This can help patients cope with negative thoughts and moods, in addition to creating appropriate health goals for prevention of future injuries. Abbasi et al. (2012) found group psychoeducation to be an effective method of delivering information about the etiology and treatment of chronic back pain. It also has the capacity to lower the number of appointments needed with pain specialists (Ballus-Creus, Penarroya, & Leff, 2016). Specifically, providers were able to utilize this method to help patients develop self-management strategies for pain such as progressive muscle relaxation, imagery, and pacing activities in a manner conducive to healing. This team of researchers also found that spouses can influence and be influenced by patients' pain-related thoughts, feelings, behaviors, concerns, and experiences. MedFTs working in or in consultation with EAP settings will want to obtain continuing education in psychoeducational approaches and mindfulness strategies, as they have been shown to be effective with a wide variety of presenting concerns, particularly pain.

Prevention

MedFTs must also be prepared to deliver prevention techniques for employees in relation to workplace stress; such services include wellness initiatives with one-on-one coaching and individualized diet, exercise, and medication adherence programs (Employer Health Asset Management, 2009). More wide-ranging research-informed interventions (e.g., Morledge et al. 2013) can also assist in promoting an enhanced work environment "in which the workplace and workforce become part of a health-promoting culture that helps the healthy people stay healthy" (Edington, 2009, p. 68).

The role of work-life stress has been getting more attention recently, particularly through studies showing that such stress is a main contributor to people's overall life stress (Hogh, Hansen, Mikkelsen, & Persson, 2012). In fact, one study that included nearly 7,000 workers found that high levels of adversity in working conditions significantly increased the risk for worker suicide (Baumert et al., 2014). Suicide prevention programs should thereby be a priority (Milner, Page, Spencer-Thomas, & Lamotagne, 2015). Other factors that increase workplace stress are workplace violence and bullying, which are often precursors to work-related anxiety and depression (O'Donnell, MacIntosh, & Wuest, 2010).

Anxiety and depression in the workplace have been an ongoing focus of researchers, because these conditions gave costly and negative impacts on performance, safety, and health (Greenberg et al., 2003). Depression, for example, impacts performance due to its negative effects on absenteeism and presenteeism and, as mentioned above, in some severe circumstances can result in suicidal ideation or suicide. Furthermore, indirect costs associated with employees' depression outweigh the employer's direct medical and pharmaceutical costs (i.e., employer sourced healthcare plans) for employees. Unfortunately, depression impacts many elements of the workforce, especially in the areas of disability. In fact, depression ranks as the second leading cause of disability worldwide (Parry & William, 2009). MedFTs should thereby help the workforce and workplace consider prevention programs that reduce the likelihood for work stress (that can lead to work-related anxiety or depression) while also helping to ensure for a work environment where people can function at their best.

One example of a prevention-based group was developed by Twemlow and Harvey (2010). They designed it to address workplace stress and helped employees understand the role of power in relation to workplace bullying. Through prevention-based programs like this, MedFTs can serve as an advocate for employee wellness and for safe work environments. In some instances, prevention programs may be available to employees via a collaborative team that can include MedFTs, nurse case managers, wellness coaches, etc. within the EAP that can address a variety of BPSS employee needs. Attending to prevention and intervention in collaboration with multiple team members will inevitably lean toward cost-effectiveness, particularly given the financial implications from the negative consequences associated with workplace stress. Prevention programs like this one are informed by research, but need to be studied for their efficacy and effectiveness with specific populations, such as those in an EAP setting.

Intervention

One in four people will be affected by some form of mental illness over their lives (Sinclair & Patel, 2012), including those who develop conditions due to complicated work circumstances. Samra and Gilbert (2009) reported that psychological disorders "are often referred to as invisible; however, their impact is anything but invisible. Psychological disorders are associated with significant impacts on the workplace including conflict, turnover, accidents and injuries" (p. 22). Therefore, it is imperative to address mental and behavioral health in the workplace through well-defined and theoretically grounded practice-based interventions.

Early intervention is an especially important staring point, given the demoralization that often occurs once a disability or pain disorder has been identified (Linton, Boersma, Traczyk, Shaw, & Nicholas, 2016). The subacute stage of disability is considered the "golden hour" for biopsychosocial intervention that will positively impact return-to-work outcomes (Loisel et al., 2003). In fact, Lamson et al. (2017) found that employees treated by a MedFT within 30 days of injury via an IBHC model had better psychosocial improvements over a series of four sessions than employees who had not received IBHC with the MedFT until 30 days after the injury. Recommended interventions in the subacute stage of care include a "reassurance of recovery, encouragement for resumption of regular activities, provision of simple exercises," and a focus on returning to work (RTW) and have been shown to reduce re-injury rates, costs, and disability duration (Loisel et al., 2003, p. 107).

Some therapy models and interventions have been connected to specific presenting concerns. For example, cognitive behavioral therapy (CBT; Beck, 1979) has emerged as a best practice for treatment during rehabilitation from musculoskeletal injuries (Marhold, Linton, & Melin, 2001). Specifically, CBT therapists who target pain, pain catastrophizing, and fear of movement or re-injury have been successful for employees with musculoskeletal injuries (Besen, Young, & Shaw, 2015). Unfortunately, these interventions have focused on individual concerns rather than relational interventions. The limitations of this individually focused only approach are discussed in the section below.

Secondly, a cognitive and problem-solving approach was found to be effective in an EAP setting with patients experiencing depression. Geraedts et al. (2014) utilized a web-based self-help intervention with employees at risk for absenteeism due to depression. The intervention was found to be effective at reducing symptoms and sustaining the reduction in symptoms and was just as effective as seeking treatment from a PCP or psychiatrist for similar services. The utilization of web-based interventions will likely be a continued trend. However, these must be further evaluated in relation to patients' risks for significant mental health concerns and confidentiality in use of such services in an EAP setting.

Solution-focused therapy (SFT; De Shazer et al., 2007) is another therapy approach that has been used to address concerns in EAP contexts. It has been adapted for use in a primary care setting (Giorlando & Schilling, 1997) and has been used by Lamson et al. (2017) when working with employees who had been injured on the job. Results from the latter project indicated many significant outcomes in relation to improving employee psychosocial health (e.g., improvements in depression, anxiety, and perceptions of pain). Initial findings suggested that SFT, along with assessing for BPSS and relational health, is an important way that MedFTs may intervene with employees in EAP contexts. Thorslund (2007) also utilized SFT group therapy with employees. She focused on what employees had done to gain control over their pain. She found that those who received the SFT group therapy intervention returned to work at a significantly faster rate, worked more days, and experienced gains in their psychological health beyond those in the control group. Fortunately, SFT is an approach that has been highly researched both with individual and relational units of analysis (Kim, 2008) and will likely gain more attention in the future as a MedFT research-informed intervention for individuals, couples, families, and larger systems in EAP contexts.

An alternative model for reaching individuals in an EAP setting is the use of peer support programs. MedFTs are well suited to implement and facilitate peer support programs for employees who experience a variety of behavioral health needs (Linnan, Fisher, & Hood, 2012). Peer supports are patients who have successfully navigated their recovery from musculoskeletal injury, depression, anxiety, or substance abuse (Linnan et al., 2012). MedFTs could use this method to connect patients to others who are facing similar experiences. Peer support interventions have a strong evidence base across multiple settings, including the workplace (e.g., Gillard, Edwards, Gibson, Owen, & Wright, 2013; Linnan et al., 2012). As mentioned, there are some research-informed interventions and resources to use with individuals seeking care in EAP settings; however, many MedFTs will also need to prepare for working with EAP patients via research-informed family therapy.

Family Approaches

Family members can often be EAP patients themselves through employee benefits or may be involved in employees' care in the EAP system. There are many tools that can be used to involve family members in EAP. One resource for MedFTs in EAP settings is a systemic family therapy interview, developed for use in a study by West, Lee, and Poynton (2012). They used it to address medical symptoms and employee relations with regard to depression in the workplace. What West et al. (2012) found is that workers often take on the instability and incoherence of the workplace, leading to outward physical and psychological expressions of distress. This interview method can help unearth these subtle changes in worker/team behavior to help prevent escalation and negative health consequences (e.g., workplace accident, injuries, and distress).

Another useful resource available to MedFTs working with families in EAP settings is the Workplace Triple P program (Sanders, Stallman, & McHale, 2011). This program is an evidence-based intervention that utilizes cognitive-behavioral and social-learning techniques (de Graaf, Speetjens, Smit, de Wolff, & Tavecchio, 2008). Workplace Triple P is specially adapted to help parents with work-life balance and highlights positive strategies to use during high-risk transition times (before and after work) and cognitive-coping skills for parents to use to manage stress (Sanders et al., 2011).

Family members should also be involved in interventions pertaining to patients' chronic pain conditions (Swift, Reed, & Hocking, 2014). Swift et al. (2014) found family members are affected by the chronic pain of the patient. When family members were not involved in the intervention, they reported increased relational tension and patients reported greater pain. Ballus-Creus et al. (2016) found some family members experienced frustration related to the employee's diagnosis, while others reported exhausted emotional states that led to reactivity toward the patient. Fortunately, family members can also be a source of support and strengthen the ways in which the patient handles an event. Regardless of the family member's stance, MedFTs should attempt to involve family members, support persons, or caregivers in group psychoeducation and therapy. Family sessions or group interventions may result in several benefits to the employee and his or her family, including increased knowledge about pain and decreased self-report in patient's pain rating.

While pain has been one area of focus for couple and family therapy, another area of concern in relation to injuries is the management of fatigue or sleep hygiene. Abbasi et al. (2012) effectively engaged patients and their spouses in sessions related to the management of fatigue by addressing effective and ineffective strategies for requesting assistance from non-patient spouse. Special attention was paid to the verbal and nonverbal expressions of fatigue, particularly to the patient's clarity in requesting help, timing of request for assistance, and the amount of assistance desired by the patient. Sessions addressed ways that spouses can provide encouragement to the patient by engaging in joint patient-spouse practice of cognitive and behavioral pain management techniques such as distractions and progressive muscle relaxation. Spouses who received psychoeducation about supportive versus unsupportive communication reported reductions in emotional contagion between the partners, and patients reported improvements in medication management, willingness to move more, and reductions in rumination about pain compared to the comparison conditions.

As a result of the research reviewed above, it appears a more complete picture of the employee's psychological and medical health condition involves incorporating family members in the prevention and intervention phases of care. This means that MedFTs must advocate for EAP programs and inventions that are family/relationally focused. MedFTs working in an EAP setting would want to advocate for (a) access to the electronic health record where they may document and collaborate with other EAP team members, (b) access to the patient portal to interact and collaborate with the employees, (c) collection of employee population health data (e.g., pharmaceutical data, medical claims, biomarkers) to track changes over time in both physical and mental health conditions, and (d) collection and evaluation of BPSS data at intake and several times points to track known presenting issues that impact treatment outcomes (e.g., work stress, family stress, depression, social support, relationship strength, trauma, anxiety, life cycle stages, and alcohol and drug abuse). This type of tracking would allow for BPSS interventions to be developed and tested by MedFTs in EAP contexts. For businesses and organizations, supporting this type of data collection could not only help track treatment outcomes better but also track the impact(s) of MedFT services on disability claims, absenteeism, and medical claims costs. MedFTs working in EAP settings need to be prepared to demonstrate the value of their work across clinical, operational, and financial levels.

Conclusion

Strategically repositioning EAP services to best introduce and capture the biopsychosocial-spiritual needs of employees is the ultimate goal of an integrated behavioral healthcare model. Given that 40–70% of employees treated for injuries, chronic diseases, and health complaints typically have a comorbid behavioral condition associated with the health issue (Fries, Coop, & Beadle, 1993; Gatchel & Oordt, 2003), MedFTs are a key contributor to the EAP team. Finding strategic ways to get trained and skilled MedFTs in front of these patients is important in the provision of BPSS and relational healthcare. While a patient treated via a traditional medical approach (i.e., linear model) could receive good services—his or her treatment could miss important psychosocial symptoms and solutions that could delay his or her return to work. Treating the employee with sensitivity to the systems in which he or she works and lives (e.g., workplace, family) could increase the likelihood for successful employee and employer outcomes. MedFTs' systemic and BPSS lenses offer an important contribution to EAP clinical practice, research, and policy efforts. Their contributions can help to ensure that an employers' costs are lowered and that employees' health and personal/professional quality of life are maximized.

Reflection Questions
1. What factors, demographics, or labs from your clinical work in an EAP system can you use to track for the purposes of constructing reports about cost-offset, cost-effectiveness, and/or reductions in healthcare utilization?
2. In working in an integrated behavioral healthcare context as part of an EAP, what do you need to do differently because of your "dual role" when an employee complains about the rough working conditions and poor pay that are causing him or her stress?
3. A manager comes in with a female employee who has bruises on her face and arms. The employee states that she fell at work, but the manager believes that the accident occurred outside of work. The employee admits that her husband is abusive and that he had threatened to come into the workplace and shoot her and/or anyone else who got in his way. What is your role?
4. An employee was just diagnosed with lung cancer. The doctor asked you to go in and talk with him and his supervisor (who is also present). How would you approach this situation?

Glossary of Important Terms in Employee Assistance Programs

Americans with Disabilities Act (ADA) A civil rights law that prohibits discrimination against individuals with disabilities in securing jobs, schools, transportation, and access to public and private places that are otherwise open to the general public.

Assessment and referral Assessment and referral are core functions of an EAP. These are not treatment or long-term counseling programs; they are proactive and accessible services for employees and their family to get basic counseling solution or referrals for long-term care. Assessment and referral EAPs also act as navigators through the complex world of behavioral health. Sessions are limited to conducting assessments and determining if the patient can benefit from short-term counseling and if not referring and navigating that member through their health system.

Brief/short-term treatment Services provided by the EAP to the employee for 1–6 sessions (some have more sessions). The basis for the number of sessions is determined by the philosophy of the organization and/or in accord with financial considerations.

Brokers Consultants who help businesses source the best possible benefits for their employees. Examples of their services include (a) helping business leaders determine what type of health coverage to purchase (e.g., where high-deductible plans would be appropriate for the business and its employees), (b) supporting businesses in establishing a culture of physical, mental, and emotional wellness, (c) advising on ways to increase employee productivity by helping to resolve employee issues that are obvious and relatively undetectable, and (d) offering strategies that may enhance managers' effectiveness in stimulating workplace performance.

Certified Employee Assistance Professional (CEAP) A specially trained and credentialed employee assistance professional who is usually licensed in a mental health or substance abuse counseling field. He or she operates in an occupational setting, and their "clients" may be both management and employees in general.

Employee assistance professional A person who assists the organization, its employees, and their family members with personal and behavioral problems. Foci of attention include (but are not limited to) health, marital, financial, alcohol, drug, legal, emotional, or other personal concerns that adversely affect employees' job performance and productivity. The specific activities of this professional may include any of the services described under the definition of EAP. If/When they provide clinical services, these professionals must be licensed or certified in the state that said services are rendered.

Employee assistance program (EAP) A worksite-based program designed to assist in the identification and resolution of work-related and nonwork-related productivity problems associated with employees who are impaired by personal concerns, including (but not limited to) health, marital, family, financial, alcohol, drug, legal, emotional, or other personal concerns which may adversely affect employee job performance. The specific core activities of EAPs include (a) services for individuals (such as identification and resolution of job performance issues related to an employee's personal concerns and assessment, referral, and follow-up), (b) services for managers and supervisors (such as assistance in referring employees to the EAP, supervisor training, and management consulting, (c) services for organizations (such as violence prevention/crisis management, group intervention, and employee orientation), and (d) administrative services such as the development of EAP policies and procedures, outreach, evaluation, and referral resources development.

EAP model The method of delivering EAP services. Typically delivered through one of three basic staffing models; these include (a) internal model, where the EAP staff is comprised of the organization's employees and there are no contractors involved; (b) external model, where the sponsoring company or organization has entered into a contract for an outside vendor to provide all EAP-related services; and (c) blended model, where both host organizations and contract personnel are involved in the delivery of EAP services.

Family and Medical Leave Act (FMLA) A labor law requiring qualifying employers to provide employees unpaid leave for serious health conditions, to care for a sick family member, or to care for a newborn or adopted child.

Management consultation Expert advice given to leaders, supervisors, human resources, and/or union representatives regarding the management of potential or actual performance and conduct concerns. One example is coaching a supervisor on how to refer an employee to the EAP.

On-site incident response An event, usually sudden, unexpected, and potentially life threatening, in which a person experiences a trauma (e.g., feels overwhelmed by a sense of personal vulnerability and/or lack of control). Examples of a need for an on-site incident include a natural disaster, serious workplace accident, hostage situation, or violence in the workplace.

Organizational development A professional process or activity designed to assist an organization, company, or office (department) to move from one level of performance or mode of operation to another in the shortest time possible.

Organizational needs assessment A systemic analysis of an organization done by collecting data through informational interviews, surveys, data, and claims analysis as to the company's needs in being more productive, safe, functional, and effective.

Risk management A systematic process for evaluating and reducing potential harm that may befall personnel, consumers of service, an organization, or a facility.

Workers' compensation service workers Workers who are either contracted by an entity embedded in occupational health/workers' compensation service or provided by the company itself when employees get injured in the workplace or while doing their job. It provides wage replacement and extends or contracts out care to employees in exchange for mandatory relinquishment of employee's rights to sue their employers for negligence.

Additional Resources

Literature

Journal of Employee Assistance. http://www.eapassn.org/JEA
Journal of Workplace Behavioral Health. http://www.tandfonline.com/toc/wjwb20/current

Partnership for Workplace Mental Health. http://www.workplacementalhealth.org/
Price, J. W. (2014). *Alcohol, drugs, and the U.S. workplace: A guide for healthcare providers, safety officers, and human resource managers.* London, England: Nova Science Publishing, Inc.
Richard, M. A., Emener, W. G., and Hutchison, W. S. (2009). *Employee assistance programs: Wellness/enhancement programming* (4th ed.). Springfield, IL: Charles C. Thomas Publishing, Ltd.

Organizations/Associations

Employee Assistance Trade Association. https://www.easna.org/
International Employee Assistance Professionals Association. http://www.eapassn.org/

References[1]

Abbasi, M., Dehghani, M., Keefe, F. J., Behtash, H., & Shams, J. (2012). Spouse-assisted training in pain coping skills and the outcome of multidisciplinary pain management for chronic low back pain treatment: A 1-year randomized controlled trial. *European Journal of Pain, 16*, 1033–1043. https://doi.org/10.1002/j.1532-2149.2011.00097.x
Attridge, M. (2016). EAP Integration with disability management. *Journal of Employee Assistance, 46*, 26–27. https://doi.org/10.1177/215824401351030
Attridge, M., Herlihy, P., Sharar, D., Amaral, T., McPherson, T., Stephenson, D., … Routledge, S. (2007). *EAP healthier, more productive employees: A report on the real potential of employee assistance programs.* Hartford, CT: The Hartford.
Attridge, M., & Vanderpol, B. (2010). The business case of workplace critical incident response: A literature review and some employer examples. *Journal of Workplace Behavioral Health, 25*, 132–145. https://doi.org/10.1080/15555241003761001
Attridge, M., & Wallace, S. (2010). *Able-minded: Return to work and accommodations for workers on disability leave for mental disorders.* Vancouver, BC: Human Solutions.
*Ballus-Creus, C., Penarroya, A., & Leff, J. (2016). How a pain management program for patients and spouses can benefit their lives? *International Journal of Social Psychiatry, 62*, 496–497. https://doi.org/10.1177/0020764016639340.
*Bankert, B., Coberley, C., Pope, J. E., & Wells, A. (2014). Regional economic activity and absenteeism: A new approach to estimating the indirect costs of employee productivity loss. *Population Health Management, 18*, 47–53. https://doi.org/10.1089/pop.2014.0025.
Baumert, J., Schneider, B., Lukaschek, K., Emeny, R., Meisenger, C., Erazo, N., … Ladgwig, K. (2014). Adverse conditions at the workplace are associated with increased suicide risk. *Journal of Psychiatric Research, 57*, 90–95. https://doi.org/10.1016/j.jpsychires.2014.06.007.
Bayer, D. L. (1995). EAP family therapy: An underutilized resource. *Employee Assistance Quarterly, 10*, 35–48. https://doi.org/10.1300/J022v10n03_03
Beck, A. T. (1979). *Cognitive therapy of depression.* New York, NY: Guilford Press.

---

[1] [Note: References that are prefaced with an asterisk are recommended readings.]

Bennet, N., Blum, T., & Roman, P. (1994). Presence of drug screening and employee assistance programs: Exclusive and inclusive human resource management practices. *Journal of Organizational Behavior, 15*, 549–560. https://doi.org/10.1002/job.4030150606

Besen, E., Young, A. E., & Shaw, W. S. (2015). Returning to work following low back pain: Towards a model of individual psychosocial factors. *Journal of Occupational Rehabilitation, 25*, 25–37. https://doi.org/10.1007/s10926-014-9522-9

Blum, T., Roman, P., & Tootle, D. (1988). The emergence of an occupation. *Work and Occupations, 15*, 96–114. https://doi.org/10.1177/0730888488015001006

Boverie, P. E. (1991). Human systems consultant: Using family therapy in organizations. *Family Therapy, 18*, 61–71. Retrieved from https://search.proquest.com/docview/1474306108?accountid=14586

Cagney, T. (2012). Supervisory and management training: Thinking outside the box. *Journal of Employee Assistance, 42*, 26–27.

*Cheing, G., Vong, S., Chan, F., Ditchman, N., Brooks, J., & Chan, C. (2014). Testing a path-analytic mediation model of how motivational enhancement physiotherapy improves physical functioning in pain patients. *Journal of Occupational Rehabilitation, 24*, 798–908. https://doi.org/10.1007/s10926-014-9515-8.

Chestnut Global Partners. (2013). *CGP workplace outcome suite.* Retrieved from http://www.eapresearch.com/documents2013/WOS_25-ItemForEAPs_2013-07-02.pdf

Cole, J. D. (1998). Psychotherapy with the chronic pain patient using coping skills development: Outcome Study. *Journal of Occupational Health Psychology, 3*, 217–226. Retrieved from https://www.ncbi.nlm.nih.gov/pubmed/9684213

Crane, D., & Christenson, J. (2014). A summary report of cost-effectiveness: Recognizing the value of family therapy in health care. In J. Hodgson, A. Lamson, T. Mendenhall, and D. Crane (Eds.), *Medical family therapy: Advanced applications* (pp. 419–436). New York, NY: Springer.

Crane, D., & Payne, S. (2011). Individual and family psychotherapy in managed care: Comparing the costs of treatment by the mental health professions. *Journal of Marital and Family Therapy, 37*, 273–289. https://doi.org/10.1111/j.1752-0606.2009.00170.x

de Graaf, I., Speetjens, P., Smit, F., de Wolff, M., & Tavecchio, L. (2008). Effectiveness of the Triple P Positive Parenting Program on behavioral problems in children: A meta-analysis. *Behavior Modification, 32*(5), 714–735. https://doi.org/10.1177/0145445508317134

De Shazer, S., Dolan, Y., Korman, H., Trepper, T. S., McCollom, E., & Berg, I. K. (2007). *More than miracles: The state of the art of solution-focused brief therapy.* Binghamton, NY: Haworth Press. https://doi.org/10.1111/j.1467-6427.2008.00419_4.x

Dewa, C. S., Hoch, J. S., Carmen, G., Guscott, R., & Anderson, C. (2009). Cost, effectiveness, and cost-effectiveness of a collaborative mental health care program for people receiving short-term disability benefits for psychiatric disorders. *Canadian Journal of Psychiatry, 54*, 379–388. https://doi.org/10.1177/070674370905400605

Duncan, B., Miller, S., & Sparks, J. (2011). *The heroic client: A revolutionary way to improve effectiveness through client-directed, outcome-informed Therapy.* San Francisco, CA: Jossey-Bass.

Edington, D. W. (2009). *Zero trends, health as a serious economic strategy.* Ann Arbor, MI: Health Management Research Center.

Employer Health Asset Management. (2009). *A roadmap for improving the health of your employees and your organization.* Retrieved from www.ihpm.org

Engel, G. L. (1977). The need for a new medical model: A challenge for biomedicine. *Science, 196*, 129–136. https://doi.org/10.1016/b978-0-409-95009-0.50006-1

Engel, G. L. (1980). The clinical application of the biopsychosocial model. *American Journal of Family Medicine, 137*, 535–544. https://doi.org/10.1176/ajp.137.5.535

Fries, J., Koop, C., & Beadle, C. (1993). Reducing health care costs by reducing the need and demand for medical services. *New England Journal of Medicine, 329*, 321–325. https://doi.org/10.1056/NEJM199307293290506

Gatchel, R. J., & Oordt, M. S. (2003). *Clinical health psychology and primary care: Practical advice and clinical guidance for successful collaboration.* Washington, DC: American Psychological Association.

Geraedts, A. S., Kleiboer, A. M., Twisk, J., Wiezer, N. M., van Mechelen, W., & Cuijpers, P. (2014). Long-term results of a web-based guided self-help intervention for employees with depressive symptoms: Randomized controlled trial. *Journal of Medical Internet Research, 16,* 1–15. https://doi.org/10.2196/jmir.3539

Gillard, S. G., Edwards, C., Gibson, S. L., Owen, K., & Wright, C. (2013). Introducing peer worker roles in UK mental health service teams: A qualitative analysis of the organizational benefits and challenges. *BMC Health Services Research, 13,* 188–201. Retrieved from http://www.biomedcentral.com/1472-6963/13/188

Giorlando, M. E., & Schilling, R. (1997). On becoming a solution-focused physician: The MED-STAT acronym. *Families, Systems & Health, 15,* 361–373. https://doi.org/10.1037/h0090137

Goldner, E., Bilsker, D., Gilbert, M., Myette, L., Corbiére, M., & Dewa, C. (2004). Disability management, return to work and treatment. *Health Care Papers, 5,* 76–90. doi: 10.12927/hcpap.16832

Gorter, J., Jacobsen Frey, J., & O'Brien, S. (2015). Broadening the value of critical incident response. *Journal of Employee Assistance, 45,* 10–13. Retrieved from https://archive.hshsl.umaryland.edu/bitstream/10713/5142/1/JEA%20-%20Critical%20Incident%20Response.pdf

Greenberg, P., Kessler, R., Birnbaum, H., Leong, S., Berglund, P., & Corey-Lisle, P. (2003). The economic burden of depression in the United States: How did it change between 1990 and 2000? *Journal of Clinical Psychiatry, 64,* 1465–1475. https://doi.org/10.4088/jcp.v64n1211

Greif, G. L. (1990). Twenty-five basic joining techniques in family therapy. *Journal of Psychoactive Drugs, 22,* 89–90. Retrieved from http://dx.doi.org/10.1080/02791072.1990.10472203

*Han, C., & Pae, C. (2015). Pain and depression: A neurobiological perspective of their relationship. *Psychiatry Investigation, 12,* 1–8. https://doi.org/10.4306/pi.2015.12.1.1.

Harris, J. (2011). Effective management consulting: Defining management consulting in employee assistance. *Journal of Employee Assistance, 41,* 20–21.

Henderson, R. M., & Bacon, S. D. (1953). Problem drinking: The Yale plan for drinking and industry. *Quarterly Studies Alcoholism., 14,* 247–262. Retrieved from https://www.ncbi.nlm.nih.gov/pubmed/?term=Problem+drinking%3A+The+Yale+plan+for+drinking+and+industry

*Hodgkin, D., Merrick, E. L., Hiatt, D., Constance, H. M., & McGuire, T. G. (2010). The effect of employee assistance plan benefits on the use of outpatient behavioral health care. *Journal of Mental Health Policy and Economics, 13,* 167–174. Retrieved from https://www.ncbi.nlm.nih.gov/pubmed/?term=The+effect++of+employee+assistance+plan+benefits+on+the+use+of+outpatient+behavioral+health+care

Hodgson, J., Lamson, A., Mendenhall, T., & Tyndall, L. (2014). Introduction to medical family therapy: Advanced applications. In J. Hodgson, A. Lamson, T. Mendenhall, and D. Crane (Eds.), *Medical family therapy: Advanced applications* (pp. 1–9). New York, NY: Springer.

*Hogh, A., Hansen, A. M., Mikkelsen, E. G., & Persson, R. (2012). Exposure to negative acts at work, psychological stress reactions and physiological stress response. *Journal of Psychosomatic Research, 73,* 47–52. https://doi.org/10.1016/j.psychores.2012.04.004.

International Employee Assistance Professionals Association (IEAPA). (2011). Definitions of an employee assistance program (EAP) and EAP core technology. Retrieved from http://www.eapassn.org/about/about-employee-assistance/eap-definitions-and-core-technology

*Intveld, R. (2013). EAP critical incident response: A multi-systemic resiliency approach. *Journal of Employee Assistance, 43,* 20–23. https://doi.org/10.1080/15555240.2015.1119655.

Joseph, B., & Walker, A. (2016). Employee assistance programs in Australia: The perspectives of organisational leaders. *Asia Pacific Journal of Human Resources, 55,* 177-191. doi http://dx.doi.org.jproxy.lib.ecu.edu/10.1111/1744-7941.12124

*Karatepe, O., & Karadas, G. (2014). The effect of psychological capital on conflicts in the work-family interface, turnover and absence intentions. *International Journal of Hospitality Management, 43,* 132–143. https://doi.org/10.1108/IJCHM-01-2014-0028.

Kim, J. S. (2008). Examining the effectiveness of solution-focused brief therapy: A meta-analysis. *Research on Social Work Practice, 18*, 107–116. https://doi.org/10.1177/1049731507307807

Korner, S. (1986). The family therapist as systems therapist: Treating the workplace. *Psychotherapy in Private Practice, 4*, 63–76. Retrieved from http://www.tandfonline.com/doi/abs/10.1300/J294v04n02_11

Kroenke, K., Spitzer, R., & Williams, J. (2001). The PHQ-9: Validity of a brief depression severity measure. *Journal of General Internal Medicine, 16*, 606–613. https://doi.org/10.1046/j.1525-1497.2001.016009606.x

Lamson, A. L., Hodgson, J., Goodman, J. & Lewis, F. (2017). *Integrated behavioral healthcare in employee assistance programs*. Unpublished manuscript, Department of Human Development and Family Science, East Carolina University, Greenville, NC.

Lerner, D., & Henke, R. M. (2008). What does research tell us about depression, job performance, and work productivity? *Journal of Occupational and Environmental Medicine, 50*, 401–410. https://doi.org/10.1097/JOM.0b013e31816bae50

Linnan, L., Fisher, E. B., & Hood, S. (2012). The power and potential of peer support in workplace interventions. *American Journal of Health Promotion, 28*, 1–6. https://doi.org/10.4278/ajhp.121116-CIT-564

Linton, S. J., Boersma, K., Traczyk, M., Shaw, W., & Nicholas, M. (2016). Early workplace communication and problem solving to prevent back disability: Results of a randomized control trial among high-risk workers and their supervisors. *Journal of Occupational Rehabilitation, 26*, 150–159. https://doi.org/10.1007/s10926-015-9596-z

Loisel, P., Durand, M., Diallo, B., Vachon, B., Charpentier, N., & Labelle, J. (2003). From evidence to community practice in work rehabilitation: The Quebec experience. *Clinical Journal of Pain, 19*, 105–113. https://doi.org/10.1097/00002508-200303000-00005

*Lund, M. (2016). *How to start, sell, and grow an EAP*. Retrieved from https://issuu.com/eapa/docs/jea_vol47no1_1stqtr2017

Macy, G., Watkins, C., Lartey, G., & Golla, V. (2017). Depression screening, education, and treatment at the workplace: A pilot study utilizing the CDC health scorecard. *Journal of Workplace Behavioral Health, 32*, 3–13. http://dx.doi.org.jproxy.lib.ecu.edu/10.1080/15555240.2017.1282826

Marhold, C., Linton, S. J., & Melin, L. (2001). A cognitive-behavioral return-to-work program: Effects on pain with a history of long-term versus short-term sick leave. *Pain, 91*, 155–163. https://doi.org/10.1016/S0304-3959(00)00431-0

Marsh, R. (2014). *How healthcare strategies impact the employer's bottom line*. Retrieved from http://inbusinessmag.com/healthcare/healthcare-strategies-impact-employers-bottom-line#.WQqrpfnyu70

Mcpherson, T. L., Goplerud, E., Derr, D., Mickenberg, J., & Courtemanche, S. (2010). Telephonic screening and brief intervention for alcohol misuse among workers contacting the employee assistance program: A feasibility study. *Drug and Alcohol Review, 29*, 641–646. https://doi.org/10.1111/j.1465-3362.2010.00249.x

Milgram, G., & McCrady, B. (1986). *Employee assistance programs (Center of Alcohol Studies Pamphlet Series)*. New Brunswich, NJ: Alcohol Research Documentation, Inc. 10.15288/jsad.2010.71.930

Milner, A., Page, K., Spencer-Thomas, S., & Lamotagne, A. D. (2015). Workplace suicide prevention: A systematic review of published and unpublished activities. *Health Promotion International, 30*, 29–37. https://doi.org/10.1093/heapro/dau085

Morledge, T. J., Allexandre, D., Fox, E., Fu, A. Z., Higashi, M. K., Kruzikas, D. T., … Reese, P. R. (2013). Feasibility of an online mindfulness program for stress management: A randomized, controlled trial. *Annals of Behavioral Medicine, 46*, 137–148. https://doi.org/10.1007/s12160-013-9490-x.

Morneau Shepell. (2014). *The integration of EAP with DM*. Retrieved from http://www.morneaushepell.com/ca-en/insights/integration-eap-disability-management-programs-fosters-better-disability-outcomes-and

Mulligan, P. M. (2007). The prevalence of employee assistance programs and the employee participation rates of Long Island companies. *Proceedings of the Northeast Business & Economics Association*, pp. 68–71. Retrieved from http://eds.b.ebscohost.com/eds/detail/detail?vid=0&sid=61551c52-5413-4cac-80de-da961e476ebd%40sessionmgr4006&bdata=JnNpdGU9ZWRzLWxpdmU%3d#AN=27535391&db=buh

Noonan, J., & Wagner, S. (2010). A biopsychosocial perspective on the management of work related musculoskeletal disorders. *AAOHN Journal, 58*, 105–114. https://doi.org/10.3928/08910162-20100224-01

O'Donnell, S., Macintosh, J., & Wuest, J. (2010). A theoretical understanding of sickness absence among women who have experienced workplace bullying. *Qualitative Health Research, 20*, 439–452. https://doi.org/10.1177/0193945910362226

Open Minds. (2000). *Yearbook of managed behavioral health market share in the United States.* Gettysburg, PA: Open Minds.

Oss, M. and Clary, J. (1998). The evolving world of employee assistance. *Behavioral Health Management*, July/August, pp. 20–27.

Parry, T., & William, M. (2009). Depression: A lot bigger than you think: The absenteeism and presenteeism- related costs of depression outweigh the medical and pharmaceutical costs and make a strong case for EAP intervention against this condition. *Journal of Employee Assistance, 39*, 18–19. Retrieved from http://directionseap.com/wp-content/uploads/2012/06/Depression-A-Lot-Bigger-Than-You-Think1.pdf

Pompe, J. C., & Sharar, D. (2014). Technology & EAP: Engaging and motivating the new workforce. *Journal of Employee Assistance, 44*, 22–24. Retrieved from https://www.highbeam.com/doc/1G1-435717807.html

Presnall, L. (1981). *Occupational counseling and referral systems.* Salt Lake City, UT: Utah Alcoholism Foundation.

*Price, J. W. (2014). *Alcohol, drugs, and the U.S. workplace: A guide for healthcare providers, safety officers, and human resource managers.* London, England: Nova Science Publishing, Inc.

*Richard, M. A., Emener, W. G., & Hutchison, W. S. (2009). *Employee assistance programs: Wellness/enhancement Programming* (4th ed.). Springfield, IL: Charles C. Thomas Publishing, Ltd.

Rollnick, S., Miller, W. R., & Butler, C. (2008). *Motivational interviewing in health care: Helping patients change behavior.* New York, NY: Guilford Press.

Roman, P. (1988). From employee alcoholism to employee assistance. *Journal of Studies of Alcohol, 42*, 244–272. Retrieved from http://www.jsad.com/doi/pdf/10.15288/jsa.1981.42.244

*Roman, P. M. (2011). *Definitions of an employee assistance program EAP and EAP core technology.* Retrieved fromhttp://www.eapassn.org/About/About-Employee-Assistance/EAP-Definitions-and-Core Technology

Samra, J., & Gilbert, M. (2009). Guarding minds @ work: A new guide to psychological safety and health. *Visions: BC's Mental Health and Addictions Journal, 5*, 22–23. Retrieved from https://www.workplacestrategiesformentalhealth.com/pdf/EE015-035_Update%20Guarding%20Minds%20at%20Work%20Brochure_English.pdf

Sanders, M. R., Stallman, H. M., & Mchale, M. (2011). Workplace Triple P: A controlled evaluation of a parenting intervention for working parents. *Journal of Family Psychology, 25*(4), 581–590. https://doi.org/10.1037/a0024148

Sharar, D. A., & DeLapp, G. P. (2016). Follow the data: New study correlates EAP to positive workplace outcomes. Employee Assistant Advisor. Retrieved from http://www.umaryland.edu

Shi, Y., Sears, L., Coberley, C. R., & Pope, L. E. (2013). The association between modifiable well-being risk and productivity. A longitudinal study in pooled employer sample. *Journal of Occupational and Environmental Medicine, 55*, 353–364. https://doi.org/10.1097/jom.ob013e3182851923

Shumway, S. T., Wampler, R. S., & Arredondo, R. (2004). A place for marriage and family services: A survey of employee assistance program client problems and needs. *Employee Assistance*

Quarterly, 19, 61–71. Retrieved from https://www.ncbi.nlm.nih.gov/pubmed/?term=A+need+for+marriage+and+family++%09services%3A+A+survey+of+employee+assistance+program+client+problems+and+needs

Shumway, S. T., Wampler, R. S., Dersch, C., & Arrendondo, R. (2004). A place for marriage and family services in employee assistance programs (EAPs): A survey of EAP client problems and needs. *Journal of Marital and Family Therapy, 30*, 71–79. https://doi.org/10.1111/j.1752-0606.2004.tb01223.x

Sinclair, J., & Patel, M. (2012). No health without mental health: Core competencies for all doctors. *Medicine, 4*, 567. https://doi.org/10.1016/j.mpmed.2012.08.004

Skidmore, R. A., & Skidmore, C. J. (1975). Marriage and family counseling in industry. *Journal of Marriage and Family Counseling, 1*, 135–144. https://doi.org/10.1111/j.1752-0606.1975.tb00077.x

Skinner, H. (1982). The drug abuse screening test. *Addictive Behaviors, 7*, 363–371. https://doi.org/10.1016/0306-4603(82)90005-3

Slawinski, T. (2005a). A strength based approach to crisis response. *Journal of Workplace Behavior Health, 21*, 79–88. https://doi.org/10.1177/0020872811435371

Slawinski, T. (2005b). Crisis response for business: More than an intervention. *Behavioral Healthcare Tomorrow, 14*, 40–41. Retrieved from https://www.ncbi.nlm.nih.gov/pubmed/15887607

Slawinski, T. (2012). Saying goodbye to the Mitchell model. *Journal of Employee Assistance, 42*, 10–13. Retrieved from https://www.highbeam.com/doc/1G1-352492037.html

Smith, T., Salts, C. J., & Smith, C. W. (1989). Preparing marriage and family therapy students to become employee assistance professionals. *Journal of Marital and Family Therapy, 15*, 419–424. https://doi.org/10.1111/j.1752-0606.1989.tb00828.x

Spitzer, R., Kroenke, K., Williams, J., & Lowe, B. (2006). A brief measure for assessing generalized anxiety disorder. *Achieves of Internal Medicine, 166*, 1092–1097. https://doi.org/10.1001/archinte.166.10.1092

Steele, P., & Trice, H. (1995). A history of job-based alcoholism programs: 1972–1980. *Journal of Drug Issues, 25*, 397–422. https://doi.org/10.1177/002204269502500211

Steenstra, I. A., Busse, J. W., Tolusso, D., Davilmar, A., Lee, H., Furlan, A. D., … Hogg Johnson, S. (2015). Predicting time on prolonged benefits for injured workers with acute back pain. *Journal of Occupational Rehabilitation, 25*, 267–278. https://doi.org/10.1007/s10926-014-9534-5.

Stewart, W. F., Ricci, J. A., Chee, E., Morganstein, D., & Lipton, R. (2003). Lost productive time and cost due to common pain conditions in the US workforce. *Journal of the American Medical Association, 290*, 2443–2454. https://doi.org/10.1001/jama.290.18.2443

Sumiec, J. (2016). Is that an elephant in the room? *Journal of Employee Assistance, 46*, 26–27. Retrieved from http://www.eapassn.org/Is-that-an-Elephant-in-the-Room

Swift, C. M., Reed, K., & Hocking, C. (2014). A new perspective on family involvement in chronic pain management programmes: Significant others in pain management programmes. *Musculoskeletal Care, 12*, 47–55. https://doi.org/10.1002/msc.1059

Thorslund, K. W. (2007). Solution-focused group therapy for patients on long-term sick leave: A comparative outcome study. *Journal of Family Psychotherapy, 18*, 11–24. https://doi.org/10.1300/J085v18n03_02

Twemlow, S. W., & Harvey, E. (2010). Power issues and power struggles in mental illness and everyday life. *International Journal of Applied Psychoanalytic Studies, 74*, 307–328. http://dx.doi.org.jproxy.lib.ecu.edu/10.1002/aps.262

von Kanel, R., van Nuffel, M., & Fuchs, W. J. (2016). Risk assessment for job burnout with a mobile health web application using questionnaire data: A proof of concept study. *BioPsychoSocial Medicine, 10*, 1–13. https://doi.org/10.1186/s13030-016-0082-4

West, L., Lee, A., & Poynton, C. (2012). Becoming depressed at work: A study of worker narratives. *Journal of Workplace Behavioral Health, 27*, 196–212. https://doi.org/10.1080/15555240.2012.701184

Willis Tower Watson (2017, January 4). Full report: 2016 21st annual Willis Towers Watson best practices in health care employer survey. Retrieved from http://www.willistowerswatson.com

Wrich, J. (1974). *The employee assistance program.* Center City, MN: Hazelden.

Wrich, J. (1980). *The employee assistance program: Updated for the 1980s.* Center City, MN: Hazelden.

Wright, L. M., Watson, W. L., & Bell, J. M. (1996). *Beliefs: The heart of healing in families and illness.* New York, NY: Basic Books.

Wynne, L. C., Weber, T. T., & McDaniel, S. H. (1986). *The road from family therapy to systems consultation.* In L. C. Wynne, S. H. McDaniel, and T. T. Weber (Eds.), *Systems consultation: A new perspective for family therapy.* New York, NY: Guildford Press.

York, D. R. (1985). The private sector: Revenue source of the 80s. *Community Mental Health Journal, 21,* 252–263. http://dx.doi.org.jproxy.lib.ecu.edu/10.1007/BF00758144

Chapter 18
Medical Family Therapy in Military and Veteran Health Systems

Angela Lamson, Meghan Lacks, Erin Cobb, and Grace Seamon

The military is the largest employer in the United States, with more than 3.5 million personnel currently serving in the Department of Defense (DoD) active duty, coast guard, and reserve (DoD, 2014a, b). As of 2017, there were 1,298,017 DoD active duty Service members, of which 1,055,972 were enlisted, 229,869 were officers, and 12,176 were cadets-midshipmen (DoD, 2017). In the reserve component, there are a total of 813,037 reservists: 131,928 officers and 681,109 enlisted (DoD, 2017). Alongside the active duty population, it is estimated that there are currently over 22 million veterans in the United States (U.S. Census Bureau, 2012). Couple these figures with the number of partners and dependents/children of current or former Service members, and the opportunity for practitioners in medical family therapy (MedFT) to extend relational care to military and veteran populations grows exponentially. To give some perspective, approximately 54% of all military personnel are married, with higher rates for men (58%) than women (45%), and just over 11% of all active duty marriages as "dual marriages" (DoD, 2015). About 45% of those in a reserve component are married, with higher percentages in the Air National Guard (56%) and Air Force Reserve (55%) than as compared to the Marine Corps Reserve (27%) (U.S. Census Bureau, 2015). Of all current veterans, about 65% of men and 49% of women identify as married (United States Department of Veterans Affairs, 2017a). Further, 2.2% of active duty men and 10.7% of active duty women identify as lesbian, gay, or bisexual (LGB) (Gates & Newport, 2012). While the true number of LGB

A. Lamson (✉) · E. Cobb · G. Seamon
Department of Human Development and Family Science, East Carolina University, Greenville, NC, USA
e-mail: lamsona@ecu.edu

M. Lacks
Goshen Medical Center, Inc., Beulaville, NC, USA

© Springer International Publishing AG, part of Springer Nature 2018
T. Mendenhall et al. (eds.), *Clinical Methods in Medical Family Therapy*, Focused Issues in Family Therapy, https://doi.org/10.1007/978-3-319-68834-3_18

veterans is unknown, it is estimated that 3% of all LGB Americans are U.S. veterans. Approximately 15,500 of active duty Service members identify as transgender, with at least 134,000 veterans who identify as transgender (Gates & Herman, 2014). Whether partnered or not, there are approximately 1.2 million dependent children in active duty families and almost 744,000 dependent children in guard and reserve families (DoD, 2012). Behind each of these statistics is a face that is situated within multiple relationships, and whose biopsychosocial-spiritual (BPSS) health is determined—at least in part—by their likelihood to sustain a career with the military.

The BPSS health (Engel, 1977, 1980; Wright, Watson & Bell, 1996) of military and veteran individuals, couples, and families is vast because it stretches across the life-span, encompasses cultural differences (e.g., diversity by ethnicity) within marked subcultures (e.g., military, reserve, veteran status, branch, hierarchy, and corresponding rules) and can be treated across a range of health-related and family-centered contexts. Attention to detail in type of military and veteran healthcare needed is necessary given that these populations may be served on military installations, in war zones, Veterans Affairs (VA) clinics, vet centers, or across civilian communities. In each of these systems, MedFTs must consider social location (e.g., unique health needs of active duty women in comparison to active duty men) because this workforce strives for sameness among its members rather than deviance (i.e., to be seen as outside of the norm) and, as such, subtle differences in health needs can be easily overlooked.

Another reason that MedFTs must attend to social location is that some social locations (such as ability) could mean the difference between maintaining and ending a military career. A similar situation with civilian careers may not result in such limited outcomes. Still another example is that life as an LGB Service member or veteran can be even more oppressive than as compared to civilian populations (see https://www.diversity.va.gov/programs/files/lgbt/fact-sheet.pdf). After all, it was not until 2011 that LGB Service members were no longer discharged from the military because of their sexual orientation. In relation to gender, more women are now serving in complex job roles within the military. As of 2017, approximately 15.8% of all enlisted Service members and 17.5% of all officers are women (DMDC, 2017), and yet many are hesitant to seek out health services to meet their BPSS needs. MedFTs' systemic training, alongside their training in cultural awareness and humility, allows them to toggle between the Service member's or veteran's BPSS and familial dynamics—while at the same time, honoring religious and ethnic diversity and duty-related experiences as U.S. -born or foreign-born active duty member or veteran.

Beyond the ability to attend to BPSS and relational needs among diverse military and veteran populations, MedFTs are able to extend prevention and intervention programs through a variety of military, reserve, and veteran health-related and family-centered systems described throughout this chapter. Below is an example of how one MedFT provided treatment for military and veteran patients through (a) an integrated behavioral healthcare (IBHC) intervention for a couple on a military installation, wherein the wife was the identified patient; (b) a family-centered agency, wherein a veteran couple was seeking treatment for complex mental health concerns and marital distress; and (c) a mobile unit that travels to military- and veteran-dense communities to extend care for homeless veterans.

Clinical Vignette
[Note: This vignette is a compilation of cases that represent treatment in military and veteran health systems. All patients' names and identifying information have been changed to protect confidentiality.]

The week began for Amy (a MedFT) in a family medicine clinic on-base. An active duty woman in her early 30s—Sally—had been telling her husband—Joe—about how much she resented coming in to see her primary care provider (PCP) (note: In military health, PCPs are often identified as primary care managers (PCMs)). On the day of Sally's first integrated behavioral healthcare visit (and the first time that Joe came with her to a visit), she was told by her PCP that she may not be able to have children because of challenges associated with body weight. After hearing this, Amy stayed with the couple to process what they had learned and to explore what they wanted to do. Sally shared that she felt overwhelmed and that she had heard this news before. Joe began to empathize with his wife and shared that he now understood better why Sally was so upset about coming in for care. He also understood better why Sally had been isolating from him prior to each healthcare visit. Together, the couple began to work with Amy and the PCP to establish realistic health goals, while also improving communication in their marriage. These goals, grounded in solution-focused brief therapy, were conjointly focused on ways that Sally could work toward improving her health. The couple discussed, too, how to collaborate with each other on meal preparation and workouts.

Amy also provided services at an off-base/post family therapy clinic. It is not uncommon to treat military or veteran couples there, particularly given that most mental health and family therapy services for these populations occurs in civilian communities. Amy engaged in a follow-up session with a young couple. The wife, Jodi, had been receiving individual therapy services for approximately 3 months prior to her husband, Mark, joining the sessions. Jodi was a non-Hispanic white female in her mid-20s who presented with depressive and post-traumatic stress (PTS) symptoms secondary to repeated sexual assaults from her stepfather that had lasted for more than 15 years. Mark was Jodi's high school sweetheart, and they had a young child together. Individual therapy for Jodi had evolved into couple's therapy because their relational health (i.e., increasing dyadic conflict) was influencing her individual progress. Mark was a non-Hispanic white male in his mid-20s. He was a disabled veteran diagnosed with a traumatic brain injury (TBI) and post-traumatic stress disorder (PTSD). He also struggled with chronic back pain. He had recently undergone surgery, but it went terribly wrong—leaving him with serious mobility issues and worsening pain. Mark's PTSD was severe; his PCP had told him that he had [potentially] experienced more TBIs than anyone she had seen before. Due to Mark's PTSD, he and Jodi did not sleep in the same bed (i.e., for safety reasons). Jodi was designated as Mark's primary caregiver through the VA. As Mark had recently begun to show improvement, however, Jodi's PTS symptoms worsened. She had become accustomed to helping her husband; by focusing on Mark's problems (e.g., disability claims, healthcare needs), Jodi had been suppressing some of her own needs. Neither partner lived near family, and Jodi had a difficult time letting their child stay with others secondary to her fear that the child would be sexually assaulted (as she had been). Also, both Mark and Jodi lived in fear that terrorists may single them out for attack and thereby worked hard to remove and/or hide evidence of their military connections (e.g., bumper stickers, clothing).

Throughout the course of therapy, Amy worked with Jodi and Mark on mindfulness, I-statements, and a variety of cognitive behavioral therapy techniques. The couple made significant progress over time. They became more involved in individual hobbies without feeling guilty for engaging in self-care. They started to communicate needs to each other more clearly (e.g., asking for personal space on a "bad" day, requesting help with a household task), and Jodi made a goal of working through what she described as shame, embarrassment, and betrayal felt from her early abuse. She learned to set boundaries and adjust expectations with family members. She also grew in her parenting skills, which eased her anxieties about their child's safety. After a series of sessions with Amy, the couple began attending a mindfulness group, during which Jodi described further improvement in managing anxiety and Mark described noticeable differences in physical pain. Before terminating with the couple, Amy also made them aware of VA respite and other services they were eligible for to include other pain management services and rehabilitation programs.

Amy also provided care through a HIPAA-approved mobile unit that drove around the state to meet with homeless veterans who needed physical, dental, and/or psychosocial health support. The unit was equipped with an interdisciplinary team that could work to assess for and respond to diverse BPSS needs. One day, Amy met John at a local homeless shelter. John was initially uncertain about whether to trust Amy, or anyone else on the mobile unit, as he expressed frustration with government systems (especially the VA). As a Vietnam-era veteran in his mid-60s, John primarily relied on the VA for his care targeting hypertension. Over the course of several weeks, John opened up to Amy and revealed that he had recently walked out of an appointment with his PCP because he had felt disrespected by his provider's use of a computer during the visit. John maintained that he had no plans to return. As a result, however, he had not taken his hypertension medication for several weeks. Amy (as the MedFT), a substance abuse counselor, and vocational rehabilitation counselor worked together to validate John's frustration and employed motivational interviewing (MI) to explore his readiness for change in managing hypertension. Their approach honored and respected John's experience, while at the same time avoided criticizing the VA or John's

> PCP. The team discussed with John current trends toward using computers and technology during healthcare visits and then role-played how he could advocate for his needs. During the session, John made an appointment with his provider at the VA and agreed to resume taking medication as prescribed. Over the next several months, the team worked with John on how to manage anger and frustration, using brief mindfulness-based interventions, with goals targeting both hypertension and interactions with the PCP. John later shared that he felt that he was better equipped to achieve these goals.

What Are Military and Veteran Health Systems?

The U.S. Military Health System (MHS) is an intricate web of healthcare led by the Office of the Assistant Secretary of Defense for Health Affairs within the Department of Defense; it includes healthcare delivery, medical education, public health, innovative military research, and collaborative efforts with private sector providers (MHS, 2017). The MHS is made up of healthcare professionals from the Army, Navy, and Air Force who extend care into both the battlefield and local healthcare systems (e.g., hospitals, clinics, dental clinics) around the world. The MHS extends care to approximately 10 million beneficiaries who are active duty and retired Service members, as well as their dependents (MHS Genesis, 2017). A primary focus of MHS is to increase military readiness and ensure that the military force is ready for deployment and prepared for a full range of military missions.

For active duty Service members, military readiness is key. In the field, care begins with a first responder (e.g., self, combat lifesaver) and then advances to higher echelons of care, including advanced trauma management and critical care transport, as needed. In 2016, injuries/poisoning, musculoskeletal diseases (e.g., back problems), and mental disorders (e.g., anxiety disorder, adjustment disorder) comprised more than half of the medical encounters for active duty Service members (Armed Forces Health Surveillance Branch, 2017a). MedFTs are called upon in these instances to assist with pain management and to assess for and treat behavioral health conditions, psychological disorders, and relational distress across both brief and traditional sessions.

As is the case with civilians, Service members and their families are more likely to seek out behavioral and relational health services (whether related to a physical concern or not) when stigma is minimized. One way that stigma may be reduced is by extending integrated behavioral healthcare services (Maguen, Cohen, et al., 2010) (i.e., services offered through a team of behavioral and primary care providers (simultaneously)). Based on recent findings, it is clear that relational health is relevant to many Service members and thus must be extended treatment and support in a stigma-free environment. In fiscal year 2013, Military OneSource provided more than 200,000 counseling sessions, with the most common concerns being partner relational problems (59%) and phase of life/religious or spiritual problems (24%), relational problem not otherwise specified (7%), parent-child relational problem (6%), and acculturation (4%). In the same year, Military Family Life Consultants provided almost 2.6 million in-person services to military Service members (not available to retirees), with the most common concerns including communication (26%), marital/relationship distress (21%), job stress (19%), general stress (13%), and problematic family dynamics (11%; Department of Defense, 2014a). Through a relational and BPSS lens, MedFTs are uniquely suited to provide care to address these issues while simultaneously assisting with the aim of military readiness on installation, in combat, or in the community.

Envisioning care delivery on an installation may seem challenging to some MedFTs, given that military installations are most commonly described as property that serves only as a command center, training grounds, and/or military housing for Service members. However, the reality is that MedFTs may find themselves delivering care in a variety of contexts on-base/on-post, including at child care centers, military treatment centers (military treatment facilities (MTFs): clinics and hospitals), family support centers (e.g., Fleet and Family Support; Army Community Service), schools, spiritual life centers, and much more. These essential services are specifically tailored to meet the needs of military personnel and their families. As evidenced by the high numbers of Service members utilizing therapy to address relational concerns (DoD, 2014a, b), it is clear that the BPSS health of military families also impacts readiness. As such, MedFTs must be in tune with both the variety of contexts for care and the unique treatment needs of military families in order to maximize Service members' and their families' well-being.

As an example, more than 200,000 children between 0 and 12 years old receive care on a daily basis from child development centers, school-age care, and family child care programs (Department of Defense, 2014a, b), and over 70,000 children are enrolled in Department of Defense schools (Department of Defense Education Activity, 2017). Among these pediatric beneficiaries, mental health issues (e.g., autism, developmental speech/language disorders, attention deficit disorder, adjustment disorders, depressive disorders, anxiety disorders) account for a significant challenge in the school system. Furthermore, these diagnoses account for the largest percentage of healthcare visits among military dependents, insofar as they reflect the reason for the highest number of pediatric medical encounters and hospital bed days (Armed Forces Health Surveillance Branch, 2017b). Through the training that MedFTs receive in BPSS care, alongside their ability to collaborate with diverse disciplines and systems (e.g., schools, healthcare), these clinicians should be on the front lines of supporting military children and families who live on military installations.

Beyond the families who live on an installation are those who have decided to move to homes in communities off-base/off-post. Approximately 80% of the 1.2 million school-aged military children attend a public school (Department of Defense, 2014a, b). Military families who live off-base/off-post are also more likely to receive their healthcare off-base/off-post. In 2016, 89.1% of non-Service beneficiaries received care in a nonmilitary medical facility (Armed Forces Health Surveillance Branch, 2017b). This figure also reflects families of active duty Service members and National Guard and Research Service members/retirees (Armed Forces Health Surveillance Branch, 2017b). It is important to clarify that many military family members (and retirees) may be receiving care through civilian providers approved by the MHS. In fact, due to the needs of the active duty population who must be seen in an MTF, in some locations, retirees and family members can only be seen in the community through the TRICARE system. In these contexts, particularly in areas with large military populations, MedFTs should be aware of the MHS structure, military culture, and ancillary services for military families as described above.

While clinics and medical centers within the MHS meet the needs of millions of beneficiaries, more than half of all veterans are likely to receive care from a civilian/community health system. Once retired or separated, veterans may opt to receive care from a civilian/community healthcare context, including community-based outpatient clinics, vet centers, specialized treatment programs for substance use disorders (SUD) or PTSD, or as described in our vignette through mobile health units (U.S. Department of Veterans Affairs, 2017b).

To clarify, veterans' healthcare is administrated through a completely separate system from those extending care to active duty, known as the Veterans Health Administration (VHA), which is part of the Department of Veterans Affairs (Military Health System, 2014)—not the DoD. Retired military members have the ability to seek services from MTF (i.e., MHS) or through the VHA, whereas veterans (i.e., members who served in the military and were released from service under conditions other than dishonorable) who are not retired are not eligible for healthcare at a MTF (Military Health System, 2014).

In 2014, there were 9.1 million veterans enrolled in the Veterans Health Administration for services. That year, veterans had 92.4 million outpatient visits and 707,400 inpatient admissions, and these numbers have all continued to increase over the past decade (U.S. Department of Veterans Affairs, 2016a). Additionally, the VA operates the Vet Center Program, which provides readjustment counseling, outreach, and referral services to veterans and their families, as well as bereavement services to parents, spouses, children, and siblings of Service members who die while on active duty (U.S. Department of Veterans Affairs, 2015). Veterans who enroll for health benefits through the U.S. Department of Veterans Affairs do so through an enrollment system that is based on priority groups (i.e., priority group 1–8; priorities are defined based on different types of needs, not on a continuum for severity of need). The priority groups are designed to assist veterans in getting services that better align to their specific needs (e.g., disability, low income, unemployable; U.S. Department of Veterans Affairs, 2016b). The average enrollee in the VA is male, 61 years old, white/non-Hispanic, and married with dependents. Approximately one-fifth of veterans receiving care from the VA stated that they were coping with memory loss, 25% reported coping with a stressful situation, and an additional one-fifth endorsed being a current smoker (Huang et al., 2017). These findings indicate that memory care support, stress management, smoking cessation, VA benefits, and an understanding of community-based services to meet their other needs (e.g., housing, financial, specialty care services, placements, etc.) are important areas for MedFTs to be trained insofar as to better support veterans and their families.

Treatment (and Support) Teams in Military and Veteran Health Systems

Due to the diversity in and between military and veteran healthcare systems, there are several potential collaborators who are important for MedFTs to be able to identify when working with military and veteran individuals, couples, families, and units. To provide clarity for MedFTs, this section is divided between (a) treatment teams that typically exist within on-base/on-post military healthcare systems and (b) treatment teams that typically exist within veteran-based healthcare systems.

Treatment Teams in Military Health Systems

The main goal for this military healthcare system section is to provide descriptions for direct patient care, readiness training, wellness education, and preventive care for members and their beneficiaries. There are several points to consider while reading this section due to the vast information that is available. First, the titles of roles may vary between Service branches; thus, if the treatment team member listed below represents a certain branch, rather than being a common role across all branches, it will be denoted accordingly: Air Force = *, Army = **, and Navy/Marines = ***. For example, all military branches use the patient-centered medical home (PCMH) model for primary care, but each branch implements their own version (Marshall et al., 2011). For example, the Navy PCMH model is called Medical Home Port (MHP), the Army model is called Army Soldier Centered Medical Home (SCMH), and the Air Force calls it the Family Health Operations. Thus, there may be roles within each of these models that are distinct to that particular branch. Second, it is important to keep in mind that across all Service branches, there are roles for officers (e.g., healthcare providers, physicians, nurses, behavioral health providers) and enlisted Service members (e.g., healthcare specialists, medical technicians). These distinctions are important to recognize because their titles may look different than as compared to civilian contexts. For example, a certified "medical assistant" in a civilian context may be referred to as "hospital corpsman" in a military setting.

Lastly, the treatment team members discussed in this chapter refer to those found in aerospace (i.e., flight) medicine, family medicine, integrated care, or pediatric primary care contexts. There is limited information below regarding military personnel injured during combat because those treatment teams vary for each branch, and that conversation goes beyond the scope of this chapter. However, it is essential for a MedFT to be knowledgeable about the process of how injured military men and women are treated on the battlefield, then transferred to a stateside hospital, because a MedFT may see these patients when said patients are receiving treatment in the United States. For example, the protocol for treating Service members who have been injured on the battlefield is guided by four levels of care, referred to as "roles" (U.S. Army Medical Department, 2013). Keep in mind, too, that these roles vary based on Service branch. The first role refers to point of injury care to triage, treat, and evacuate the patient with the goal to return the Service member to duty or get him or her stabilized and transported to the second role. The second role refers to providing basic primary care but could also include limited optometry, combat and operational stress control, dental, laboratory, radiographic, and/or surgical services. The third role expands the support provided in the second role and refers to patients transported to medical treatment facilities (typically located in the theater of operations) who are not stable enough to be transported over long distances. The care in this role includes resuscitation, initial wound surgery, damage control surgery, and postoperative treatment. The final role is when Service members have been transported to medical care provided in continental U.S.-based hospitals or other safe havens, including hospitals in the Department of Veterans Affairs and those in the National Disaster Medical System (U.S. Army Medical Department, 2013). For a more detailed description of these roles, refer to the U.S. Army Medical Department (2013).

Treatment and Support Teams for Military Populations and Their Dependents

Teams that serve military populations and their dependents via treatment or support services include the following:

Aerospace medical service specialists*. Specialists enlisted as personnel who assist medical providers in a variety of ways, such as administrating immunizations, assembling/operating/maintaining medical equipment, and assisting in aeromedical evacuations.

Aerospace medicine specialists/flight surgeons*. Providers who are primary care physicians with either a Doctor of Medicine (MD) or Doctor of Osteopathic Medicine (DO) degree; they treat pilots and crew members traveling in air or space.

Behavioral healthcare facilitators (BHCF). These professionals are registered nurses who act as liaisons between the external behavioral health consultant (EBHC) and the primary care team. The BHCF reinforces, encourages, checks, and supports the treatment plan created by the primary care manager (PCM) and the internal behavioral health consultant.

Behavioral health technicians***. These technicians aid medical officers in the care and treatment of mental health patients, administrative procedures, and maintaining clinic equipment. They also observe and report patient symptoms to the medical officer.

Beneficiary counseling and assistance coordinators (BCAC). Professionals who are located at military treatment facilities (MTFs) and TRICARE regional offices; they assist beneficiaries in accessing medical and dental care.

Case managers. Professionals who assist patients in developing plans to control their illness or injury, especially those with complex medical, social, financial, and/or mental health issues. Case managers in the military may help with linking patients to helpful community or federal support systems, coordinate services among providers, and/or schedule said services.

Certified alcohol and drug abuse counselors (CADAC)*. Mental health technicians who serve as alcohol and drug counselors. Officers can also be CADACs; they are responsible for screening, intake, orientation, assessment, treatment planning, counseling, case management, crisis intervention, education, referral, report/record keeping, and consultation with patients.

Exceptional family member program (EFMP) staff. Staff who facilitate initial enrollment into the EFMP (a mandatory program for someone identified as having a special need) and guide families to additional services. They also assist in referrals, individualized service plans, and case management from one duty station to the next. "Special needs" refer to any special medical, dental, mental health, developmental or educational requirement, wheelchair accessibility, adaptive equipment, or assistive technology devices and services.

External behavioral health consultants (EBHC). Consultants who assist the primary care manager and behavioral healthcare facilitator regarding psychotropic medications for patients by providing verbal and/or written consultation on medication decisions, changing medications, and managing side effects.

Hospital corpsmen*.** Professionals who assist healthcare providers in delivering medical care to Service members and their families. They may act as a clinical or specialty technician at a MTF or as a battlefield corpsman with the Marine Corps, providing emergency medical services in combat. Hospital corpsmen also help maintain treatment records, administer injections, and perform clinical tests.

Internal behavioral health consultants. Consultants who function as mental health providers embedded in primary care settings to assist primary care managers in helping patients with a wide range of behavioral health conditions, chronic medical problems, and adverse health behaviors. These consultants assist patients with issues related to anxiety, depression, grief, increasing exercise, managing home or work stress, quitting smoking, cholesterol and blood pressure management, weight management, improving sleep, chronic pain management, and managing diabetes.

Medical corps officers.** Graduates of an American Medical Association or American Osteopathic Association accredited medical school; these officers are responsible for the overall health of Service members and those eligible to receive care in the military community.

Medical evaluation board case managers. Professionals who do initial counseling with Service members before being entered into the Disability Evaluation

System, signed up for an Integrated Disability Evaluation System Consultation Course (ICC), or given contact information for a Physical Evaluation Board Liaison Officer (PEBLO).

Mental health service specialists*. Specialists who work with psychiatrists, psychologists, and/or other providers to help formally assess and provide behavioral healthcare to Service members in order to get them back to their jobs.

Mental health specialists**. Specialists who are enlisted personnel; they assist with inpatient and outpatient treatment of psychiatric, drug, and alcohol patients. They are also responsible for collecting and recording patients' psychosocial and physical data.

Military family life consultants (MFLC). Consultants who have at least a master's degree in mental health (e.g., marriage and family therapy, counseling, social work, psychology); they provide confidential nonmedical therapy or counseling services related to deployment stress, reintegration, relocation adjustment, separation, anger management, conflict resolution, parenting, and relationship issues. Meetings are face-to-face and can be held on- or off-military installation

Military service coordinators (MSC). Coordinators who function as essential representatives throughout the Integrated Disability Evaluation System process; they act as a liaison between the Service member and the Department of Veterans Affairs. The MSC helps patients with their VA claims and keep them and the Physical Evaluation Board Liaison Officer informed of all VA processes.

Patient advocates. Professionals who respond to patient grievances and complaints. They also assist obtaining information or services for Service members and their families and help increase communication among clinic staff and patients and their families regarding wait issues, scheduling problems, billing matters, and physician concerns.

Patient relations representatives (PRR)***. Representatives who act as liaisons between clinic staff and patients and their families; they also aid in resolving conflicts or areas of concerns from patients and families.

Physical evaluation board liaison officers (PEBLO). Professionals who assist Service members in their fitness for duty, rights, and entitlement to benefits and ensure that they are aware of options and required decisions through the Integrated Disability Evaluation System (IDES) process.

Primary care managers (PCM). Professionals who provide all routine, non-emergency, and urgent healthcare to patients. If PCMs are unable to provide the level of care needed, the patient will be referred to a specialist.

Privileged mental health providers*. Active duty military, reservists, and civilian personnel who have privileges to diagnose, initiate, alter, or terminate healthcare treatment plans within the scope of their license, certification, or registration.

Resiliency staff. Specifically focus on resiliency related to vicarious traumatization and stress management.

Sexual assault response coordinators (SARC). Professionals who serve as a single point of contact to coordinate sexual assault response when a sexual assault is reported. They are available 24 hours per day/7 days per week to assist victims of sexual assault and report the information to the installation commander.

Victim advocates. Professionals who provide nonclinical advocacy services and support to Service members and their families who are experiencing domestic abuse. They are on-call 24 hours per day/7 days per week to provide immediate assistance, safety planning, nonjudgmental support, and information about available resources. They can also help victims and families find shelter and support, secure a military protective order (MPO), and assist with locating clinical counseling services.

Treatment and support teams in veteran facilities. Teams that function within veteran facilities are extensive (including a variety of providers who treat military sexual trauma, polytrauma, and TBI via rehabilitation services) as well as the following staff and provider types.

Mental health intensive case management (MHICM) staff. A multidisciplinary team that provides a variety of services (e.g., crisis intervention, medication management, socialization skills, transportation, family/caregiver support) to veterans with mental illness to maintain their independence through intensive case management services.

Mental health treatment coordinators (MHTC). Professionals who ensure that all veterans who receive specialty mental health services have continuity through their mental healthcare/transitions. MHTCs are assigned to veterans in order for the veteran to have a continuous point of contact while the veteran is receiving mental health services.

Military service coordinators. Coordinators who assist Service members in the IDES process by guiding and counseling them and by helping them file their VA benefits in a timely manner in order to receive benefits as soon as possible after separating from the service.

Patient advocates. Professionals who collect and manage feedback from veterans and their families regarding their experiences at the clinic. Patient advocates assist with complaints or concerns regarding patients' quality of medical care.

Patient aligned care teams (PACTs). Primary care medical teams that include behavioral health professionals. Primary care providers utilize these team members to coordinate appropriate services for patients. For example, the PCP can manage a veteran's mental health problems with the collaboration of a behavioral health provider, but if more intensive treatment is necessary, he or she will refer the veteran to a specialized mental health program. The VA also has Geriatric Patient Aligned Care Teams (GeriPACT).

Peer support specialists. Individuals with a mental health struggle and/or co-occurring condition who have been trained to work with others with similar conditions. Peer support specialists aid others by sharing their personal experiences and by helping veterans navigate the VA system.

Primary care-mental health integration (PC-MHI) staff. Staff who work in the primary care-mental health integration program who are fully licensed behavioral health professionals; they are embedded in a primary care setting as part of an interdisciplinary team delivering brief consultation services to veterans. Veterans meet with the behavioral health provider as part of their routine primary care service to identify, treat, and manage behavioral conditions.

Readjustment counselors. Licensed mental health providers who work in community-based counseling vet venters. They provide free services to all veterans who have served in any combat zone.

Fundamentals of Care in Military and Veteran Health Systems

MedFTs may typically focus their sessions on ways in which physical health conditions influence psychosocial functioning or vice versa, but it is essential in military and veteran healthcare systems that they have a fundamental understanding of military culture. Understanding this culture helps MedFTs to build credibility and advance joining efforts as they address BPSS concerns of military/veteran patients, couples, and/or families. While there are many cultural dynamics that are unique to military service (e.g., geographic mobility, periodic or enduring separations, unpredictable duty hours), this section focuses primarily on requisite knowledge regarding the roles of deployment, combat, and reintegration in the lives of active duty and veteran populations. We also highlight several BPSS health factors experienced by these groups. MedFTs working in a military and veteran contexts should also be aware of common health concerns experienced by Service members, including alcohol and tobacco use, intimate partner violence, military sexual trauma, moral injuries, post-traumatic stress, traumatic brain injuries, sexual health, and suicide.

Deployment

Deployments have received considerable attention in military and veteran research because they have immediate- and long-term effects on relationships, which are at least partly due to the gaps in communication and increases in anxiety between couples and families that they bring (Lowe, Adams, Browne, & Hinkle, 2012). Investigators have reported that families are not the only ones stressed by deployments, either: Service members who deploy also show an increase in work- and family-related stress (Deployment Information and Resources, 2010) than as compared to non-deployed personnel.

For every branch of the military, family stress is significantly higher for members who had deployed than members who had not deployed (Bray et al., 2010). However, it is possible that after a certain length of time deployed, military spouses adapt to the stressors brought on from deploying. For example, Karney and Crown (2007) found that for every branch except the Air Force, the longer the military spouse was deployed, the more stable his or her relationship. On the other hand, researchers have suggested that military spouses often experience loneliness, anxiety, and depression (MacGregor, Han, Dougherty, & Galarneau, 2012; Makin-Byrd, Gifford, McCutcheon, & Glynn, 2011; Mansfield et al., 2010) throughout the deployment cycle. Researchers have also found that spouses tend to experience more emotional stress during deployments if the Service member is of lower rank, the Service member has less military experience and social support, and the non-deployed spouse is unemployed (Allen, Rhoades, Stanley, & Markman, 2010).

Although military Service members and their families commonly experience stress during times of deployment, the literature is inconsistent about the impact of multiple deployments (MacGregor et al., 2012). For example, the "healthy warrior effect" is a term used for Service members who are deemed healthier prior to a deployment and who go on to deploy or who may be more likely to experience multiple deployments in comparison to those who do not deploy (Larson, Highfill-Mcroy, & Booth-Kewley, 2008). The use of this term implies that the more psychologically resilient Service members are, the more likely they are to deploy (and then asked to redeploy). This sequence is less likely for Service members who experience more serious illnesses, such as depression or bipolar disorder (MacGregor et al., 2012).

Combat

Since the introduction of PTSD to the *Diagnostic and Statistical Manual of Mental Disorders* (DSM) in the 1980s, researchers have continued to find positive relationships between combat exposure and high levels of psychological distress (McCuaig-Edge & Ivey, 2012). Service members, especially those who have recently returned from combat, often experience difficulties coping with daily life, significant emotional distress, increases in risk-taking behaviors, relationship distress with spouses and families, and significantly more health concerns than as compared to their civilian counterparts (Allen, Rhoades, Stanley, & Markman, 2010; Brooks, 2005; Fischer, 2007; Jordan, 2011).

Although PTSD continues to plague veterans (and is discussed in more detail later in this chapter), it is important for MedFTs to understand that the stress of combat does not always lead to PTSD. In fact, research continues to show that the unpredictable and persistent potential for imminent danger which accompanies deployment to a combat zone is often the prominent source of distress upon returning home (Junger, 2010; Van Der Kolk, 2015). This is mainly caused by the hardening of neuro-pathways in the brain, which strengthen the fight-or-flight response and cause a significant increase in baseline levels of stress hormones (Van Der Kolk, 2015). More specifically, the chronic anxiety and fear that comes from being deployed to a combat area cause the body to maintain a heightened state of arousal, regardless of whether the Service member ever experiences contact or a life-threatening (or otherwise "traumatic") situation.

Thus, much of the emotional, behavioral, and relational distress that researchers have found to correlate with combat exposure has an inherently biological component. Because of this, MedFTs should garner skills in behavioral medicine (e.g., treatment for insomnia, pain) and in providing psychoeducation about the biological implications related to combat stress to both veterans and their families as a way to normalize and depersonalize any sudden and significant changes in personality, mood, or behaviors. Similarly, as PTSD and combat-related stress continue to carry stigma in the military, reframing the biological alterations associated with combat stress as the body's natural survival response has the potential to relieve Service members of feelings of personal weakness or shame (Fox & Pease, 2012; Lorber & Garcia, 2010).

Reintegration

In the military community, reintegration applies to two important life phases: (a) reintegration back into the family following deployment and (b) reintegration back into the civilian world following military service. Although the levels of distress that result from each type of reintegration are subject to the uniqueness of each Service member's personality, military career, and family dynamics, it is clear from the literature that stress paired with reintegration is predominantly caused by role change (Marek, Stetzer, Adams, Popejoy, & Rantz, 2012).

For example, when a Service member deploys, his or her spouse is left to run the household (e.g., functioning as a single parent, being responsible for all bill payments and household chores, and adjusting to a new duty station with little to no community or family support). Spouses of deployed Service members, as a consequence, often feel high levels of stress, anxiety, depression, sleep disturbance, and grief (Makin-Byrd, Gifford, McCutcheon, & Glynn, 2011; Mansfield et al., 2010; Steelfisher, Zaslavsky, & Blendon, 2008). Also significant is that these symptoms are often exacerbated when the Service member returns home. Through this reintegration process, both partners typically struggle to restructure the altered family dynamics that occurred during deployment. Each partner must also adapt to and cope with any personality or mood changes (e.g., irritability, unable to concentrate, violent episodes) that the Service member or spouse may exhibit secondary to combat or deployment stress (Makin-Byrd et al., 2011; Marek et al., 2012). Similarly, veterans reintegrating into the civilian world may experience an increase in stress across both their family and personal life as they struggle to "fit" in a civilian society that is less structured and stable than the military culture from whence they came.

Due to multiple levels of stress and distress, ambiguity of roles, and constantly changing family dynamics, MedFTs working with veterans and their families through any period of reintegration should rely on skills gained through their systemic family therapy training. Assessing for rigid and permeable boundaries; highlighting problematic communication patterns, comradery, and alliance with other veterans to the exclusion of family members; and altering triangulated relationships are all effective skills for reducing ambiguity and role uncertainty in family units and larger societal systems (Greenman & Johnson, 2012; Guay, et al., 2011; Johnson, 2005; Shapiro, 2007; Weissman et al. 2011). Interventions pertaining to these presenting problems are further discussed in the research-informed practices described later in this chapter. Additionally, because reintegration impacts more people than the Service member, couples therapy and family therapy should be considered when treating BPSS concerns (Greenman & Johnson, 2012; Johnson, 2005; Sayers, 2011; Shapiro, 2007; Weissman et al., 2011). Below are just some of the complex BPSS concerns that tend to become more evident in times of deployment, combat, and/or reintegration.

Tobacco and Alcohol Use

Despite the fact that physical fitness is required in the military, many Service members still take part in activities that are detrimental to their physical health. For example, Smith and Malone (2014) found that military members risk the negative health consequences of tobacco use because it helps relieve stress and allows individuals to take "breaks" from work. MedFTs should be knowledgeable about the effects of tobacco use and nicotine, alongside evidence-based options for reducing and/or stopping it. In addition, since Smith and Malone (2014) found that most Service members did not report alternative ways to manage stress, MedFTs should be equipped with skills and knowledge about how stress impacts one's body. They should be able to teach healthier techniques (e.g., deep breathing, muscle relaxation, guided imagery) to manage stress, rather than resorting to the use of substances.

Men who serve in the military drink alcohol at higher rates compared to civilian men, whereas military women drink less alcohol compared to civilian women (Teachman, Anderson, & Tedrow, 2015). Similar to tobacco use, researchers have found that the culture of the military promotes alcohol use because it has traditionally been used to promote bonding and unit cohesion (Teachman et al., 2015). Sadly, the trend does not change once becoming a veteran; McCauley, Blosnich, and Dichter (2015) found that veterans were significantly more likely (24.9%) than non-veterans (17.4%) to use substances. MedFTs must be knowledgeable about the connections, too, between tobacco and alcohol use and other biopsychosocial concerns. For example, both tobacco and alcohol use increase when PTSD symptoms are present (Hermes et al., 2012; Marshall et al., 2012). Also, MedFTs should use their systemic training to recognize how the military organization as a larger system impacts substance use; alternative techniques to reduce stress have yet to be endorsed by the military, and the myth of tobacco as effective at reducing stress is still pervasive (Smith & Malone, 2014).

Intimate Partner Violence

Although intimate partner violence (IPV) affects both civilian and military families, military stressors such as multiple deployments, family separation and reintegration, work demands, previous head traumas, mental illness, and substance abuse can increase the risk for IPV (Gierisch et al., 2013). In fact, researchers have found that IPV in military families is more severe than in civilian families (Rentz et al., 2006). This is a significant health concern because of its impact on victims (Anderson, 2002), children in the home (Kitzmann, Gaylord, Holt, & Kenny, 2003), and the economic burden that IPV has on society as a whole (National Center for Injury Prevention and Control, 2003). It is essential to remember that there are several factors that correlate with IPV (e.g., childhood trauma, relationship adjustment, psychopathology, substance abuse, military factors, etc.), but discussing these confounding factors in depth goes beyond the scope of this chapter. With that said, MedFTs must be knowledgeable about these risk factors in order to understand how they interact with one another and could lead to violent behaviors in military families.

It is essential that MedFTs have a thorough understanding of the military structure and the options available to military families in order to know how to best assess and intervene in IPV cases. For example, every branch of the military has a Family Advocacy Program (FAP) that offers a variety of services to IPV victims (Military OneSource, 2016). However, it is important to recognize that IPV in a military context presents unique challenges; if the perpetrator is a Service member, there could be negative career consequences like reassignment or discharge (Klostermann, Mignone, Kelley, Musson, & Bohall, 2012). Since researchers report rates of IPV up to three times higher in military families compared to civilian counterparts and there is no standardized way to measure IPV in military settings (Klostermann et al., 2012), MedFTs can play an important role in identifying, preventing, and helping treat both perpetrators and victims of IPV. MedFTs are experts in collaborating with a variety of providers on the interconnectedness between biopsychosocial issues; they are thereby able to identify the BPSS repercussions of IPV and communicate those health issues to the treatment team as indicated.

Military Sexual Trauma

Although sexual assault in general is not unique to the military community, it is more common for those in the military than as compared to civilians (Bostock and Daley, 2007). More specifically, military sexual trauma (MST) refers to sexual assault that occurs while the individual is in the military; it includes any and all incidents ranging from harassment to violent rape. It is important to know, too, that sexual harassment is not only more common for Service members, but it is complicated by the fact that it is often perpetrated by another Service member within the context of work (Zinzow, Grubaugh, Monnier, Suffoletta-Maierle, & Frueh, 2007). This is an important distinction compared to sexual assault in the civilian world, because the military is often seen as a family—especially when preparing for or during deployments. The military member often seeks support and stability from the military family instead of his or her family at home (Goodcase, Love, & Ladson, 2015). There are several benefits to being a part of the "military family" (e.g., successful missions), but when MST occurs the detrimental effects that ensue can look similar to a child experiencing incest (Goodcase et al., 2015). It is not surprising, then, that the negative effects of MST are best understood and treated through a systemic and BPSS lens. MedFTs working in military settings must be equipped to assess for prior trauma, especially MST, and be able to provide sensitive, inclusive, and comprehensive support to victims (Holland, Rabelo, & Cortina, 2016). For more specific guidance on how to assess MST from both individual and systemic perspectives, see Goodcase et al. (2015).

Moral Injuries

According to the National Center for Posttraumatic Stress, moral injury is defined as any act, or the witnessing of any act, which fundamentally transforms moral and ethical expectations that are rooted in religious, spiritual, cultural, organizational, and/or group-based rules (Maguen & Litz, 2016). To put concisely, moral injury typically occurs when a veteran perpetrates, fails to prevent, bears witness to, or learns about instances which violate and permanently alter previously held beliefs and expectations of humanity and/or society as a whole (Litz et al., 2009; Maguen & Litz, 2012). Examples of experiences which typically lead to moral injury include witnessing or perpetrating disproportionate acts of violence, being betrayed by peers or leadership, witnessing or perpetrating any act of violence toward civilians, and witnessing or perpetrating violence within peer groups (e.g., sexual assault) (Maguen & Litz, 2012).

Moral injury results in a negative altering of a one's world view, and as such many veterans often present to primary care, behavioral health providers, or spiritual leaders with feelings of anhedonia, difficulty relating to others, relationship distress, emotional avoidance, feelings of numbness, and/or intrusive thoughts (Maguen & Litz, 2016; Maguen & Litz, 2012). Veterans may also report self-harming behaviors and/or experiencing overwhelming suicidal thoughts in context of a moral injury. In particular, veterans who have experienced a moral injury after taking another person's life are more likely to screen positive for PTSD; they are also more likely to abuse substances (Maguen & Litz, 2012; Maguen, Lucenko, et al., 2010).

It is important to note, however, that while a veteran struggling with moral injury may be diagnosed with PTSD, not all veterans with PTSD have sustained moral injury (just as veterans with moral injury may not have PTSD or may have never experienced combat). In fact, the distinguishing factor between PTSD and moral injury is that a diagnosis of PTSD requires that veterans experience or witness a life-threatening incident linked to feelings of helplessness and loss of safety (American Psychiatric Association, 2013), whereas moral injury requires that veterans witness or perpetrate an act that alters their worldview and, thus, beliefs about the goodness and purpose(s) of life. More specifically, veterans suffering from PTSD may exhibit thoughts such as "bad things happened to me and I cannot control them," while veterans suffering from moral injury may exhibit thoughts such as "bad things have happened because I did not control them." Beliefs such as these often cause deep shame and guilt or survivor guilt, alongside losses of hope (Maguen & Litz, 2012).

Due to the overwhelming similarities in symptom presentation and comorbidity of PTSD and moral injury, MedFTs must be diligent in the assessment of negative beliefs, grief, and loss vis-à-vis biological and behavioral impacts and impairments expressed by the patient. Although little research has been done on best practices for treating moral injury, existing studies suggest that multimodal interventions that include experiential techniques, cognitive behavioral therapies, bilateral simulation, and co-occurring couples therapy have proven to be most effective in ameliorating shame, anhedonia, and relational sabotage common to moral injuries (e.g., Johnson, 2005; MacIntosh & Johnson, 2008; Forrest & Shapiro, 1998; Maguen & Litz, 2012; Van Der Kolk, 2015; Wiebe & Johnson, 2016).

Post-Traumatic Stress and Traumatic Brain Injuries

Soldier's heart, shell shock, combat fatigue, and post-traumatic stress are common terms that have been used over decades of research related to traumatic exposure and experiences that influence the mental health of service men and women. Recently, researchers have become more attuned to the ways in which physical trauma to the brain—called traumatic brain injury (TBI)—interfaces with post-traumatic stress symptoms (PTS) or post-traumatic stress disorder (PTSD). Untangling TBI and PTS/PTSD symptoms experienced by Service members or veterans— alongside those perceived or observed by others—has not been an easy task for clinicians or researchers. We are continuing to learn about how these fit together and about what ways to best advance care.

Post-Traumatic Stress

Post-traumatic stress has become one of the most common conditions associated with military Service members. Approximately 8% of those who were deployed to the Iraq and Afghanistan conflicts were diagnosed with PTSD (Institute of Medicine [IOM], 2014). And even though PTSD has received a lot of attention among military and veteran healthcare providers and populations for decades, a chasm still exists in continuity of care (i.e., gaps in treatment stability between cares as an active Service member versus retired military or veteran). These gaps make it difficult to track the quality of care for those with PTSD (IOM, 2014). This also makes it difficult to track health outcomes for active duty Service members versus veterans who are experiencing PTS or PTSD. Since PTSD impairs an individual's physical, psychological, social, and occupational functioning, MedFTs must be sure to assess how each of these areas is impacting one another in order to provide quality BPSS treatment. In fact, the Institute of Medicine recommended an integrated and comprehensive approach to preventing and treating PTSD in active duty members and veterans (IOM, 2014). Relatedly, Bohnert, Sripada, Mach, and McCarthy (2016) also found that same-day integrated mental health services in primary care settings increased the odds of accurately diagnosing PTSD and initiating treatment for it. MedFTs are uniquely trained to such models of integrated behavioral healthcare secondary to their systemic and BPSS training, ability to diagnose, and philosophical beliefs regarding the importance of interdisciplinary collaboration.

MedFTs working in military contexts should not only be skilled at assessing for PTSD and providing comprehensive, evidence-based treatment options; they should also be knowledgeable about the BPSS impacts of PTSD on military members' partners and children throughout the treatment process. MedFTs can use a relational lens to find predictor variables (as well as mediators and moderators) that can minimize the likelihood for PTSD for active duty Service members, veterans, and their families (Campbell & Renshaw, 2013). It is not uncommon for family members (who share a home with a veteran or Service member who is experiencing PTS/PTSD) to experience post-traumatic symptoms at levels equal to or beyond those of their loved one. For this reason, MedFT's BPSS and systemic clinical skills are essential to the future of PTSD research and treatment. For a comprehensive summary about current evidence-based practice, the VA and DoD have released a pocket guide to aid primary care and behavioral health providers in the treatment of PTS and PTSD (see Defense Centers of Excellence for Psychological Health & Traumatic Brain Injury, 2013).

Traumatic Brain Injuries

Traumatic brain injuries are primarily caused direct or indirect blast impacts to the head from improvised explosive devices (IEDs), motor vehicle accidents (MVAs), and/or gunshot wounds (Summerall, 2017). Though the cause of most TBIs suggests severe bodily harm, the majority of Service members who qualify for a TBI diagnosis appear healthy to the outsider's eye—i.e., with no physical wounds or obvious cognitive deficits (Jordan, 2011). Additionally, many symptoms of TBI—including irritability, anger/outbursts, trouble concentrating, fatigue, hyperarousal, insomnia, difficulty with balance or mobility, general feelings of anxiety, and depression (Morissette et al., 2011; Stein & McAllister, 2009)—overlap with other frequently occurring diagnoses such as PTSD, major depressive disorder, and generalized anxiety disorder (American Psychiatric Association, 2013). These similarities can easily lead to misdiagnoses that leave the TBI untreated. Providers must thereby be diligent in utilizing all axioms of care in order to ensure accurate identification and quality treatment. Examples of such should include involving the patient's family members during assessment phases of care; after all, many patients who have a TBI are not aware of recent changes in personality and neurological impairments that those close to said patients can more readily see (Jordan, 2011).

Collaboration with healthcare personnel (e.g., neurologists, primary care physicians, and polytrauma care teams) is an especially important skill set for MedFTs in the case of TBI, particularly because the timeline for assessment, diagnosis, and indicated care for TBIs is an essential ingredient toward the healthiest outcomes for Service members or veterans (Summerall, 2017). According to research, untreated TBI can lead to seizures, infections, pneumonia, olfactory impairment, perilous falls, and significant neurodegeneration. These sequelae can result in impairment to executive functioning, memory loss, and continued behavioral changes (CDC, 2017; McKee & Robinson, 2014; Ruff, Riechers, Wang, Piero, & Smith-Ruff, 2012). Providing systemic therapy and BPSS treatment to patients and their families is paramount. In particular, reframing symptoms as a neurological condition, rather than a temporary shift in mood or an adverse reaction to current relationship dynamics, provides an opportunity for spouses and families to view TBI as a diagnosis which they can face together—rather than a demon of sorts that pulls them apart (Greenman & Johnson, 2012; Johnson, 2005; Jordan, 2011).

Sexual Health

Sexual health refers to both positive and negative experiences around sexuality, including foci related to overall reproductive health. Sexual health is important to understand in the military community, because military-specific factors are readily able to impact it. For example, researchers have found that Service members who had experienced military sexual trauma (MST) reported higher rates of sexually transmitted diseases and sexually transmitted infections compared to those who had not experienced MST (Turchik et al. 2012). Also, although there is a lack of research on the sexual health of lesbian, gay, and bisexual military members, some evidence exists that demonstrates how military members who were unable to share their sexual identity at work experienced greater symptoms of depression and PTSD (Cochran. Balsam, Flentje, Malte, & Simpson, 2013) and increased suicidal ideation compared to heterosexual counterparts (Blosnich, Bossarte, & Silenzio, 2012). Good sexual health is associated with good mental health and good well-being in general. Thus, in order to promote good sexual health, MedFTs working in military contexts should use assessments that include questions about sexual orientation; gender identity; role of physical, emotional, and sexual safety in intimate relationships (including an understanding of the presence/use of pornography); and healthy sexual practices (Kauth, Meier, & Latini, 2014). MedFTs can play a role in assessing for sexual health practices and address health disparities; this is important because only 57.6% of primary care providers feel confident in addressing and treating patients' concerns about sexual health (Wittenberg & Gerber, 2009). MedFTs should acquire training in relation to sexual health, sexual pathology, and intimacy across casual and committed relationships in order to adequately and accurately address these issues with military members, veterans, dependents, and healthcare collaborators. This knowledge will also assist in reducing common disparities that exist as Service members become veteran patients in VA clinics and community health systems.

Suicide

Suicide remains a major concern for our military community (Lineberry & O'Connor, 2012). According to the Armed Forces Medical Examiner System, there were 438 suicide deaths from active, reserves, and guard components in 2014 (Pruitt et al., 2014). When taking a closer look at those who took their own lives, most were non-Hispanic white males under 30 years of age and of enlisted rank (E1–E9; Pruitt et al., 2014). MedFTs working in military and veteran healthcare contexts must be aware of the risk factors associated with suicide and use their systemic skills and training when assessing for it. This is especially important for relationally trained providers, insofar as 42% of suicide deaths and 42.9% of suicide attempts involved "failed relationships" within 3 months of the attempt or death (Pruitt et al., 2014). MedFTs are in a unique position to intervene with Service members and veterans at risk for suicide, especially in light of the influence(s) that relationships have on individuals contemplating or completing a suicide.

MedFTs should also expand their knowledge and training beyond what they know about suicide among civilian populations because military-specific factors, such as deployments and combat exposure, may also contribute to risk. For example, over half of Service members who had completed suicide in 2014 had experienced at least one deployment (Pruitt et al., 2014). LeardMann et al. (2013) found that untreated mental illness (mood disorders) and substance abuse disorders were considerable risk factors for current and former military members who had completed suicide. This finding, coupled with results from a review conducted by Harmon, Cooper, Nugent, and Butcher (2016), suggested that 33% of military members who had completed a suicide had not come in contact with a behavioral health provider after being deployed. This outcome signals that MedFTs must be proficient in assessing for suicidal ideations even in sessions wherein the presenting concern is more benign or biological/physical in nature. Furthermore, MedFTs must be prepared to extend research-informed interventions (such as those described later in this chapter) and collaborate with larger systems to reach beyond the therapy room. They must recognize when commanders, unit leaders, chaplains, family members, healthcare providers, and community members can be helpful in the care of patients who are struggling.

Military and Veteran Health Across the MedFT Healthcare Continuum

Whatever their level of involvement in the military and veteran community, all MedFTs who encounter Service members or veterans and their families must have a basic understanding of military culture. Further, MedFTs must familiarize themselves with an entire subculture of American society that is steeped in hierarchy, social class division, heroic morals and values, unique bonds of brotherhood and sisterhood, and constantly changing family roles and dynamics. Because of this, MedFTs working in the military community should approach learning military culture as they would approach learning about any other foreign culture—i.e., by seeking to understand social norms, cultural quirks, and, to some extent, a new language.

Additionally, MedFTs working in the military community must understand trauma and the effects that it has on all BPSS domains. While different levels of MedFTs will have varying experience and knowledge about trauma treatment, all MedFTs working with the military should able to identify symptoms of PTSD and be familiar enough with PTSD and trauma-based care modalities so that they can provide informed referrals. This same level of understanding should also apply to TBI and substance use disorders. With that said, the levels described in Hodgson, Lamson, Mendenhall, and Tyndall's (2014) MedFT Healthcare Continuum serve to illustrate a range of knowledge and skills for providers; see Tables 18.1 and 18.2.

MedFTs working at *Level 1* are typically clinicians positioned in a private practice or agency unaffiliated with military organizations and installations. MedFTs working at this level should have a basic understanding of military culture, the effects of deployment on family relationships, and stressors associated with combat and military service. *Level 1* MedFTs should also be able to diagnose PTSD and identify possible signs of TBI. Although MedFTs working at *Level 1* may not have the expertise to treat PTSD (and certainly not TBI), they should be familiar with local resources that offer research-informed or evidence-based care in order to make appropriate referrals and treatment recommendations. *Level 1* MedFTs should also be able to use the BPSS model in order to provide education about, and normalize the effects of, deployment, combat, and reintegration back into civilian life and the impact(s) that each has on family and couple dynamics.

MedFTs functioning at *Level 2* should be further able to advance, collaborate, and/or coordinate treatment with other clinicians, healthcare professionals, and military family support and relief organizations (like those described in the second and third cases of our vignette above) in order to ensure that both the patient and/or partner are receiving quality care.

MedFTs functioning at *Levels 3* and *4* of the healthcare continuum will likely be working on a military installation or for a military/veteran organization. They are more apt to interact with active duty Service members and/or veterans and their families on a regular basis. Performance at these levels will require MedFTs to have full knowledge of military rank and command structures, as well as special populations such as SEALS, Green Berets, and rangers. MedFTs will need to be prepared to collaborate with a Service member's chaplain, chain of command, and possibly the mental health unit at the military hospital (as was the case described in the first couple in our vignette). As chaplains, chain of commands, and military hospital mental health are all held to different levels of confidentiality (chaplains are the only providers with absolute confidentiality), MedFTs need to be knowledgeable of their clinic's, hospital's, or organization's policies surrounding release of information sequences. They must be prepared to advocate and coordinate services for their patients when their commanders are hesitant to allow participation in care.

Table 18.1 MedFTs in Military and Veteran Health Systems: Basic Knowledge and Skills

MedFT Healthcare Continuum Level	Level 1	Level 2	Level 3
Knowledge	Basic understanding of military culture to include the effects of deployment on family relationships and stressors associated with combat and military service. Familiar with interventions used to provide relief to individuals, families, and couples struggling with varying levels of multisystemic stress. Familiar with resources that offer TBI and PTSD treatment.	Familiar with the benefits of ongoing couple and family therapy in conjunction with individual trauma treatment. Ability to differentiate between depression and anxiety symptoms from those of PTSD and TBI.	In-depth understanding of military culture and military installation policies and procedures. Understanding of limits of confidentiality and policies surrounding release of information when collaborating with other providers. Basic understanding of treatment options for PTSD, TBI, and substance use for active duty military. Basic understanding of different medication and physical therapy options available for patients who have experienced trauma.
Skills	Ability to diagnose PTSD and refer patients to appropriate resources. Ability to identify possible signs of TBI and refer patients to treatment resources. Can use BPSS model to provide education on, and normalize the effects of, deployment, combat, and reintegration back into civilian life. Minimal collaboration with other providers and resources located on military installations.	Ability to collaborate with resources within both the civilian and military community in order to ensure both veterans and their families are taken care of in the event of veteran admission to an inpatient facility or the family's relocation to another duty station. Knowledgeable about how to apply systemic interventions in practice but does it occasionally; capable of assessing patients BPSS and invite support system members to be present for background health issues such as family history and risk-related factors, as well as treatment planning.	Can discuss treatment options with patients and their families as well as patient's chain of command. Frequently collaborates with healthcare professionals for purposes of medication management. Skilled with standardized measures to track patients' individual and relational strengths and challenges (e.g., depression, PTSD, anxiety, pain, social support).

Table 18.2 MedFTs in Military and Veteran Health Systems: Advanced Knowledge and Skills

MedFT Healthcare Continuum Level	Level 4	Level 5
Knowledge	Understands the different levels of trauma and types of trauma as well as different trauma diagnoses. Is aware of different mental health clinics, treatment groups, and education programs that are available on the military installation for Service members and their families or in the community for veterans. Knowledgeable about benefits and risks of associated treatments for multiple complex conditions (e.g., pain, PTSD, TBI, musculoskeletal injuries, depression, anxiety). Understands how to collaborate with other disciplines to implement evidence-based BPSS and family therapy protocols in traditional and integrated behavioral healthcare military and veteran health contexts.	Understands and educates others about treatment and care sequences for unique and/or challenging topics in military and veteran healthcare practice (e.g., pain management, comorbidities); can consult proficiently with professionals about BPSS topics from other fields. Proficient understanding in policies, procedures, and available treatment options for veteran, retired, and active duty Service members. Has an understanding of the physical and neurobiological changes that can occur after experiencing combat, sexual assault, and other traumatic events. Knowledgeable about BPSS research designs and execution, policies, and advocacy needs as relevant to military and veteran care. Proficient in developing a curriculum on integrated behavioral healthcare, BPSS applications, MedFT, etc. to behavioral health and other health professionals employed in a military or veteran healthcare setting. Understands leadership and supervision strategies for building integrated behavioral healthcare teams in a military or veteran healthcare setting.

(continued)

Table 18.2 (continued)

MedFT Healthcare Continuum Level	Level 4	Level 5
Skills	Able to deliver seminars and workshops about the BPSS complexities of a variety of commonly reported diagnoses injuries to a variety of professional types (e.g., behavioral health, biomedical). Can apply several BPSS interventions in care (including most types of brief interventions); can administer mood- and disease-specific assessment tools as the military and veteran health context requires. Can independently and collaboratively construct research and program evaluation studies that study the impact of BPSS interventions with a variety of diagnoses and patient/family units of care. Ability to advocate for treatment for active duty Service members in seeking research-informed treatment. Ability to provide continuity of care for Service members and their families who have experienced trauma until specialized trauma treatment becomes available.	Certified in at least one trauma-focused intervention (e.g., EMDR, CPT, PE). Ability to advocate for BPSS treatment plans in context of the level of collaboration existing among mental and physical health specialists. Ability to provide research-informed relational practices in integrated mental healthcare in both primary care and traditional therapy settings for military and veteran couple and family systems. Leads, supervises, and/or studies success of the implementation and dissemination of BPSS curriculum on integrated behavioral healthcare, BPSS applications, MedFT, etc. for military and/or veteran healthcare contexts. Routinely engages as an administrator/leader and supervisor in a team-based approach to inpatient and/or outpatient care, with consistent communication through electronic health records, patient introductions, curbside consultations, and team meetings and visits. Works proficiently as a MedFT and collaborates with other providers from a variety of disciples.

Additionally, clinicians operating at *Levels 3* and *4* should be familiar with the symptoms of PTSD, TBI, and substance use, as well as an understanding of the needs of amputees and burn survivors—alongside organizations and specialty clinics and services within the military installation and VA system that exist to treat these conditions. It is also at these levels that MedFTs may need to be well versed in research-informed or evidence-based methods of trauma treatment so that they are able to provide interim care to Service members (most active duty trauma treatment programs lack immediate availability for Service members' entry).

MedFTs functioning at the highest level of the healthcare continuum, *Level 5*, will typically be working in a military hospital, VA facility, or MHS/VA clinic.

They will usually function, too, in the capacity of an integrated behavioral healthcare clinician, care coordinator/case manager, supervisor, and/or director. MedFTs at *Level 5* should have an in-depth understanding about military culture and should be able to confidently collaborate and coordinate care with veteran organizations, healthcare staff and trauma treatment teams, spiritual leaders, military commands, and veteran and active duty case managers. These MedFTs should understand the changes in biology, neurobiology, psychology, and behavior that occur after a TBI, combat deployment, sexual assault, or traumatic combat experience—and should thereby be prepared to educate Service members and their families about these effects. MedFTs should also be trained and certified in at least one research-informed trauma intervention—e.g., eye movement desensitization and reprocessing (EMDR; Shapiro, 1989), cognitive processing therapy (CPT; Resick et al., 2008), and prolonged exposure therapy (Foa, Rothbaum, & Hembree, 2007)—and be able to coordinate care with psychiatrists, neurologists, physical therapists, and other marriage and family therapists in order to ensure the best possible care is advanced. Further, *Level 5* MedFTs should be able to advocate for BPSS-based treatment plans for veterans and their families, even if integrated behavioral healthcare policies and treatment teams do not yet exist in the facility in which the MedFT functions. MedFTs working at this level of care must also be prepared to face challenges related to the bureaucracy and policy restrictions that come with military and veteran healthcare and health systems and be willing to use innovation and creativity vis-à-vis these restrictions so as to ensure that patients receive high-quality care.

Research-Informed Practices

For military and veteran populations, MedFT services that are brief and integrated into healthcare contexts may be critical in reducing barriers to treatment and receiving mental healthcare in tandem with acute and complex physical health concerns (Zinzow, Britt, McFadden, Burnette, & Gillispie, 2012). MedFTs' systemic and BPSS perspectives make them ideal collaborators for addressing common concerns experienced by military Service members and veterans (e.g., depression, anxiety, trauma, substance abuse). While there is extensive research on evidence-based practices for working with the military and veteran populations in traditional care settings, some of these treatments have only begun to be adapted for integrated behavioral healthcare models. The DoD (2014b) recently released guidelines for behavioral health interventions in primary care; these include recommendations for four or fewer sessions with appointment durations of 15 to 30 minutes. Fortunately, MedFTs are trained to offer both traditional and IBHC sessions that span from 15 to 30 minutes for brief encounters and up to 50 minutes for traditional encounters. While MedFTs are commonly trained first as family therapists, all are well trained in extending BPSS and relational care to individuals, couples, families, and other communities of interest.

Individual Approaches

When serving any context, MedFTs should be cognizant of their patients' culture(s). As stigma regarding mental health issues is often cited as a barrier in treatment engagement (e.g., Zinzow et al., 2012), some researchers recommend avoiding terms such as "patient," "PTSD," "therapy," and "treatment" (Steenkamp et al., 2017). Due to the prevalence of such stigma among military and veteran populations, some programs have implemented universal screenings for depression and PTSD in primary care as part of standard of care (Engel et al., 2008) and resiliency staff. The prevailing evidence-based treatments for PTSD include prolonged exposure therapy (PE; Foa et al., 2007), CPT (Resick et al., 2008), and EMDR (Van der Kolk, et al., 2007). Core elements of these treatments (and others) have been adapted for brief, integrated delivery formats. Cigrang et al. (2011) utilized PE, combined with aspects of CPT, to treat PTSD in a brief, four-session format. Their intervention included homework via a workbook format, in which patients wrote their trauma narratives and self-monitored their emotional responses. Throughout treatment, the clinician served as a collaborator and assisted patients with implementation. Glover et al. (2016) applied focused acceptance and commitment therapy (FACT; Strosahl, Robinson, & Gustavsson, 2012), an abbreviated version of acceptance and commitment therapy (ACT; Hayes, Strosahl, & Wilson, 1999, 2011), to create a four-session group at the VA. This intervention, which included mindfulness and cognitive exercises, was effective in the reduction of depression, anxiety, and stress. Further, cognitive behavioral therapy (CBT) techniques have demonstrated effectiveness for the treatment of insomnia in primary care (Edinger & Sampson, 2003; Edinger et al., 2009).

While some brief interventions may have the primary goal of symptom reduction, others—such as Steenkamp et al. (2017)—aim to "plant seeds" for new, more adaptive ways of coping with trauma. Their exposure-based treatment for active duty Service members with PTSD combined elements of PE, CPT, CBT, EMDR, as well as Gestalt therapy (Perls, Hefferline, & Goodman, 1957), through imaginal exposure, interpersonal sharing, increasing Service members' awareness of personal meaning-making regarding traumatic events, and a modified empty chair technique. In particular, the modified empty chair technique was used to address concerns related to moral injury. Other brief interventions with demonstrated efficacy in treating PTSD and common comorbid concerns include behavioral activation, relaxation techniques, written exercises, and creating impact statements (e.g., Corso et al., 2009).

Brief interventions may have long-term effects for Service members and veterans. In an outcome study in a primary care setting that served military Service members, veterans, and their families, Ray-Sannerud et al. (2012) found that patients improved over the course of treatment and that these improvements were maintained 2 years posttreatment. Common presenting concerns included insomnia, depression, stress/anxiety, and panic, with interventions including psychoeducation, mindfulness training, diaphragmatic breathing, and behavioral activation. While

MedFTs should be adept at implementing individual BPSS psychotherapy approaches, they are also uniquely positioned to promote relational change.

Couple and Family Approaches

In recent years, numerous programs have been implemented to support the relational health of Service members and veterans. However, many of these programs are in the form of traditional therapy or weekend retreats. Recently, Cigrang et al. (2016) adapted the Marriage Checkup (MC; Cordova, 2009) for primary care, which MedFTs may find helpful in their service delivery. The adapted MC takes place over the course of three 30-minute sessions, with the goals of prevention, detection, and early intervention of relational health concerns to promote long-term marital health. This brief intervention encompasses a relationship history interview, the assessment of relational strengths and concerns, and motivational feedback with specific therapeutic techniques consisting of uncovering "soft" emotions (e.g., sadness, loneliness), discovering understandable reasons, and identifying patterns and themes. While brief couples interventions are relatively new in this context, military and veteran couples have additional resources available to them (Lewis, Lamson, & Lesueur, 2012).

The Strength at Home Couples program is a CBT-informed, 10-week couples group for the prevention of IPV among veteran and Service member couples (Taft et al., 2016). This intervention includes psychoeducation, strategies to improve emotional expression, and skill building in conflict management, assertiveness, listening, and communication. While this program does not punctuate BPSS health per se, MedFTs who deliver such programs must be proficient at knowing signs of PTSD and TBI, among other diagnoses, that could influence the physical or psychosocial dynamics of couples. Having a MedFT skill set can allow the MedFT to access knowledge beyond what may be provided in the intervention manual; it can assist in knowing when an intervention should be concluded in order to turn to more serious physical or psychosocial concerns.

Army couples have the opportunity to participate in weekend retreat-style programs such as PREP (Prevention and Relationship Education Program) for Strong Bonds (Allen, Rhoades, Markman, & Stanley, 2015). These programs are typically facilitated by Army chaplains. Aspects of this 14+ hour intervention include communication skills, emotion regulation, relaxation, core beliefs, and forgiveness. The Navy also offers a couple's retreat, CREDO (Chaplain Religious Enrichment Development Operation (Department of the Navy, 2017)). These retreats have demonstrated effectiveness in reducing divorce and breakup rates for minority couples, couples experiencing financial strain, and precommitment cohabiting couples. MedFTs are commonly great leaders or coleaders for programs such as these, because of their training with and awareness for diverse social locations (i.e., factors that are influential in significant findings from this program).

For many couples, outcomes from relational (Baptist & Nelson Goff, 2012) and BPSS assessments may become influential in the interventions they receive and may open the door for more targeted treatments if indicated. Relational-focused assessment and treatment, particularly in primary care contexts, have important implications for Service members' readiness. Trump, Lamson, Lewis, and Muse (2015) highlighted the interplay between partners' physical health (e.g., pain), mental health (e.g., depression), and marital satisfaction, underscoring the importance of BPSS assessments as a part of IBHC couples' treatment in primary care and other health-related contexts (e.g., the Army Child and Family Services). Some of the most common challenges cited by other authors and tied to education or intervention with military and veteran populations include amputations, TBI, insomnia, chronic pain, IPV, MST, substance use, and relational distress (Blaisure, Saathoff-Wells, Pereira, MacDermid-Wadsworth, & Dombro, 2016; Goff, Crow, Reisbig, & Hamilton, 2007; Mansfield, Kaufman, Marshall, Gaynes, Morrissey, & Engel, 2010; Trump, Lamson, Lewis & Muse, 2015).

Only minimal research exists about the BPSS needs of dual military couples (Lacks, Lamson, Lewis, White, & Russoniello, 2015) and LGB military and veteran couples (Johnston, Webb-Murphy, & Bhakta, 2016). More interventions must thereby be developed, implemented, and evaluated for these couples. For more information about interventions that have been tested with military or veteran dyads, see Lewis, Lamson, and White (2016).

For military and veteran families with children, interventions that attend to BPSS and relational needs of both the caregiver/parent/guardian and child are important (Chandra et al., 2010). Many family therapy interventions have emerged over the past decade for military and veteran families. These interventions commonly consist of psychoeducation, self-monitoring, relaxation training, and altering maladaptive beliefs (Friedberg & Brelsford, 2011; Kortla & Dyer, 2008; Murphy & Fairbank, 2013). Given the volume of family-based programs that may be available in military and veteran communities, MedFTs should take time to review systematic reviews and meta-analyses that offer a consolidated perspective on promising and research-informed interventions (Creech, Hadley, & Borsari, 2014). Below are examples of some of the promising interventions delivered to military and veteran families with children and adolescents.

FOCUS (Families OverComing Under Stress; Beardslee et al., 2011) is a program that is theoretically grounded in individual and family resilience and has received national recognition for its success. It is an eight-session resiliency training program for military children and families that aims to improve emotion regulation, honor family members' multiple perspectives on deployment, enhance family strengths and coping skills, engage community supports and services, create a family narrative about the deployment experience, strengthen parental leadership, and advance collaborative problem solving and goal setting. MedFTs would serve as an asset to a FOCUS team, given their training in parent psychological health, child behavioral health, and family functioning.

For reserve component and National Guard families, the After Deployment Adaptive Parenting Tools Program (Gewirtz, Erbes, Polusny, Forgatch, & DeGarmo, 2011; ADAPT), an extension of Parent Management Training-Oregon (Forgatch & Martinez, 1999; PMTO), may be useful. In this 14-week multifamily sessions program, parents learn emotion regulation and parenting skills with a focus on deployment-related issues through role-plays and group discussions. Again, MedFTs' prevention and intervention skills in relational health would offer a strong contribution to any ADAPT team.

Passport to Success (Wilson, Wilkum, Chernichky, MacDermid-Wadsworth, & Broniarczyk, 2011) is a research-informed program that was constructed for adolescent dependents of reservists. The program was developed as part of the Department of Defense's Yellow Ribbon Program. MedFTs who collaborate with program leaders would assist in focusing on challenges associated with PTS that exist with parents or are intergenerationally transmitted. While many other family-based programs have been developed over the years for these populations, MedFTs must become good consumers of research in order to recognize what is best indicated for the social locations of the potential participants.

Community Approaches

Limited outcome research exists regarding interventions for community-dwelling members of the military and veteran populations (Murphy & Fairbank, 2013). Vet centers are located throughout the country and may assist veterans and their families with mental health needs. Standard group psychotherapy for PTSD at vet centers is emotion focused and centered on the impact of symptoms on current functioning; group member input, feedback, and disclosures are also encouraged (Daniels, Boehnlein, & McCallion, 2015). While this approach produces some benefits, the inclusion of a "life-review" component was found to significantly improve PTSD symptoms in a small sample of older veterans (Daniels et al., 2015). For the structured life-review component, MedFTs should collaborate with group members on best ways to share content associated with premilitary history, military/war zone history, and post-military history.

More recently, researchers have initiated interventions for the partners of Service members. HomeFront Strong (Kees & Rosenblum, 2015) is an 8-week community-based group intervention for military spouses that emphasizes self-care, building community, stress management, re-authoring narratives, allowing emotions, and building positive coping skills. Though the sample size in this initial pilot study was small, spouses reported reductions in stress and anxiety, but not depression, as well as increases in life satisfaction and engagement. Research on interventions for community-dwelling children is very limited, but it is notable that nonmilitary providers deliver physical and mental healthcare to more than 50% of military children (particularly those of activated Service members in the National Guard and Reserve; Gorman, Eide, & Hisle-Gorman, 2010). For this reason, even if a MedFT is not working in a context that primarily serves Service members, veterans, or their families, MedFTs should strive to be military informed. Military-informed MedFTs should consistently ask patients: "Have you or a member of your family ever served in the military?" (Brown, 2012; Murphy & Fairbanks, 2013; Siegel, Davis, & the Committee on Psychosocial Aspects of Child and Family Health and Section on Uniformed Services, 2013).

Veterans may also benefit in peer-to-peer models of care. Matthias et al. (2015) found that veterans with chronic pain reported reduced pain severity and interference after receiving phone and/or in-person meetings at least twice per month with a trained "peer coach." Coaches are trained in areas such as communication, cultural competence, crisis management, and motivational strategies, alongside basics of chronic pain, relaxation, self-care, cognitive behavioral skills, and interpersonal functioning. In a study of peer-led pain self-management groups, Baur et al. (2016) recommended that peers focus on goal setting, and how to make goals measurable, when working with veterans. It is important that MedFTs be aware of such programs in the community given that "experience with mental health" and "barriers to treatment" were two concerns that National Guard soldiers mentioned would be harder to discuss with a peer (Pfeiffer et al., 2012).

Research has also shown that peer-to-peer models in military and veteran healthcare increase utilization of psychotherapy services and reduce dropout. Goetter et al. (2017) found that after trained non-clinician veterans performed a telephone check-in with prospective veteran patients (1 week after a clinical evaluation and 1 month after the initial session), patients were likely to attend more psychotherapy sessions and had lower dropout rates than those who had received only one or zero check-ins.

Another peer-to-peer network that should include MedFTs is one that targets healthcare provider burnout and vicarious traumatization, which is a common concern for those who provide care to military and veteran populations. Among behavioral health providers serving Operation Enduring Freedom (OEF) and/or Operation Iraqi Freedom (OIF) veterans, researchers found that the more confidants a provider had at work, the lower the burnout rates (Ballenger-Browning et al., 2011). MedFTs are commonly trained in how to maintain awareness of their own self-of-the-therapist needs and can raise that awareness further through initiatives that focus on provider to provider well-being. MedFTs must recognize their own risks for burnout, as well as the risks for providers on the care team. Given MedFTs' training in larger systems, an (additional) important role awaits them in improving provider/staff quality of life. Initiatives that address prevention of or solutions to burnout can increase the wellness of the integrated behavioral healthcare team, both personally and professionally (Ballenger-Browning, Schmitz, Rothacker, Hammer, Webb-Murphy, & Johnson, 2011).

Conclusion

The Department of Defense is the largest employer in the United States, and it is clear that this workforce and its retirees be a prime focus for MedFT practice, research, training, and advocacy. BPSS conditions experienced by civilians may be more acute and/or complicated in the military by nature of the variety of job duties, risks, and social locations associated with active duty or veteran patients. MedFTs must be on the front lines of creating and implementing research-informed interventions that can maximize relational and BPSS health for diverse military personnel and veterans, alongside their dependents and communities. Furthermore, MedFTs can strengthen the well-being of the provider workforce and sustainability of the integrated behavioral healthcare team by using their systemic lenses to identify risks to productivity (e.g., burnout) and then offering strength-based solutions that promote workforce success.

Reflection Questions
1. What are some of the BPSS factors that must be taken into consideration when assessing, diagnosing, or treating a military or veteran individual, couple, or family that may be different from civilian counterparts?
2. What are some of the research-informed practices that MedFTs may use to improve mental health symptoms when working with military or veteran couples and families facing challenges after a combat injury?
3. What programs could be implemented by a MedFT in a military or veteran healthcare context, or in the community, that could help to reduce military or veteran health disparities?

Glossary of Important Terms in Military and Veteran Health Systems

AD Active duty; refers to Service members who serve full time in the armed forces.
ADAPT Air Force Alcohol and Drug Abuse Prevention and Treatment Program.
AMEDD Army Medical Department of the United States of America; refers to the Army's healthcare organization.
ASAP Army Substance Abuse Program; the anti-substance abuse program in the U.S. Army.
BHIP Behavioral Health Integration Program; the U.S. Navy's model for embedding behavioral health providers into primary care settings.
BHOP Behavioral Health Optimization Program; the U.S. Air Force's model for embedding behavioral health providers into primary care settings.
BUMED Bureau of Medicine and Surgery; the organization that manages healthcare services for the U.S. Navy and U.S. Marine Corps.

CAC Common Access Card; the standard identification for active duty personnel, selected reserve, DoD civilian employees, and eligible contractor personnel. It also allows the card holder to have access to buildings, controlled areas, and DoD computer systems.

CAF Comprehensive Airman Fitness; refers to the well-being of Airmen from a four-pillar approach (mental, physical, social, and spiritual).

CBOC Community-based outpatient clinics; created by the VA to expand healthcare services to veterans in rural areas and/or those without access to the larger VA medical centers.

CHAMPVA Civilian Health and Medical Program of the Department of Veterans Affairs; refers to a health benefits program.

CSF2 Army's Comprehensive Soldier and Family Fitness; uses five areas (physical, social, family, spiritual, and emotional) to promote resiliency and performance enhancement in soldiers, their families, and civilians.

DEERS Defense Enrollment Eligibility Reporting System; the database of military members and their beneficiaries to receive TRICARE benefits.

Deployment A long-term assignment, often situated in a combat zone.

DoD Department of Defense; a branch of the federal government that oversees national security and the U.S. Armed Forces.

EBHP Embedded behavioral healthcare providers; professionals who work in units to help in preventing behavioral health issues from becoming a serious issue for the Service member or unit. They tend to teach classes on behavioral health and coordinate referrals to those who have a need for specialty services.

Fleet and Family Support Services The Navy's Family Readiness programs that include services for work and family life, counseling, advocacy, and prevention, as well as sexual assault prevention programs.

IDES Integrated Disability Evaluation System; a joint process between the Department of Defense (DoD) and Department of Veterans Affairs (VA) to determine if a Service members have sustained wounds that may prevent them from performing their duties and their ability to continuing serving in the armed forces.

Installation Generic term used for a military facility (e.g., base, camp, post, fort, or station).

MEB Medical Evaluation Board; recommends whether a Service member's medical condition prevents him/her from performing assigned work duties.

MHS Military Health System; the organization within the DoD that provides healthcare to active duty and retired military personnel and their dependents.

MOS Military occupational specialty; code used to identify a specific job in the military.

MST Military sexual trauma; refers to sexual assault or repeated harassment that occurs during military service.

MTF Military treatment facilities; military hospitals and clinics at military installations around the world.

OEF Operation Enduring Freedom; began in 2001 when the U.S. military deployed to Afghanistan to combat terrorism. The conflict ended in 2014.

OIF Operation Iraqi Freedom; began in 2003 when the U.S. military deployed to Iraq. The initiative ended in 2011.
PCS Permanent change of station; the mandatory relocation of an active duty service member to a different duty location.
PDHRA Post-Deployment Health Reassessment; a comprehensive health screening that examines physical and behavioral health concerns associated with deployment, 3 to 6 months after return from deployment.
PEB Physical Evaluation Board; reviews the findings from the MEB to determine the Service member's ability to perform his/her work duties.
PHA Periodic Health Assessment; an annual health screen to evaluate medical readiness.
Profile An official document that prohibits a Service member from certain types of military duty due to injury or disability; can be temporary or permanent.
SARP Substance Abuse Rehabilitation Program; the anti-substance abuse program for all active duty members.
SCMH Army Soldier Centered Medical Home; the U.S. Army's version of the patient-centered medical home (PCMH).
TDY Temporary duty assignment; refers to a travel assignment to a location other than the permanent duty station.
Transitioning The readjustment period of transitioning from military back into civilian life; also known as "reintegration."
Veteran Someone who has served in the military.
VA Veterans Administration.
VHA Veterans Health Administration.

Additional Resources

Literature

Anderson, W. (2015). *Battlefield doc: Memoirs of a Korean war combat medic*. St. Louis, MO: Moonbridge Publications.
Benimoff, R. (2010). *Faith under fire: An Army chaplain's memoir*. New York, NY: Three Rivers Press.
Hegar, M. (2017). *Shoot like a girl*. New York, NY: Berkley.
Johnson, S. (2005). *Emotion focused couples therapy with trauma survivors: Strengthen in attachment bonds*. New York, NY: Guilford Press.
Junger, S. (2010). *War*. New York, NY: Grand Central Publishing.
Junger, S. (2016). *Tribe*. New York, NY: Grand Central Publishing.
Klay, P. (2014). *Redeployment*. New York, NY: Penguin Books.
Van Der Kolk, B. (2015). *The body keeps the score: Brain, mind, and body in the healing of trauma*. New York, NY: Penguin Books.

Measurements/Questionnaires

Alcohol Use Disorders Identification Test (AUDIT). http://www.integration.samhsa.gov/AUDIT_screener_for_alcohol.pdf
CAGE Alcohol Questionnaire. http://www.integration.samhsa.gov/images/res/CAGEAID.pdf
Clinician-Administered PTSD Scale for DSM-5 (CAPS-5). http://www.ptsd.va.gov/professional/assessment/adult-int/caps.asp
Generalized Anxiety Disorder. http://www.integration.samhsa.gov/clinical-practice/GAD708.19.08Cartwright.pdf
Patient Health Questionnaire (PHQ-9). http://www.integration.samhsa.gov/images/res/PHQ%20-%20Questions.pdf
Sexual Harassment Scale. http://www.ptsd.va.gov/professional/assessment/deployment/sexual-harassment.asp
Suicide Risk: Columbia-Suicide Severity Rating Scale (C-SSRS). http://cssrs.columbia.edu/the-columbia-scale-c-ssrs/about-the-scale/, http://www.integration.samhsa.gov/clinical-practice/Columbia_Suicide_Severity_Rating_Scale.pdf

Organizations/Associations

After Deployment. http://afterdeployment.dcoe.mil/
Center for Deployment Psychology. http://deploymentpsych.org/
Department of Defense. https://www.defense.gov/
Family Advocacy Program. http://www.militaryonesource.mil/phases-military-leadership?content_id=266712
Military Family Research Institute. https://www.mfri.purdue.edu/
Military OneSource. http://www.militaryonesource.mil/
National Center for PTSD. http://www.ptsd.va.gov/
National Child Traumatic Stress Network. http://www.nctsn.org/
National Military Family Association. http://www.militaryfamily.org/
SAMHSA Military Families. http://www.samhsa.gov/MilitaryFamilies/
Veterans Affairs. https://va.gov/

References[1]

Allen, E. S., Rhoades, G. K., Markman, H. J., & Stanley, S. M. (2015). PREP for strong bonds: A review of outcomes from a randomized clinical trial. *Contemporary Family Therapy, 37*, 232–246. https://doi.org/10.1007/s10591-014-9325-3

---

[1] [Note: References that are prefaced with an asterisk are recommended readings.]

*Allen, E. S., Rhoades, G. K., Stanley, S. M., & Markman, H. J. (2010). Hitting home: Relationships between recent deployment, posttraumatic stress symptoms, and marital functioning for Army couples. *Journal of Family Psychology, 24*, 280–288. https://doi.org/10.1037/a0019405.

American Psychiatric Association. (2013). *Diagnostic and statistical manual of mental disorder* (5th ed.). Washington, DC: Author.

Anderson, K. L. (2002). Perpetrator or victim: Relationships between intimate partner violence and well-being. *Journal of Marriage and the Family, 64*, 851–863. https://doi.org/10.1111/j.1741-3737.2002.00851.x

*Anderson, W. (2015). *Battlefield doc: Memoirs of a Korean war combat medic.* St. Louis, MO: Moonbridge Publications.

Armed Forces Health Surveillance Branch. (2017a). Absolute and relative morbidity burdens attributable to various illnesses and injuries, active component, U.S. Armed Forces, 2016. *Medical Surveillance Monthly Report, 24.* Retrieved from https://www.health.mil/Military-Health-Topics/Health-Readiness/Armed-Forces-Health-Surveillance-Branch/Reports-and-Publications/Medical-Surveillance-Monthly-Report

Armed Forces Health Surveillance Branch. (2017b). Absolute and relative morbidity burdens attributable to various illnesses and injuries, non-service member beneficiaries of the Military Health System, 2016. *Medical Surveillance Monthly Report, 24.* Retrieved from https://www.health.mil/Military-Health-Topics/Health-Readiness/Armed-Forces-Health-Surveillance-Branch/Reports-and-Publications/Medical-Surveillance-Monthly-Report

Ballenger-Browning, K. K., Schmitz, K. J., Rothacker, J. A., Hammer, P. S., Webb-Murphy, J. A., & Johnson, D. C. (2011). Predictors of burnout among military mental health providers. *Military Medicine, 176*, 253–260. https://doi.org/10.7205/MILMED-D-10-00269

Baptist, J. A., & Nelson Goff, B. S. (2012). An examination of broaden-and-build model of positive emotions in military marriages: An actor-partner analysis. *Journal of Couple & Relationship Therapy, 11*, 205.220. https://doi.org/10.1080/15332691.2012.692942

Baur, S. M., McGuire, A. B., Kukla, M., McGuire, S., Bair, M. J., & Matthias, M. S. (2016). Veterans' pain management goals: Changes during the course of a peer-led pain self-management program. *Patient Education and Counseling, 99*, 2080–2086. https://doi.org/10.1016/j.pec.2016.07.034

Beardslee, W., Lester, P., Klosinski, L., Saltzman, W., Woodward, K., Nash, W., ... Leskin, G. (2011). Family-centered preventive intervention for military families: Implications for implementation science. *Prevention Science, 12*, 339–348. doi: https://doi.org/10.1007/s11121-011-0234-5.

*Benimoff, R. (2010). *Faith under fire: An Army chaplain's memoir.* New York, NY: Three Rivers Press.

Blaisure, K. R., Saathoff-Wells, T., Pereira, A., MacDermid-Wadsworth, S., & Dombro, A. L. (2016). *Serving military families* (2nd ed.). Florence, GA: Routledge.

Blosnich, J., Bossarte, R., & Silenzio, V. (2012). Suicidal ideation among sexual minority veterans: Results from the 2005–2010 Massachusetts Behavioral Risk Factor Surveillance Survey. *American Journal of Public Health, 102*, S44–S47. https://doi.org/10.2105/ajph.2011.300565

*Bohnert, K. M., Sripada, R. K., Mach, J., & McCarthy, J. F. (2016). Same-day integrated mental health care and PTSD diagnosis and treatment among VHA primary care patients with positive PTSD screens. *Psychiatric Services, 67*, 94–100. https://doi.org/10.1176/appi.ps.201500035.

Bostock, D. J., & Daley, J. G. (2007). Lifetime and current sexual assault and harassment victimization rates of active-duty United States Air Force women. *Violence Against Women, 13*, 927–944. https://doi.org/10.1177/1077801207305232

Bray, R. M., Pemberton, M. R., Lane, M. E., Hourani, L. L., Mattiko, M. J., & Babeu, L. A. (2010). Substance use and mental health trends among U.S. Military active duty personnel: Key findings from the 2008 DoD health behavior survey. *Military Medicine, 175*, 390–399. https://doi.org/10.7205/milmed-d-09-00132

Brooks, G. R. (2005). Counseling and psychotherapy for male military veterans. In G. E. Good and G. R. Brooks (Eds.), *The new handbook for psychotherapy and counseling with men:*

A comprehensive guide to settings, problems, and treatment approaches (pp. 206–225). San Francisco, CA: Jossey-Bass.

Brown, M. (2012). *Enlisting masculinity: The construction of gender in U.S. military recruiting advertising during the all-volunteer force*. New York, NY: Oxford University Press.

Campbell, S. B., & Renshaw, K. D. (2013). PTSD symptoms, disclosure, and relationship distress: Explorations of mediation and associations over time. *Journal of Anxiety Disorders, 27*, 494–502. https://doi.org/10.1016/j.janxdis.2013.06.007

Center for Disease Control. (2017). *TBI: Get the facts*. Retrieved from https://www.cdc.gov/traumaticbraininjury/get_the_facts.html

Chandra, A., Lara-Cinisomo, S., Jaycox, L. H., Tanielian, T., Burns, R. M., Ruder, T., & Han, B. (2010). Children on the homefront: The experience of children from military families. *Pediatrics, 125*, 16–25. https://doi.org/10.1542/peds.2009-1180

Cigrang, J. A., Cordova, J. V., Gray, T. D., Najera, E., Hawrilenko, M., Pinkley, C., ... Redd, K. (2016). The marriage checkup: Adapting and implementing a brief relationship intervention for military couples. *Cognitive and Behavioral Practice, 23*, 561–570. https://doi.org/10.1016/j.cbpra.2016.01.002.

Cigrang, J. A., Rauch, S. A. M., Avila, L. L., Bryan, C. J., Goodie, J. L., Hryshko-Mullen, A., ... STRONG STAR Consortium (2011). Treatment of active-duty military with PTSD in primary care: Early findings. Psychological Services, 8, 104–113. doi: https://doi.org/10.1037/a0022740.

Cochran, B. N., Balsam, K., Flentje, A., Malte, C. A., & Simpson, T. (2013). Mental health characteristics of sexual minority veterans. *Journal of Homosexuality, 60*, 419–435. https://doi.org/10.1080/00918369.2013.744932

Cordova, J. V. (2009). *The marriage checkup: A scientific program for sustaining and strengthening marital health*. New York, NY: Jason Aronson.

Corso, K. A., Bryan, C. J., Morrow, C. E., Kanzler Appolonio, K., Dodendorf, D. M., & Baker, M. T. (2009). Managing posttraumatic stress disorder symptoms in active-duty military personnel in primary care settings. *Journal of Mental Health Counseling, 31*, 119–137. 10.17744/mehc.31.2.1m2238t85rv38041

Creech, S. K., Hadley, W., & Borsari, B. (2014). The impact of military deployment and reintegration on children and parenting: A systematic review. *Professional Psychology: Research and Practice, 45*, 452–464. http://dx.doi.org/10.1037/a0035055

Daniels, L. R., Boehnlein, J., & McCallion, P. (2015). Aging, depression, and wisdom: A pilot study of life-review intervention and PTSD treatment with two groups of Vietnam veterans. *Journal of Gerontological Social Work, 58*, 420–436. https://doi.org/10.1080/01634372.2015.1013657

*Defense Centers of Excellence for Psychological Health and Traumatic Brain Injury. (2013). *Post-traumatic stress disorder pocket guide*. Retrieved from http://www.healthquality.va.gov/guidelines/MH/ptsd/PTSDPocketGuide23May2013v1.pdf

Defense Manpower Data Center. (2017). *DoD personnel workforce reports & publications*. Retrieved from https://www.dmdc.osd.mil/appj/dwp/dwp_reports.jsp

Department of Defense. (2015). *2015 demographics: Profile of the military community*. Retrieved from http://download.militaryonesource.mil/12038/MOS/Reports/2015-Demographics-Report.pdf

Department of Defense. (2014a). *Annual report to the congressional defense committee on the plans for the Department of Defense for the support of military family readiness: Fiscal year 2013*. Retrieved from http://download.militaryonesource.mil/12038/MOS/Reports/FY2013-Report-MilitaryFamilyReadinessPrograms.pdf

Department of Defense. (2014b). *Instruction*. Retrieved from http://www.dtic.mil/whs/directives/corres/pdf/649015p.pdf

Department of Defense. (2012). *2012 Demographics report: Profile of the military community*. Retrieved from http://military.sla.org/2012-demographics-report-profile-of-the-military-community/

Department of Defense Education Activity. (2017). *Enrollment data*. Retrieved from http://www.dodea.edu/datacenter/enrollment.cfm

Department of the Navy. (2017). *Chaplain religious enrichment development operation*. Retrieved from http://www.navy.mil/local/chaplaincorps/CREDO-Map.html

Deployment Information and Resources. (2010). *Deployment: An overview*. Retrieved from http://www.military.com/deployment

Edinger, J. D., Olsen, M. K., Stechuchak, K. M., Means, M. K., Lineberger, M. D., Kirby, A., & Carney, C. E. (2009). Cognitive behavioral therapy for patients with primary insomnia or insomnia associated predominantly with mixed psychiatric disorders: A randomized clinical trial. *Sleep, 32*, 499–510. https://doi.org/10.1093/sleep/32.4.499

Edinger, J. D., & Sampson, W. S. (2003). A primary care "friendly" cognitive behavioral insomnia therapy. *Sleep, 26*, 177–182. https://doi.org/10.1093/sleep/26.2.177

Engel, C. C., Oxman, T., Yamamoto, C., Gould, D., Barry, S., Stewart, P., ... Dietrich, A. J. (2008). RESPECT-MIL: Feasibility of a systems-level collaborative care approach to depression and post-traumatic stress disorder in military primary care. *Military Medicine, 173*, 935–940. https://doi.org/10.7205/MILMED.173.10.935.

Engel, G. L. (1980). The clinical application of the biopsychosocial model. *American Journal of Family Medicine, 137*, 535–544. https://doi.org/10.1176/ajp.137.5.535

Engel, G. L. (1977). The need for a new medical model: A challenge for biomedicine. *Science, 196*, 129–136. https://doi.org/10.1016/b978-0-409-95009-0.50006-1

Fischer, H. (2007). United States military casualty statistics: Operation Iraqi Freedom and Operation Enduring Freedom. *CRS Report for Congress*. Retrieved from https://contextualscience.org/publications/hayes_strosahl_wilson_1999

Foa, E. B., Rothbaum, B. A., & Hembree, E. A. (2007). *Prolonged exposure therapy for PTSD: Emotional processing of traumatic experiences: Therapist guide*. New York, NY: Oxford University Press.

Forgatch, M. S., & Martinez, C. R., Jr. (1999). Parent management training: A program linking basic research and practical application. *Parent Management Training, 36*, 923–937. Retrieved from https://www.researchgate.net/profile/Marion_Forgatch/publication/229633106_Parent_management_training_A_program_linking_basic_research_and_practical_application/links/0912f50104c96205fc000000/Parent-management-training-A-program-linking-basic-research-and-practical-application.pdf.

Forrest, M. S., & Shapiro, F. (1998). *EMDR: The breakthrough eye movement therapy for overcoming anxiety, stress, and trauma*. New York, NY: Basic Books.

Fox, J., & Pease, B. (2012). Military deployment, masculinity, and trauma: Reviewing the connections. *Journal of Men's Studies, 20*, 16–31. https://doi.org/10.3149/jms.2001.16

Friedberg, R. D., & Brelsford, G. M. (2011). Using cognitive behavioral interventions to help children cope with parental military deployment. *Journal of Contemporary Psychotherapy, 41*, 229–236. https://doi.org/10.1007/s10879-011-9175-3

Gates, G. J., & Herman, J. L. (2014). *Transgender military service in the United States*. Los Angeles, CA: Williams Institute/UCLA School of Law.

Gates, G. J., & Newport, F. (2012). *Special report: 3.4% of US adults identify as LGBT. Politics*. Retrieved from http://www.gallup.com/poll/158066/special-report-adults-identify-lgbt.aspx

Gewirtz, A. H., Erbes, C. R., Polusny, M. A., Forgatch, M. S., & DeGarmo, D. S. (2011). Helping military families through the deployment process: Strategies to support parenting. *Professional Psychology: Research and Practice, 42*, 56–62. https://doi.org/10.1037/a0022345

*Gierisch, J.M., Shapiro, A., Grant, N. N., King, H. A., McDuffie, J. R., & Williams Jr., J. W. (2013). *Intimate partner violence: Prevalence among U.S. military veterans and active duty service members and a review of intervention approaches*. Retrieved from http://www.hsrd.research.va.gov/publications/esp/partner_violence.cfm

Glover, N. G., Sylvers, P. D., Shearer, E. M., Kane, M.-K., Clasen, P. C., Epler, A. J., ... Jakupcak, M. (2016). The efficacy of focused acceptance and commitment therapy in VA primary care. *Psychological Services, 13*, 156–161. doi: https://doi.org/10.1037/ser0000062.

Goetter, E. M., Bui, E., Weiner, T. P., Lakin, L., Furlong, T., & Simon, N. M. (2017). Pilot data of a brief veteran peer intervention and its relationship to mental health treatment engagement. *Psychological Services*, 1–4. Advance online publication. https://doi.org/10.1037/ser0000151.

Goff, B. S. N., Crow, J. R., Reisbig, A. M. J., & Hamilton, S. (2007). The impact of individual trauma symptoms of deployed soldiers on relationship satisfaction. *Journal of Family Psychology, 21*, 344–353. https://doi.org/10.1037/0893-3200.21.3.344

*Goodcase, E. T., Love, H. A., & Ladson, E. (2015). A conceptualization of processing military sexual trauma within the couple relationship. *Contemporary Family Therapy, 37*, 291–301. https://doi.org/10.1007/s10591-015-9354-6.

Gorman, G., Eide, M., & Hisle-Gorman, E. (2010). Wartime military deployment and increased pediatric mental and behavioral health complaints. *Pediatrics, 126*, 1058–1066. http://dx.doi.org/10.1542/peds.2009-2856

Greenman, P., & Johnson, S. (2012). United we stand: Emotionally focused therapy for couples in the treatment of posttraumatic stress disorder. *Journal of Clinical Psychology, 68*, 561-569. doi:10.1002/jclp.21853

Guay, S., Beaulieu-Prévost, D., Beaudoin, C., St-Jean-Trudel, J., Nachar, N., Marchand, A., & O'Connor, K. P. (2011). How do social interactions with a significant other affect PTSD symptoms? An empirical investigation with a clinical sample. *Journal of Aggression, Maltreatment & Trauma, 20*, 280–303. https://doi.org/10.1080/10926771.2011.562478

*Harmon, L. M., Cooper, R. L., Nugent, W. R., & Butcher, J. J. (2016). A review of the effectiveness of military suicide prevention programs in reducing rates of military suicides. *Journal of Human Behavior in the Social Environment, 26*, 15–24. https://doi.org/10.1080/10911359.2015.1058139.

Hayes, S. C., Strosahl, K. D., & Wilson, K. G. (1999). *Acceptance and commitment therapy: An experiential approach to behavior change*. New York, NY: Guilford Press.

Hayes, S. C., Strosahl, K. D., & Wilson, K. G. (2011). *Acceptance and commitment therapy: The process and practice of mindful change* (2nd ed.). New York, NY: Guilford Press.

*Hegar, M. (2017). *Shoot like a girl*. New York, NY: Berkley.

Hermes, E. D. A., Wells, T. S., Smith, B., Boyko, E. J., Gackstetter, G. G., Miller, S. C., ... Millennium Cohort Study Team. (2012). Smokeless tobacco use related to military deployment, cigarettes and mental health symptoms in a large, prospective cohort study among US service members. *Addiction, 107*, 983–994. https://doi.org/10.1111/j.1360-0443.2011.03737.x

Hodgson, J., Lamson, A., Mendenhall, T., & Tyndall, L. (2014). Introduction to medical family therapy: Advanced applications. In J. Hodgson, A. Lamson, T. Mendenhall, and D. Crane (Eds.), *Medical family therapy: Advanced applications* (pp. 1–9). New York, NY: Springer.

Holland, K. J., Rabelo, V. C., & Cortina, L. M. (2016). Collateral damage: Military sexual trauma and help-seeking barriers. *Psychology of Violence, 6*, 253–261. https://doi.org/10.1037/a0039467

Huang, G., Kim, S., Gasper, J., Xu, Y., Bosworth, T., & May, L. (2017). *2016 survey of veteran enrollees' health and use of health care*. Westat. Retrieved from https://www.va.gov/HEALTHPOLICYPLANNING/SoE2016/2016_Survey_of_Veteran_Enrollees_Health_and_Health_Care.pdf

Institute of Medicine [IOM]. (2014). *Treatment for posttraumatic stress disorder in military and veteran populations*. Retrieved from http://www.nationalacademies.org/hmd/Reports/2014/Treatment-for-Posttraumatic-Stress-Disorder-in-Military-and-Veteran-Populations-Final-Assessment/Report-Brief-062014.aspx

*Johnson, S. (2005). *Emotion focused couples therapy with trauma survivors: Strengthening attachment bonds*. New York, NY: Guilford Press.

Jordan, K. (2011). Counselors helping service veterans re-enter their couple relationship after combat and military services: A comprehensive review. *The Family Journal: Counseling and Therapy for Couples and Families, 19*, 263–273. https://doi.org/10.1177/1066480711406689

Johnston, S., Webb-Murphy, J., & Bhakta, J. (2016). Lesbian, gay, and bisexual service members. In N. Ainspan, C. Bryan, and W. Penk (Eds.), *Handbook of psychosocial interventions for veterans and service members: A guide for the non-military mental health clinician (pp. 45–52). New York, NY: Oxford University Press.

*Junger, S. (2010). War. New York, NY: Grand Central Publishing.

*Junger, S. (2016). Tribe. New York, NY: Grand Central Publishing.

Karney, B. R., & Crown, J. S. (2007). Families under stress: An assessment of data, theory, and research on marriage and divorce in the military. Santa Monica, CA: RAND.

*Kauth, M. R., Meier, C., & Latini, D. M. (2014). A review of sexual health among lesbian, gay, and bisexual veterans. Current Sexual Health Reports, 6, 106–113. https://doi.org/10.1007/s11930-014-0018-6.

Kees, M., & Rosenblum, K. (2015). Evaluation of a psychological health and resilience intervention for military spouses: A pilot study. Psychological Services, 12, 222–230. https://doi.org/10.1037/ser0000035

Kitzmann, K., Gaylord, N., Holt, A., & Kenny, E. (2003). Child witnesses to domestic violence: A meta-analytic review. Journal of Consulting and Clinical Psychology, 71, 339–352. https://doi.org/10.1037/0022-006X.71.2.339

*Klay, P. (2014). Redeployment. New York, NY: Penguin Books.

Kortla, K., & Dyer, P. (2008). Using marriage education to strengthen military families: Evaluation of the activity military life skills program. Social Work and Christianity, 35, 287–311. Retrieved from http://www.nacsw.org/Publications/Proceedings2007/KotrlaKMarriageEducationE.pdf

Klostermann, K., Mignone, T., Kelley, M. L., Musson, S., & Bohall, G. (2012). Intimate partner violence in the military: Treatment considerations. Aggression and Violent Behavior, 17, 53. https://doi.org/10.1016/j.avb.2011.09.004

Lacks, M., Lamson, A. L., Lewis, M., White, M., & Russoniello, C. (2015). Reporting for double duty: A dyadic perspective on the biopsychosocial health of dual military couples. Contemporary Family Therapy, 37, 302–315. https://doi.org/10.1007/s10591-015-9341-y

Larson, G. E., Highfill-Mcroy, R. M., & Booth-Kewley, S. (2008). Psychiatric diagnoses in historic and contemporary military cohorts: Combat deployment and the healthy warrior effect. American Journal of Epidemiology, 167, 1269–1276. https://doi.org/10.1093/aje/kwn084

LeardMann, C. A., Powell, T. M., Smith, T. C., Bell, M. R., Smith, B., Boyko, E. J., & Hoge, C. W. (2013). Risk factors associated with suicide in current and former US military personnel. Journal of American Medical Association, 310, 496–506. https://doi.org/10.1001/jama.2013.65164

Lewis, M., Lamson, A. L., & Leseuer, B. (2012). Health dynamics of military and veteran couples: A biopsychorelational overview. Contemporary Family Therapy, 34, 259–276. https://doi.org/10.1007/s10591-012-9193-7

Lewis, M., Lamson, A., & White, M. (2016). The state of dyadic methodology: An analysis of the literature on interventions for military couples. Journal of Couple & Relationship Therapy, 15, 135–157. https://doi.org/10.1080/15332691.2015.1106998

Lineberry, T. W., & O'Connor, S. S. (2012). Suicide in the US Army. Mayo Clinic Proceedings, 87, 871–878. https://doi.org/10.1016/j.mayocp.2012.07.002

Litz, B. T., Stein, N., Delaney, E., Lebowitz, L., Nash, W. P., Silva, C., & Maguen, S. (2009). Moral injury and moral repair in war veterans: A preliminary model and intervention strategy. Clinical Psychology Review, 29, 695–706. https://doi.org/10.1016/j.cpr.2009.07.003

Lorber, W., & Garcia, H. A. (2010). Not supposed to feel this: Traditional masculinity in psychotherapy with male veterans returning from Afghanistan and Iraq. Psychotherapy: Therapy, Research, Practice, Training, 47, 296–305. https://doi.org/10.1037/a0021161

Lowe, K. N., Adams, K. S., Browne, B. L., & Hinkle, K. T. (2012). Impact of military deployment on family relationships. Journal of Family Studies, 18, 17–27. https://doi.org/10.5172/jfs.2012.18.1.17

MacGregor, A. J., Han, P. P., Dougherty, A. L., & Galarneau, M. R. (2012). Effect of dwell time on the mental health of US Military personnel with multiple combat tours. American Journal of Public Health, 102, S55–S59. https://doi.org/10.2105/AJPH.2011.300341

MacIntosh, H., & Johnson, S. (2008). Emotionally focused therapy for couples and childhood sexual abuse survivors. *Journal of Marital and Family Therapy, 34,* 298–315. https://doi.org/10.1111/j.1752-0606.2008.00074.x

Makin-Byrd, K., Gifford, E., McCutcheon, S., & Glynn, S. (2011). Family and couples treatment for newly returning veterans. *Professional Psychology: Research and Practice, 42,* 47–55. https://doi.org/10.1037/a0022292

Maguen, S., Cohen, G., Cohen, B., Lawhon, G., Marmar, C., & Seal, K. (2010). The role of psychologists in the care of Iraq and Afghanistan veterans in primary care settings. *Professional Psychology: Research and Practice, 41,* 135–142. https://doi.org/10.1037/a0018835

Maguen, S., & Litz, B. T. (2012). Moral injury in veterans of war. *PTSD Research Quarterly, 23,* 1–6. Retrieved from http://vva1071.org/uploads/3/1/6/2/3162163/moral_injury_in_veterans_of_war.pdf

Maguen, S., & Litz, B. (2016). *Moral injury in the context of war.* Retrieved from https://www.ptsd.va.gov/professional/co-occurring/moral_injury_at_war.asp

Maguen, S., Lucenko, B. A., Reger, M. A., Gahm, G. A., Litz, B. T., Seal K.H., ... Marmar, C.R. (2010). The impact of reported direct and indirect killing on mental health symptoms in Iraq War veterans. *Journal of Traumatic Stress, 23,* 86–90. https://doi.org/10.1002/jts.20434.

Mansfield, A. J., Kaufman, J. S., Marshall, S. W., Gaynes, B. N., Morrissey, J. P., & Engel, C. C. (2010). Deployment and the use of mental health services among U.S. Army wives. *New England Journal of Medicine, 362,* 101–109. https://doi.org/10.1056/nejmoa0900177

Marek, K. D., Stetzer, F., Adams, S. J., Popejoy, L. L., & Rantz, M. (2012). Aging in place versus nursing home care: Comparison of costs to medicare and medicaid. *Research in Gerontological Nursing, 5,* 123–129. http://dx.doi.org.jproxy.lib.ecu.edu/10.3928/19404921-20110802-01

Marshall, R. C., Doperak, M., Milner, M., Motsinger, C., Newton, T., Padden, M., ... Mun, S. K. (2011). Patient-centered medical home: An emerging primary care model and the military health system. *Military Medicine, 176,* 1253–1259. https://doi.org/10.7205/MILMED-D-11-00109.

Marshall, B. D., Prescott, M. R., Liberzon, I., Tamburrino, M. B., Calabrese, J. R., & Galea, S. (2012). Coincident posttraumatic stress disorder and depression predict alcohol abuse during and after deployment among Army National Guard soldiers. *Drug Alcohol Dependency, 124,* 193–199. https://doi.org/10.1016/j.drugalcdep.2011.12.027

Matthias, M. S., McGuire, A. B., Kukla, M., Daggy, J., Myers, L. J., & Blair, M. J. (2015). A brief peer support intervention for veterans with chronic musculoskeletal pain: A pilot study of feasibility and effectiveness. *Pain Medicine, 16,* 81–87. https://doi.org/10.1111/pme.12571

McCauley, H. L., Blosnich, J. R., & Dichter, M. E. (2015). Adverse childhood experiences and adult health outcomes among veteran and non-veteran women. *Journal of Women's Health, 24,* 723–729. https://doi.org/10.1089/jwh.2014.4997

McCuaig Edge, H. J., & Ivey, G. W. (2012). Mediation of cognitive appraisal on combat exposure and psychological distress. *Military Psychology, 24,* 71–85. https://doi.org/10.1080/08995605.2012.642292

McKee, A. C., & Robinson, M. E. (2014). Military-related traumatic brain injury and neurodegeneration. *Alzheimer's & Dementia, 10,* 242–253. https://doi.org/10.1016/j.jalz.2014.04.003

Military Health System. (2014). *Final report to the Secretary of Defense: Military health system review.* Retrieved from http://archive.defense.gov/pubs/140930_MHS_Review_Final_Report_Main_Body.pdf

Military Health System. (2017). *About the military health system.* Retrieved from https://www.health.mil/About-MHS

Military Health System Genesis. (2017). *MHS genesis factsheet.* Retrieved from https://health.mil/Reference-Center/Fact-Sheets?page=1#pagingAnchor

Military OneSource. (2016). *The family advocacy program.* Retrieved from http://www.militaryonesource.mil/phases-military-leadership?content_id=266712

Morissette, S. B., Woodward, M., Kimbrel, N. A., Meyer, E. C., Kruse, M. L., Dolan, S., & Gulliver, S. (2011). Deployment-related TBI, persistent postconcussive symptoms, PTSD, and depression in OEF/OIF veterans. *Rehabilitation Psychology, 56,* 340–350. https://doi.org/10.1037/a0025462

Murphy, R. A., & Fairbank, J. A. (2013). Implementation and dissemination of military informed and evidence-based interventions for community dwelling military families. *Clinical Child and Family Psychology Review, 16,* 348–364. https://doi.org/10.1007/s10567-013-0149-8

National Center for Injury Prevention and Control. (2003). *Cost of intimate partner violence against women in the United States.* Retrieved from https://www.cdc.gov/violenceprevention/pdf/ipvbook-a.pdf

Perls, F. S., Hefferline, R. F., & Goodman, P. (1957). *Gestalt therapy.* New York, NY: Dell.

Pfeiffer, P. N., Blow, A. J., Miller, E., Forman, J., Dalack, G. W., & Valenstein, M. (2012). Peers and peer-based interventions in supporting reintegration and mental health among National Guard soldiers: A qualitative study. *Military Medicine, 177,* 1471–1476. https://doi.org/10.7205/MILMED-D-12-00115

Pruitt, L. D., Smolenski, D. J., Reger, M. A., Bush N. E., Skopp, N. A., & Campise, R. L. (2014). *Department of Defense suicide event report.* Retrieved from http://www.dspo.mil/Portals/113/Documents/CY%202014%20DoDSER%20Annual%20Report%20-%20Final.pdf

Ray-Sannerud, B. N., Dolan, D. C., Morrow, C. E., Corso, K. A., Kanzler, K. E., Corso, M. L., & Bryan, C. J. (2012). Longitudinal outcomes after brief behavioral health intervention in an integrated primary care clinic. *Families, Systems & Health, 30,* 60–71. https://doi.org/10.1037/a0027029

Rentz, E. D., Martin, S. L., Gibbs, D. A., Clinton-Sherrod, M., Hardison, J., & Marshall, S. W. (2006). Family violence in the military: A review of the literature. *Trauma, Violence & Abuse, 7,* 93–108. https://doi.org/10.1177/1524838005285916

Resick, P. A., Galovski, T. E., Uhlmansiek, M. O., Scher, C. D., Clum, G. A., & Young-Xu, Y. (2008). A randomized clinical trial to dismantle components of cognitive processing therapy for posttraumatic stress disorder in female victims of interpersonal violence. *Journal of Consulting and Clinical Psychology, 76,* 243–258. https://doi.org/10.1037/0022-006X.76.2.243

Ruff, L. R., Riechers, R. G., Wang, X. F., Piero, T., & Smith-Ruff, S. (2012). A case control study examining weather neurological deficits and PTSD in combat veterans are related to episodes of mild TBI. *BMJ Open, 2,* 1–12. https://doi.org/10.1136/bmjopen-2011-000312

Sayers, S. (2011). Family reintegration difficulties and couple therapy for military veterans and their spouses. *Cognitive and Behavioral Practice, 18,* 108–119. https://doi.org/10.1016/j.cbpra.2010.03.002

Siegel, B. S., Davis, B. E., & Committee on Psychosocial Aspects of Child and Family Health and Section on Uniformed Services. (2013). Health and mental health needs of children in US military families. *Pediatrics, 131,* e2002–e2015. https://doi.org/10.1542/peds.2013-0940

Shapiro, F. (2007). EDMR and emotionally focused couple therapy for war veteran couples. In *Handbook of EMDR and family therapy processes* (pp. 202–220). Hoboken, NJ: John Wiley & Sons.

Shapiro, F. (1989). Efficacy of the eye movement desensitization procedure in the treatment of traumatic memories. *Journal of Traumatic Stress, 2,* 199–223. https://doi.org/10.1002/jts.2490020207

Smith, E. A., & Malone, R. E. (2014). Mediatory myths in the U.S. military: Tobacco use as "stress relief". *American Journal of Health Promotion, 29,* 115–122. https://doi.org/10.4278/ajhp.121009-QUAL-491

SteelFisher, G. K., Zaslavsky, A. M., & Blendon, R. J. (2008). Health related impact of deployment extensions on spouses of active duty Army Personnel. *Military Medicine, 173,* 221–229. https://doi.org/10.7205/MILMED.173.3.221

Steenkamp, M. M., Schlenger, W. E., Corry, N., Henn-Haase, C., Qian, M., Li, M. ... Marmar, C. (2017). Predictors of PTSD 40 years after combat: Findings from the National Vietnam Veterans longitudinal study. *Depression and Anxiety, 34*(8):711–722. https://doi.org/10.1002/da.22628.

Stein, M. B., & McAllister, T. W. (2009). Exploring the convergence of posttraumtic stress disorder and mild traumatic brain injury. *American Journal of Psychiatry, 166*, 768–776. https://doi.org/10.1176/appi.ajp.2009.08101604

Strosahl, K., Robinson, P., & Gustavsson, T. (2012). *Brief interventions for radical change: Principles & practice of focused acceptance & commitment therapy*. Oakland, CA: New Harbinger Publications.

Summerall, E. L. (2017). *Traumatic brain injury and PTSD*. Retrieved from https://www.ptsd.va.gov/professional/co-occurring/traumatic-brain-injury-ptsd.asp

Taft, C. T., Creech, S. K., Gallagher, M. W., Macdonald, A., Murphy, C. M., & Monson, C. (2016). Strength at Home Couples program to prevent military partner violence: A randomized controlled trial. *Journal of Consulting and Clinical Psychology, 84*, 935–945. https://doi.org/10.1037/ccp0000129

Teachman, J., Anderson, C., & Tedrow, L. M. (2015). Military service and alcohol use in the United States. *Armed Forces & Society, 41*, 460–476. https://doi.org/10.1177/0095327X14543848

Trump, L. J., Lamson, A. L., Lewis, M., & Muse, A. (2015). His and hers: The interface of military couples' biological, psychological, and relational health. *Contemporary Family Therapy, 37*, 316–328. https://doi.org/10.1007/s10591-015-9344-8

Turchik, J. A., Pavao, J., Nazarian, D., Iqbal, S., McLean, C., & Kimerling, R. (2012). Sexually transmitted infections and sexual dysfunctions among newly returned veterans with and without military sexual trauma. *International Journal of Sexual Health, 24*, 45–59. https://doi.org/10.1080/19317611.2011.639592

U.S. Army Medical Department. (2013). Roles of medical care (United States). In U.S. Army, *Emergency war surgery* (4th ed., pp. 17–28). Retrieved from http://www.cs.amedd.army.mil/FileDownloadpublic.aspx?docid=1a73495d-1176-4638-9011-9e7f3c6017d8

U.S. Census Bureau. (2012). *Section 10: National security and veterans affairs* (Report No. Statistical Abstract of the United States: 2012 [131st ed.]). Retrieved from https://www.census

U.S. Census Bureau. (2015). *Veteran poverty trends*. Retrieved from https://www.va.gov/vetdata/docs/specialreports/veteran_poverty_trends.pdf

U.S. Department of Veterans Affairs. (2015). *Vet center program*. Retrieved from https://www.vetcenter.va.gov/

U.S. Department of Veterans Affairs. (2016a). *Health benefits*. Retrieved from https://www.va.gov/healthbenefits/resources/priority_groups.asp

U.S. Department of Veterans Affairs. (2016b). *National Center for Veterans Analysis and Statistics*. Retrieved from https://www.va.gov/vetdata/Utilization.asp

U.S. Department of Veterans Affairs. (2017a). *Profile of veterans: 2015 data from the American Community Survey*. Retrieved from https://www.va.gov/vetdata/docs/SpecialReports/Profile_of_Veterans_2015.pdf

U.S. Department of Veterans Affairs. (2017b). *Veterans Health Administration*. Retrieved from https://www.va.gov/health/

*Van der Kolk, B. A. (2015). The *body keeps the score: Brain, mind, and body in the healing of trauma*. New York, NY: Penguin Books.

Van der Kolk, B., Spinazolla, J., Blaustien, M., Hopper, J., Hopper, E., Korn, D., & Simpson, W. B. (2007). A randomized clinical trial of EMDR, fluoxetine and pill placebo in the treatment of PTSD: Treatment effects and long-term maintenance. *Journal of Clinical Psychiatry, 68*, 37–46. https://doi.org/10.4088/JCP.v68n0105

Weissman, N., Batten, S. V., Dixon, L., Pasillas, R. M., Potts, W., Decker, M., & Brown, C. H. (2011). The effectiveness of emotionally focused couples therapy (EFT) with veterans with PTSD. *Poster presented at the Veterans Affairs National Annual Conference: Improving Veterans Mental Health Care for the 1st Century*. Baltimore, MD.

Wiebe, S. A., & Johnson, S. M. (2016). A review of the research in emotionally focused therapy for couples. *Family Process, 55*, 390–407. https://doi.org/10.1111/famp.12229

Wilson, S. R., Wilkum, K., Chernichky, S. M., MacDermid Wadsworth, S. M., & Broniarczyk, K. M. (2011). Passport toward success: Description and evaluation of a program designed to help children and families reconnect after a military deployment. *Journal of Applied Communication Research, 39,* 223–249. https://doi.org/10.1080/00909882.2011.585399

Wittenberg, A., & Gerber, J. (2009). Recommendations for improving sexual health curricula in medical schools: Results from a two-arm study collecting data from patients and medical students. *Journal of Sexual Medicine, 6,* 362–368. https://doi.org/10.1111/j.1743-6109.2008.01046.x

Wright, L. M., Watson, W. L., & Bell, J. M. (1996). *Beliefs: The heart of healing in families and illness.* New York, NY: Basic Books.

Zinzow, H. M., Britt, T. W., McFadden, A. C., Burnette, C. M., & Gillispie, S. (2012). Connecting active duty and returning veterans to mental health treatment: Interventions and treatment adaptations that may reduce barriers to care. *Clinical Psychology Review, 32,* 741–753. https://doi.org/10.1016/j/cpr.2012.09.002

Zinzow, H. M., Grubaugh, A. L., Monnier, J., Suffoletta-Maierle, S., & Frueh, B. C. (2007). Trauma among female veterans: A critical review. *Trauma, Violence & Abuse, 8,* 384–400. https://doi.org/10.1177/1524838007307295

Chapter 19
Innovations in MedFT: Pioneering New Frontiers!

Jennifer Hodgson, Tai Mendenhall, Angela Lamson, Macaran Baird, and Jackie Williams-Reade

The principal advantages for pioneering new territory lay in both the creativity for courageous individuals and opportunities for those who follow. The West was settled on inspiration (and perspiration) fueled by a desire for a better way, a better life, and a more hopeful future. Likewise, the development of medical family therapy (MedFT) grew from a need in health care for a more collaborative, relationally based, and systemic system. Today, it is finding its place. Much like pioneering settlers, MedFTs have moved from the most populated areas to those in need of more development. With each step, there is continued learning and growing appreciation for each setting's unique populations, needs, diverse cultures, and resources. In McDaniel, Hepworth, and Doherty's (1992) early primer, primary care was described as an ideal environment for MedFT. Over the years, this scope and attention has evolved to include secondary and tertiary care settings. This book attempts to serve as a learning tool for new and experienced professionals wanting to develop as MedFTs and who wish to expand into new territories for which they were not formally trained.

J. Hodgson (✉) · A. Lamson
Department of Human Development and Family Science, East Carolina University, Greenville, NC, USA
e-mail: hodgsonj@ecu.edu

T. Mendenhall
Department of Family Social Science, University of Minnesota, Saint Paul, MN, USA

M. Baird
Department of Family Medicine and Community Health,
University of Minnesota Medical School, Minneapolis, MN, USA

J. Williams-Reade
School of Behavioral Health, Loma Linda University, Loma Linda, CA, USA

Throughout this text, contributors have highlighted how MedFTs can find professional homes in a variety of settings where healthcare is practiced. Each chapter introduced the contexts, foundational knowledge and skills, research-informed interventions, and ways that MedFTs can enhance and expand their skills. We also showcased the diversity of skills that MedFTs have in working with individuals, couples, families, and groups and through community engagement. While the chapters included were chosen by our editorial team, the directions that MedFT can be taken are expanding every day.

This chapter highlights the work of MedFTs who are pioneering in a variety of health-related contexts. It was written for those who ask: "What can I do with MedFT training?" It is our hope that this chapter will light a fire by reading the stories of those who have pioneered before you. The contributors below responded to a call for submissions to write about the innovative ways that they are using MedFT in their work. Their contributions provide evidence of what some MedFTs are doing with their expertise. Submissions are presented according to the following groupings/headings, albeit many could easily fit into multiple categories: (a) interdisciplinary research; (b) training innovations and health specializations; (c) faculty appointments in primary, secondary, and tertiary care departments; and (d) policy and leadership.

MedFT Interdisciplinary Research

The MedFT Healthcare Continuum (Hodgson, Lamson, Mendenhall, & Tyndall, 2014) showcases how MedFTs work in interdisciplinary teams to conduct research across a variety of healthcare settings. Examples of this span decades and represent advancements that include the integration of relational health into mainstream healthcare. In Hodgson, Lamson, Mendenhall, and Crane's (2014) text, *Medical Family Therapy: Advanced Applications*, several authors collected research showcasing the empirical reach of MedFT into areas such as scientist-practitioner studies (Zak-Hunter et al., 2014); qualitative, quantitative, and mixed-method research (Mendenhall, Pratt, Phelps, Baird, & Younkin, 2014); community-engaged scholarship (Mendenhall, Berge, & Doherty, 2014); program evaluation studies (Williams-Reade, Gordon, & Wray, 2014); dissemination and implementation science (Polaha & Nolan, 2014); and research to advance health equity (Lewis, Myhra, & Walker, 2014).

While the authors below were all active MedFT researchers well before the 2014 text, their contributions here highlight new growth and potential applications for interdisciplinary scholarship that lies ahead:

Jerica Berge, Ph.D., MPH, LMFT, CFLE. I am a tenured faculty member at the University of Minnesota's Medical School. I also hold adjunct appointments in the Department of Family Social Science and the School of Public Health. I am both a MedFT clinician and researcher. A clinical expertise of mine is group-based integrated care for women's health. On a weekly basis, I co-facilitate a prenatal group with an obstetrics nurse, a lactation specialist nurse, and a physician. This interdisciplinary team has been highly successful in attracting and providing prenatal care for our high needs, underserved minority, and low-income populations. As part of the group, patients learn to take their own vitals, use a support group effectively, discuss a topic of the week related to pregnancy (e.g., breastfeeding, postpartum depression, labor/delivery), and receive an individual doctor visit—all within 90 minutes. When developing the prenatal group model, we built in an evaluation component with a control group. We have replicated findings to other prenatal group studies and extended prior findings (e.g., overutilization patterns decreased in prenatal group patients compared to control). These prenatal groups are run through a residency clinic, which advances prior research as well. We conducted focus groups with prenatal group participants; they shared that they loved several things about group, including how (a) providers spent more time with them, (b) team facilitation of the group was crucial for addressing all of their needs (e.g., medical and behavioral health), (c) other women were a part of the support group, (d) they learned more in a group format and felt like they could ask questions comfortably, and (e) they understood their bodies better as a result of prenatal group. Facilitating this model of group-based care puts MedFTs on the cutting-edge of healthcare delivery in Family Medicine. Additionally, since many MedFTs have been trained in evaluation, this skill reinforces the need for them to function in healthcare settings.

A second area of my expertise is in conducting National Institutes of Health (NIH) research on risk and protective factors for childhood obesity in the home environment. I carry several NIH grants, including traditional epidemiological cohort studies, mixed-method (e.g., ecological momentary assessment, video-recorded tasks) in-home studies, and interventions. A common factor among the studies is a reliance on the strengths of the fields that I work within (i.e., Family Medicine, Family Science, Public Health). For example, a current R01 grant of mine uses a mixed-method two-phased incremental approach. In Phase I, in-home observations of diverse families ($n = 150$; African American, American Indian, Hispanic, Hmong, White) were conducted and included: (a) an interactive observational family task; (b) ecological momentary assessment (EMA) of parent stress, mood, and parenting practices; and (c) child accelerometry and 24-hour dietary recalls. Data from Phase I informed Phase II, where an epidemiological cohort study is now being carried out with a large representative sample of caregivers with children ages 5–7 years ($n = 1200$) from diverse backgrounds. Recruitment for both phases occurred in Family Medicine clinics. The R01 study will collect individual, dyadic (e.g., parent/child, sibling), and familial data to characterize associations between the home environment and child body mass index (BMI) z-score and weight-related behaviors to inform the development of culturally tailored interventions to be carried out in partnership with families and their Family Medicine physicians. Carrying out NIH-funded research increases the prominence of MedFTs in healthcare as they are seen as innovative and invaluable contributors to creating a culture of health.

Jerica Berge, Ph.D., MPH, LMFT, CFLE
Associate Professor
Family Medicine and Community Health
University of Minnesota (UMN) Medical School
Adjunct Faculty, Family Social Science, UMN
Adjunct Faculty, School of Public Health, UMN

Dixie Meyer, Ph.D., NCC, LPC. My research seeks to uncover the underlying mechanisms explaining why relationships are beneficial or detrimental to health. My specific focus is romantic relationships, but I also have measured the intersections between childhood traumas and current romantic couple functioning. This path leads me down to several avenues of investigation. My scholarship supports the notion that people can regulate health and wellness in their romantic partners. One study demonstrated females' mental, physical, and romantic relationship health may regulate their male partners' respective cortisol levels. Due to the sex differences present, I am also investigating the role of the menstrual cycle in this regulatory process. My other studies demonstrated that individuals with a history of childhood traumas experience fewer depressive and anxious symptoms if they are in a romantic relationship. The data suggest a possible buffering effect whereby romantic partners may be helping to heal past traumas to support healthy functioning. One of my key research collaborators, Dr. Tony Buchanan, is an associate professor of Psychology. His expertise on stress responses helped to identify the stress hormone, cortisol, as a potential outcome variable that explains the power of relationships in health. This research will help to inform the field of Medical Family Therapy of the biological mechanisms influenced by relationships. The purpose of this work is to create MedFT interventions that enhance relationships to promote health.

Dixie Meyer, Ph.D., NCC, LPC
Assistant Professor
Medical Family Therapy Program
Family and Community Medicine
School of Medicine
Saint Louis University

Mary Lisa Pories, Ph.D., LCSW. I returned to school for my Ph.D. in Medical Family Therapy in order to become a better biopsychosocial researcher. I currently work as a Research Administrator at East Carolina University. This position allows me to work with faculty members to hone their research agendas and seek out funding. I oversee all grants and sponsored program submissions in our college, from working with the primary investigator on the budget and other pieces of the grant to navigating the university and funder systems to submit proposals. While we all understand the importance and value of our research, the realities of searching for and securing funding, especially as new Ph.D.s, can be daunting. Understanding the challenges of initiating a research stream, the intricacies of finding and securing funding, and navigating the institutional systems are paramount to becoming a successful scholar. Many of us are exposed to pieces of this in our doctoral programs, but having the opportunity to assist other researchers as they begin this journey allows me the opportunity to help others advance science and their careers. This role also allows me to nurture my own research around the impact of bariatric surgery on the family, and on rural farm women's health.

Mary Lisa Pories, Ph.D., LCSW
Research Administrator
College of Health and Human Performance
East Carolina University

Keeley J. Pratt Ph.D., LMFT. I am a faculty member at the Ohio State University (OSU) Wexner Medical Center in the Department of Surgery, wherein I oversee the behavioral health and family therapy programming for adult weight management and bariatric surgery patients. I serve as coordinator for a newly approved, campus-wide Graduate Interdisciplinary Specialization in Obesity Sciences. Over the past decade, I have worked with pediatric obesity treatment centers, residential healthy lifestyle camps, adult outpatient weight management and bariatric surgery, and school-based settings as a therapist and researcher. I currently train students at OSU to work as MedFTs in Pediatrics and Weight Management placements. My research aims to determine which family, couple, and parent-child variables predict short- and long-term behavior change and weight loss in pediatric and adult weight management programs. Understanding this enables us to develop effective family-based interventions grounded in family systems theory. Specifically, I am conducting research to: (a) describe family outcomes from integrated, multidisciplinary care models in the treatment of childhood obesity; (b) develop culturally tailored treatment interventions for racial/ethnic minority and underserved families in obesity treatment; (c) determine how to include partners/spouses and family members in adult weight management and bariatric surgery treatment; and (d) expand mental and behavioral health education to include clinician training for the treatment of clients and families with overweight and obesity.

Keeley Pratt Ph.D., LMFT
Assistant Professor
Human Development and Family Science Program
Couple and Family Therapy Specialization
Department of Human Sciences
The Ohio State University

While the evidence mounts for how family-based interventions can help advance healthcare (Crane & Christianson, 2014; Crane & Payne, 2011), MedFT scholars must continue to secure and function in prominent roles on interdisciplinary research teams. Expanding on this body of work will help build effective bodies of knowledge that demonstrate MedFT's effectiveness and efficacy on healthcare teams and as healthcare leaders. It will showcase their advanced training and degrees as they stand shoulder-to-shoulder with other behavioral health disciplines (e.g., Psychiatry, Psychology, Social Work, Professional Counseling) who seek employment opportunities in healthcare settings. Ideally, all health-related fields (e.g., Medicine, Dentistry, Nursing, Behavioral Health, Nutrition, Pharmacy) will move past the outdated models that we employ currently and instead begin to train alongside each other to provide patient- and family-centered care and research.

MedFT Training Innovations and Health Specializations

Medical Family Therapy grew primarily from the fields of Psychiatry, Family Medicine, Family Psychology, and Marriage and Family Therapy (McDaniel, Doherty, & Hepworth, 2014). Some of the earliest training was done during summer institutes like that offered by the University of Rochester in New York by Susan McDaniel and colleagues and by John Rolland through the Chicago Center for Family Health. Now, there are multiple locations and opportunities for professionals to obtain training in MedFT. Table 19.1 includes known training programs and institutes where MedFT training is offered. All schools on the list met the minimum qualification of having at least one course specifically devoted to MedFT, families and health, and/or integrated care. The programs denoted in Table 19.1 were identified through using the MedFT Facebook page and by emailing all program directors of accredited programs during the months of July–August 2017.

Examples of longstanding training locations and innovations are described below. Each innovator describes how he or she has designed MedFT training opportunities and/or how they have expanded MedFT into specific areas of health specialization. Their combined work has resulted in invaluable training and healing opportunities for others.

Table 19.1 MFT Programs Offering Training in Medical Family Therapy, Families and Health, and/or Integrated Care

Medical Family Therapy degrees	*Website or contact information*
East Carolina University (Ph.D.)	https://hhp.ecu.edu/hdfs/phd/
St. Louis University (Ph.D.)	https://sites.google.com/a/slu.edu/medical-family-therapy-program/
Doctoral programs	*Website or contact information*
Drexel University	http://drexel.edu/cnhp/academics/doctoral/PHD-Couple-Family-Therapy/
Loma Linda University	http://behavioralhealth.llu.edu/programs/counseling-and-family-sciences
Northcentral University	http://www.ncu.edu/school-of-marriage-and-family-sciences/doctor-of-philosophy-in-marriage-and-family-therapy/medical-family-therapy
Ohio State University	https://ehe.osu.edu/human-sciences/hdfs/couples-and-family-therapy-licensure
Texas Woman's University	http://catalog.twu.edu/graduate/professional-education/family-sciences/family-therapy-phd/
University of Minnesota	http://www.cehd.umn.edu/FSoS/programs/phd-cft.asp
Master programs	*Website or contact information*
Drexel University	http://drexel.edu/cnhp/academics/graduate/MFT-Family-Therapy/
East Carolina University	https://hhp.ecu.edu/hdfs/ms-mft/

(continued)

Table 19.1 (countinued)

Jefferson School of Health Professions	http://www.jefferson.edu/university/health-professions/departments/couple-family-therapy/degrees-programs/ms-family-therapy.html
Loma Linda University	http://behavioralhealth.llu.edu/programs/counseling-and-family-sciences
Mercer University	https://medicine.mercer.edu/admissions/mft/
Northcentral University	http://www.ncu.edu/school-of-marriage-and-family-sciences/master-of-arts-in-marriage-and-family-therapy
Regis University	http://www.regis.edu/RHCHP/Academics/Degrees-and-Programs/Graduate-and-Doctorate-Programs/MA-Marriage-and-Family-Therapy.aspx
San Diego State University	http://go.sdsu.edu/education/csp/mft.aspx
Seattle Pacific University	http://spu.edu/academics/school-of-psychology-family-community/graduate-programs/medical-family-therapy
St. Louis University	https://www.slu.edu/programs/graduate/family-therapy-ma.php
Texas Woman's University	http://catalog.twu.edu/graduate/professional-education/family-sciences/family-therapy-ms/
University of Oregon	https://education.uoregon.edu/couples-and-family-therapy/program-information
University of Rochester	https://www.urmc.rochester.edu/psychiatry/institute-for-the-family/family-therapy.aspx
University of San Diego	https://www.sandiego.edu/soles/academics/ma-marital-family-therapy/
Post-degree certificates	*Website or contact information*
Abilene Christian University	http://www.acu.edu/graduate/academics/medical-family-therapy.html
Northern Illinois University	http://catalog.niu.edu/preview_program.php?catoid=15&poid=2571&returnto=457
Nova Southeastern	http://cahss.nova.edu/departments/ft/graduate/familysystems/index.html
Oklahoma Baptist University	http://www.okbu.edu/graduate/certificate/medical-family-therapy
Seattle Pacific University	http://spu.edu/academics/school-of-psychology-family-community/graduate-programs/medical-family-therapy
University of Nebraska Medical Center	http://www.unl.edu/gradstudies/prospective/programs/Cert_MedicalFamilyTherapy
University of Rochester	https://www.urmc.rochester.edu/psychiatry/institute-for-the-family/family-therapy/post-degree.aspx
Postdoctoral internships/fellowships	*Website or contact information*
Dartmouth Family Practice Residency, Concord Hospital, Concord, NH	http://www.concordhospital.org/healthcare-professionals/nh-dartmouth-family-medicine-residency/
Duke/Southern Regional Area Health Education Center Medical Family Therapy Residency Program, Fayetteville, NC	http://www.ncahec.net/graduate-medical-support/nc-ahec-residency-programs/southern-regional-ahec-residency-programs/

(continued)

Table 19.1 (continued)

Families, Illness, and Collaborative Healthcare Doctoral Fellowship, Chicago Center for Family Health, University of Chicago, Chicago, IL	http://ccfhchicago.org/training/fichprogram/
MedFT Fellowship/Internship, Saint Mary's Family Medicine Residency, Grand Junction, CO	https://www.sclhealth.org/locations/st-marys-medical-center/for-healthcare-professionals/family-medicine-residency-program/medical-family-therapy-fellowship/
MedFT Internship, Behavioral Medicine Faculty In-Training University of Nebraska Medical Center, Omaha, NE	Contact Jennifer Harsh at: jennifer.harsh@unmc.edu or 402-595-1424

This list was compiled through emailing program directors listed on the AAMFT directory, using feedback from members of the Medical Family Therapy Facebook page, and word-of-mouth. All institutions were reviewed to determine they met the minimum qualification of having at least one course specifically devoted to issues of medical family therapy, families and health, and/or integrated care and at least one internship in a medical setting. Institutional offerings are often changing and those interested in receiving this training are advised to contact the programs directly to inquire about active opportunities.

Christine Borst, Ph.D., LMFT. As a faculty member and clinical assistant professor with the Doctor of Behavioral Health (DBH) program at Arizona State University, I help prepare graduate students for careers in integrated healthcare with concentrations in both clinical and management perspectives. I develop and teach graduate courses, mentor students, provide service to the program and University, and work with healthcare system partners on integration initiatives. I am able to collaborate with my integrated colleagues across the country to pursue scholarly endeavors and research, in conjunction with preparing the future workforce in integrated care. Working in a variety of settings during my MedFT training (which included helping to set up a fully integrated clinic during my doctoral internship) gave me exposure to a myriad of foci and aspects of healthcare. The knowledge gained during these experiences informs the work I do to this day.

Christine E. W. Borst, Ph.D., LMFT
Clinical Assistant Professor
Doctor of Behavioral Health Program
College of Health Solutions
Arizona State University
christine.borst@asu.edu

Jennifer Hodgson, Ph.D., LMFT, and **Angela Lamson, Ph.D., LMFT.** In 2004, East Carolina University (ECU) was granted permission to establish the first Medical Family Therapy doctoral program in the nation. Since that time, the program has graduated 24 doctoral students and has maintained its accreditation through the Commission on Accreditation for Marriage and Family Therapy Education (COAMFTE). Doctoral students who want to learn about integrated behavioral healthcare, make a difference in reducing health disparities, and train in advanced theories pertaining to diverse healthcare fields, statistics and research methods, dyadic analyses, biopsychosocial-spiritual (BPSS) research, program evaluation, and health informatics have opportunities to excel in these areas within this program. They also have opportunities to teach at the undergraduate, medical student, and medical resident levels.

In addition to doctoral preparation, master's students in Marriage and Family Therapy (MFT) at ECU have opportunities to work in a variety of primary, secondary, and tertiary care settings throughout the university's inpatient and outpatient systems, at a number of hospitals and school health systems in our region. There are also clinical placements available for masters and doctoral students in our local community healthcare centers, wherein we have established an integrated behavioral healthcare model.

Lastly, we have been successful in providing doctoral internship and postdoctoral fellowship training in community healthcare centers (i.e., IBHC with underserved populations in primary care, dental, outreach with migrant farm workers, and school health systems) and supporting students as they stand up new MedFT research, policy, and practice internship sites all around the world. These training opportunities support students and learners to advance their research, teaching, clinical, policy, and leadership skills. It is through successful partnerships like these that MedFT training has thrived in our program(s).

Jennifer Hodgson, Ph.D., LMFT
Professor and Director
Medical Family Therapy Doctoral Program
Department of Human Development and Family Science
East Carolina University

Angela Lamson, Ph.D., LMFT, CFLE
Professor and Associate Dean
College of Health and Human Performance
Department of Human Development and Family Science
East Carolina University

Tina Sellers, Ph.D., LMFT. After over 20 years in the medical field, much has changed and much has remained the same. Back in the mid-1990s, we were just beginning to amass the research showing profound psychosocial impact(s) of integrating behavioral health into standard care. Those of us doing it could see the difference it made for patients, families, and providers—and we knew that the future of healthcare was in this work. Now research is plentiful and conclusive, and more and more large health systems across the United States have behavioral health integrated into primary care. However, many specialty care clinics (e.g., Oncology, Nephrology, Infertility, Cardiology, genetic testing, high risk maternity, and postpartum)—wherein there are significant behavioral health indicators—are still practicing in the old biomedical model. Their patients and families flounder.

The Medical Family Therapy program at Seattle Pacific University has placed our externs in outpatient community-based primary care and specialty care clinics since 2000. It is here where we have learned how important it is to attend to the psychosocial needs of these patients and their families. We have witnessed how these clinic cultures have changed and how clear they have become that they do not want to go back to the ways they functioned before (i.e., unable to address the psychosocial burdens of their patients and the heavy hearts of their providers).

Another shift I have emphasized with our MedFT students that grew out of my work in Women's Health, Oncology, and with patients suffering from severe sexual shame was the lack of training in sexual health of allopathic and psychotherapeutic providers—of all types. I found that patients with a sexual dysfunction issue went to see their doctors or their therapists and far too often were given misinformation that often made their situation worse. The doctor or therapist commonly did not know that the information they provided was, in fact, wrong and/or informed by myth or bias—not by empirical knowledge. Patients assumed—and rightly so, I believe—that the clinician had received adequate training in sexual health and in confronting their sexual biases. But the reality is psychotherapeutically and allopathically trained clinicians do not get adequate training in sexual health or in spiritual intimacy.

I also found Sexology clinicians far too often had no training in working with relationship systems. And neither set of clinicians had training in the cultural competence of working with those from religiously conservative backgrounds, or working with the spiritual sides of sexuality—both of which come up frequently in therapy when couples are seeking more intimacy. This creates a whole new set of problems.

In Washington State, in 2013, we were down to five certified sex therapists and two certified sex therapy supervisors (of which, I was one). This was, in part, because there were no American Association of Sexuality Educators, Counselors, and Therapists (AASECT) certified training centers in the Northern quadrant of the United States. To solve this dilemma, in 2015, I launched the Northwest Institute on Intimacy, with three distinct missions: (a) to provide efficient and effective AASECT training for clinicians; (b) to raise the bar in the field of Psychotherapy; and (c) to educate the public on how to choose a comprehensively trained clinician. We partnered with physician and physical therapy groups who treated complex sexual dysfunction patients and collaborated closely. We advertised those therapists who were trained in the domains of individual, couple, family, sex, and spiritual intimacy therapy to the community, and many would go out to train physicians in local residency programs in sexual health and treating sexual dysfunction.

We also began to reach out to pediatricians and family physicians regarding how they could integrate sexual health education into their well-child visits via the concept of 100 1-minute conversations (versus one 100-minute conversation) with your children as they grow, providing handouts about books that parents can have sitting out as children are growing and what sexual health resources there might be in the community. Another one of our therapists began working with young families, midwives, doulas, obstetricians, and pediatricians around how she could support young parents on adjusting to the changes that marriages endure as they are adjusting to becoming parents. She hosted mini-parenting retreats focusing on intimacy and tricks about how to stay connected as young parents. I also developed a 4-day intimacy retreat for couples, now run through the institute that is conducted several times a year in multiple locations around the United States to help educate couples about how a fast-paced child- and career-focused, technology-driven culture can impact marriage. The retreat, while providing information about sexuality, gender, and culture heretofore not available, is about sacred touch practices that transform couples' relationships and their understanding of the purpose of sexuality in their lives. Connection and pleasure are restored, as is "spark." It is truly revolutionary for nearly all the couples who have experienced this retreat.

Tina Sellers, Ph.D., LMFT
Associate Professor
Marriage and Family Therapy Program
Director of Medical Family Therapy Certificate Program
School of Psychology, Family, and Community
Seattle Pacific University

Lisa Tyndall, Ph.D., LMFT. As a technical assistant/integration consultant, I am part of a team that works in varying capacities with practices and training agencies across the state of North Carolina to help integrate behavioral/mental health and physical health. Our team is part of a larger health foundation that works to improve the health of the whole person through a whole-community approach. Through grants and contracts, we are able to work at the broader system level with healthcare administration to talk about policy and protocol changes necessary to ensure a paradigm shift from siloed healthcare to integrated care. Clinically, we work one on one with all staff and providers to ensure a successful transition to integrated care (from the patient perspective as well). A good portion of my work has involved training and teaching the existing workforce in areas that are critical to integrated care such as communication, team-based care, patient- and family-centered care, successful program implementation, and clinical competencies needed. My training in Medical Family Therapy allowed me to see the levels of systems, both within a practice and external to that practice that need to work together for successful implementation of new programs and models—and to have a good understanding of the point and process of the intervention(s) needed. Additionally, my clinical and supervisory training allows me to work directly with practicing clinicians on their patient-level work and interventions.

Lisa Tyndall, Ph.D., LMFT
Technical Assistant
Center of Excellence for Integrated Care
Foundation for Health Leadership & Innovation
2401 Weston Parkway, Suite 203, Cary, NC 27513

Jonathan Wilson, Ph.D., LMFT. Since graduating from East Carolina University's (ECU) Medical Family Therapy program in 2014, I have sought to pioneer MedFT training programs in Oklahoma, as none existed upon my arrival to Oklahoma Baptist University. Along with Dr. Grace Wilson, I cofounded Oklahoma's only clinical certificate training program in MedFT. OBU's certificate, which consists of three 8-week classes, is an advanced training certificate program offered entirely online and is designed for licensed behavioral and medical professionals. Since its inception, 17 students have completed the training certificate, including every behavioral healthcare provider currently employed within the Chickasaw Nation Healthcare System across the state. These students and faculty are helping to reduce health disparities and advance the health and well-being of Native American members of Chickasaw Nation.

Jonathan Wilson, Ph.D., LMFT
Assistant Professor
Marriage and Family Therapy Program
College of Humanities and Social Sciences
Oklahoma Baptist University

Max Zubatsky, Ph.D., LMFT. At Saint Louis University, we have been integrating MedFTs in a variety of educational and clinical areas. As part of a federally funded grant, I help coordinate a cross-training curriculum with MedFT graduate students and Family Medicine residents to improve collaborative skills and practice outcomes. One of the activities that I have supervised is "continuity of care month," wherein MedFTs help direct patients' transitions of care from the hospital to primary care. On this rotation, MedFTs collect data regarding family history (via genograms), health literacy, depression, and hospitalization readmissions. As part of this cross-training, we are piloting the Family-Centered Observation Form (FCOF); this is a tool to evaluate and provide feedback to residents working with families in routine practice. Additionally, we are conducting a quality improvement project on the impact of MedFT services in primary and tertiary care settings. This project will assess for how behavioral health services can improve underlying health issues, reduce patient costs, and improve overall satisfaction of providers in the healthcare system. I also oversee and supervise the Memory Clinic service provided by the Center for Counseling and Family Therapy at Saint Louis University. This clinic is a comprehensive care service that addresses the needs of individuals with dementia and their families. A range of services are offered to meet the emotional, physical, and familial challenges that go along with this diagnosis.

Max Zubatsky, Ph.D., LMFT
Assistant Professor
Medical Family Therapy Program
Family and Community Medicine
School of Medicine
Saint Louis University

Ruth McKay, MA, LMFT, SP. For 12 years I worked as a MedFT embedded in a Pediatric Oncology-Hematology practice at a Children's Hospital. I already had more than two decades of experience as a marriage and family therapist when I entered the position and became certified early on as a Sandplay Practitioner by the Sandplay Therapists of America. Integrating sandplay therapy into family therapy in this unique setting brought me some of the most meaningful experiences of my career. One example was the use of the modality by a family (father, mother, survivor, and sibling) for their termination of therapy session. I set up three trays and each family member chose five or so miniatures for each tray to represent (a) what their family had been like before cancer entered their lives, (b) what it was like to go through treatment, and (c) what they were taking forward from their experience. In earlier sessions the couple's relationship, the siblings' relationship (8-year old survivor and 6-year old brother), the family's frequent separations for out-of-state treatments, and the survivor's uniquely painful treatments were addressed. Sand trays were often catalysts for discussion, as well as powerful, visually metaphoric experiences within the sessions. The family was able to show in their trays the creative ways that they had personally ritualized their experiences throughout treatment and honored how well they had made cancer a "whole family" experience. The modality of sandplay therapy allowed them to see and listen to each other's experiences and to behold within each tray how their experiences fit together. The last session was the most touching for me when the father remarked how they had taken everything from the "before" tray into the "future" tray, except for one miniature. He told how that represented their "innocence." Never again would they think that "bad things" could not happen to them. As a family proud of their means and achievements, they no longer saw themselves as untouchable by suffering. Acknowledging their resources as gifts supported their sense(s) of empathy toward and commonality with others going through pediatric cancer. Their experience of cancer, and of the therapy, helped them to find deeper and broader connections to each other and to their community of support.

Ruth McKay, MA, LMFT, SP
Medical Family Therapist
Center for Children's Cancer and Blood Disorders

It is a goal of our editing team to promote different methods of training to help with workforce development of behavioral health providers. The growth in degree granting programs in MedFT, since the McDaniel et al.'s (1992) primer text, are one indication that there is a need for these graduates in the job market. Programs such as the doctoral programs in Medical Family Therapy at East Carolina University and Saint Louis University report 100% job placement rates. In fact, ECU reported that over 50% of its graduates since the program's establishment in 2005 hold faculty positions in university settings (e.g., medical schools, residency programs, marriage and family therapy master's and doctoral programs, MedFT master's and doctoral programs).

MedFT Faculty Appointments in Primary, Secondary, and Tertiary Care Departments

Early on, the most common placements for MedFTs were in Family Medicine residency settings. This is where MedFT's pioneering authors McDaniel et al. (1992) all worked at the time they first envisaged the field. Since then, doctoral-level MedFTs have come to hold faculty appointments across an increasingly diverse range of medical, medical school, and medical residency settings. They are recognized for their unique knowledge and skills as researchers, clinicians, leaders, and training innovators (Hodgson, Lamson, Mendenhall, & Crane, 2014). A few of those settings, although not an exhaustive representation, are described below:

Jennifer Harsh, Ph.D., LIMFT. I recently added Director of Resident Wellness to my current position as Director of Behavioral Medicine for the Division of General Internal Medicine at the University of Nebraska Medical Center. In this role, I am responsible for co-developing and facilitating a wellness program that has been crafted to meet residents' unique needs. Stemming from residents' reported desire for an increased focus on well-being, the wellness program was developed using a biopsychosocial-spiritual (BPSS) lens and extant literature regarding resident burnout and resilience. The program in its current form is the result of purposeful collaboration between residents, behavioral medicine faculty and interns, medical faculty, and program administration. Program components include a beginning of residency day-long retreat, a bi-monthly lecture series on wellness topics (e.g., wellness goal setting, resilience, second-victim distress, relationship health), noon hours set aside for residents to take part in informal conversation with co-residents, and resident-to-resident mentorship. A resident wellness advisory board that consists of five current residents, three chief residents, a MedFT doctoral intern, and myself, now oversees the program and modifies program components based on formal evaluation and informal resident feedback.

Jennifer Harsh, Ph.D., LIMFT
Assistant Professor
Director of Behavioral Medicine
Director of Resident Wellness
Division of General Internal Medicine
Department of Internal Medicine
University of Nebraska Medical Center

Patrick Meadors, Ph.D., LMFT. Levine Cancer Institute (LCI) is an eight-hospital network of cancer centers within the Carolinas' Healthcare System (which includes over 25 practice locations across North and South Carolina). Within the Department of Supportive Oncology, I serve in an administrative role that is responsible for the provision of psychosocial care to the over 10,000 cancer patients and their families. We have a team of 15 licensed clinical social workers, two psychotherapists, two psychiatrists, one registered nurse program coordinator, and four support staff with aggressive growth plans to meet increased psychosocial needs over the next 2 years.

A significant portion of my role stems from collaboration with other leaders and providers to successfully integrate services while aligning with the overall strategic direction of our institution to effectively manage the psychosocial needs of our patients. Through these collaborative efforts, we integrated an electronic screening method in all practices that identifies various symptoms early in the care process to connect patients to various resources. When these symptoms are properly managed, our department can have a significant impact on clinical outcomes, quality of life, and overall survival. Additionally, it is expected that we initiate and present/publish research from our respective areas across the local, national, and international level. Overall, I am accountable for the development of a sustainable model for psychosocial care delivery, programmatic development, fiscal and budgetary oversight, strategic business planning, psychosocial research initiatives, and personnel management with the Section of Psycho-Oncology.

Patrick Meadors, Ph.D., LMFT
Manager, Section of Psycho-Oncology
Department of Supportive Oncology
Levine Cancer Institute
Carolinas HealthCare System

Kenneth Phelps, Ph.D., LMFT. As a faculty member in both Departments of Neuropsychiatry and Pediatrics, I have developed a sub-specialty in the treatment of youth and families living with neurologic, neurodevelopmental, and psychiatric conditions. On a typical week, children, adolescents, and their parents present to our collaborative team with complaints related to autism spectrum disorders, obsessive-compulsive disorder, epilepsy, multiple sclerosis, headache, and functional neurologic symptoms. I primarily treat those living with Tic Disorders, including Tourette's Disorder, through one of the few Tourette Centers of Excellence (see https://www.tourette.org/about-tourette/overview/centers-of-excellence/). I collaborate with pediatric movement specialists, occupational therapists, child psychologists, and child psychiatrists to deliver cohesive care to families. Given this specialization, I am currently a national faculty member through the Tourette Association of America's Behavioral Therapy Institute, which disseminates education on the evidence-based approach of Comprehensive Behavioral Intervention for Tics (CBIT). Beyond these clinical responsibilities, I teach in three psychiatric residency programs and serve as a support staff at a summer camp for children living with neurologic illness. My background working in an array of settings (OB-GYN, Family Medicine, NICU, PICU) during my MedFT rotations prepared me to partner with a range of healthcare providers. This collaboration extends beyond the clinical consultation room to grand rounds presentations, scientific inquiry, and Board or committee service.

Kenneth Phelps, Ph.D., LMFT
Associate Professor of Clinical Neuropsychiatry
Adjunct Associate Professor of Clinical Pediatrics
School of Medicine
University of South Carolina

From the examples above, it is clear that MedFTs are marketable across a wide variety of academic settings. Their diverse skill sets and training permit them to work in primary, secondary, and tertiary specialty academic departments, as well as in traditional behavioral health training programs (e.g., Marriage/Couple and Family Therapy, Medical Family Therapy, Psychiatry, Psychology, Social Work, Counseling). Advancements in training MedFTs to lead, research, execute, and fund integrated behavioral healthcare (IBHC) programs add to their marketability in these settings and beyond.

MedFT Policy and Leadership

Leadership is a *Level 5* skill on the MedFT Healthcare Continuum (Hodgson, Lamson, Mendenhall, & Tyndall, 2014). MedFTs at this level are innovators in healthcare research, administration, policy, and behavioral health programming. They advocate for patient- and family-centered care policies, alongside policies that advance parity among the behavioral health professions (e.g., reimbursement, employment prospects, grant/funding opportunities). Parity is critical for successfully run IBHC services and in systems wherein behavioral health work is carried out. It removes barriers so that employers may hire the most qualified professional for the position.

Additionally, MedFTs have held prominent roles in professional associations and organizations that are in pursuit of a better healthcare system. For example, many of the founders of the Collaborative Family Healthcare Association (CFHA) were MedFTs, licensed as marriage and family therapists and/or psychologists. The CFHA is a non-guild organization wherein membership is composed of those aligned with many different healthcare disciplines—all unified to help advance collaborative research, training, policies, and healthcare models. Examples of MedFTs who have assumed leadership positions to advance their profession include:

Randall Reitz, Ph.D., LMFT. Training in Medical Family Therapy prepared me for a diverse career that crosses clinical, administrative, advocacy, scientific, and teaching domains. In the clinical areas, I have chosen to only practice in primary care settings, providing family therapy, behavioral health consultation, group medical visits, and supervision of peer support services. I have had the fortune to practice in safety net medical clinics, inpatient hospital wards, and population-specific clinics for migrant farmers and people living with HIV. From an administration perspective, I have served as the CEO of a community health center where I led the expansion of an all-volunteer evening clinic into a full-time healthcare operation that integrated behavioral health and dental services. I also served as the executive director of the Collaborative Family Healthcare Association (CFHA), the national organization that has led the movement for collaborative- and family-oriented primary care services since 1992. In advocacy, I have led numerous healthcare transformation initiatives at the state, regional, and county levels. These include lobbying efforts that successfully passed a Colorado law that promotes integrated behavioral health services as a statewide best practice in Colorado. Within 5 years of passing this law, Colorado was the recipient of a $65 million CMMS grant to ensure that 80% of Coloradans had an integrated primary care office. At the county level, I chaired numerous governmental and citizen committees that organize healthcare services and promote best practice standards. I have also overseen several grant-funded projects that advance integration at the county and regional levels. My advanced training as a Ph.D. has allowed me many opportunities to supervise and publish clinical and professional development research and to lead numerous quality improvement projects. And finally, the broad expertise of a MedFT has served me well in my current role as the Director of Behavioral Medicine in a program where I teach family medicine residents and medical family therapy fellows.

Randall Reitz, Ph.D., LMFT
Director of Behavioral Sciences
Saint Mary's Family Medicine Residency

Ryan Anderson, Ph.D., LMFT. I graduated as part of East Carolina University's (ECU) first class of doctoral MedFT students. Since then, my career has gone through a number of twists and turns. Last year, I teamed up with a group of partners to open an innovative treatment center for young adults. Telos U—located in Orem, Utah—is a school designed to help young adults with learning disabilities, autism spectrum disorder, ADHD, process addictions, and other information processing disorders transition successfully into adult roles. The team is interdisciplinary (including couple/marriage and family therapists, social workers, substance use counselors, nurses, psychiatrists, educators, advisers, executive function coaches, residential staff, and more) and highly collaborative in nature. While the work I am doing may not be strictly conceptualized as MedFT, the training I received at ECU in integrated healthcare and fostering autonomy and community as a part of treatment is central to the philosophy and the practices of Telos U. In fact, you could accurately say that Telos U utilizes a Medical Family Therapy approach, even though it is not a classic healthcare setting.

Ryan Anderson, Ph.D., LMFT
Executive Director for Telos Discovery Space Center and
Process Addiction Specialist for Telos Companies

Jackie Williams-Reade, Ph.D., LMFT. Following internship and postdoctoral training in Pediatric Palliative Care (Johns Hopkins University), I joined the faculty at Loma Linda University in the School of Behavioral Health as the MedFT program coordinator. In this role, I have furthered the work of MedFT through training and supervising students, developing relationships and internship sites across our health sciences campus, and publishing and presenting nationally on topics including family systems interventions with pediatric chronic or life-threatening illnesses, enhancing medical professionals' compassionate communication, and the use of narrative therapy in medical settings. I have served our respective organizations through being a member of the AAMFT Elections Council, a board member for the California Division of AAMFT, and representing MedFTs on the

Collaborative Family Healthcare Association (CFHA) conference planning committee. I have also developed the MedFT Facebook page to serve as a convening tool and opportunity to share information relevant to the field of MedFT. One of my career goals is to help grow MedFT on a national and international level, with a special focus on specialty care areas. Through both my training and current roles, I am able to contribute to the field in these ways while at the same time mentoring future MedFT pioneers.

Jackie Williams-Reade, Ph.D., LMFT
Associate Professor
Department of Counseling and Family Services
Loma Linda University

The advancement of doctoral degrees and specialists in MedFT has led to positions in leadership and advocacy in a wide variety of settings. MedFTs are now serving in executive roles and leading national healthcare organizations, research teams, and healthcare entities. Whether leading or advocating for patient systems or healthcare systems, MedFTs are prepared, trained, and sought after for their relational and systemic skill sets.

Conclusion

Opportunities for MedFTs are limited only by one's passion and willingness to be told "no" at least once along the way. It may take time to acquire parity in reimbursement, correct the misinformation that is published in texts and peer reviewed articles (e.g., about diagnostic skills, research training, and/or scope of practice), amend job announcements to be written more inclusively, and motivate the federal government to allocate money for MedFT workforce development. This chapter serves as an example of what MedFTs have more recently done to advance the field. They benefited from people who believed in them, their ideas, and their abilities. They sought specialized training and opportunities to learn as much as they could about MedFT. As a result, they are now in positions such as (a) university and hospital administration; (b) health foundation administrators; (c) technical assistance specialists for integrated care; (d) grant administrators; (e) directors of institutional assessment; (f) innovators in school, law, and law-enforcement health services; and (g) leaders at the local, state, regional, and national levels—many of which were addressed in this chapter and more broadly in this text.

We encourage you, our readers, to push the boundaries of what MedFTs can do. Along the way, we hope that you will pursue training beyond this book's foci and scope. We invite you to promote workforce development, and look forward to hearing about your contributions in pioneering new territories and innovations in this exciting field. Onward!

References

Crane, D., & Christenson, J. (2014). A summary report of cost-effectiveness: Recognizing the value of family therapy in health care. In J. Hodgson, A. Lamson, T. Mendenhall, and D. Crane (Eds.), *Medical family therapy: Advanced applications* (pp. 419–436). New York, NY: Springer.

Crane, D., & Payne, S. (2011). Individual and family psychotherapy in managed care: Comparing the costs of treatment by the mental health professions. *Journal of Marital and Family Therapy, 37*, 273–289. https://doi.org/10.1111/j.1752-0606.2009.00170.x

Hodgson, J., Lamson, A., Mendenhall, T., & Crane, D. (Eds.). (2014). *Medical family therapy: Advanced applications*. New York, NY: Springer.

Hodgson, J., Lamson, A., Mendenhall, T., & Tyndall, L. (2014). Introduction to medical family therapy: Advanced applications. In J. Hodgson, A. Lamson, T. Mendenhall, and D. Crane (Eds.), *Medical family therapy: Advanced applications* (pp. 1–9). New York, NY: Springer.

Lewis, M., Myhra, L., & Walker, M. (2014). Advancing health equity in medical family therapy research. In J. Hodgson, A. Lamson, T. Mendenhall, and D. Crane (Eds.), *Medical family therapy: Advanced applications* (pp. 319–340). New York, NY: Springer.

McDaniel, S., Doherty, W., & Hepworth, J. (2014). *Medical family therapy and integrated care* (2nd ed.). Washington, DC: American Psychological Association.

McDaniel, S., Hepworth, J., & Doherty, W. (1992). *Medical family therapy: A biopsychosocial approach to families with health problems*. New York, NY: Basic Books.

Mendenhall, T., Berge, J., & Doherty, W. (2014). Engaging communities as partners in research: Advancing integrated care through purposeful partnerships. In J. Hodgson, A. Lamson, T. Mendenhall, and D. Crane (Eds.), *Medical family therapy: Advanced applications* (pp. 259–282). New York, NY: Springer.

Mendenhall, T., Pratt, K., Phelps, K., Baird, M., & Younkin, F. (2014). Advancing medical family therapy through qualitative, quantitative, and mixed-methods research. In J. Hodgson, A. Lamson, T. Mendenhall, and D. Crane (Eds.), *Medical family therapy: Advanced applications* (pp. 241–258). New York, NY: Springer.

Polaha, J., & Nolan, B. (2014). Dissemination and implementation science: Research for the real-world medical family therapist. In J. Hodgson, A. Lamson, T. Mendenhall, and D. Crane (Eds.), *Medical family therapy: Advanced applications* (pp. 301–318). New York, NY: Springer.

Williams-Reede, J., Gordon, B., & Wray, W. (2014). A primer in program evaluation for MedFTs. In J. Hodgson, A. Lamson, T. Mendenhall, and D. Crane (Eds.), *Medical family therapy: Advanced applications* (pp. 283–300). New York, NY: Springer.

Zak-Hunter, L., Berge, J., Lister, Z., Davey, M., Lynch, L., & Denton, W. (2014). Medical family therapy scientist-practitioners. In J. Hodgson, A. Lamson, T. Mendenhall, and D. Crane (Eds.), *Medical family therapy: Advanced applications* (pp. 219–240). New York, NY: Springer.

Index

A

Absenteeism, 339, 498, 507, 512, 513, 519, 522, 523, 525
Abstinence, 190, 326, 327, 334, 339, 341, 343–346, 483
A1c, 24, 28, 62, 97, 294, 360, 402
Academic, 1–3, 8, 10, 45, 67, 116–118, 120, 210, 217, 232, 413, 598
Academy of Nutrition and Dietetics, 82
Action Learning, 404
Action Research, 404
Active duty (AD), 537–539, 541, 543, 547, 556, 559, 562, 569–571
Active listening skills, 438, 441
Acute, 22, 23, 25, 30, 47, 67, 76, 87, 88, 98, 99, 105, 113, 123, 125–127, 130, 133, 151, 166, 181, 184–187, 190, 193, 196, 197, 199–201, 207, 219, 220, 234, 252, 253, 265, 293, 294, 304, 333, 362, 369, 370, 443–445, 447–451, 563, 569
Acute myocardial infraction, 126–127
Addiction, 10, 40, 102, 155, 166, 322, 325, 329, 333, 336–340, 343, 346, 483, 599
Adherence, 24, 31, 40, 63, 76, 88, 102, 105, 134, 153, 297, 375, 386, 483, 505, 521
Adolescent psychiatrists, 68, 155, 234, 248
Adolescents, 21, 22, 27, 41, 42, 47, 61, 62, 64, 65, 67–69, 76, 120, 151, 153, 155, 196, 199, 217, 218, 233, 234, 248, 249, 251, 274, 302, 310, 334, 342, 367, 408, 409, 412, 418, 566, 567, 597
Adult intensive care unit (AICU), 126–128, 138
Adults, 20–22, 24–28, 37, 40, 42, 61, 76, 87, 90, 113, 119, 124, 137, 138, 151, 182, 213, 217, 221, 225, 234, 268, 274, 281, 283, 296, 300, 302, 310, 334, 342, 343, 367, 368, 375, 385, 408, 418, 443, 451, 465, 482, 599
Advanced life support (ALS), 201, 269
Advanced practice providers (APPs), 91
Advanced practice registered nurses (APRN), 153, 467
Aerospace medical service specialists, 545
Aerospace medicine specialists/flight surgeons, 545
African American, 18, 75, 335, 360, 585
Agnostics, 483, 484
Agonal, 200
Airway with cervical spine control, breathing, circulation with control of bleeding (ABCs), 190, 200
Alanine aminotransferase (ALT), 30
Al-Anon, 345, 401
Albumin, 30
Alcohol, xiv, 40, 95, 121, 186, 195, 252, 302, 324, 346, 347, 368, 445, 502, 503, 509, 525, 527, 546, 552
Alcohol and Drug Abuse Prevention and Treatment (ADAPT) program managers, 567, 569
Alcohol/drug abuse and dependency, 190
Alcoholics Anonymous (AA), 251, 329, 344, 401, 482, 485
Alcohol Use Disorders Identification Test (AUDIT), 339, 368

Alkaline phosphatase (ALP), 30
American Academy of Pediatrics (AAP), 61, 62, 64, 65, 78
American Association of Diabetes Educators, 303, 314
American Association for Marriage and Family Therapy (AAMFT), 5, 9, 11, 157, 198, 590, 599
American Association of Pastoral Counselors, 488
American Cancer Society, 207
American College of Emergency Physicians, 184
American College of Physicians, 106
American College of Surgeons Commission on Cancer (COC), 210
American Diabetes Association (ADA), 24, 296, 299–304, 309, 509, 510, 526
American Indian (AI), 296, 303, 311, 371, 389, 402, 403, 407, 416, 585
American Medical Association (AMA), 27, 69, 190, 201, 546
American Psycho-Oncology Society, 227
American Red Cross (ARC), 437, 440
Anabolic steroids, 332
Anderson, R., 599
Anticipatory guidance, 64–67, 77
Anxiety, 26, 27, 29, 35, 39, 41, 42, 62, 87, 88, 90, 93, 97, 101–103, 119, 134, 151, 156, 158–160, 164, 166, 168–170, 172, 181, 194–196, 199, 209, 212, 214, 219, 224, 234, 238–240, 248, 250, 251, 253, 277, 278, 294, 301, 304, 310, 325, 330, 331, 341, 347, 360, 361, 364, 368, 371, 379, 381, 383, 386, 387, 440, 447, 452, 468, 474, 482, 500, 516, 517, 522–525, 540–542, 546, 549, 551, 556, 563, 564, 567
Apnea, 80, 123, 124, 308
Arterial catheterization, 138
Aspartate aminotransferase (AST), 30
Assessment and referral, 527
Assessments, 34, 36, 38, 43, 62, 64, 65, 68, 69, 78, 88, 93, 94, 97, 100, 101, 103–105, 118–120, 128–130, 133, 134, 147, 153, 154, 158, 159, 164–166, 168, 169, 172, 183, 187, 194–196, 212, 213, 215, 216, 224, 233, 234, 236, 241, 243, 245, 249, 271, 272, 277, 282, 298, 306, 307, 322–325, 336–338, 340, 345, 358, 359, 365, 367–369, 371, 372, 376, 378, 380, 382, 417, 442, 443, 446, 466–470, 472, 474, 476, 480, 481, 484, 497, 501, 504, 505, 508–510, 512, 514, 516–518, 520, 521, 527, 528, 546, 555–557, 565, 566, 585, 600
Assessment skills, 189–190
Asthma, 26, 27, 35, 61, 69, 71, 72, 76–78, 80, 125, 127, 186, 371, 418, 519
Atheists, 483, 484
Attachment-based family therapy (ABFT), 41, 42, 251
Attending physicians, 47, 96, 105, 118, 120, 185, 186, 189, 195, 196, 402, 466
Attention deficit hyperactivity disorder (ADHD), 26, 27, 41, 234, 250, 327, 331, 368, 480, 599
Atypical antipsychotic, 252, 253
Audit of Diabetes-Dependent Quality of Life, 313
Australian Journal of Pastoral Care and Health, 487

B
B12, 29
Basic life support (BLS), 190, 201
Behavioral health, 2, 17, 62–64, 67, 68, 70–77, 87, 181, 207, 263, 293, 357–359, 361–363, 365, 367–370, 372, 373, 375, 376, 379–384, 386, 388, 389, 403, 431, 466, 467, 469, 470, 472, 474–477, 585, 587, 591, 592, 594, 595, 598, 599
Behavioral healthcare facilitators (BHCF), 545
Behavioral health providers (BHPs), 12, 18–22, 34, 36, 46, 47, 63, 67, 68, 72, 76, 93, 96, 150, 152, 153, 166, 184, 187, 190, 191, 200, 211, 215, 224, 268, 277, 279, 298, 321, 324, 328, 329, 333–335, 338, 340, 341, 343, 361–363, 376, 380, 382, 408, 436, 438, 445, 466, 510, 544, 549, 568
Behavioral health technicians, 237, 545, 546
Behavioral therapy, 39, 41, 42, 76, 170, 240, 247, 343, 345, 446
Bell, J.M., 3, 20, 35, 71, 147, 193, 212, 236, 297, 322, 358, 365, 407, 434, 466, 504, 538
Beneficiaries, 541, 543, 544, 546, 570
Beneficiary counseling and assistance coordinators (BCAC), 546
Benzodiazepines, 248, 252, 330
Bereavement, 155, 170, 171, 224, 271, 272, 276, 465, 543
Berge, J., 72, 74, 77, 414, 415, 419, 584, 585
Biopsy, 225

Biopsychosocial, 2, 70, 91, 96, 98, 99, 134, 147, 149–151, 153, 159, 163, 165–167, 170, 171, 220, 221, 268, 276, 297, 305, 407, 434, 504, 520, 523, 552, 553
Biopsychosocial-spiritual (BPSS), xiii, 2, 3, 20, 26, 68, 71, 77, 118, 122, 125, 126, 130–132, 137, 147, 149, 150, 153, 159, 163, 165, 166, 193, 212, 235, 263, 275, 297, 322, 325, 339, 346, 358, 359, 362, 365, 377–384, 387, 389, 407, 434, 440, 443, 444, 446–449, 451–453, 465, 466, 468, 469, 471–477, 484, 504, 513–519, 521–523, 525, 526, 538, 591, 596
Bipolar disorder, 41, 160, 239, 240, 249, 252, 253, 368
Blood glucose, 30, 293, 300–302, 305, 306, 309, 312, 364, 365, 403
Blood glucose monitoring, 301
Blood urea nitrogen (BUN), 30
Borst, C., 590
Breech presentation, 173
Brief treatment, 26, 103, 153, 521
Bright Futures™ guidelines, 65
Bubble CPAP, 138
Buddhism, 469, 484
Burnout, 114, 115, 124, 131, 282, 447, 507, 508
Burn surface area (BSA), 201

C
CAGE Alcohol Questionnaire, 202, 572
Canadian Association for Spiritual Care, 488
Cancer, 31, 40, 115, 125, 207, 209–211, 213–215, 217, 220, 223–226, 239, 269, 281, 479
Cancer care trajectory, 7, 17, 208, 210–215, 219–222, 225
Cannabis, 332
Cao Dai, 484
Carcinoma, 225
Cardiopulmonary resuscitation (CPR), 201, 283
Cardiovascular illness, 23, 44, 88, 123, 126, 127, 302, 336, 480
Care/case manager, 119, 132
Care coordinators, 155, 236, 264, 408
Case managers, 92, 99, 166, 187, 328, 362, 476, 505, 522, 546, 563
Care managers/coordinators, 363, 546
Catheters, 126, 138
CC nurses, 120
Central nervous system depressants, 331
Central nervous system stimulants, 331
Cerebral infarction, 24, 126, 127

Cerebral palsy, 78, 125
Certified Alcohol and Drug Abuse Counselors (CADAC), 546
Certified Employee Assistance Professional (CEAP), 514, 527
Cervix, 174
Chaplains, 114, 119, 121, 132, 153, 187, 194, 195, 213, 242, 245, 267, 268, 271, 279, 436, 437, 444, 446, 464–468, 471, 474, 475, 483, 484, 559
Chemical dependency, 329, 346
Chemotherapy, 208, 210, 217, 218, 264, 278
Chest film, 201
Chest tube thoracostomy, 138
Child-centered medical home (CCMH), 64, 72, 73, 75, 78
Childhood cancer, 125
Child life specialists, 47, 119, 120, 132, 187, 268
Child psychologists, 68
Children, 22, 26, 61, 62, 64–70, 75–80, 114, 119, 120, 124–126, 131, 132, 135, 136, 187, 218, 223, 235, 274, 302, 367, 387, 403, 480, 481, 538, 542, 553, 566, 567
ChooseMyPlate.gov, 71, 72
Christianity, 469, 478, 484–486
Chronic, 25, 36, 69–70, 95, 105, 151, 245, 269, 271, 307, 382, 451–452
Chronic health conditions, 27, 90, 161, 359, 361, 369, 519
Chronic obstructive pulmonary disease (COPD), 35, 90, 95, 127, 186, 269, 386
Chronic pain, 24, 25, 88, 90, 96, 308, 408, 416, 520, 524, 546, 566, 568
Citizen health care (CHC), 405–407
Citizen professionals, 406, 409–410, 414
Civilians, 538, 539, 541, 543, 547, 551–554, 558, 559, 569–571
Classroom Action Research, 404
Clinical/organizational team, 165, 504
Clinicians, 5, 9, 11, 22, 35, 38, 46, 47, 128, 129, 131, 137, 163, 166, 168, 170, 171, 192, 196, 215, 232, 246, 247, 264, 278, 281, 305, 337, 358, 431, 443, 446, 451, 469, 471, 480, 481, 506, 514, 542, 559, 563, 568, 592, 593, 596
Closed ICUs, 118
Coag panel, 190, 201
Cognitive behavioral conjoint therapy, 451
Cognitive behavioral couples therapy (CBCT), 42, 172, 251, 342
Cognitive behavior therapy (CBT), 25, 39, 41, 42, 127, 164, 167–170, 196, 199, 212, 240, 248, 250, 252, 310, 341, 386, 390, 446, 449, 450, 478, 481, 523, 540, 564, 565

Collaboration, 2, 21, 39, 67, 74, 91, 98, 115, 118, 120, 121, 126, 128–131, 134, 163, 165, 197, 215, 231, 278, 297, 322, 359, 376–378, 404, 447, 464, 473, 474, 508, 522, 548, 596, 597
Collaborative care, 47, 67, 151, 390, 498
Collaborative Family Healthcare Association (CFHA), 6, 9, 11
Co-located care, 20, 38, 47, 91, 211, 278, 298, 358, 362, 472, 475, 516
Colorado School of Public Health's Rocky Mountain Prevention Research Center, 420
Columbia-Suicide Severity Rating Scale (C-SSRS), 454
Combat, 152, 263, 375, 541, 542, 544, 546, 549–552, 554, 555, 559, 570
Communication, 33, 34, 62–67, 70, 79, 96, 104, 119, 124–126, 130, 131, 135, 136, 151, 152, 157, 164, 167, 168, 170, 171, 188, 195, 209–211, 213, 220, 223, 233, 242, 245, 249, 267, 268, 274, 307, 337, 358, 387, 446, 474, 476, 477, 481, 499, 510, 511, 515, 516, 518, 525, 539, 542, 547, 549, 565, 568
Community, 6, 20, 63, 87, 115, 165–167, 172, 187, 218, 235, 265, 297, 328, 357, 401, 432, 467, 470, 476, 481–483, 486, 503, 542, 584, 591–593, 595, 598, 599
  approaches, 44–46, 104, 164, 172–173, 251–252, 281, 308, 311, 344–345, 388, 389, 481–483, 567–568
  engagement, 44, 401–419
  health centers, xiv, 363–365, 368, 372, 379, 380, 382, 388, 389
  health workers, 408
  professionals, 409
Community-based Participatory Action Research, 404–405
Community-based Participatory Research (CBPR), 44, 47, 311, 388, 389, 401, 404–423
Community-based Research, 404
Community-oriented primary care, 401
Compassionate presence, 188, 438, 441, 443, 444
Compassion fatigue, 7, 114, 115, 124, 131, 157, 165, 275, 445, 446
Compensation benefits, 508
Complementary and alternative medicine, 25
Complementary and alternative treatments, 269
Complete blood count (CBC), 30, 31
Confidentiality, 216, 232, 339, 359, 366, 367, 374, 375, 464, 466, 499, 506, 523, 560

Congenital heart abnormalities/diseases (CHDs), 125
Congestive heart failure (CHF), 90, 95, 269
Consent, 31, 73, 115, 274, 366, 367, 374, 375, 377, 412
Coronary care (CCU), 113
Corporate safety officers, 504, 505
Cost-effectiveness, 38, 41, 135, 384, 510, 522, 526
Cost report, 390
Countertransference, 252
Crasher, 201
Creatinine, 30
Critical care settings, 212
Critical care/units/teams, 113, 114, 116–122, 124, 126, 128, 131–134, 137, 215, 541
Critical Incident Stress Management (CISM), 448, 449
C-section (Cesarean birth), 161, 174
Cultures, 65, 93, 104, 124, 165, 217, 240, 273, 274, 281, 303, 363, 403, 407, 408, 411, 412, 414, 441, 470, 471, 480, 481, 486, 498, 499, 510, 521, 527, 543, 549, 552, 558–560
Curative care, 266
Curative treatment, 226, 266

D
Daoism, 485
Dead body (DB), 433
Dead on arrival (DOA), 201
Death, 19, 24, 114, 115, 121, 123, 125, 126, 128–130, 137, 148, 149, 153, 173, 174, 187, 197, 207, 209, 224, 265, 271–275, 277, 278, 301, 302, 374, 437, 442, 446, 468, 485, 558
De-escalation skills, 191
Delirium, 121, 183, 234, 244, 270
Delivering bad news, 191–192, 198
Department of Defense (DOD), 537, 542, 543, 556, 563
Department of Homeland Security (DHS), 434
Dependents, 66, 169, 198, 323, 411, 412, 537, 538, 543, 545–549, 557, 567
Deployments, 446, 447, 541, 547, 549–553, 559, 566
Depression, 19, 24, 26–29, 35, 39, 41, 42, 44, 62, 87, 88, 90, 93, 94, 97, 102, 125–127, 156–160, 165, 166, 168, 169, 172, 181, 189, 194, 196, 199, 212, 217, 223, 233, 239, 240, 246, 249, 251, 271, 277, 294, 296, 304, 305, 310, 331, 360, 361, 364, 368, 370, 372, 379, 381, 386,

387, 440, 452, 468, 474, 478, 479, 482, 498, 500–504, 512, 516, 517, 519, 522–525, 546, 551, 556, 557, 563, 564, 566, 567, 585, 594
Detroit Community-Academic Urban Research Center, 420
Developmentally and age-appropriate care, 78
Diabetes, 23, 24, 27, 29, 43, 44, 66, 69, 72, 76–79, 88, 89, 92, 99–102, 125, 127, 194, 198, 239, 242, 294–311, 360, 361, 363, 369, 371, 372, 379, 381, 385, 387, 389, 402, 403, 405–410, 412, 416, 418, 464, 472, 483
   educators, 92, 298, 303, 363
   health educators, 363
   health profile, 313
   management, 92, 297, 300–303, 309–311, 363, 387, 406, 408, 410
Diabetes Quality Of Life Measure, 313
Diabetes Self-Management Questionnaire, 313
Diabetic ketoacidosis, 312
Diagnosis, 24, 27, 28, 31, 40, 62, 64, 69, 73, 79, 80, 87, 90, 105, 121, 123, 125–128, 155, 161, 162, 186, 191, 207, 208, 210, 212–214, 218, 220, 233, 234, 236–239, 241, 266, 271, 280, 283, 295, 298, 300, 301, 323–325, 330, 337, 359, 365, 368, 369, 381, 383, 509, 525, 554, 556, 557, 594
Dialectical-Behavioral Therapy (DBT), 248
Dieticians, 23, 36, 73, 92, 100, 298, 382, 403
Differential diagnosis, 105
Dilation and curettage (D&C), 174
Directors of occupational health, 505
Direct patient care, 67, 115, 544
Disaster-preparedness, xiv, 444–446, 452
Discrimination, 157, 158, 241
Disease-free survival (DFS), 226
Disorder(s), 20, 26, 27, 31, 35, 39–43, 64, 67, 68, 75, 79, 80, 94, 96, 116, 123, 125, 151, 155, 156, 158–162, 168, 170, 189, 193, 224, 231, 233, 234, 238–240, 244, 247–253, 266, 293, 296, 298, 299, 305–307, 312, 321, 322, 324–327, 329, 330, 333, 336, 339, 340, 343, 344, 360, 370, 371, 379, 381, 386, 387, 440, 443, 451, 479, 508, 509, 522, 523, 541, 542, 558, 597, 599
Diversity, 23, 32, 97, 124, 138, 185, 198, 273, 303, 335, 358, 403, 442–443, 470, 478, 538, 544, 584
Documentation, 187, 371, 373, 384, 506, 516
Do not resuscitate (DNR), 194, 283
Doulas, 154

Drug Abuse Screening Test (DAST-7), 520
Drugs, 128, 138, 161, 321, 322, 328, 337, 341
Dual roles, 502, 509
Dyadic coping inventory, 314
Dynamics, xiii, 2, 37, 42, 62, 66, 67, 72–74, 128, 167, 211, 220–222, 235, 236, 246, 278, 335, 343, 499, 517, 538, 542, 549, 551, 559
Dyspnea, 190

E

Early-intervention, 64
Ectopic pregnancy, 149, 174
Ego-dystonic, 160, 170, 233, 252
Elderly, 26, 28, 87, 183, 263
Electroconvulsive therapy (ECT), 240, 253
Electronic health record (EHR), 19, 33, 361, 365, 368, 369, 372–375, 379, 472
Emergency department physicians, 185
Emergency management, 435–438, 445–447, 505
Emergency medical technicians (EMTs), 186, 196
Emergency medicine, xiv, 21, 120, 184, 194, 195, 431, 466
Emergency medicine clerks, 188, 436
Emergency planning coordinators, 505
Emergency room technicians (ERTs), 186
Emotionally focused couples therapy (EFT), 42, 171, 172, 223, 250, 251, 451
Emotionally focused therapy (EFT), 42
Emotional regulation, 248, 253
Empathy, 102, 131, 135–137, 156, 164, 191, 275, 280, 471, 482, 595
Employee assistance professional, 527
Employee assistance programs (EAP), 466, 467, 497–507, 515–518
   directors, 505
   model, 499, 528
Employees, 409, 467, 497–499, 503–509, 512–514, 519–528
Enabling, 73, 253, 312, 357
Encounter rate, 390
Encounters, 64, 70, 99, 101, 102, 131, 135, 162, 167, 188, 200, 369–372, 377, 390, 468, 472, 516, 541, 542, 563
Endocrine disorders, 125, 296, 305–307, 312
Endocrinologists, 67, 77, 296, 298, 302, 408
Endocrinology, xiv, 27, 61, 63, 74, 125, 155, 293–313
Engel, G., 2, 3, 20, 35, 71, 91, 113, 114, 118, 147, 193, 212, 236, 241, 263, 297, 322, 325, 358, 365, 407, 434, 441, 466, 504, 538, 564, 566

Ergonomists, 506
Ethics, 167, 173, 222, 277, 279, 304, 374, 412–413, 470, 485
Eucharist, 464, 485
Exceptional Family Member Program (EFMP) Staff, 546
Exposure and response prevention (E/RP), 160, 170, 233, 240, 246, 247, 250
Expressed emotion (EE), 249, 253
External behavioral health consultants (EBHC), 545, 546
Eye movement desensitization and reprocessing (EMDR), 196, 446, 449, 450, 563, 564

F
Faculty appointments, xv, 584, 596–598
Familismo, 45, 335
Family(ies), 2, 17, 18, 62, 87, 88, 113, 115, 118, 119, 121–126, 128–137, 147, 148, 181, 207, 208, 231, 263, 293, 321, 358, 401, 403, 431, 434, 463–478, 480–484, 497–499, 504, 507, 508, 513–520, 524–528, 537, 538, 584, 585, 587–590, 592–594, 596, 597
Family accommodation, 250, 253
Family and Medical Leave Act (FMLA), 510, 528
Family approaches, 40–44, 101–103, 135–137, 171–172, 249–251, 280–281, 310–311, 342–344, 386–389, 480–481, 524–525, 565–567
Family-based approaches, 43, 310, 342
Family-based care, 62, 64, 65, 78, 137
Family-centered, 2, 9, 65, 211, 212, 222, 225, 252, 278, 357, 383, 418, 538
Family-centered care, 3, 65, 77, 78, 119, 131, 135, 136, 212, 221, 225, 302, 587, 593, 598
Family cognitive behavioral therapy, 41, 42
Family-focused care, 78
Family focused grief therapy (FFGT), 223, 224, 280
Family medicine, xiv, 7, 8, 11, 12, 36, 46, 183–185, 294, 297, 409, 431, 466, 539, 585, 588, 594, 596, 597, 599
Family medicine provider, 17, 21, 22, 24, 26–28, 31, 409
Family Relationships Index (FRI), 224
Family therapy, xiii–xv, 2, 4–6, 8, 10, 11, 36, 46, 61–77, 88, 98, 99, 116, 129, 130, 132–134, 138, 147–155, 164, 165, 169, 181–202, 209, 213, 231, 242, 244–247, 249, 251, 252, 368, 372, 379, 380, 382, 389, 414, 415, 419, 444–446, 452, 463–467, 470, 473–476, 497–507, 537, 538, 540–559, 561, 563–567, 583, 586–595, 598, 599
Fasting blood sugar, 300
Federal Emergency Management Administration (FEMA), 437, 438
Federally qualified health center (FQHC), 390
Fellowship training, 21, 22, 47, 234, 591
Fertility, 27, 148, 149
FICA Spiritual History Tool, 470
Financial, xiii, 12, 37, 46, 93, 97, 100, 152, 157, 187, 197, 211, 245, 246, 268, 308, 324, 326, 328, 338, 346, 362, 366, 375, 378, 384, 388, 435, 497, 499, 503, 508, 510–512, 522, 525, 527, 544, 546
Financial teams, 187
Forensic interviewing, 253
Forgiveness, 223, 272, 465, 482, 485
Front desk staff, 363
Functional family therapy (FFT), 41, 42, 250, 343

G
General internists, 90, 105
Generalized Anxiety Disorder (GAD), 26, 34, 42, 159, 199, 240, 243, 276, 360, 368, 386, 556
Generalized Anxiety Disorder 7-item scale (GAD-7), 520
General pediatrician, 4, 22, 44, 61–63, 66, 67, 72, 75–78, 218
Genetic counselors, 93, 154, 166, 213
Gestational diabetes, 24, 164, 166, 296, 298, 300, 309
Glucagon, 301
Glucagon administration, 302
Glucose, 24, 28, 29, 79, 127, 301, 312
Glycated hemoglobin (A1c) test, 28, 30, 62, 94, 97, 300, 305, 312, 402, 403
Glycemic index, 76, 309, 312
God, 184, 274, 441, 463, 464, 470, 478, 484–486
Grace, 485
Green Cross Academy of Traumatology, 454
Grief, 114, 115, 124, 128, 129, 131, 155, 168, 187, 192, 209, 214, 223–225, 271, 272, 275, 276, 280, 546, 551, 555
Gunshot wound (GSW), 190, 194, 201
Gynecology, xiv, 21, 22, 147–155, 164, 165, 169, 173

H

Hallucinogens, 332
Harsh, J., 88, 89, 98, 99, 596
Health, 2, 17, 87, 147, 211, 231, 263, 293, 321, 357, 463, 537, 538, 540–559, 563–567
 behavior changes, 65, 72, 73, 94, 95, 98, 100, 102, 369, 384, 483
 behaviors, 66, 88, 94, 99, 100, 198, 243, 363, 364, 371, 384, 388, 390, 483, 546
 centers, 239, 362–384, 389
 disparities, 32, 131, 165–167, 303, 375, 376, 390, 416, 557
 educators, 76, 92, 281, 298, 303, 363, 408
 literacy, 31, 32, 371, 376
 risks, 364, 498, 512
Health and Social Care Chaplaincy Journal, 488
Healthcare, 2, 3, 5, 7, 11, 17, 61, 89, 91–93, 96, 97, 99, 103, 105, 113, 118, 119, 121–126, 128, 130, 131, 135–137, 181, 219, 241, 263, 273, 275, 276, 296, 357, 404, 434, 463–469, 471–477, 479, 480, 482–484, 539, 559, 583, 584
 professionals, 3, 22, 91, 118, 124, 131, 153, 275, 283, 297, 405, 445, 473, 479, 498, 541
 team, 20, 23, 33, 37, 38, 62–64, 67, 73, 74, 77, 78, 92, 97, 99, 100, 102–104, 114, 123, 126, 129–131, 136, 149, 154, 155, 242, 246, 265, 271, 272, 274, 276–278, 338, 339, 366, 367, 369, 370, 375–379, 383, 389, 390, 466, 468, 472, 475, 498–502, 514, 517
Health coaches (HCs), 68, 359, 360, 363, 364
Health unit coordinators (HUCs), 188, 363, 408, 436
Healthy eating, 23, 42, 44, 297, 364, 369, 372
Healthy people 2020, 71, 72
Heart disease, 23, 24, 90, 95, 97, 98, 125, 163, 313
Hematocrit, 30
Hemoglobin, 30, 300
Hemoglobin A1c (A1c), 24, 28, 30, 62, 94, 97, 360, 402, 403
Hepworth, J., 6, 11
Higher power, 345, 358, 470, 478, 480, 484–486
High-frequency oscillation, 138
Hinduism, 469, 484, 485
Hispanic, 296, 335, 391, 585
History and Physical (H&P), 105
Hodgson, J., 5, 7–9, 11, 12, 36, 46, 231, 368, 372, 379, 380, 382, 389, 463–467, 470, 473–476, 497–507, 584–600
Holistic care, 17, 46, 68, 77, 187, 305, 311
Home health aides (Hospice), xiv, 28, 80, 211, 214, 266–269, 276, 464
Homicidality, 160, 166, 187, 189, 233, 237, 378, 443, 444
HOPE Approach to Spiritual Assessment, 488
Hospice care, 211, 263, 265–273, 275–282
Hospital corpsmen, 546
Hospitalists, 90–92, 101
Hotspotting, 45–47
HR knowledge, 510, 511
Human resource managers, 511
Human subjects protection, 216, 412–413
Hyperglycemia, 30, 301
Hypertension, 23–26, 31, 33, 35, 88, 90, 92, 97, 105, 127, 161, 313, 371, 379, 381, 540
Hypoglycemia, 29, 125, 301, 302, 306
Hysterectomy, 174

I

ICU acquired weakness, 138
Illness, 6, 17, 62, 87, 113, 153, 185, 207, 231, 263, 296, 325, 358, 418, 436, 468, 503, 546, 590
Immigrant, 45
Impaired fasting glucose (IFG), 312
Incident Command, 432, 435–437, 443, 444, 446
Industrial Action Research, 404
Infertility, 152, 155, 160, 164, 165, 171, 172, 217, 592
Inhalants, 332
Innovations in MedFT, 583–600
Inpatients, 25, 26, 38, 40, 43, 44, 95, 102, 120, 132, 133, 153, 173, 194, 198, 208, 237, 272, 296, 302, 306, 378, 414, 463, 479, 500, 591, 598
Installation, 538, 542, 547, 548, 559–562
Insulin, 24, 78, 79, 89, 94, 296, 298–301, 305–307, 309, 371
Insulin administration, 302
Integrated behavioral health care (IBHC), xv, 3, 18, 19, 36, 70, 73, 74, 122, 123, 130, 137, 147, 151, 159, 165–168, 173, 241, 321, 322, 324, 326, 327, 334, 335, 340, 344, 345, 359, 362, 365, 367, 370, 373–377, 384, 386, 477, 498, 500, 502, 504, 507, 512, 513, 516–519, 523, 526, 538, 563, 566, 569, 591, 598
Integrated care, 10, 21, 32, 166, 232, 358, 360, 377, 584, 588–590, 593, 600
Integrative behavioral couple therapy (IBCT), 250

Intensive care unit (ICU), 113, 116–122, 126–138
Intensive outpatient treatment (IOP), 334
Intensivists, 117, 118, 120, 121, 133
Interdisciplinary, 10, 11, 17, 43, 64, 70, 118, 126, 166, 167, 197, 222, 231, 235, 237, 263, 266, 295, 308, 324, 329, 338, 339, 361, 418, 431, 438, 447, 465, 467, 504, 540, 549, 556, 584–587, 599
Interdisciplinary research, xv, 584–587
Internal behavioral health consultants, 546
Internal medicine, xiv, 22, 88, 98, 99, 596
International Committee of the Red Cross, 454
International Critical Incident Stress Foundation (ICISF), 438
International Diabetes Federation, 314
International Psycho-Oncology Society, 227
Internists, 87, 90, 105
Interpersonal psychotherapy (IPT), 39, 164, 168–170, 249
Interprofessional collaboration, 38, 131, 165
Interventions, 17, 64, 93, 116, 147, 186, 208, 233, 265, 298, 324, 363, 405, 433, 469, 499, 538, 584
  brief, 24, 26, 36, 101, 103, 190, 245, 279, 307, 363, 382, 476, 501, 564, 565
  family-based, 40, 43, 76, 199, 222, 386, 587
Intervention crisis, 219, 237, 251, 328, 370, 371, 499, 546, 548
Intimacy-Enhancing Couples Therapy (IECT), 223
Intimate partner violence (IPV), 553, 565, 566
Intracranial hemorrhage, 123, 126, 127
Intrauterine fetal demise (IFUD), 161
Intraventricular hemorrhage (IVH), 123
Intubation, 138
Involuntary commitment, 253
Islam, 328, 469, 484–486

J

Jaundice, 123
Jesus Christ, 484–486
Joining behaviors, 366
Joint Commission on Accreditation of Healthcare Organization (JCAHO), 467
Journal of Health Care Chaplaincy, 488
Judaism, 469, 484, 486
Juvenile Diabetes Research Foundation, 314

K

Ketone monitoring, 302
Knowledge, xiv, 3, 18, 26, 33, 35, 37, 38, 66, 68–70, 72–74, 77, 90, 97–100, 114, 117, 122, 123, 128–130, 133, 137, 156, 163–165, 171, 173, 190, 194, 195, 220, 222, 232, 242, 244, 246, 249, 251, 272, 276, 277, 281, 298, 304–308, 311, 335, 336, 339, 340, 342, 363, 365, 372, 378–384, 389, 390, 517, 552, 559

L

Lab technicians, 364
Lactation consultants, 154
Latina/Latino, 32, 45, 75, 136, 296, 376, 391
Lamson, A., 1–13, 116, 129, 130, 132–134, 138, 147–155, 164, 165, 169, 357–390, 497–507, 537, 538, 540–559, 563–567, 584–587
Lantus, 309, 313
Latino families (Latino), 45, 136
Leadership, xv, 2, 3, 35, 244, 304, 363, 381, 414, 416, 421, 445, 467, 475, 477, 504, 507–511, 514, 517, 554, 566, 584, 591, 593, 598–600
Leave/disability managers, 505, 506
Lesbian, gay, bisexual (LGB), 537, 566
Lesbian, gay, bisexual, and transgender (LGBT), 157–159
Life cycle, 150, 152, 167
Life events checklist (LEC), 454
Lifemaps, 480, 481
Lifespan, 23, 26, 28, 35, 41, 136, 147, 154, 165, 365, 381, 417, 538
Lifestyle habits, 40, 296, 298, 310
Linking human systems approach, 452
Literacy, 363, 376
Localized, 223, 434
Lord's Prayer, 464, 486
Loss, 6, 104, 114, 115, 124, 129–131, 137, 148–150, 152, 155, 161, 162, 164, 165, 167–169, 171, 174, 187, 224, 249, 263, 265, 270, 271, 275, 276, 280, 328, 358, 435, 451, 465, 511, 554, 555
Loss of consciousness (LOC), 201

M

Malignant, 226
Malnutrition, 23, 61, 79, 124, 134, 270
Management consultation, 503, 528
Maudsley family therapy, 41
McDaniel, S., 6, 8, 11, 588
Meadors, P., 596
Meaning-making, 265, 271, 278, 387
Mechanical ventilation, 116, 126, 127

Index 611

MedFT healthcare continuum, xiv, xv, 3, 12, 34–38, 46, 70–72, 74, 97–101, 128–134, 163–167, 193–197, 219–222, 241–247, 275–279, 305–308, 335–340, 378–384, 413–417, 443–447, 471–477, 502, 513–515, 517, 558–563
Medical assistants (MAs), 22, 182, 185, 237, 373, 377, 544
Medical corps officers, 546
Medical directors, 268, 324, 505, 506
Medical evaluation board case managers, 546
Medical family therapy (MedFT), 1, 2, 6, 7, 10, 11, 17–46, 72, 74, 77, 87–104, 113–137, 147–173, 184, 207–227, 231, 263, 296, 322, 368, 372, 379, 380, 382, 389, 414, 415, 419, 431–452, 463–484, 497–528, 537, 538, 540–559, 563–567, 588–590
Medically unexplained symptoms (MUS), 95, 96
Medical office assistants (MOA), 364
Medical oncologists, 210
Medical receptionists, 92
Medical residents, 185, 197, 436
Medical–surgical include coronary care (MSICU), 113
Medication management, 40, 133, 233, 247, 371, 525, 560
Medications, 22–25, 31, 33, 43, 63, 70, 73, 74, 88–92, 96, 97, 99, 100, 102, 105, 117, 119, 128, 133, 153–155, 161, 162, 183, 185, 195, 196, 210, 212, 233, 236, 237, 239, 240, 242–244, 246, 265, 268, 270, 283, 296, 300, 307–310, 327, 329, 331, 339, 363–365, 371
Meditative prayer, 478
Menarche, 150, 151, 164
Mendenhall, T., xiii–xv, 12, 192, 304, 414, 415, 419, 444–446, 452, 584–587
Menopause, 151–153, 155, 162–164, 167, 171
Mental health, 9, 17, 20, 22, 26, 27, 29, 32, 35–38, 40–44, 46, 62, 65, 68, 69, 79, 114, 128, 151, 153, 156, 158, 164, 167, 170, 172, 181, 211, 242–246, 251, 276, 295, 304, 305, 307, 337, 357, 359–365, 367–372, 375, 381–387, 389, 431–432, 440, 444, 463, 475, 476, 503, 517, 521, 523, 525, 527, 539, 546–549, 555, 557, 566, 567, 593
　service specialists, 547
　specialists, 268, 547
　technicians, 237
Mental health treatment coordinators (MHTC), 548

Metabolic syndrome, 313
Metastasis, 264
Metformin, 24, 62, 305
Meyer, D., 586
Military, xiv, 7, 166, 435, 537, 538, 540–559, 563–567
Military family life consultants (MFLC), 542, 547
Military health system (MHS), 541, 543–545, 562
Military service coordinators (MSC), 547
Military service members, 550, 555, 564
Military sexual trauma (MST), 553, 557, 566
Mindfulness, 25, 31, 115, 160, 172, 248, 479, 480, 482, 484, 498, 501, 502, 521, 540, 564
Mindfulness-based interventions, 172, 479–480, 541
Mixed-methods approaches, 410
Mood, 29, 125, 151, 158–160, 167–169, 194, 233, 238, 239, 249, 278, 306, 325, 371, 444, 521, 551, 558, 585
Mood stabilizer, 240
Moral injuries, 554–555
Motivational interviewing (MI), 102, 248, 309, 338, 341, 384, 540
Motor vehicle accident (MVA), 183, 190, 194, 198
Muism, 486
Multidimensional family therapy (MDFT), 41, 342
Multi-family groups, 43
Muslim, 464, 478, 486

N

Narcotics, 252, 331, 345
National Cancer Institute (NCI), 207, 210
National Child Traumatic Stress Network (NCTS), 438
National Comprehensive Cancer Network Distress Thermometer, 226
National Incident Management System (NIMS), 434, 444
Necrotizing enterocolitis, 123, 124
Neonatal, 22, 113, 115, 122–124, 135, 137, 138
Neonatal intensive care unit (NICU), 7, 48, 61, 79, 113–115, 119, 122–124, 128, 131, 154, 597
Neonatologists, 154
Neonatology, 61
Neuromuscular blockers, 138
Nonacademic, 117, 118

Normal saline (NS), 190, 201
Nurse practitioners (NPs), 22, 33, 63, 91, 116, 133, 153, 185, 236, 298, 364, 379, 408
Nurses, 99, 113, 114, 116–118, 120, 133, 209, 215, 221, 236, 242, 245, 252, 305, 338, 373, 377, 409, 501, 504, 506, 518, 522, 584, 596
Nurses/medical assistants (MAs), 2, 22, 36, 43, 47, 67, 92, 114, 117, 118, 120, 121, 133, 153–155, 183, 185, 186, 211, 212, 221, 222, 236, 267, 268, 298, 324, 334, 335, 344, 345, 362, 364, 372, 376, 379, 382, 383, 403, 408, 436, 467, 471, 544, 545, 599
Nutrition, 23, 40, 67, 69, 70, 78, 79, 92, 116, 122, 134, 161, 193, 269, 298, 303, 304, 308, 325, 369, 371, 408, 587
Nutritionist, 27, 33, 68, 324, 328, 336–338, 340, 345, 362, 379, 408

O

Obesity, 26, 27, 45, 61, 62, 65, 66, 69–72, 74, 76–80, 88, 94, 100, 161, 303, 313, 360, 369, 371, 387, 412, 416, 418, 519, 585, 587
Obesity Action Coalition, 82
Obsessive Compulsive Disorder (OCD), 42, 156, 160, 168, 232–234, 240, 246, 247, 250, 252, 253, 597
Obstetrics, xiv, 21, 22, 147–155, 164, 165, 169, 584
Occupational health, 499–502, 504–506, 528
Occupational therapists, 92, 121, 237, 268, 597
Oncologists, 207, 208, 210, 211, 213, 215, 217, 219, 221, 222, 264, 268
Oncology, 155, 184, 208, 268, 592, 596, 597
  nurses, 210, 212, 264
  social workers, 211
  team, 212, 220–222, 225
On-site incident response, 528
Open ICU, 116–118
Operational, 35, 37, 46, 73, 131, 133, 135, 197, 245, 246, 279, 308, 359, 384, 484, 510–512, 525, 545
Organizational development (OD), 499, 505–507, 528
Organizational development directors, 505
Organizational needs assessment, 528
Organizations, xv, 8, 11, 12, 32, 44, 45, 65, 251, 265, 269, 277, 279, 283, 308, 345, 389, 401, 404, 409, 413, 416, 421, 434–438, 440, 443, 482, 483, 497–499, 502–513, 525, 527, 528, 552, 554, 559, 562, 598–600

Outpatient, 21, 31, 35, 68, 87, 90, 91, 99, 117, 132, 152, 153, 187, 213, 215, 221, 232–234, 239, 241, 244–246, 248, 249, 252, 253, 267, 324, 328, 333, 338–340, 342, 344, 464, 466, 476, 518, 519, 543, 547, 587, 591, 592
Overweight/obesity, 23, 44, 79

P

Pain, 23–25, 40, 44, 88, 90, 94, 96, 102, 103, 121, 132, 134, 148, 151, 152, 155, 164–166, 168, 170, 171, 174, 208, 214, 265, 266, 270, 273, 301–303, 308, 331, 408, 416, 480, 500, 502, 513, 516, 517, 520, 521, 523–525, 539–541, 546, 566
Palliative care, xiv, 21, 123, 126, 131, 208, 209, 211, 215, 219, 224, 264, 266, 267, 269–272, 276–278, 281, 466
  coordinators, 155
  nurses, 268
  physicians, 211
  specialists, 211
  teams, 123
Palliative/Hospice physician/medical directors, 268
Palliative treatment, 226
Panic, 159, 169, 181, 238
Parenting interventions, 43
Participatory Action Development, 404
Participatory Action Learning, 404
Participatory Action Research, 404
Participatory Research, 388–390, 404–409
Patient advocates, 547, 548
Patient aligned care teams (PACTs), 548
Patient care technicians, 92
Patient-centered, 359, 369, 386, 387, 389
  approach, 25, 39, 119, 384
  communication, 387
Patient Health Questionnaire (PHQ/PHQ9), 304, 360, 501, 520
Patient Health Questionnaire-9 (PHQ-9), 106, 520
Patient relations representatives (PRR), 547
Patients, 2, 17, 61, 62, 64, 65, 67, 70, 71, 73–78, 87, 113–128, 130–138, 147, 181, 207, 231, 263, 293, 321, 357, 372, 379–382, 401, 436, 464, 498, 501, 514–517, 525, 538, 585, 587, 592, 594, 596, 597
Patient sitters, 188
Pediatricians, 67, 72, 73
Pediatric Intake Form, 81
Pediatric intensive care (PICU), 7, 61, 113–115, 119, 122, 124–126, 128, 131, 136, 597

Pediatric patient-centered medical homes (PPMH), 61
Pediatric primary care medical home (PCMH), 75, 544, 571
Pediatrics, xiv, 7, 22, 64–70, 72–74, 77, 154, 184, 185, 268, 380, 587, 597
  asthma, 69, 76
  audiology, 79
  audiology and speech pathology, 61
  behavioral health providers, 68
  diabetes, 76, 387
  dietician and/ nutritionists, 68
  endocrinology, 61, 63, 79
  gastroenterology, 61
  hematology, 61, 79
  nephrology, 61, 79
  obesity, 66, 69, 74, 76, 77, 79, 587
  oncology, 61, 79, 212, 215, 595
  orthopedics, 61, 80
  palliative care, 61, 274, 599
  PEDS, 115
  pulmonary, 61, 80
  rheumatology, 61, 80
  social workers, 68
  speech pathology, 79
  subspecialists, 67
  urology, 61, 80
Pediatric Symptom Checklist (PSC), 27, 368
Peer support specialists, 548
Perinatal distress, 156–158, 160, 164, 168, 170
Perinatologists, 149, 155
Peri/post-partum, 592
Personalismo, 45
Personal physicians, 268
Petitionary prayer, 478, 479
Pharmacists, 23, 33, 36, 43, 92, 117, 118, 121, 133, 185, 237, 268, 298, 379, 382, 436
Pharmacology, 234, 239–243, 309
Pharmacotherapy, 121, 133, 169, 239, 327, 337, 340, 346
Phelps, K., 147–155, 164, 165, 169, 231, 597
Physical activity, 25, 40, 44, 63, 69, 70, 77, 78, 95, 296, 297, 300–303, 308–310, 364, 369, 371, 372, 385, 387, 402, 410, 412
Physical and occupational therapists, 92, 268
Physical dependence, 332, 339, 346, 347
Physical Evaluation Board Liaison Officers (PEBLO), 547
Physical therapists, 23, 33, 92, 118, 121, 134, 379, 476
Physician(s), 5, 7, 10–12, 18, 20–23, 26–28, 32, 33, 43, 47, 67, 68, 78, 88, 89, 91, 93, 96, 105, 114, 116–118, 120, 124, 136, 153–155, 185, 186, 188, 189, 194–196, 208, 210, 231, 234–236, 267, 268, 273, 277, 294, 305, 364, 376, 379, 402, 403, 408, 436, 466, 467, 544, 547, 584, 585, 592, 593
Physician assistants (PAs), 22, 91, 116, 153, 155, 183, 185, 436, 466
Physician extenders, 20, 136, 185, 186, 403, 408, 436
Physiology/physiological, 121, 147, 156, 190, 247, 248, 295, 296, 299, 321, 323–325, 328, 330, 331, 335, 337, 498
Placenta previa, 161, 174
Plainviews E-Newsletter, 488
Platelet count, 31
Police and other security personnel, 186, 436
Policy, xiii–xv, 2, 3, 5–7, 9, 12, 33–35, 37, 71, 130, 131, 134, 135, 137, 163–166, 193, 195, 241, 242, 244, 246, 275, 281, 305, 307, 337, 339, 340, 370, 379, 383, 384, 443, 445, 447, 471–474, 497, 504, 506, 510, 514–517, 519, 526, 563, 584, 591, 593, 598–600
Polydrug abuse, 346
Polysubstance abuse, 330
Population health, 26, 33, 45, 46, 92, 379, 390, 483, 525
Pories, M.L., 586
Postpartum psychosis, 160, 169
Post-traumatic stress (PTS), 125, 137, 189, 193, 247, 250, 443, 447, 500, 501, 539, 549, 555–557, 567
Post-traumatic stress disorder (PTSD), 162, 194, 199, 217, 218, 368, 440, 444, 448–452, 481, 543, 550, 552, 554–557, 559, 560, 564, 565, 567
Post-treatment phase of cancer, 217–219
Pratt, K., 72, 74, 77
Prayer, 193, 213, 273, 464, 465, 469, 471, 477–479, 486
Pre-Diabetes Screening Test, 313
Preeclampsia, 161, 164, 174
Pregnancy, 28, 125, 148, 149, 151–158, 160–164, 171–174, 300, 309, 409, 585
Pregnancy loss, 152, 161, 164, 167
Preterm delivery, 174
Preterm labor, 161, 174
Prevention, 45, 64, 65, 68, 69, 71, 72, 75, 76, 87, 90, 95, 121, 147, 150, 160, 162, 173, 207, 231, 234, 263, 296, 298, 337, 340, 363, 409, 410, 412, 436, 450, 521–522, 525, 538, 553, 565
Preventive care, 22, 24, 26, 44, 544
Previable delivery, 174

Primary care, xiv, 3, 17, 20–28, 32, 34, 36, 38–45, 47, 61, 62, 64, 67, 69–73, 75, 77, 78, 88, 90–93, 95, 97, 99, 147, 148, 154, 156, 187, 234, 239, 296–298, 305, 357, 359, 360, 365, 367, 371, 380, 382, 384, 386, 387, 389, 391, 401, 408, 417, 465, 470, 498, 499, 512, 523, 544, 546, 549, 554, 556, 564, 565, 583, 591, 592, 594, 598, 599
Primary care manager (PCM), 545–547
Primary Care-Mental Health Integration (PC-MHI) Staff, 549
Primary care providers (PCPs), 20, 22, 28, 34, 36, 43, 62, 70, 71, 89–92, 95, 99, 101, 118, 119, 147, 154, 239, 243, 268, 295–297, 299, 303, 304, 307, 311, 322–324, 328, 332, 343, 345, 359, 360, 364, 367, 371, 377, 380, 382, 402, 409, 446, 516, 539, 541, 545, 548, 557
Privileged Mental Health Providers, 547
Probation officers, 10, 322, 324, 327–329, 333, 334, 337, 338, 345
Procedures, 23, 28–31, 37, 45, 66, 119, 131, 136, 153, 155, 185–187, 199, 210, 213, 246, 301, 359, 364, 374, 413, 435, 467, 503–505, 507, 528, 545, 560
Professional Quality of Life Measure (Version 5), 454
Progress/encounter note, 277, 372
Progressive care units (PACUs), 113
Promoting health project (PHP), 45
Promotoras, 362, 391, 408
Psychiatric care coordinators, 236
Psychiatric illnesses, 158, 238–240, 242
Psychiatric-mental health nurse practitioners, 236
Psychiatrists, 8, 10, 77, 155, 211, 212, 231–239, 242, 245, 264, 324, 326, 327, 334–336, 338, 339, 343–345, 466, 523, 547, 596, 597, 599
Psychiatry, xiv, 10, 150, 155, 185, 199, 208, 231, 362, 363, 587, 588, 598
Psychoactive substances, 331, 332
Psychoeducation, 36, 40, 72, 114, 115, 127, 134, 152, 167–171, 185, 211, 216, 218, 219, 222, 233, 236, 240, 244, 248, 251, 276, 278–280, 310, 333, 337, 370, 381, 382, 408, 414, 438, 444, 445, 451, 452, 475–477, 482–483, 517, 518, 521–525, 551, 565, 566
Psychological anxiety, 158
Psychological debriefing (PD), 448
Psychological decompensation, 181
Psychological dependence, 332
Psychological depression, 158
Psychological distress, 88, 152, 153, 158–160, 167, 170, 188, 212, 223–224, 449, 480, 550
Psychological First Aid (PFA), 187, 193–195, 200, 431, 432, 438, 440–445, 447, 448, 509
Psychological testing, 236
Psychologists, 10, 22, 43, 68, 93, 153, 187, 211, 212, 236, 298, 326, 408, 466, 471, 597, 598
Psycho-oncology, 207, 208, 213, 597
Psychosis, 160, 169, 181, 235, 336, 387
Psychosocial, 2, 20, 40, 46, 62, 67, 87–91, 93, 95–101, 103, 104, 113, 114, 125–130, 137, 151, 157, 163, 165, 166, 168–170, 173, 192, 207, 211, 213–215, 220–222, 239, 240, 247, 265, 267, 268, 272, 276, 277, 279, 281, 295, 298, 309, 312, 358, 378, 432, 434, 445, 447, 466, 472, 477, 498, 510, 513, 520, 523, 526, 540, 549, 565, 568, 592, 596, 597
Psychosocial care, 99–101, 213, 219, 270–272, 596
Psychospiritual, 2, 3, 26, 68, 71, 77, 118, 122, 125, 126, 130–132, 150, 159, 163, 165, 166, 212, 220, 275, 305, 322, 339, 358, 407, 434, 465, 466, 526, 538, 596
Psychotherapy, 36, 38, 39, 93, 98–101, 155, 164, 169, 212, 222, 233, 234, 236, 237, 239–241, 248, 249, 362, 378, 471, 478, 482, 521, 567, 568, 592
Public action, 410
Public conversations, 410–412
Public health, 103, 417, 436, 439, 446, 541, 584, 585
Pulmonary, 33, 90, 95, 127, 266, 386

Q

Quality of life, 18, 19, 25, 40, 44, 69, 78, 80, 88, 92, 95, 97, 126, 137, 158, 159, 211, 250, 263, 264, 266, 270, 281, 283, 386, 468, 479, 481, 482, 526
Questionnaire on Stress in Diabetic Patients-Revised, 314
Qur'an, 464, 485, 486

R

Radiation oncologists, 210, 264
Radiologists, 186, 213, 436
Radiology technicians, 186, 213
Random blood sugar test, 300

Rape kit, 201
Readiness, 39, 70, 333, 334, 338, 341, 385, 509, 540–542, 566, 570, 571
Readjustment counselors, 549
Receptive prayer, 478
Recreational therapists, 235, 237, 242
Red blood cell count (RBC), 30
Referral specialists, 364
Registered dieticians, 122, 134, 298
Registered nurses (RNs), 22, 92, 153, 155, 186, 236, 268, 377
Reimbursement, 20, 34, 241, 268, 359, 390, 510
Reitz, R., 9, 598, 599
Relational, 3, 12, 20, 33, 41, 68, 71–73, 128–130, 137, 151–153, 156–160, 163–168, 170–173, 197, 200, 211, 216, 222, 232, 242, 243, 246, 247, 275, 324, 358, 378, 379, 419, 449, 504, 510, 511, 513–517, 519, 523–526, 537, 584, 600
Relationship Dynamics Scale, 34
Relaxation strategies, 102, 103
Religions, 65, 124, 132, 273, 437, 463, 468–470, 477, 481, 482, 484–486
Religiously integrated cognitive behavioral therapy, 478–479
Remission, 218, 226, 251
Reserve component, 537, 567
Residency, 10, 11, 18, 21, 22, 47, 105, 124, 154, 155, 234, 466
Resident, 47
Resident physicians, 18, 96, 105, 155
Respeto, 45, 335
Respiratory diseases, 125–127
Respiratory distress syndrome (RDS), 123–125
Respiratory therapists (RTs), 134, 186
Retirees, 542, 543, 569
Risk management, 510, 528
Rural health clinics, 391
Rural populations, 32, 391

S

Schizophrenia, 189, 232, 239, 249, 251, 252, 296, 330, 370
School-based interventions, 450, 452
Screening, Brief Intervention, and Referral to Treatment (SBIRT) approach, 103, 190, 521
Screening for Child Anxiety Related Disorders (SCARED), 81
Screening tools, 27, 159, 224, 368, 474, 520
Scribes, 188, 436
Scripture, 465, 479, 486
Secondary care, xiv, 48

Secondary traumatic stress, 114
Security chiefs, 505, 507
Selective serotonin reuptake inhibitors (SSRIs), 128, 239, 248, 253, 465
Self-care, 115, 137, 159, 169, 172, 192–193, 253, 275–277, 279, 282, 298, 304, 310, 439, 447, 540, 567, 568
Self-management, 25, 27, 127, 309, 345, 483, 521, 568
Sellers, T., 592, 593
Sepsis, 123, 124, 126, 127, 131
Septicemia, 126, 127
Serotonin and norepinephrine reuptake inhibitors (SNRIs), 128, 239
Service branches, 544
Service member, 537, 538, 541–553, 555–559, 561–571
Sexual assault, 539, 553, 554
Sexual assault nurse examiners (SANEs), 186
Sexual assault response coordinators (SARC), 548
Sexual dysfunctions, 152, 163, 171, 592
Sexual health, 150, 151, 162, 171, 173, 549, 557, 592, 593
Sexually transmitted infections (STI), 162, 174, 557
Shintoism, 486
Sikhism, 486
Silos, 7, 12, 48, 511, 512
Single-issue medicine, 184, 200
Skills, 3, 12, 18, 21, 22, 33–38, 41, 43, 44, 46, 68, 70, 72–74, 88, 89, 92, 93, 97–99, 114, 117, 120–124, 128–130, 135–137, 150, 156, 157, 163–165, 167, 168, 170, 173, 189, 191, 193–196, 200, 201, 213, 216, 219, 220, 222, 223, 225, 233–236, 241, 246–248, 252, 263, 268, 274–278, 280, 281, 297, 305–307, 310, 335–339, 343, 344, 364, 376, 378–384, 386, 405, 406, 408–410, 413–416, 419, 422, 438, 441, 443–446, 451, 452, 463, 471–477, 482, 483, 504, 507–519, 524, 540, 552, 556, 558–560, 568, 584, 591, 594, 596, 600
Sleep, 27, 40, 80, 88, 103, 155, 159, 160, 167, 169, 193, 237, 273, 308, 360, 369, 371, 383, 480, 500, 539, 546, 551
  apnea, 88
  hygiene, 40, 46, 193, 361, 364, 387, 525
SMART goals, 373
Smoking cessation, 40, 360, 369, 409, 418
Social determinants of health, 32, 391

Social locations, 158, 239, 358, 366, 384, 385, 538, 565, 567, 569
Social workers, 10, 22, 43, 93, 153, 187, 197, 211, 235–237, 264, 267, 298, 322, 408, 436, 466, 471, 596, 599
Society for Behavioral Medicine, 227
Society of General Internal Medicine, 106
Solution focused family therapy (SFBT)/ solution focused (SFT), 38, 41, 42, 102, 103, 280, 344, 387, 390, 523, 539
Solvents, 332
Spiritual care, xiv, 119, 125, 463–467, 470, 473–476
Spiritual competencies, 471
Spiritual ecomaps, 480
Spirituality, 17, 38, 65, 187, 263, 271, 335, 345, 358, 403, 463, 465–471, 474, 476–484, 486
Spouses, 44, 136, 186, 218, 246, 299, 311, 403, 408, 521, 525, 543, 551, 567, 587
Stability, 172, 191, 200, 236, 417, 440, 555
Stigma, 20, 28, 32, 171, 207, 241, 243, 362, 367, 541, 551, 564
Stress, 39, 88, 89, 95, 122, 124–126, 130, 135, 137, 152, 159, 162, 170, 172, 186, 187, 189, 193–196, 199, 212, 216, 217, 234, 237, 247, 265, 275–277, 293, 295, 301, 304, 308, 310, 311, 325, 326, 338, 341, 343, 345, 360, 361, 364, 369, 371, 372, 411, 434, 437, 438, 440, 443–445, 447–450, 452, 480–482, 484, 498, 500, 501, 503, 508, 512, 519–522, 524–526, 542, 543, 546, 547, 549–552, 554, 559, 564, 566, 585, 586
Stress management, 31, 46, 187, 195, 237, 248, 304, 364, 369, 445, 448, 449, 503, 543, 547, 567
Structured approach therapy, 451
Subcultures, 538, 558
Substance abuse, 17, 40–42, 46, 91, 98, 100, 102, 166, 187, 190, 234, 235, 245, 248, 253, 326, 339, 342–346, 357, 364, 370, 371, 466, 503, 524, 527, 540, 558, 563, 569, 571
Substance-induced mental disorders, 330
Substance use, 41–43, 101, 103, 104, 124, 133, 166, 189, 190, 238, 304, 321, 322, 324–328, 330, 333–336, 339–344, 346, 368, 389, 519, 521, 552, 566, 599
Substance use behaviors, 42, 325, 341–343
Substance use disorders (SUD), 41, 43, 239, 250, 252, 325, 326, 329, 330, 333, 335–339, 344, 379, 381, 519, 521, 543, 559

Suicidality, 181, 183, 187, 189, 194, 195, 235, 239, 378, 438, 442–445
Suicide, 41, 160, 169, 196, 198, 232, 374, 432, 522, 549, 558
  disability, 239, 522
  ideation assessment, 442
  prevention, 251, 522
Suicide Assessment Five-step Evaluation and Triage (SAFE-T), 454
Super-utilizers, 46
Surgical oncologists, 210
Sutra, 478, 486
Symptoms, 19, 20, 26, 27, 29, 30, 35, 36, 39, 42, 63, 73, 74, 78, 79, 88, 94–96, 99–103, 105, 124, 126, 127, 137, 152, 156, 158–160, 162, 163, 167–170, 174
Systemic, xiii, 2, 20, 27, 34, 35, 41, 70, 73, 74, 98–101, 103, 104, 118, 123, 125, 127–131, 150, 152, 159, 163, 164, 167, 168, 193, 194, 196, 208, 221, 237, 243, 247, 249, 250, 263, 275, 277, 278, 282, 306, 310, 324, 335–340, 344, 358, 359, 362, 378, 380, 381, 389, 434, 451, 467, 468, 473, 474, 499, 504, 514, 516, 519, 524, 526, 528, 538
Systemic therapy, 168, 250, 557

T
Taoism, 484, 485
Tertiary care, xiv, xv, 21, 61, 69, 70, 72, 74, 77, 275, 279, 281, 296–298, 305, 306, 310, 324, 327, 329, 336, 338, 466, 467, 583, 591, 594, 596–598
Tests, 23, 26, 28–31, 67–68, 99, 222, 236, 300, 323, 364
Three world view, 197, 308
Thromboembolic disease, 161, 174
Thyroid stimulating hormone (TSH), 29, 33, 379
Tobacco, 25, 45, 95, 385, 408, 549, 552
Tolerance, 330, 336, 337
Total bilirubin, 30
Tracheostomy, 138
Traditional psychotherapy, 36, 38, 241
Trained volunteers (Hospice), 269
Training innovations, xv, 584, 588–595
Training managers, 505, 507
Transference, 249
Transtheoretical model for change, 385
Trauma, 113–116, 125, 128, 130, 131, 133, 368, 444–446, 452, 553–554
  response teams, xiv
  surgeons, 186
  teams, 186

Trauma intensive care unit (TICU), 113
Traumatic brain injury (TBI), 242, 539, 548, 556, 559, 560, 565, 566
Treatment plans, 3, 34, 37–39, 63, 64, 68, 76, 91, 99–101, 134, 135, 159, 164, 165, 167, 212, 213, 220, 234, 235, 243, 245, 247, 264, 276, 278, 295, 297, 298, 300, 305, 306, 336, 338, 358, 359, 363, 365, 373, 377, 380, 382, 385, 387, 408, 466, 472, 474, 475, 478, 484, 516, 545, 547
Treatment teams, 12, 21–23, 27, 38, 62–68, 71–74, 91–93, 114, 118–122, 129, 153–155, 157, 164, 170, 185–188, 209–213, 233, 235–237, 263, 266–270, 276–278, 297–298, 303, 321, 323, 326–329, 334, 336–344, 362–364, 372, 373, 375, 464, 466–468, 473–475, 504–507, 515, 544, 553
Tricyclic antidepressants, 128, 240, 253
Tumor markers, 226
Tyndall, L., 593
Type 1 diabetes, 24, 78, 298, 299, 309
Type 2 diabetes, 24, 43, 44, 78, 88, 90, 125, 298, 300, 309, 483
Typical antipsychotic, 253

U

UCLA child/adolescent PTSD reaction index for DSM-5, 454
Unintentional injury, 126
University of Chicago's Institute for Translational Medicine, 420
University of Minnesota's (UMN) Citizen Professional Center, 420
University of New Mexico's (UNM) Center for Participatory Research, 420
Urine toxicology screen (UTOX), 253
Utilization reports, 512

V

Vanderbilt ADHD Diagnostic Rating Scale, 81
Veteran, xiv, 234, 251, 537, 538, 540–560, 563–567
Victim advocates, 548
Vital signs, 22, 92, 105, 154, 185, 268
Vitamin D, 29, 299

W

Watson, W.L., 3, 20, 35, 71, 118, 147, 193, 212, 236, 297, 322, 358, 365, 407, 434, 466, 504, 538
Wellness coach, 501, 512, 522
White blood cell count (WBC), 31
Whole health, 20, 469
Williams-Reade, J., 263, 584–587, 599, 600
Wilson, J., 463–467, 470, 473–476, 594
Withdrawal, 214, 232, 235, 273, 322–324, 326, 328, 330–334, 336–339, 361, 442
Workers compensation, 476, 498–500, 502, 504, 506, 508, 512, 514, 517, 519
Workers compensation service workers, 528
Workplaces, xiii, 2, 3, 475, 477, 498, 499, 502–505, 508–511, 513, 514, 517, 518, 521–524, 526–528
Wright, L.M., 3, 20, 71, 118, 147, 193, 212, 236, 297, 322, 358, 365, 407, 434, 466, 504, 538

X

X-ray technicians, 365

Z

Zubatsky, M., 296, 594